MEDICAL RADIOLOGY

Diagnostic Imaging and Radiation Oncology

Springer
Berlin
Heidelberg
New York
Barcelona
Budapest
Hong Kong
London
Milan
Paris
Santa Clara
Singapore
Tokyo

Spiral CT of the Chest

With Contributions by

J.E. Aldrich · A.A. Bankier · C. Beigelman · P. Costello · D. Fleischmann · P. Grenier
C.J. Herold · W.A. Kalender · J.R. Mayo · R. Meuli · D.P. Naidich · M. Prokop · J. Rémy
M. Rémy-Jardin · G.D. Rubin · C.M. Schaefer-Prokop · P. Schnyder · M.W. Vannier
J.A. Verschakelen · P. Vock · G. Wang · S. Wicky

Edited by

M. Rémy-Jardin and J. Rémy

Foreword by

Albert L. Baert

With 243 Figures in 540 Separate Illustrations, Some in Color

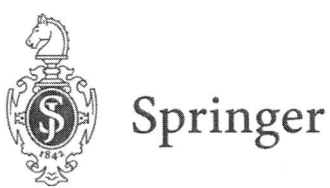

Springer

MARTINE RÉMY-JARDIN, MD, PhD
JACQUES RÉMY, MD, Professor

Department of Radiology
Hospital Calmette
Boulevard Jules Leclerc
59037 Lille Cédex
France

ISBN-13: 978-3-540-41176-5

MEDICAL RADIOLOGY · Diagnostic Imaging and Radiation Oncology

Continuation of
Handbuch der medizinischen Radiologie
Encyclopedia of Medical Radiology

ISSN 0942-5373

ISBN-13: 978-3-540-41176-5   e-ISBN-13: 978-3-642-60349-5
DOI: 10.1007/978-3-642-60349-5

Library of Congress Cataloging-in-Publication Data. Spiral CT of the chest/with contributions by J.E. Aldrich ... et al.: edited by M. Rémy-Jardin and J. Rémy: foreword by Albert L. Baert. p. cm. – (Medical radiology) Includes bibliographical references and index. ISBN-13: 978-3-540-41176-5   1. Chest – Tomography.   2. Spiral computed tomography.   I. Aldrich, J.E. (John E.) II. Rémy-Jardin, Martine. III. Rémy, J. (Jacques), 1933– . IV. Series. [DNLM: 1. Thoracic Diseases – radiography.   2. Thoracic Radiography.   3. Tomography, X-Ray Computed – methods.   WF 975 S759 1996] RC941.S65 1996 617.5′407572 – dc20   DNLM/DLC for Library of Congress 96-19321

© Springer-Verlag Berlin Heidelberg 1996

Softcover reprint of the hardcover 1st edition 1996

Cover design: E. Kirchner, Springer-Verlag

Typesetting: Best-set Typesetter Ltd., Hong Kong

SPIN: 10474552   21/3135/SPS – 5 4 3 2 1 0 – Printed on acid-free paper

Foreword

The advent of spiral CT has dramatically changed the practice of x-ray computed tomography. Fast and volumetric data acquisition has allowed not only the procurement of more diagnostic information in the axial plane by providing more thin and overlapping sections but also new applications, such as the acquisition of a three-dimensional data set with 3D surface shaded display (SSD), projective images by maximal intensity projection (MIP), and better multiplanar reformatting. In addition, spiral CT allows optimal use of contrast media, resulting in a reduction in the total amount of contrast medium administered for a particular clinical purpose, as well as in optimal and selective depiction of specific phases of vessel or organ contrast enhancement. By taking advantage of some of these features, spiral CT allows one to depict selectively the vessels of the body following simple intravenous contrast administration. CT angiography has therefore become an alternative to intra-arterial digital subtraction angiography in some instances. The advantages of spiral CT can be exploited optimally in anatomical areas subject to physiological motion, which is the reason why the method has been applied so successfully in the chest.

This book is edited by two internationally well-known chest radiologists, Martine Rémy-Jardin and Jacques Rémy. They were personally involved at a very early stage in the use of spiral CT in the chest and have contributed three chapters as the fruit of their exceptional personal expertise with this method. The editors have also been very successful in engaging in this project a large number of internationally leading chest radiologists with particular experience in computed tomography of this anatomical region. The result is a very comprehensive and up-to-date overview, spread over 15 chapters, of the principles, radiation exposure, techniques, clinical applications, and future developments of this method for the study of chest dieases.

I am convinced that readers will use this book both as a learning base and as a reference text. It will provide them with correct answers to their questions and with solutions to the problems that they will encounter in performing spiral CT of the chest in their daily clinical practice.

Leuven   ALBERT L. BAERT

Preface

First introduced into clinical practice in 1990, spiral CT constitutes a major technological advance which has dramatically enhanced our ability to detect and characterize abnormalities in the chest. Essentially, it allows the rapid acquisition of a continuous set of CT scan data, greatly improving image quality in regions with physiologic motion and high blood flow. Ideally suited to the chest, this technique permits truly contiguous volumetric scanning of the thorax during a single breath-hold. In cooperative patients, respiratory motion misregistration artifacts are essentially eliminated. The continuous nature of the data acquisition allows the production of multiple overlapping images without additional radiation exposure, resulting in enhanced spatial resolution in the longitudinal axis. These overlapping reconstructions have greatly improved the quality of multiplanar and three-dimensional reformations.

Although new applications for spiral CT and further refinements in technique are being developed at a rapid pace, there exists a need to place the large amount of accumulated data into clinical perspective. This textbook succeeds in that task, summarizing the current information in an accessible and pragmatic format which is relevant to the practicing radiologist. The authors include the main individuals who were responsible for developing the clinical applications of spiral CT in the chest. The editors, Martine Rémy-Jardin and Jacques Rémy, are world leaders in chest radiology and individually responsible for major applications of the technique. Their comprehensive knowledge of this field and their meticulous attention to detail are reflected throughout the text.

It has been my pleasure and a learning experience to review the page proofs of this book. I am sure this volume will be regarded as a standard reference for all who perform spiral CT of the chest.

Vancouver

N. MÜLLER

Contents

1 Principles of Spiral CT

M.W. Vannier and G. Wang

CONTENTS

1.1 Introduction

Spiral/helical x-ray computed tomography (CT) is an important recent advance for volumetric medical imaging. The spiral CT concept was first presented in the patent literature in 1987 (MORI 1987). Related work began in Japan in the late 1980s and was reported in Japanese language publications (KATAKURA et al. 1989; IDA et al. 1990). Physical performance measurements and clinical studies using spiral CT were first presented at the 1989 Radiological Society of North America meeting (KALENDER et al. 1989; VOCK et al. 1989a,b). Interpolation methods associated with spiral scanning were studied in detail (SKRABACZ 1988; BRESLER and SKRABACZ 1989; CRAWFORD and KING 1990).

The development of spiral CT was motivated by improvements in electronics and computers as well as requirements for fewer motion artifacts. In spiral CT, x-ray source rotation and patient table translation are performed simultaneously, as illustrated in Fig. 1.1. Consequently, raw data acquisition time is greatly reduced, transverse slices can be reconstructed at a consistent respiratory level, and misregistration between adjacent slices is eliminated.

Figure 1.2 compares various scanning sequences, including (a) multislice scanning, (b) rapid-sequence scanning, and (c) spiral scanning. Note that both multislice and rapid-sequence scanning involve incremental stepping and shooting while spiral scanning is continuous. Fig. 1.3 is a schematic representation of a raw data set for a scan period. Reconstructions can be done with a variable time interval and a variable reconstruction window. Figure 1.4 illustrates single versus multiple spiral scans. Some scanners are restricted to a single preprogrammed spiral scan while others permit multiple sequential spiral scans separated by short breathing intervals, allowing patients with diminished breath-holding capability to undergo spiral scanning.

Spiral scanning introduces two additional imaging parameters: helical pitch and reconstruction interval. The pitch is defined as the ratio of table increment to detector collimation. The reconstruction interval is the longitudinal distance between reconstructed adjacent transverse slices. An important feature of spiral CT is that retrospective reconstruction may be performed; that is, spiral raw data are collected first, and any transverse slice can be specified for reconstruction afterwards regardless of the pitch. Recently, it was established that for a given x-ray dose and with overlapping reconstruction spiral CT allows substantially better longitudinal resolution than conventional CT (WANG and VANNIER 1994a; WANG et al. 1994; KALENDER et al. 1994). It becomes clear that in spiral CT, improved longitudinal resolution due to overlapping reconstruction is as important as improved temporal resolution due to fast data acquisition. Both advantages make spiral CT the method of choice for volumetric imaging, as

M.W. VANNIER, MD, Mallinckrodt Institute of Radiology, Washington University School of Medicine, 510 South Kingshighway Blvd., St. Louis, MO 63110, USA
G. WANG, PhD, Mallinckrodt Institute of Radiology, Washington University School of Medicine, 510 South Kingshighway Blvd., St. Louis, MO 63110, USA

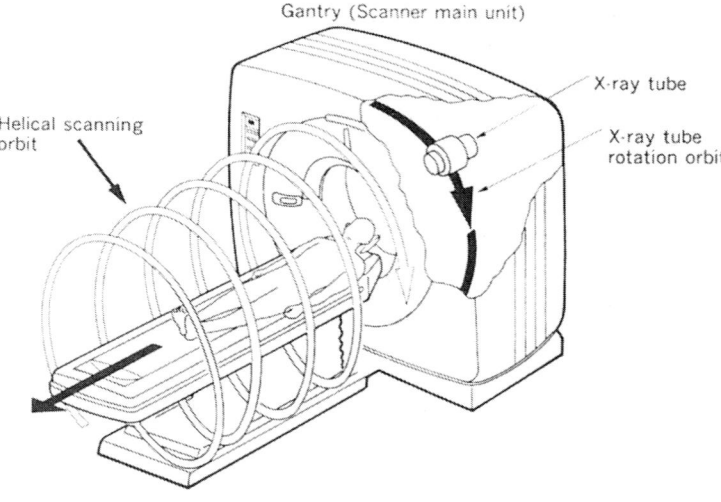

Gantry (Scanner main unit)

Helical scanning orbit

X-ray tube

X-ray tube rotation orbit

Patient couch

Fig. 1.1. Simultaneous translation of the patient couch and orbit of the x-ray tube and detector assembly within the gantry results in the spiral/helical scanning orbit (from Tohki 1993)

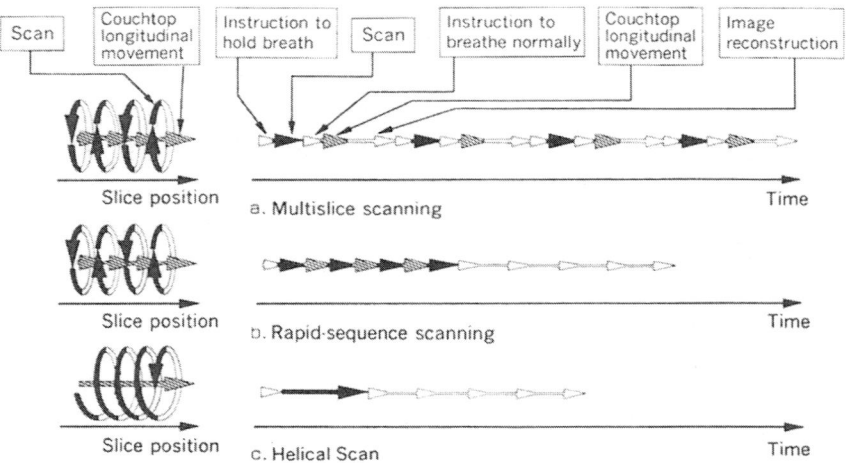

Fig. 1.2. Comparison of temporal sequences contrasts **a** multislice scanning, **b** rapid-sequence scanning, and **c** spiral/helical scanning. Note that both multislice and rapid-sequence scanning involve incremental "step and shoot" scanning while the spiral scanning process is continuous. (From Tohki 1993)

outlined in Fig. 1.5. Since its introduction in 1989 (Kalender et al. 1989; Vock et al. 1989a,b), spiral CT has gained general acceptance as the standard medical CT mode.

Temporal CT image resolution has been optimized using the e-beam technique (Boyd and Lipton 1983). In the e-beam CT scanner developed at the Imatron Company, mechanical movement usually needed for tomographic scanning is completely eliminated for subsecond cross-sectional imaging. The primary application of the e-beam scanner is cardiac imaging. Currently, CT detectors are arranged along a one-dimensional arc, resulting

in fan-beam imaging geometry. Cone-beam spiral CT using a two-dimensional detector array was first reported in 1991 (Wang et al. 1991, 1993). Earlier work on cone-beam tomography led to this development (Feldkamp et al. 1984; Tuy 1983; Smith 1985; Grangeat 1991; Jaszczak et al. 1988; Gullberg and Zeng 1992). A cone-beam x-ray imaging system for angiography was recently implemented (Saint-Félix et al. 1994). These topics are beyond the scope of this chapter.

The CT process – in which projection data are collected by means of scanning x-rays across a patient from different orientations, and an image is

Fig. 1.3. Schematic representation of a raw data set for a scan period T_M. Reconstructions with variable time interval (Δt) and variable reconstruction window (R) are possible. (From RIGAUTS et al. 1990)

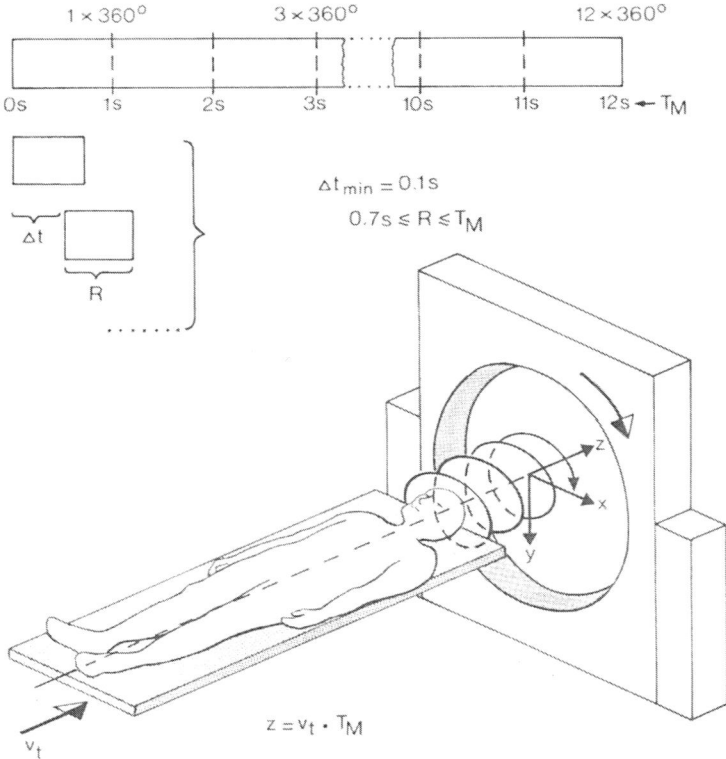

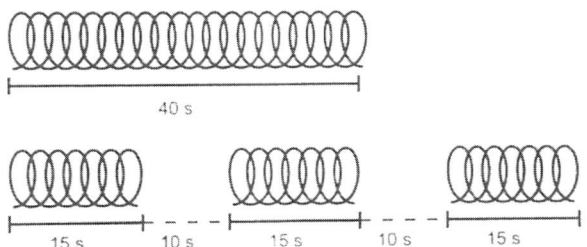

Fig. 1.4. Single versus multiple spiral scans. Some scanners are restricted to a single preprogrammed spiral scan while others permit multiple sequential helical scans separated by short breathing intervals. (From BRINK et al. 1994)

resolution for differentiating large areas similar in gray-scale. Image noise imposes a grainy appearance due to random fluctuations of x-ray photon flux. Image artifacts are structured or patterned interference. Stair-step, blurring, metal, and motion artifacts are the four most important types encountered in spiral CT. We will address these aspects in this chapter.

1.2 Computed Tomography Process

As the first step in the CT process, raw projection data are acquired when a patient is probed with x-ray beams from various directions, and line integrals of x-ray attenuation in the patient are recorded. Basically, there are four generations of CT scanning geometries as shown in Fig. 1.6. The first-generation scanner is characterized by an assembly of an x-ray source and a single detector. A parallel-beam projection profile is collected with the assembly being translated along a straight line segment after each incremental rotation of the assembly. The second-generation scanner is also a translation-rotation device but multiple detectors are employed, which

mathematically reconstructed from the projections using computing technology – is now well understood. In spiral CT, planar projection sets are synthesized from spiral raw projection data via interpolation, and then reconstructed via filtered backprojection. Therefore, raw data interpolation is central to spiral CT. As in conventional CT, image quality in spiral CT also has three components: resolution, noise, and artifacts. Image resolution contains two major categories: spatial resolution for distinguishing small adjacent objects and contrast

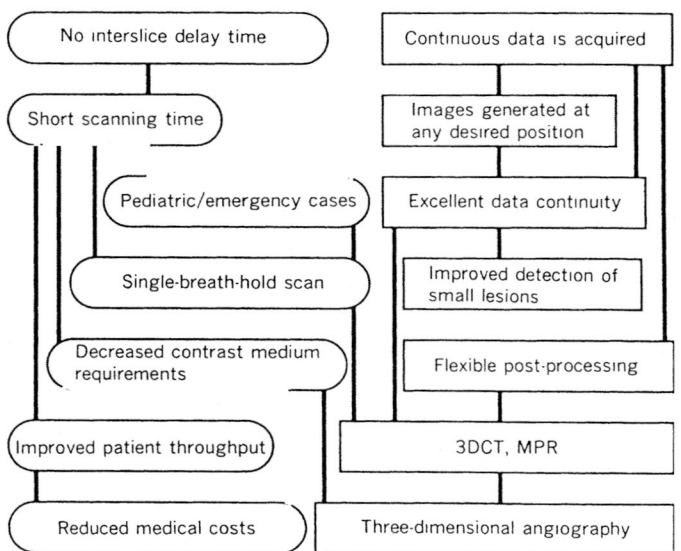

Fig. 1.5. Advantages of spiral/helical CT scanning are outlined diagrammatically. The simultaneity of transaxial and longitudinal data collection reduces interslice delays and provides a continuous stream of projection data. (From KATADA 1993)

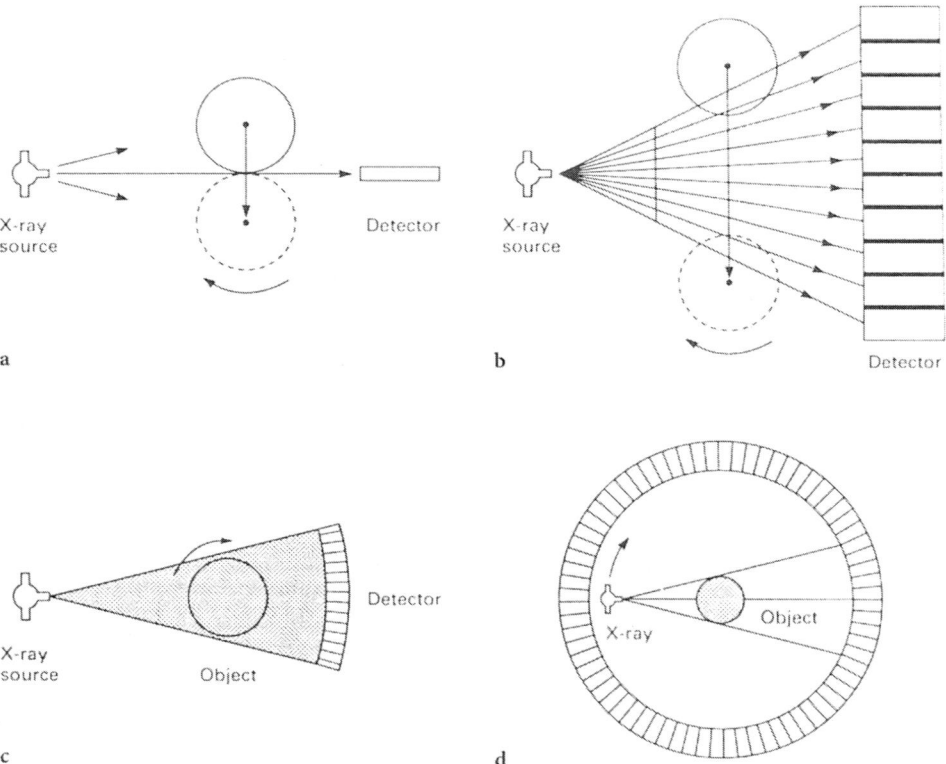

Fig. 1.6a–d. Basic CT scanning geometries. **a** Single-detector translate-rotate, first-generation system; **b** multidetector translate-rotate, second-generation system; **c** rotate-only (rotate-rotate), third-generation system; **d** stationary detector rotate-only, fourth-generation system. In medical systems, the source and detectors are manipulated while the object remains stationary. (From DENNIS 1989)

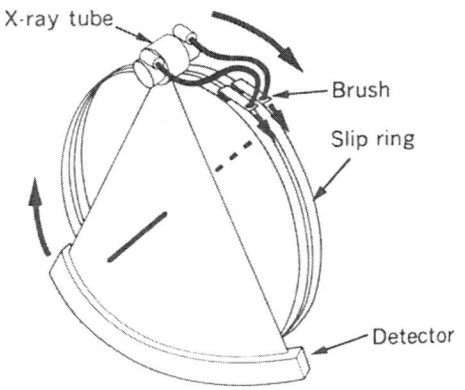

Fig. 1.7. Slip ring in a third-generation CT geometry allowing continuous x-ray tube (source) and detector rotation. The slip-ring mechanism is essential for continuous multiple rotation scanning. The brush slides along a slip ring as the assembly rotates to supply the power continuously to the x-ray tube. (From TOHKI 1993)

extends a small fan-beam angle. The third-generation scanner utilizes fan-beam imaging geometry. Many detectors are used so that all x-rays from a source through a cross-section of the patient can be detected. In this mode, there is no need for translating the source-detector assembly; in other words, the assembly works in a rotation-rotation fashion. Twin-beam scanning is a novel third-generation design developed at the Elscint Company (ELSCINT 1992). This technology is based on scanning two contiguous transaxial sections simultaneously. In the fourth mode, detectors are distributed along

a full circle, and only an x-ray source is orbited. Evolution of these imaging geometries was largely motivated by the requirement of fast scanning, but has a cost of increased scattering. The scattering problem can be greatly reduced by using x-ray collimators.

The third-generation scanners are the most popular. The slip-ring technique of the third-generation CT geometry is fundamental to spiral scanning. As shown in Fig. 1.7, a slip ring allows continuous rotation of the x-ray tube and detector array assembly. The key element in the slip-ring technique is the power supply which operates over an extended scanning period. Conceptually, a brush slides along a slip ring as the assembly rotates so that electrical energy is provided to the x-ray tube during continuous scanning. The maximum scanning time with the slip-ring technique is mainly determined by the thermal limitation of the x-ray tube. Typically, in the x-ray tube assembly, relatively low voltages are transformed into high voltages for operating the tube.

It is the slip-ring technique that makes spiral scanning possible. Figure 1.8 illustrates the coordinate system for spiral CT with a fan beam geometry. In spiral CT, an x-ray source illuminates a detector array distributed along an arc. The helical scanning locus lies outside the plane of the slice to be reconstructed except for a single point of intersection. The x-y plane contains the slice to be reconstructed. The z-axis indicates the direction of table motion. Note that spiral CT in the fourth-generation

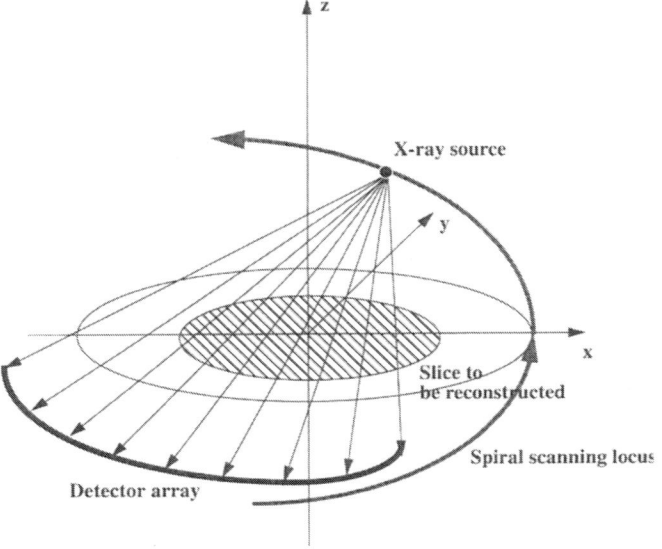

Fig. 1.8. Coordinate system for spiral CT with a fan-beam geometry. The x-ray source illuminates a detector array along an arc. The helical scanning locus lies outside the plane of the slice to be reconstructed except for a single point of intersection. The x-y plane contains the slice to be reconstructed. The table motion is along the z-axis

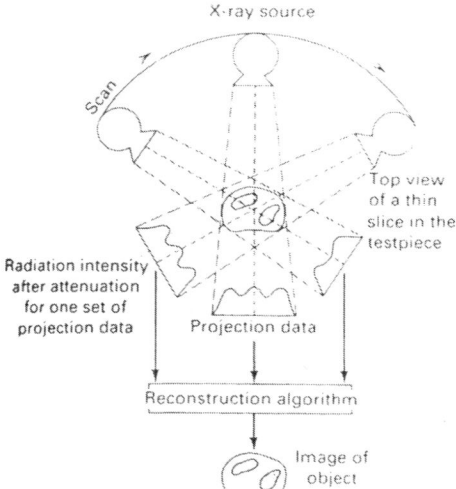

Fig. 1.9. Schematic of a CT process where a moving x-ray source illuminates an object and generates projection data through a set of detectors, which may be stationary or moving. Projection data are input to a computational algorithm for image reconstruction. (From DENNIS 1989)

scanning mode differs from conventional CT in the same fashion as with the third-generation scanning mode. Therefore, in the following we will assume that the third-generation scanning mode is used. Both the methodology and the results can

be extended to spiral CT in the twin-beam third-generation mode or in the fourth-generation scanning mode.

A schematic of the conventional CT process is shown in Fig. 1.9, where a moving x-ray source illuminates a patient and generates fan-beam projection data through a set of detectors, which may be stationary or moving. The projection data are input to a computational reconstruction algorithm that results in formation of a digital image for a corresponding slice taken from the patient. Filtered backprojection is a well-established method for image reconstruction. As shown in Fig. 1.10, simple backprojection cannot exactly recover an image from its projections because of the smearing effect; however, filtered backprojection reproduces the actual image as the blurring from simple backprojection is cancelled in filtered backprojection.

There is a rigorous mathematical foundation for the filtered backprojection method. This can be best explained in both the projection and the Fourier domains in Fig. 1.11. An elegant relationship was derived that the Fourier transform of a parallel-beam projection profile obtained in the orientation shown in Fig. 1.11a is equal to the data points on one spoke in the two-dimensional Fourier transform space in Fig. 1.11b (NATTERER 1986; KAK and SLANEY 1987). If all parallel-beam projection profiles

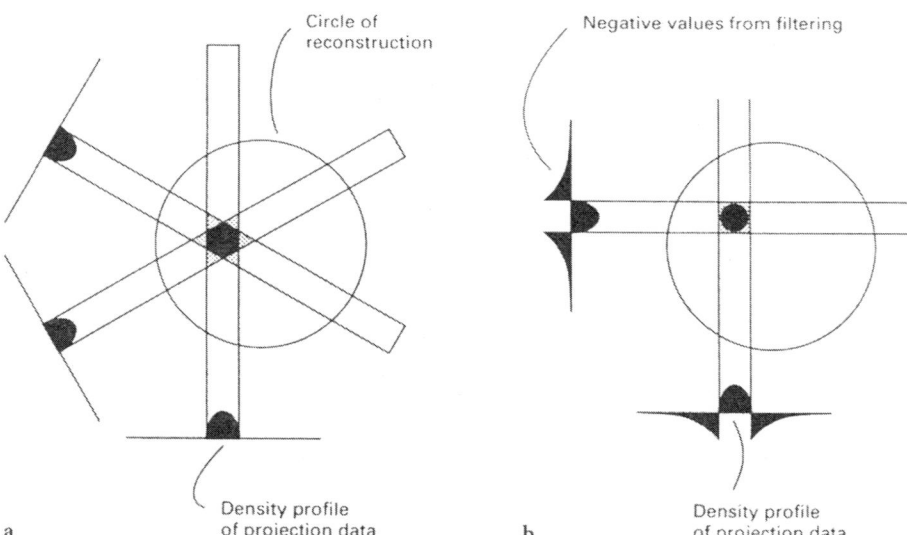

Fig. 1.10. Schematic of CT image reconstruction by **a** simple backprojection and **b** filtered backprojection. Simple backprojection produces a blurred and broadened image. Fil-

tering can eliminate the smearing effect from simple backprojections. (From DENNIS 1989)

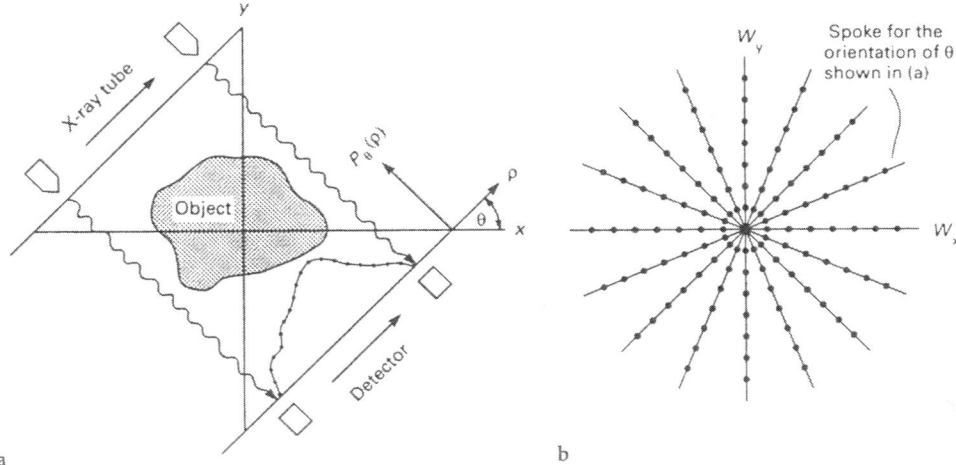

Fig. 1.11a,b. Relationship between projection data and the Fourier transform of an image to be reconstructed. The projection data points in the orientation shown in **a** correspond to the data points on one spoke in the two-dimensional Fourier space shown in **b**. (From Dennis 1989)

are available, the corresponding spokes will completely cover the two-dimensional Fourier transform space. Hence, the inverse Fourier transform will reconstruct the image exactly. It can be mathematically demonstrated that this Fourier reconstruction process is equivalent to filtered backprojection (Natterer 1986; Kak and Slaney 1987). Although what is described above is for parallel-beam geometry, the filtered backprojection mechanism is also established in fan-beam geometry (Natterer 1986; Kak and Slaney 1987). Because only one fan-beam projection profile is acquired within any transaxial plane in spiral CT, sufficient projection data are not available for reconstruction of any transaxial slice, and planar projection sets must be produced from raw spiral scan data prior to filtered backprojection.

1.3 Raw Data Interpolation

Figure 1.12 illustrates different scanning areas covered in conventional and spiral scanning. Conventional scanning creates slices which lie entirely within a right circular cylinder bounded by two planes while the spiral scan is offset by continuous table motion. As a result, image quality using direct reconstruction of the spiral data as opposed to reconstruction using interpolation is substantially different, as shown in Fig. 1.13, where the streak artifacts are removed by interpolation.

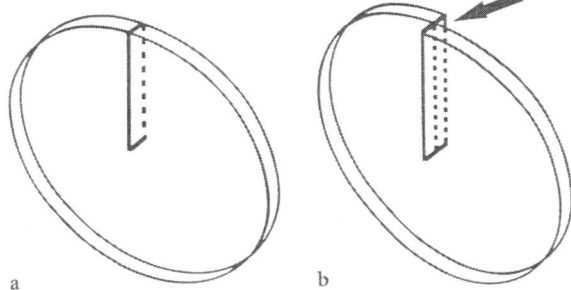

Fig. 1.12a,b. Different scanning areas are used in **a** conventional and **b** spiral scanning. Conventional scanning creates slices which lie entirely within a right circular cylinder bounded by two planes while the spiral scan is offset by continuous table motion. (From Tohki 1993)

Among various spiral raw projection data interpolation techniques, linear interpolation is usually preferred due to its efficiency and performance (Crawford and King 1990; Kalender and Polacin 1991; Polacin et al. 1992). Typical linear interpolation techniques include full-scan (FS), under-scan (US), full-scan with interpolation (FI), half-scan (HS), half-scan with interpolation (HI), and half-scan with extrapolation (HE) methods. In the FS method, raw projection data collected at an angular range of 360° undergo no modification before convolution and backprojection. Hence, the FS is the simplest interpolation algorithm. The US and HS methods require the angular range to be 360° and

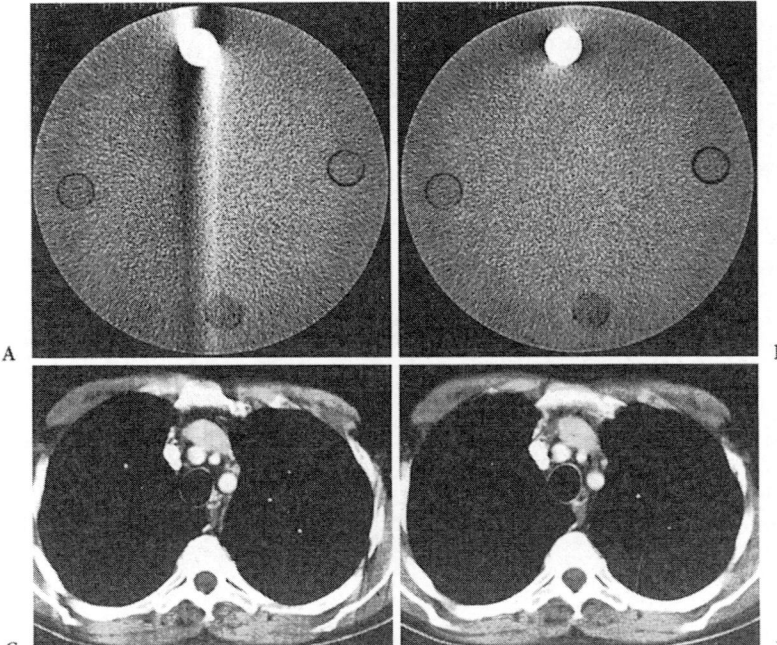

Fig. 1.13. Comparison of image quality using direct reconstruction of spiral data (**A,C**) as opposed to reconstruction using interpolation (**B,D**) for phantom (**A,B**) and mediastinal (**C,D**) studies. Note that the streak artifacts are removed when interpolation is used. (From KALENDER et al. 1990)

180° plus a fan-angle, respectively. In both the US and the HS methods, raw projection data are underweighted near the beginning and end of a scan, compensated by overweighting projection data near the middle of the scan. In the FI method, a set of planar projection data in a 360° angular range is obtained via linearly interpolating neighboring raw projection data at the same orientation as shown in Fig. 1.14; hence the raw data involved span a 720° angular range. The HI method utilizes the redundancy of raw fan-beam data, interpolates neighboring raw data at opposite directions, and thus reduces the angular range from 720° required by the FI method to 360° plus two fan-angles. The HE method eliminates the condition required by the HI method that the projection rays must be from different sides of a reconstruction plane. In the HE method, if the opposite rays are from the same side of the plane, extrapolation is performed to estimate the corresponding projection value; otherwise, interpolation is done as described for the HI method. Using the notations chosen by Kalender et al. (KALENDER and POLACIN 1991; POLACIN et al. 1992), the FI and HI methods are equivalent to the 360° LI and 180° LI methods, respectively.

All of the above methods perform interpolation longitudinally and thus, in cases of structures discontinuous in the z direction, produce vertical blurring in synthesized projection data. This blurring process

and periodically varying interpolation geometry may also distort structures in a transverse plane. Noting this limitation, an adaptive interpolation method was suggested to perform linear interpolation along inclined paths to improve current spiral CT interpolation methods (WANG and VANNIER 1994c). The adaptive interpolation concept can be described as follows. Suppose that an elongated structure is inclined with respect to the longitudinal axis, then there will be a relative displacement between the neighboring projections of the same orientation. This mismatch can be estimated with the traditional correlation technique and used to define the interpolation paths. For multiple differently inclined structures, an interpolation path originating from a projection position may be determined by correlating a short series of projection data centered at this position with the neighboring projection data of the same orientation. Other techniques are also possible for this purpose, such as use of wavelet decomposition for structure identification in the projection domain (KAISER and STREATER 1992).

These typical linear interpolation methods are summarized in Fig. 1.15. Among these linear interpolation methods, the HI and HE methods are widely favored; they efficiently utilize raw data, reliably synthesize planar projections, and generally result in satisfactory reconstructed images.

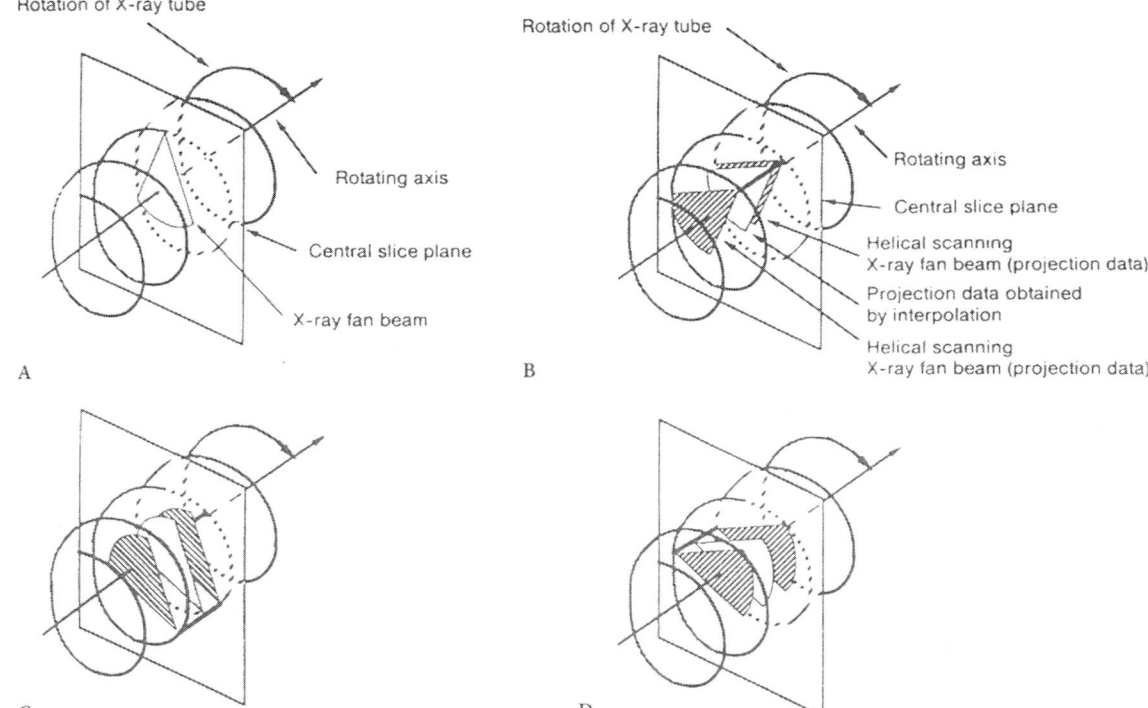

Fig. 1.14A–D. Diagrammatic representation of an interpolation algorithm. **A** The arbitrary slice and spiral data intersect only at one point, which means that there is only a single profile of true projection data in the planar image. **B** The projection data in the planar slice are obtained by interpolating the spiral data at two points at the same rotational phase on either side of the planar slice. **C,D** This procedure is repeated for successive rotational phases to obtain interpolated data for 360°, sufficient to reconstruct the transaxial slice. (From TOHKI 1991)

1.4 Image Resolution

Several studies have shown that in-plane spatial resolution in spiral CT with the HI/HE method is quite similar to that in conventional CT (CRAWFORD and KING 1990; POLACIN et al. 1992; BRINK et al. 1992). Longitudinal spatial resolution in spiral CT differs from that in conventional CT. Longitudinal resolution is closely related to the slice sensitivity profile (SSP).

1.4.1 Slice Sensitivity Profile

The SSP can be defined as the longitudinal central profile of a CT scanner point spread function (PSF) and is commonly measured along the longitudinal axis that passes through the geometric center of the gantry aperture. The SSP is important for both high-contrast and low-contrast longitudinal image resolution. As shown in Fig. 1.16, the SSP affects imaging of small lesions. The contrast, that is, the ratio between the CT values of a small lesion and its background,

will be reduced when its diameter is smaller than the slide width. This effect is increased further when the SSP deviates from the ideal rectangular shape. As compared with the SSP in conventional CT (zero table feed), spiral CT causes some SSP blurring, as shown in Fig. 1.17. This becomes quite pronounced with the FI (360° LI) method at higher table speeds. However, this effect is largely reduced with the HI (180° LI) method; even table speeds greater than the detector collimation appear practical.

Clearly, an SSP is dependent on the transverse position of an associated longitudinal line, due to asymmetry of the spiral CT interpolation geometry. The SSP spatial variation was recently investigated (WANG and VANNIER 1994b). Let us assume that detectors in a transverse array are densely arranged, and detector characterization is only needed in the longitudinal direction. Under this assumption a detector response to a point source is also a function of the longitudinal relative distance between the detector center and the point source. We model the detector response as a rectangular function:

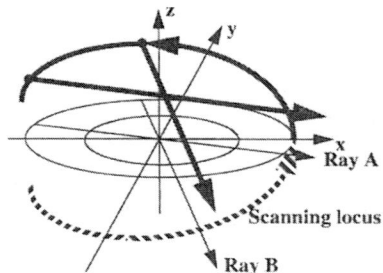

* 360 Degrees
* No Modification on Projections

a

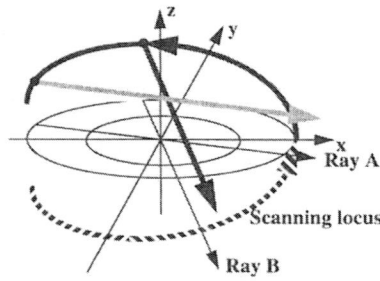

* 360 Degrees
* Under-/Over-Weighting Projections

b

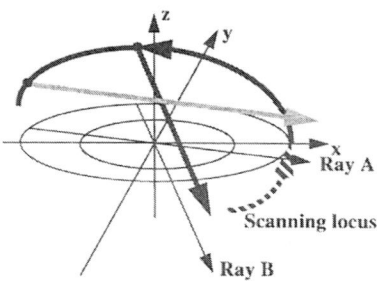

* 180 Degrees + Fan-Angle
* Under-/Over-Weighting Projections

c

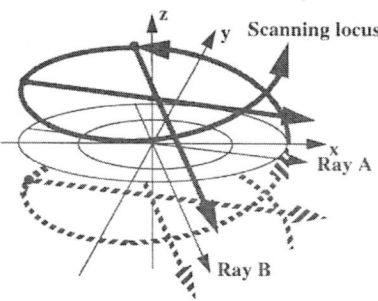

* 720 Degrees
* Interpolation with Rays at Same Orientation

d

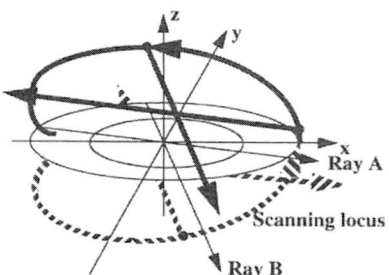

* 360 Degrees + 2 Fan-Angles
* Interpolation with Opposite Rays

e

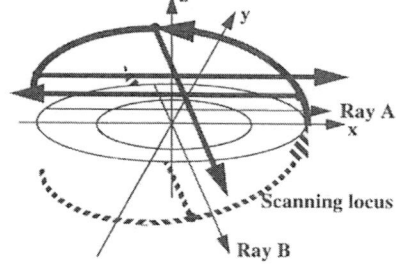

* 360 Degrees
* Extrapolation/Interpolation with Opposite Rays

f

* 720 Degrees
* Directional Interpolation

g

$$r(d) = \frac{1}{D}rect\left(\frac{d}{D}\right), \qquad (1.1)$$

where d is the longitudinal relative distance between the detector center and the point source, D is the longitudinal dimension of the detector collimation, and $rect(.)$ is the rectangular function:

$$rect(x) = \begin{cases} 1, & x \in \left[-\frac{1}{2}, \frac{1}{2}\right]; \\ 0, & \text{otherwise.} \end{cases}$$

In conventional CT, if the longitudinal relative distance between a point source and a transaxial plane is not greater than $D/2$, the reconstructed image using projection data from the point source should recover the same point source independent of its position. Therefore, the SSP in conventional CT, $p_c(z)$, is directly obtained below:

$$p_c(z) = r(z), \qquad (1.2)$$

where z is the longitudinal coordinate.

Due to the interpolation process, the SSP in spiral CT is degraded compared to $p_c(z)$. We assume that the HI method is used in spiral CT. Figure 1.18 shows the reconstruction system and variables used in HI. If an ideal impulse is located at a point $(r, \phi, 0)$ in cylindrical coordinates, ϕ is measured with respect to the axis from the gantry center to the x-ray source position in the plane at $z = 0$, and the table feed is equal to the detector collimation, then the SSP at (r, ϕ) can be expressed as follows (WANG and VANNIER 1994b):

$$p_x(r, \phi, z) = \frac{1}{\pi}\int_{\theta_0}^{\theta_0+\pi}\left[\omega(\theta)r\left(z - \frac{D}{2\pi}\beta_1(\theta)\right)\right.$$

$$\left. +\left(1-\omega(\theta)\right)r\left(z - \frac{D}{2\pi}\beta_2(\theta)\right)\right]d\theta, \qquad (1.3)$$

where θ_0 is the normal direction of the upper projection ray in the plane $z = 0$, θ is the normal direction of a projection ray l passing through the point $(r, \phi, 0)$, and β_1 and β_2 are the gantry rotation angles associated with the opposite ray pair of ray l,

◀───────────────────────────────

Fig. 1.15a–g. Interpolation schemes for spiral CT: a full-scan (FS), b under-scan (US), c half-scan (HS), d full-scan interpolation (FI or 360° LI), e half-scan interpolation (HI or 180° LI), f half-scan extrapolation (HE), and g adaptive interpolation (AI)

$$\omega(\theta) = \frac{\beta_2(\theta)}{\beta_2(\theta) - \beta_1(\theta)}.$$

It was proven (WANG and VANNIER 1994a) that:

$$p_s(0, 0, z) = g(z) * p_c(z), \qquad (1.4)$$

where $g(.)$ is referred to as the table motion function associated with the HI method,

$$g(z) = \begin{cases} \dfrac{2}{D} + \dfrac{4z}{D^2}, & z \in \left[-\dfrac{D}{2}, 0\right]; \\ \dfrac{2}{D} - \dfrac{4z}{D^2}, & z \in \left[0, \dfrac{D}{2}\right); \\ 0, & \text{otherwise.} \end{cases}$$

In other words, the SSP at the gantry center in spiral CT is the convolution of detector response and table motion functions.

Equation 1.3 is the basis for the analysis of the SSP spatial variation over a scan field. Interestingly, the mean of the SSP was shown to be always equal to zero, although the profile is generally asymmetric with respect to the z-axis. The mean of the SSP can be explained as the local longitudnal position of a transverse slice. The zero mean over the scan field indicates that a transverse slice is not distorted in longitudinal direction in spiral CT. Numerical simulation shows that the variation of the SSP standard deviation is up to about 10% for a 50° fan-angle and within about 5% for a 40° fan-angle. Figure 1.19 illustrates SSPs at four representative positions in the x-y plane for fan angles of 50° (a) and 40° (b), respectively. If the fan-angle is not too large, the SSP at the gantry center, $p_s(0, 0, z)$ or simply $p_s(z)$, is a satisfactory representation of the SSP family.

1.4.2 Slice Thickness

Slice thickness does not have a unique definition. As a result, derivation of the slice thickness from the SSP does not produce a unique result. In addition to the popular full-width at half-maximum (FWHM) and full-width at tenth-maximum (FWTM) (CRAWFORD and KING 1990; BRINK et al. 1992; POLACIN et al. 1992), the standard deviation of the SSP is also a good alternative, because the use of the standard deviation is the standard statistical method to quantify the deviation of a distribution. In the preceding subsection, the standard deviation was used for a relative assessment of spiral CT SSP transverse variation

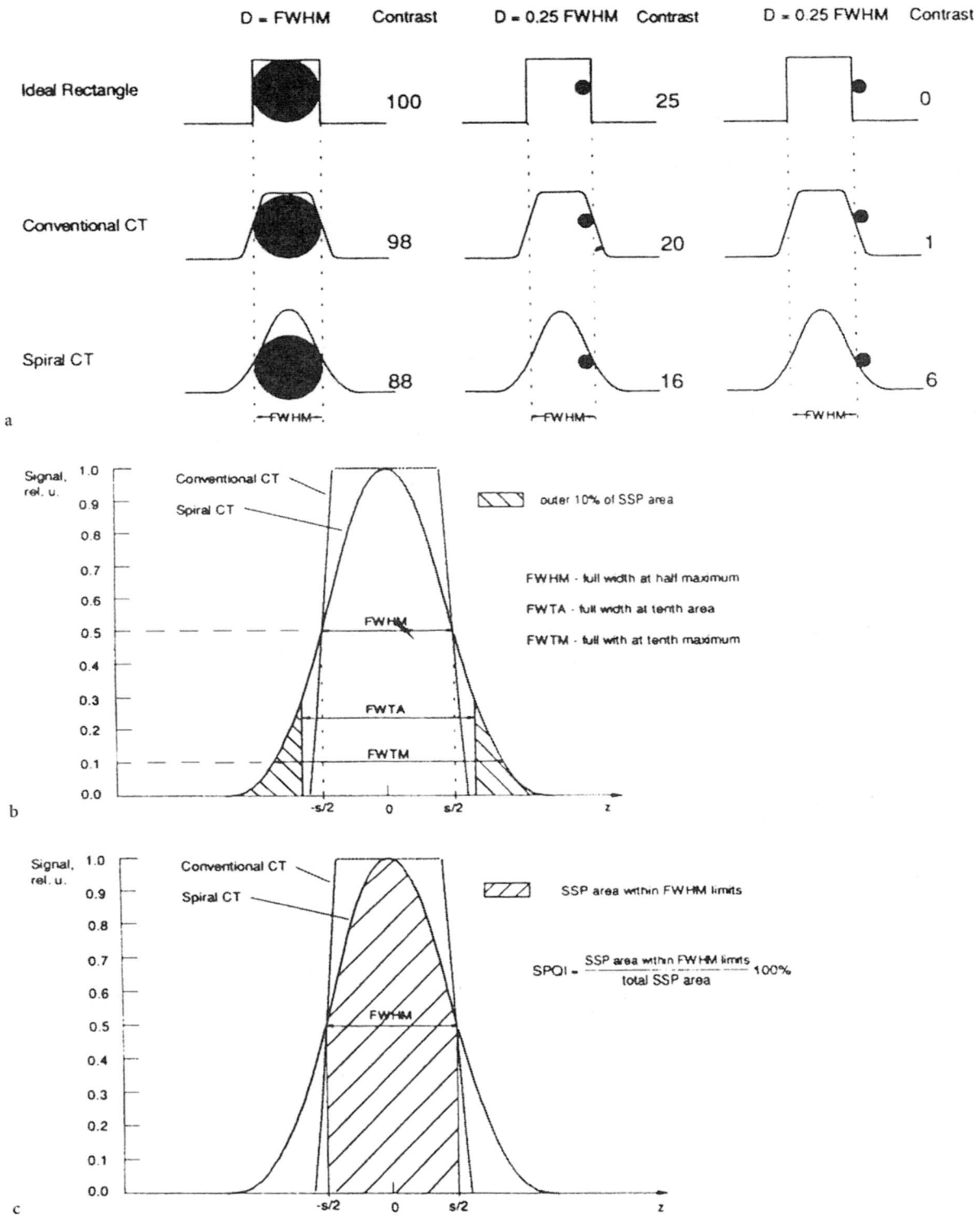

Fig. 1.16a–c. Influence of the SSP shape on the imaging of small lesions. **a** The contrast of a small lesion will be reduced when its diameter is smaller than the slide width; this effect is increased further when SSPs deviate from the ideal rectangular shape (**b,c**). (From KALENDER 1995)

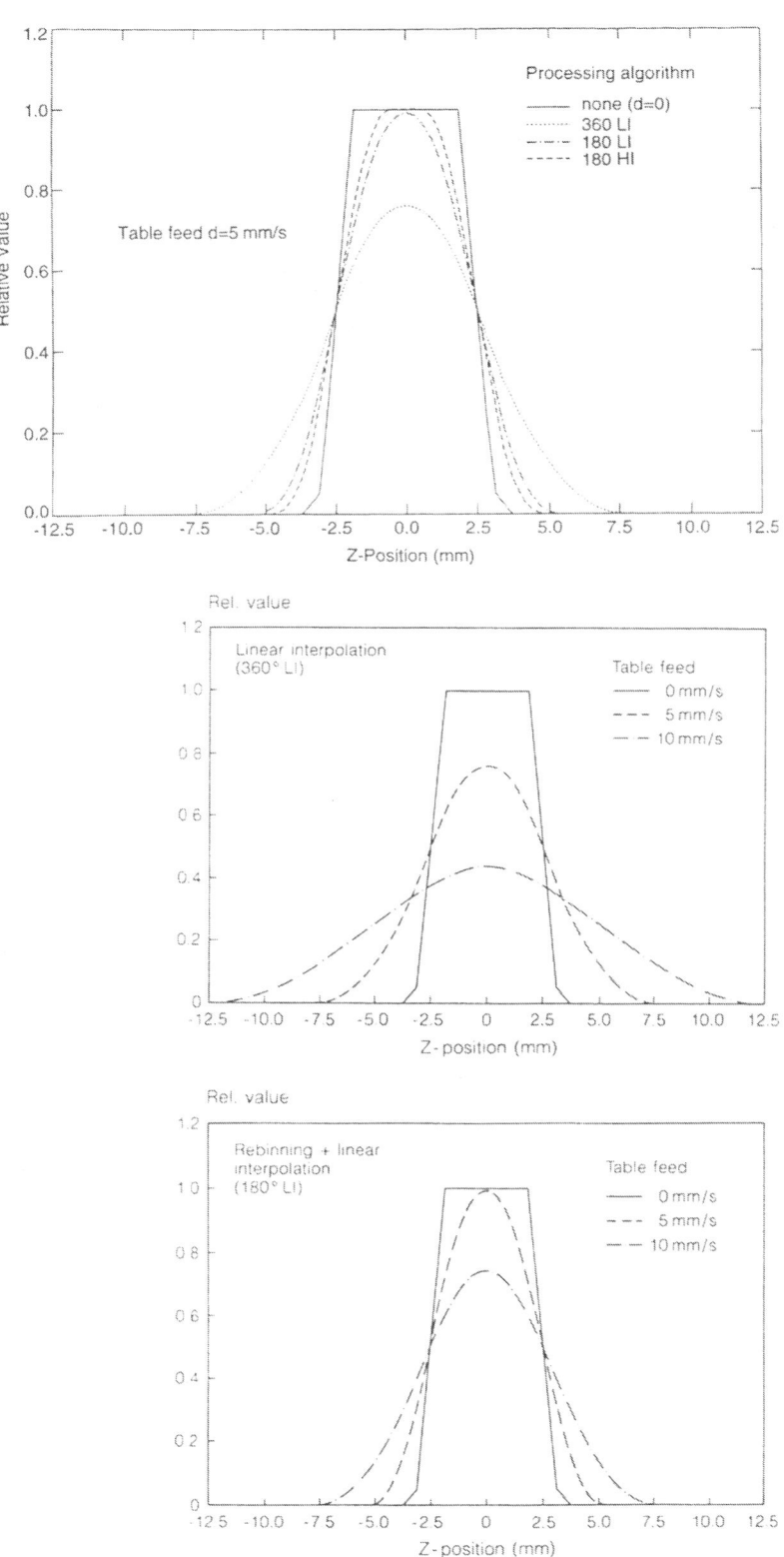

Fig. 1.17a,b. Slice sensitivity profiles in spiral CT. As compared with the conventional SSP (table feed = 0 mm/s), spiral CT causes some SSP blurring. This becomes quite pronounced for FI (360° LI) at higher table speeds (**a**. With HI (180° LI) this effect is largely reduced (**b**); even table speeds greater than the detector collimation appear practical. (From KALENDER et al. 1992)

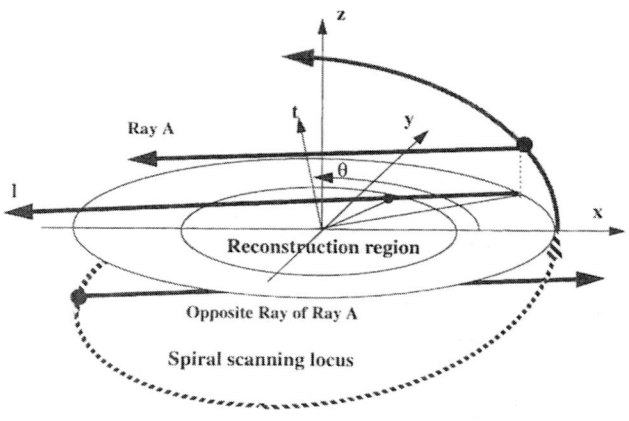

Fig. 1.18. Reconstruction coordinate system and variables used in the HI (180° LI)

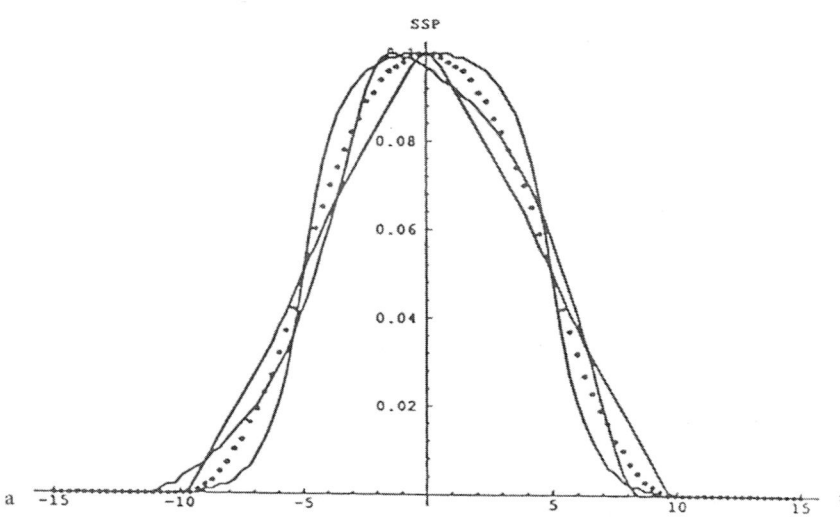

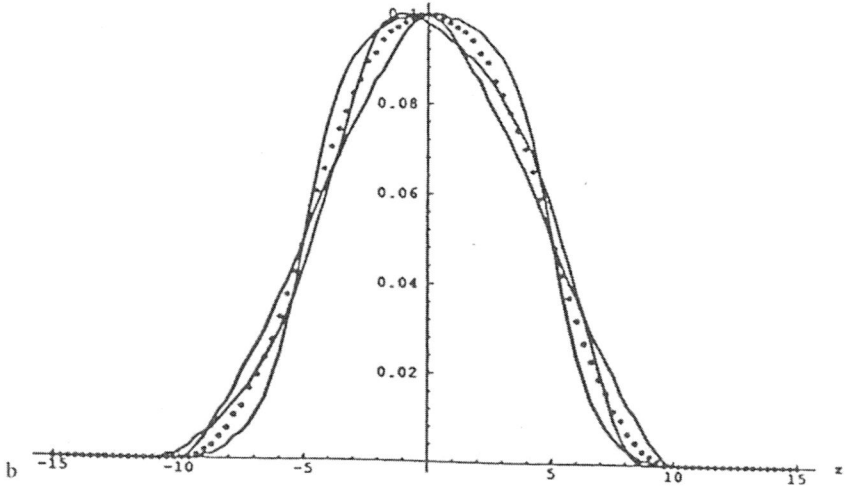

Fig. 1.19. SSPs at four representative positions in the x-y plane are plotted for fan angles of 50° (**a**) and 40° (**b**). The dotted profiles were computed at the gantry iso-center (0, 0), the asymmetric curves at (0, r), where $r = 32.6$ cm is the radius of the field of view, and the two solid symmetric curves at (r,0) and ($-r$, 0), shown as the flatter and sharper peaks, respectively

(WANG and VANNIER 1994b). Actually, the standard deviation is strongly correlated with either the FWHM or the FWTM. In the case of a Gaussian SSP $\dfrac{1}{\sqrt{2\pi}\sigma}e^{-\frac{z^2}{2\sigma^2}}$, the full-width at p-percentage-maximum (FWpM) equals $2\sqrt{2}\sigma\sqrt{|\log p|}$. Therefore, a given slice thickness in FWHM or FWTM can be directly translated into a specific SSP standard deviation σ.

Based on the spiral CT SSP formula (Eq. 1.4), it was proven (WANG and VANNIER 1996a) that:

$$\sigma^2 = \frac{T^2}{24} + \frac{D^2}{12}, \tag{1.5}$$

where T and D are the table increment and detector collimation, respectively. This relationship may be referred to as *the spiral CT slice thickness formula*, since it directly relates the standard deviation of the spiral CT SSP to the two key imaging parameters: the table increment and the detector collimation. Interestingly, it can be observed that to reduce the spiral CT slice thickness, narrowing the detector collimation is twice as important as slowing the table advancement.

1.4.3 Longitudinal Bandwidth Comparison

In the preceding two subsections, the SSPs in conventional and spiral CT are given under the following conditions: (1) in conventional CT, a very fine table increment is used, and the reconstruction interval is therefore sufficiently small; (2) in spiral CT, the table increment is equal to the detector collimation, but the reconstruction interval is made sufficiently small, since retrospective reconstruction can be performed to produce overlapped transverse slices.

If the reconstruction interval is not sufficiently small, the ideal SSP can be modified into a convoluted version: the convolution of the ideal SSP and a low-pass filter, $\dfrac{1}{kD}\operatorname{sinc}\left(\dfrac{\pi z}{kD}\right)$, determined by the reconstruction interval kD (the longitudinal sampling step) (WANG and VANNIER 1994a; WANG et al. 1994). That is, in conventional CT with a table increment kD the low-pass filtered SSP $p_{c,k}(z)$ is:

$$p_{c,k}(z) = \frac{1}{kD^2}\operatorname{sinc}\left(\frac{\pi z}{kD}\right)*rect\left(\frac{z}{D}\right), \tag{1.6}$$

where:

$$\operatorname{sinc}(x) = \frac{\sin x}{x}. \tag{1.7}$$

Similarly, in spiral CT with a reconstruction interval kD the low-pass filtered SSP $p_{s,k}(z)$ is:

$$p_{s,k}(z) = \frac{1}{kD}\operatorname{sinc}\left(\frac{\pi z}{kD}\right)*g(z)*p_c(z). \tag{1.8}$$

Strictly speaking, the real system response to an impulse (a tiny ball) is nonstationary along the z axis due to the aliasing effect. The rationale for use of the low-pass filtered SSPs is as follows. When a finite longitudinal sampling is performed, it is usually assumed that the sampling rate is sufficiently high, that is, greater than the Nyquist rate associated with an object image, so that the spectrum aliasing is not a problem. With the low-pass filtered SSPs, a proper longitudinal cutoff frequency of an object (patient) image is implied, since in reality the interpolation (using a finite number transverse slices to obtain a volumetric image) is performed on the discretized convolution of the SSP and the volumetric image instead of the discretized SSP itself. In this sense, no aliasing effect is involved, and the low-pass filtered SSPs describe the system longitudinal response to a low-pass filtered impulse. Spatial image resolution is typically parameterized as spatial frequency bandwidth for an imaging system. Longitudinal bandwidths in conventional and spiral CT can be computed from the Fourier transforms of the low-pass filtered SSPs. The meaning of the longitudinal bandwidth is that an original longitudinal signal can be exactly recovered from its discretized version if its maximum frequency stays within the system bandwidth. If the aliasing effect is taken into account in the bandwidth determination, the original physical meaning of the bandwidth will be lost. On the other hand, if a sampling rate is less than the Nyquist rate (a tiny ball and a large reconstruction interval), the aliasing effect will cause errors in the interpolation. In this case, our low-pass filtered SSPs are approximations to nonstationary profiles and should provide a reasonable basis for performance evaluation.

A Fourier transform pair is denoted as:

$$f(x) \Leftrightarrow F(u), \tag{1.9}$$

with the definitions

$$F(u) = \int_{-\infty}^{\infty} f(x)e^{-i2\pi ux}dx, \tag{1.10}$$

and

$$f(x) = \int_{-\infty}^{\infty} F(u)e^{i2\pi ux} du. \qquad (1.11)$$

The Fourier transforms $P_c(u)$, $P_{c,k}(u)$, $P_s(u)$, and $P_{s,k}(u)$, corresponding to $p_c(z)$, $p_{c,k}(z)$, $p_s(z)$, and $p_{s,k}(z)$ respectively, can be shown to be the following:

$$P_c(z) = \mathrm{sinc}(\pi Du), \qquad (1.12)$$

$$P_{c,k}(u) = \mathrm{sinc}(\pi Du)\,rect(kDu), \qquad (1.13)$$

$$P_s(u) = \mathrm{sinc}^2\left(\frac{\pi Du}{2}\right)\mathrm{sinc}(\pi Du), \qquad (1.14)$$

$$P_{s,k}(u) = \mathrm{sinc}^2\left(\frac{\pi Du}{2}\right)\mathrm{sinc}(\pi Du)\,rect(kDu). \qquad (1.15)$$

The mean-square-root of a Fourier power spectrum is a reasonable measure of the bandwidth. The mean-square-root bandwidth $\bar{u}$ for $F(u)$ is defined as:

$$\bar{u}^2 = \frac{\int_0^{\infty} u^2 |F(u)|^2 du}{\int_0^{\infty} |F(u)|^2 du}. \qquad (1.16)$$

Table 1.1 lists the bandwidth in conventional and spiral CT as a function of k; kD is the reconstruction interval in conventional and spiral CT (WANG and VANNIER 1994a).

The longitudinal resolution depends on both the detector collimation and the table increment. Suppose that in conventional CT the table increment is a very small fraction of the collimation, the longitudinal resolution is solely determined by the detector response function and reaches its theoretically possible maximum. With the table increment being equal to the collimation in spiral CT, even if the reconstruction interval is sufficiently small, the longitudinal resolution in spiral CT would not be as good as the maximum permissible in conventional CT, since $p_s(z)$ is the convolution of $p_c(z)$ and a low-pass filter. Also, if the table increments in both conventional and spiral CT are the same and equal to the

reconstruction interval in spiral CT, the spiral CT SSP would not be favorably compared to that in conventional CT, because of the table motion function in the spiral CT SSP.

These facts could lead to the erroneous impression that the longitudinal resolution in conventional CT is superior. However, the above arguments overlook two important factors. First, a sufficiently small table increment results in a very large x-ray dose, which is impossible in practice. As a result, the maximum possible longitudinal resolution in conventional CT is seldom reachable, and the real longitudinal resolution is then the low-pass filtered version ($\bar{u}_{c,k}$) instead of the maximum possible one ($\bar{u}_{c,0}$). Second, the reconstruction interval in spiral CT can be made sufficiently fine only at the cost of computing resources. Setting the reconstruction interval to the table increment is just one possible choice. To compare longitudinal resolution in conventional and spiral CT, it is only fair to require that not only the collimation but also the x-ray dose be the same. Identical x-ray dose means equal table increments. In conventional CT, the reconstruction interval is the same as the table increment, and the retrospective reconstruction can be achieved via interpolation. In spiral CT, the reconstruction interval is arbitrary, and it is feasible to reach the maximum possible spiral CT longitudinal bandwidth. Therefore, in evaluating the longitudinal resolution, it is $\bar{u}_{c,1}$ (the conventional CT bandwidth with the same table increment as the detector collimation) and $\bar{u}_{s,0}$ (the maximum possible bandwidth in spiral CT) that should be compared. Based on the bandwidth computation, the longitudinal resolution in spiral CT is superior to that in conventional CT, as the spiral CT bandwidth is substantially larger than the conventional CT counterparts [$\bar{u}_{s,0}(0.297) > \bar{u}_{c,1}(0.256)$].

Therefore, in addition to the advantage of faster projection data acquisition, another major advantage of spiral CT is better image longitudinal resolution, compared to conventional CT (WANG and VANNIER 1994a; WANG et al. 1994). Intuitively, spiral CT allows that a transverse slice can be freely specified for reconstruction, and thus have a greater capability to capture longitudinal details than con-

Table 1.1. Mean-square-root bandwidth in conventional and spiral CT as a function of the reconstruction interval kD, where D is the detector collimation and was set to 1

k	0.0	0.2	0.4	0.6	0.8	1.0	1.2	1.4	1.6	1.8	2.0
$\bar{u}_{c,k}$	∞	0.514	0.349	0.331	0.296	0.256	0.222	0.194	0.173	0.155	0.14
$\bar{u}_{s,k}$	0.297	0.296	0.294	0.291	0.272	0.242	0.213	0.189	0.169	0.152	0.138

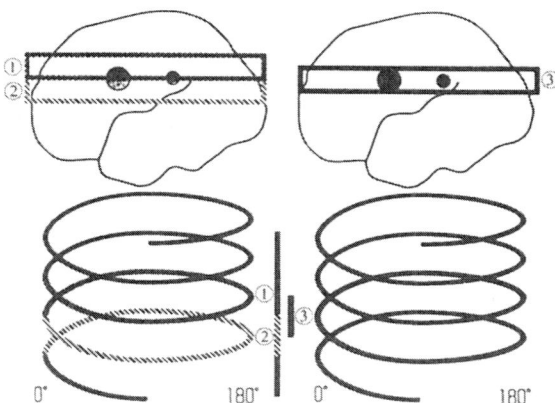

Fig. 1.20. Transaxial image reconstruction is possible at any desired position along the longitudinal axis. An intermediate slice is easily generated by reconstructing spiral scan data corresponding to the desired slice position, and the target lesion or anatomical structure can always be situated at the center of a slice. (From KATADA 1993)

Table 1.2. FWTM values as a function of pitch (p, the first column) and reconstructed slice number (n, the first row) per collimation length

p/n	1	2	3	4	5
0.33	9.9	6.9	6.5	6.2	6.0
0.67	10.1	7.5	6.9	6.9	6.7
1.0	10.3	7.9	7.7	7.7	7.7
1.33	10.6	8.7	8.7	8.7	8.7
1.67	11.0	9.9	9.9	9.9	9.9
2.0	11.8	11.0	11.2	11.2	11.2

ventional CT, in which a much smaller number of reconstructed slices may miss or distort features with sizes comparable to the table increment, as illustrated in Fig. 1.20.

1.4.4 Overlapping Slice Reconstruction

Based on the low-pass filtered spiral CT SSP formula (Eq. 1.8), FWTM values are tabulated in Table 1.2 as a function of pitch $p = \dfrac{T}{D}$ and reconstructed slice number n per collimation length (WANG et al. 1994). In the computation, D was set to 5. For each combination of p and n, the functions $\sin c$, g, and p_c were generated in one-dimensional arrays of 512 elements and 50 in length. The convolutions were implemented via fast Fourier transform. The z coordinates corresponding to the one-tenth of the SSP maximum were found via an automatic search process. Experimental FWTM values in spiral CT for $D = 5$, $p = 1$ and 2 are 8.0 and 11.3, respectively (POLACIN et al. 1992;

BRINK et al. 1992). They are consistent with our theoretical values, which are 7.7 and 11.2, respectively. The tendency of slight underestimation mainly arises from the idealized shape of the *rect* function, which results in less blurring in the theoretical SSP. Note that as n increases, the SSP will be narrowed, and its maximum be increased at the same time. The FWTM as a function of n does not always decrease monotonically. It can be observed that the minimum FWTM for $p = 2$ was reached at $n = 2$, which reflects the fact that the FWTM is only an approximate descriptor of the longitudinal image resolution. According to Table 1.2, the less p is, the more slices should be reconstructed to make full use of spiral raw projection data. Generally, it seems that three to five slices should be reconstructed for $p \leqslant 1$, and two slices for $p > 1$. Figure 1.21 shows spatial resolution in the z-direction in spiral CT. A test pattern with 1-mm holes oriented along the z-axis was reconstructed with respect to various combinations of imaging parameters. With 1-mm collimation, 1-mm table feed and 0.2-mm reconstruction interval, the holes are well resolved when using the HI (180° LI) algorithm.

Alternatively, overlapping reconstruction may be considered in the following way. Assuming that the SSP can be approximated as a Gaussian distribution and that the standard deviation of the SSP can be computed according to our slice-thickness formula (Eq. 1.5), the standard deviation Σ of the Fourier transform of the SSP can be directly derived:

$$\Sigma = \frac{1}{2\pi\sigma} = \frac{1}{2\pi\sqrt{\dfrac{D^2}{12} + \dfrac{T^2}{24}}}, \tag{1.17}$$

where D and T are detector collimation and table feed, respectively. Further assuming that the cutoff frequency f_{max} of the Fourier spectrum is given by tripling Σ, we have:

$$f_{max} = 3\Sigma = \frac{3}{2\pi\sqrt{\dfrac{D^2}{12} + \dfrac{T^2}{24}}}. \tag{1.18}$$

Hence, the longitudinal sampling step Δ, that is, the reconstruction interval between adjacent transverse slices, can be estimated by meeting the Nyquist sampling requirement:

$$\Delta = \frac{1}{2f_{max}} = \frac{\pi}{3}\sqrt{\dfrac{D^2}{12} + \dfrac{T^2}{24}}. \tag{1.19}$$

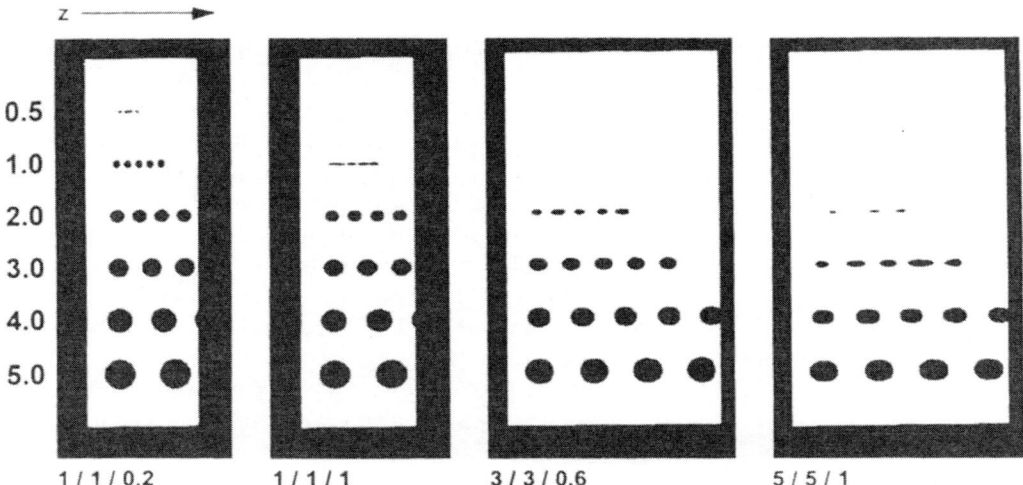

Fig. 1.21. Spatial resolution in the z-direction. Measurement of a test pattern with holes oriented along the z-axis with different parameters. With 1-mm detector collimation, 1-mm table feed, and 0.2-mm reconstruction interval, the 1-mm holes are well resolved when using the HI (180° LI) algorithm. (From KALENDER 1995)

Table 1.3. Recommended number of reconstructed slices per collimation according to the Nyquist sampling criterion

p	0.1	0.3	0.5	0.7	0.9	1.1	1.3	1.5	1.7	1.9
n	3.30	3.12	3.12	2.97	2.79	2.61	2.44	2.27	2.12	1.98
N	4	4	4	3	3	3	3	3	3	2

In other words, the number n of reconstructed slices per collimation is:

$$n = \frac{D}{\Delta} = \frac{3}{\pi\sqrt{\frac{1}{12}+\frac{p^2}{24}}}. \tag{1.20}$$

Roughly, overlapping reconstruction number N in integer per collimation is:

$$N = \left\lceil \frac{D}{\Delta} \right\rceil = \left\lceil \frac{3}{\pi\sqrt{\frac{1}{12}+\frac{p^2}{24}}} \right\rceil. \tag{1.21}$$

n and N are tabulated in Table 1.3 with respect to various typical p. Clearly, to avoid aliasing the SSP Fourier spectrum, at least four, three, and two transverse slices should be reconstructed per collimation in the cases of pitch substantially less than 1, around 1, and close to 2, respectively. This is consistent with what we discussed in the preceding paragraph. Overlapping reconstruction leads to improved longitudi-nal image resolution, which can be translated into better diagnostic performance in various applications, for example, detection of pulmonary nodules (RÉMY-JARDIN et al. 1993).

Overlapping reconstruction is important not only for high-contrast resolution but also for low-contrast resolution (KALENDER et al. 1994). Figure 1.22 shows comparison of contrast and spatial resolution for conventional and spiral CT. Performance in conventional CT varies with the random relationship of scan pattern and lesion location in Fig. 1.22a while spiral CT can always offer optimal performance in Fig. 1.22b. Phantom experiments verified that spiral CT gives significantly better contrast and spatial separation of spheres than does conventional CT (Fig. 1.22c,d). The tumor contrast as a function of tumor and spiral CT parameters was also studied with clinically interesting cases and physical phantom measurements (HU and FOX 1993, 1995). It was found that both the detector collimation and the table feed should be comparable to the tumor radius and that overlapping reconstruction should be performed to reduce the nonuniformity of the contrast sensitivity.

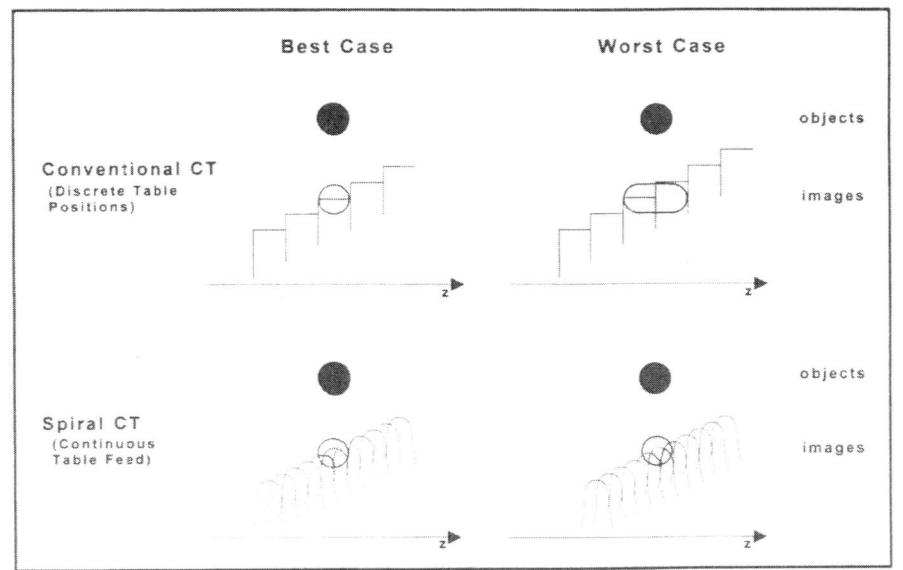

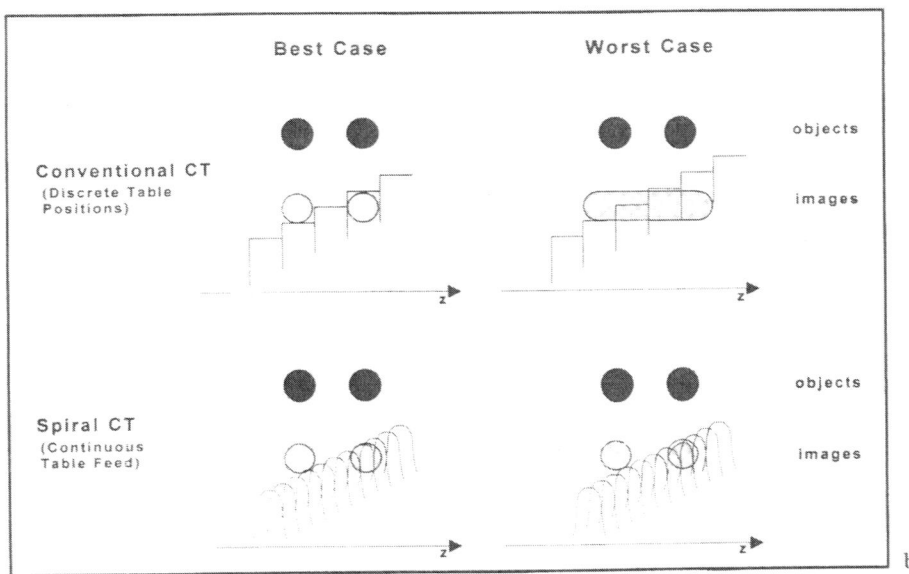

Fig. 1.22a–d. Comparison of contrast and spatial resolution for conventional and spiral CT. **a,b** Schematic presentation of the dependence of resolution on sampling along the z-axis (the number of images available per collimation). Performance in conventional CT varies with the random relationship of scan pattern and lesion location while spiral CT can always offer optimal performance. **c,d** Phantom experiments verified that contrast and spatial separation of spheres are significantly better in spiral CT. (From KALENDER et al. 1994)

1.4.5 Optimal Scanning Pitch

X-ray tube and dose considerations limit spiral CT volume coverage (ZEMAN et al. 1994) and spatial and contrast resolution during a single scan. In what follows, the slice thickness formula (Eq. 1.5) is applied to determine the detector collimation, table incre-ment, and scanning pitch for the maximum volume coverage in spiral CT (WANG and VANNIER 1996a).

Rewriting the spiral CT slice thickness formula (Eq. 1.5), we have:

$$T^2 = 24\left(\sigma^2 - \frac{D^2}{12}\right), \tag{1.22}$$

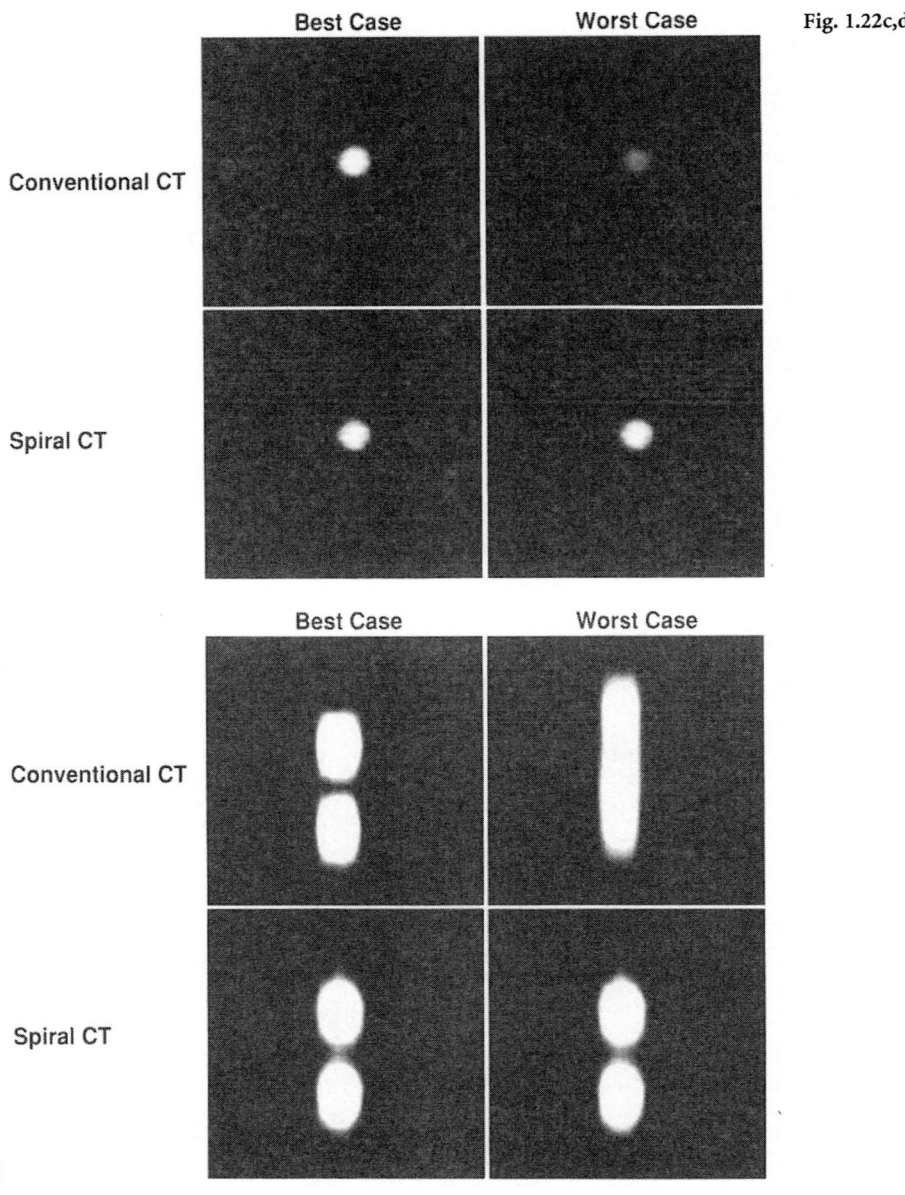

Fig. 1.22c,d

c

d

where D and T are detector collimation and table feed, respectively. A key fact is that the total volume coverage during a spiral scan is proportional to both T and D. It is evident that the volume coverage is proportional to T; that is, the greater T is, the larger the volume that will be covered. On the other hand, if D is increased, the tube current must be proportionally decreased to maintain the same photon statistics so as to achieve the same image noise level. As a result, the total continuous scanning time is proportionally increased if we work at the limit of the x-ray tube heat capacity. Because the volume coverage is proportional to the total scanning time, the volume coverage is also proportional to D. Consequently, the

optimization yields $\hat{D} = \sqrt{6}\sigma$ and $\hat{T} = 2\sqrt{3}\sigma$. That is, the optimal pitch is:

$$\hat{P} = \frac{\hat{T}}{\hat{D}} = \sqrt{2}. \tag{1.23}$$

In other words, given SSP and image noise variance, the maximum volume coverage in spiral CT is reached by setting the pitch to $\sqrt{2}$.

Similarly, the following three optimization problems can be defined, which are clinically significant:

1. Given a scanning coverage L and an image noise level η, minimize the slice thickness σ.

2. Given a scanning coverage L and a slice thickness σ, minimize the image noise level η.
3. Given a scanning coverage L, minimize the product of slice thickness and image noise, which is equivalent to minimize $\sigma^2\eta^2$, so that the conflicting requirements for slice thickness and image noise can be optimally balanced.

Actually, the third optimization problem is also to maximize the signal-to-noise ratio in the sense that the signal strength is measured as being proportional to $1/\sigma$ and the noise as proportional to η. The rationale for quantifying the signal strength in this manner can be explained as follows. Since our SSP profile contains a unit area with the horizontal axis, the smaller σ is, the narrower the SSP, and the greater the peak of the SSP. Clearly, the peak of the SSP may represent the signal strength. Interestingly, in all the three cases the optimal pitch is still $\sqrt{2}$ (WANG and VANNIER 1996b). With the pitch being set to $\sqrt{2}$, other imaging parameters, such as detector collimation and table increment, can be readily determined in specific applications.

Note that what we optimized are mathematically well-defined quantities. Their relevance to diagnostic performance needs to be evaluated further. For example, what the best indicator is for the slice thickness is still an open question.

1.5 Image Noise

Previous studies on the relationship between spiral CT image noise and linear interpolation schemes were done either numerically or experimentally (CRAWFORD and KING 1990; POLACIN et al. 1992; BRINK et al. 1992). We analytically obtained image noise variance with linear interpolation methods (WANG and VANNIER 1993). Assume that the parallel-beam projection $P_\theta(t)$ is corrupted by an additive white noise $v_\theta(t)$, then the measured projection $P_\theta^m(t)$ is expressed as:

$$P_\theta^m(t) = P_\theta(t) + v_\theta(t), \tag{1.24}$$

and the correlation function as:

$$E\left[v_{\theta_1}(t_1)v_{\theta_2}(t_2)\right] = S_0\delta(\theta_1 - \theta_2)\delta(t_1 - t_2), \tag{1.25}$$

where S_0 is the noise spectrum density. Since spiral CT raw data linear interpolation and subsequent filtered backprojection are well-defined linear processes, the image noise variance associated with various interpolation methods can be derived. It was found that the spiral CT image noise after longitudinal integral is independent of the transaxial position, proportional to the raw projection noise, and not affected by the fan-angle (approximately true for the HE method). Also, the spiral CT image noise variance is proportional to the area under the square of the reconstruction filter. Image noise deviation ratios of spiral CT to conventional 360° reconstruction (CR) are tabulated in Table 1.4 (WANG and VANNIER 1993), and are consistent with previously reported simulation results at the gantry center (CRAWFORD and KING 1990). In several spiral CT applications including lesion detection, volume estimation, and image restoration, the theoretical characterization of the noise performance is important to model the imaging process.

Note that the above conclusions on spiral CT image noise are insightful in theory but are approximate in practice. If we model the projection noise in other ways, the image noise would have different characteristics; in particular, it would no longer be spatially invariant in general. Recently, spiral CT image noise was studied under the assumption that the fan-beam projection is corrupted by an additive white noise (CRAWFORD et al. 1994). An equation was derived for noise at any location in an image. Simulations and experiments demonstrated a 40% variation in the standard deviation of the noise over a 48-cm field of view. The image noise in a given transverse slice can be locally reduced by starting data collection at an angle equal to the polar angle of the center of a region of interest.

Table 1.4. Image noise deviation ratios of spiral CT to conventional 360° reconstruction for the conventional 360° reconstruction (CR), full-scan (FS), under-scan (US), full-scan with interpolation (FI), half-scan (HS), half-scan with interpolation (HI), and half-scan with extrapolation (HE). σ and σ' denote theoretical and measured deviations, respectively

Method	CR	FS	US	FI	HS	HI	HE
$\dfrac{\sigma}{\sigma_{CR}}$	1.00	1.00	$\sqrt{1+\dfrac{26}{35}\dfrac{\beta_u}{\pi}} \approx 1.09$	$\sqrt{\dfrac{2}{3}} \approx 0.817$	$\sqrt{2} \approx 1.41$	$\dfrac{2}{3}\sqrt{3} \approx 1.16$	$1.16 \sim 1.23$
$\dfrac{\sigma'}{\sigma'_{CR}}$	1.0	1.0	1.1	0.83	1.4	1.2	1.2

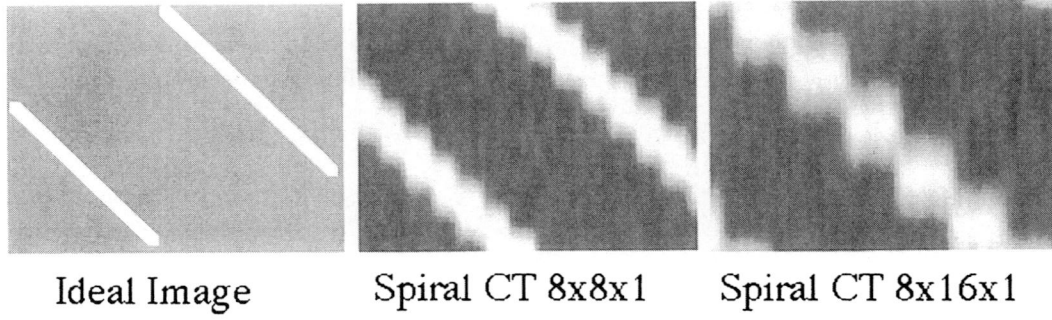

Ideal Image   Spiral CT 8x8x1   Spiral CT 8x16x1

Aluminum Ramps @ 45° relative to table motion

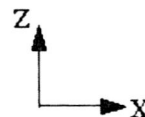

Fig. 1.23. "Stair-step" artifact seen in longitudinal reformations from spiral CT [8-mm collimation, 8- and 16-mm table increment (*middle* and *right*, respectively), 1-mm reconstruction interval] of thin aluminum plates oriented oblique to the patient travel direction. These should appear as straight lines in ideal reformations (*left*), but are discontinuous "stairsteps" (*middle, right*). (From BRINK 1995)

1.6 Image Artifacts

Image artifacts are defined as structured or patterned interference in reconstructed images. A good portion of research effort in CT is devoted to overcoming or suppressing various image artifacts. Here, we only discuss the characteristics and correction of stair-step, blurring, metal and motion artifacts, which are the most important image artifacts in practice.

1.6.1 Stair-step Artifacts

Stair-step artifacts in spiral CT images are associated with inclined surfaces in reformatted longitudinal slices, as shown in Fig. 1.23. The origin of these artifacts, dependencies on imaging parameters, and means of suppressing them were investigated (WANG and VANNIER 1994c).

A spiral CT scanner (Siemens Somatom PLUS-S, Siemens Medical Systems, Iselin, N.J., USA) was employed in this study. This system produces up to 30 consecutive 1-s scans. The detector collimation is selectable from 1 mm to 10 mm. The table increment per gantry rotation can be from 1 to 20 mm. The reconstruction matrix is 512 by 512 pixels with 4096 gray-levels (12 bits). The maximum spatial resolution at high contrast is approximately 14 lp (line pair) per cm (at the 2% cut-off frequency of modulation transfer function). The cross-field uniformity is ±2 HU. A research spiral CT software package is available with the scanner for raw data interpolation and three-dimensional image visualization. A hollow Plexiglas cone phantom and an adult skull were used as test objects. The cone phantom has minimum external and internal diameters of 7 cm and 6 cm, and the maximum counterparts are 34 cm and 33 cm, respectively. Its height is 16 cm. The side surface makes a tilt angle of about 45° with respect to the bottom surface. The principal axis of the cone phantom is defined as the axis passing through the centers of its top and bottom circles. The side surface of the cone phantom is used to model an inclined organ surface in the human body. The skull is similar to the cone phantom since it is roughly circularly symmetric about its principal axis; on the other hand, its irregularities make it more suitable for simulation of clinical scenarios.

Stair-step artifacts, strong or weak, were perceived in reformatted images for most parameter combinations. It was found that the stair-step artifacts were due to a large reconstruction interval (aliasing effect) and asymmetric spiral CT interpolation (rotation effect). Generally speaking, the height of the stair-steps due to the rotation effect depends on the pattern of asymmetry in the transverse image, which is determined by the interpolation method, the object to be reconstructed, and the imaging and reformation parameters. In reality, the artifacts due to both aliasing and rotation effects may be mixed, resulting in irregular stair-step artifacts. Even if the reconstruction interval is sufficiently small, the stair-step artifacts will appear so long as the object cross-section varies longitudinally. This is demonstrated in Fig. 1.24.

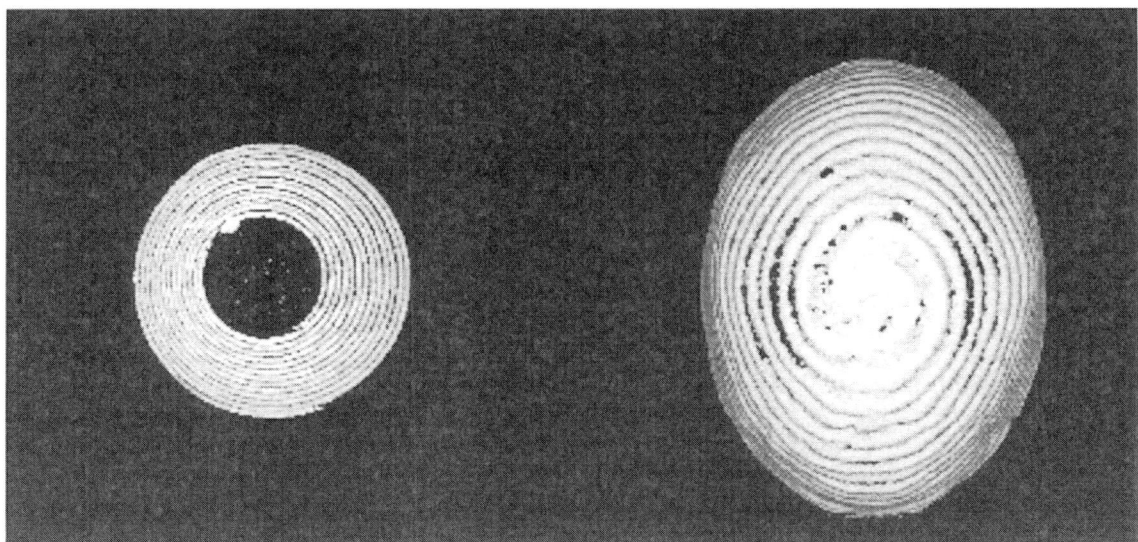

Fig. 1.24. Three-dimensional axial views of images (5-mm collimation, 10-mm table feed, and 1-mm reconstruction interval) of the cone phantom (*left*) and skull (*right*). Because the reconstruction interval is small and the table increment is large, the rotation effect dominates. Spiral-like patterns can be seen

The stair-step artifacts will be more remarkable if the surface tilt angle is reduced with respect to the transverse plane, the surface thickness is decreased, or the contrast is increased, because these changes strengthen the interpolation asymmetry. Another important factor related to the stair-step artifacts is the zoom or magnification factor. As the zoom factor increases, voxel edge length decreases, and more pronounced stair-step artifacts will be observed.

For minimal stair-step artifacts, both the detector collimation and the table increment in spiral CT should be less than the longitudinal dimension of features of interest. Also, the adaptive interpolation scheme discussed earlier may suppress the stair-step artifacts.

1.6.2 Blurring Artifacts

No imaging system is perfect. A common phenomenon is that sharp edges in an image look blurred due to a degraded system high-frequency response. The blurring or volume averaging artifacts are certainly undesirable when details are examined. For example, spiral CT is advantageous in visualizing and measuring bony structures of the middle and inner ear and geometric features of implanted devices compared with other imaging modalities; however, blurring in spiral CT images limits the *in situ* study of cochlear implant electrode arrays (VANNIER and WANG 1993; SKINNER et al. 1994).

Digital deblurring is an established approach to undo image blurring retrospectively. A pilot study was performed on longitudinal spiral CT image deblurring for abdominal imaging (SCHLUETER et al. 1994). In that study longitudinal blurring in spiral CT images was approximated as a one-dimensional spatially invariant linear system. The one-dimensional PSF of the system was experimentally determined. With the measured PSF, phantom and clinical images were deconvolved using Wiener filtering and constrained iteration methods. The FWHM of the SSP was significantly decreased after deconvolution, and anatomical boundaries in clinical images were more clearly delineated.

After the pilot study, a methodology for volumetric image deblurring in spiral CT was developed to improve the quality of temporal bone image volumes (WANG et al. 1996a). Assuming that the spiral CT imaging process is a three-dimensional linear spatially invariant system, the key step in deblurring an image is to estimate the three-dimensional system PSF. To the first-order approximation, we model the spiral CT PSF as a separable Gaussian function. Spiral CT image resolution is anisotropic; specifically, longitudinal resolution is worse than in-plane resolution. Accordingly, the Gaussian blurring in a volumetric spiral CT image is decomposed into transverse and longitudinal components that can be respectively characterized by standard deviations and independently estimated.

The formulas used in estimating standard deviations of the Gaussian PSF of the spiral CT system are summarized below. During the CT monthly quality test, the modulation transfer function (MTF) of a thin wire is imaged to determine the in-plane resolution in terms of frequencies at typical fall-offs, for example, 50%, 10%, and 2%. These experimental values can be used to determine the in-plane PSF in a Gaussian form. It can be shown that the in-plane standard deviation σ_{xy} of the PSF can be expressed as:

$$\sigma_{xy} = \frac{\sqrt{-2\ln m_0}}{2\pi u_0}, \qquad (1.26)$$

where m_0 is the MTF value at frequency u_0. Regarding the longitudinal standard deviation σ_z of the PSF, it can be shown that:

$$\sigma_z = \frac{\sqrt{2}}{4} D, \qquad (1.27)$$

where D is again the detector collimation.

There are various image deblurring algorithms available. In this study we employed Wiener filtering and maximum likelihood (or expectation maximization) deconvolution methods that were implemented in the ANALYZE image analysis and visualization software system developed at the Mayo Clinic (ROBB 1995). Wiener filtering is a well-known linear deblurring method. The maximum likelihood method can be roughly described as follows. In each iteration, a previous guess is convolved with a system PSF. Then, an observed image is point by point divided by the convolved guess. Third, the ratio image is convolved

again with the PSF. Finally, the convolved ratio image is point by point multiplied by the previous guess to obtain an updated guess. A reconstructed image can be used as an initial guess.

In our study, the in-plane and longitudinal deviations of the Fourier transform of the system PSF were theoretically derived. Then, a constant ratio of noise and image power spectrum components was interactively determined from experiments. The criterion was to maximize image clarity without introducing substantial image noise and edge ringing. With the same criterion and the optimal constant ratio of noise and image spectra, the theoretically derived standard deviations in the discrete Fourier domain were adjusted via perturbation using the Wiener filtering method. In our experiments, greater image clarity is achieved after deblurring. The maximum likelihood method produced more deblurring improvement but took a longer processing time than the Wiener filtering method. Figure 1.25 shows original and three-dimensionally deblurred temporal-beam images using the maximum likelihood method.

The maximum likelihood method has attractive theoretical advantages (HOLMES 1989; SNYDER et al. 1992). To appreciate them, we may consider image deblurring as estimating the true image from an observed image with a known system PSF, and evaluating the result with a measure of discrepancy between the true and deblurred images. Given a discrepancy

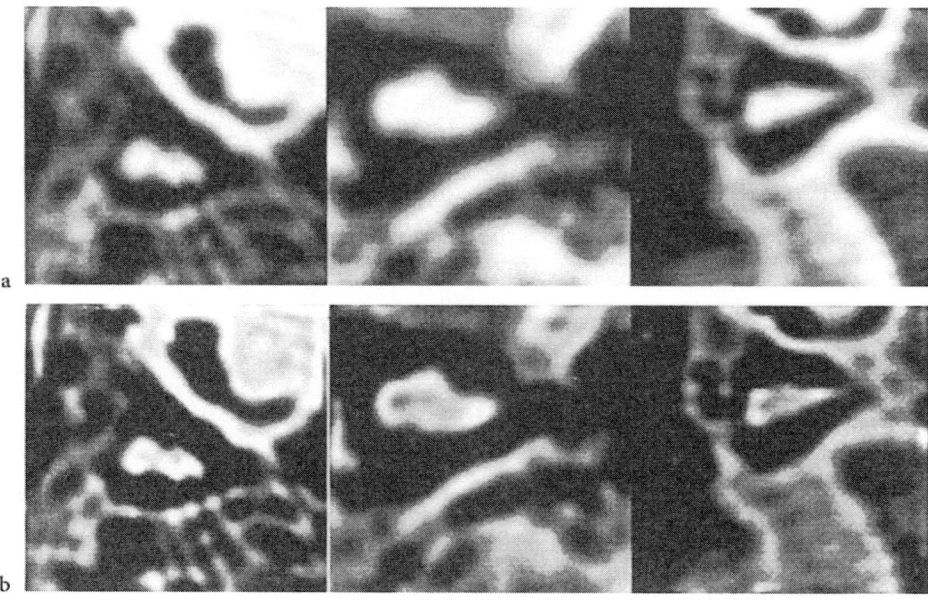

a

b

Fig. 1.25a,b. Spiral CT temporal bone image deblurring using the expectation maximization (EM) method. **a** Original temporal bone spiral CT transaxial slices of 1 cm² in area and 1 mm in thickness, and **b** deblurred images using the EM method. (Original slice data courtesy of Dr. ESSELMAN)

measure, the optimal deblurring method produces the solution minimizing the discrepancy. There are many discrepancy measures. However, CSISZÀR (1991) proved that to be consistent with his axioms, which any good discrepancy measure should satisfy, the least square measure and the Csiszàr's *I*-divergence are the only choices for real and nonnegative functions, respectively. SNYDER et al. (1992) proved under some conditions that the maximum likelihood method deblurs an image so as to minimize Csiszàr's *I*-divergence. HOLMES (1989) showed restoration of missing Fourier components by this method, even in the presence of noise. This spectral-extrapolation property makes this method superior to any linear methods, including Wiener filtering. These findings distinguish the maximum likelihood method from other deblurring methods.

The volumetric spiral CT image deblurring methodology we developed (WANG et al. 1996a) can be applied to other kinds of CT images. Generally speaking, higher image resolution always translates into better diagnosis and finer assessment. Alternatively, for a specified resolution, x-ray dose can be decreased with deblurring techniques.

1.6.3 Metal Artifacts

A major limitation with x-ray CT is that metal artifacts compromise image quality. Because of their higher atomic number, metals attenuate x-rays in the diagnostic energy range much more than soft tissues and bone. The most severe effect of metals is missing data. The x-ray beam is attenuated so strongly by metals that almost no photons reach the detectors. In other words, when metal objects are presented, projections are no longer complete. Pronounced dark and bright streaks are thus produced in reconstruction using conventional filtered backprojection. Metal artifacts seriously degrade image quality, particularly with reconstruction errors near the surface of orthopedic implants and dental restorations. Figure 1.26 shows typical metal artifacts in a CT image due to a prosthesis.

Various methods have been proposed to suppress metal artifacts. There are basically two types of algorithms that are based on either correction in the projection domain or iteration in the spatial and frequency domains. LEWITT and BATES (1978) developed an algorithm for image reconstruction from hollow projections, in which data gaps are either bridged by polynomial interpolations or filled with data satisfying consistency criteria. HINDERLING et al. (1979) applied Lewitt and Bates' data gap bridging technique for in vivo evaluation of artificial hip joints. KALENDER et al. (1987) investigated suppression of streak artifacts by linearly fitting raw data in the shadows of a metal object with adjacent raw data which do not involve the metal. LONN and CRAWFORD (1988) improved the linear fitting method by estimating the contributions from other high density structures with a high-resolution reprojector. These interpolation methods have met with varying degrees of success and appear to de-

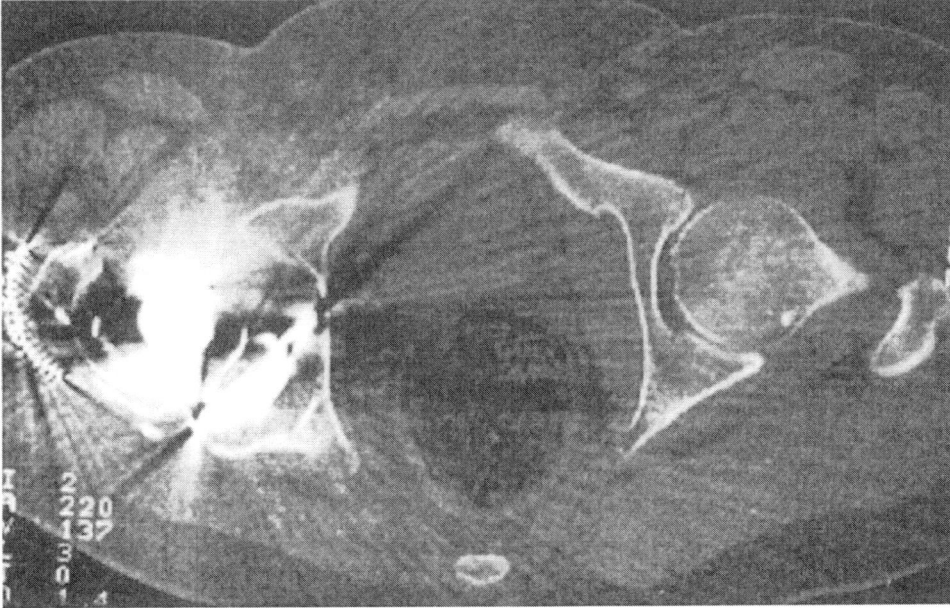

Fig. 1.26. Metal artifacts caused by a prosthesis (original slice data courtesy of Dr. ROBERTSON)

pend on the complexity of the structures examined. Highly complex structures may generate additional new artifacts.

Development of iterative algorithms was to a large degree motivated by studies on extrapolation of a band-limited function. Briefly speaking, iterative algorithms go back and forth between spatial and frequency domains and apply constraints. Gerchberg and Papoulis studied iterative extrapolation of a band-limited function (GERCHBERG 1974; PAPOULIS 1975). MEDOFF et al. (1983) proposed a framework that allows all types of limited data and incorporates a priori information using constraint operators. From this framework they derived an iterative filtered backprojection algorithm. SEZAN and STARK (1984) addressed the incomplete data problem using the method of projections onto convex sets (POCS). Due to the ill-posedness in reconstruction from incomplete data and the complexity of actual structures, reconstruction with these iterative algorithms is often unsatisfactory. In particular, noise and distortion introduced in the extrapolation procedure may be severe.

To suppress metal artifacts, an iterative deblurring method (SNYDER et al. 1992; CSISZÀR 1991) was adapted (WANG et al. 1995b, 1996) that minimize I-divergence and converges monotonically. The mathematical structure of this method is very similar to that of the maximum likelihood method. From a theoretical viewpoint, this method produces the optimal results given a set of incomplete projection data. This method can be roughly described as follows. First, an initial guess, typically a constant, is made about an image to be reconstructed. Second, a current guess in each iteration is projected along x-ray paths to obtain estimated projection profiles. Third, every physically measured projection profile is point by point divided by the estimated counterpart. Fourth, the ratio profiles are backprojected onto the field of view. Finally, the backprojected image is point by point multiplied by the current guess image to produce a better guess.

Mathematically, this method can be described below. Following SNYDER et al. (1992), the deblurring problem is formulated as the inversion of the equation:

$$\int_{\bar{x} \in X} h(\bar{y}|\bar{x}) c(\bar{x}) d\bar{x} = a(\bar{y}), \tag{1.28}$$

where $a(\bar{y})$, $\bar{y} \in Y$, is an observed function, $h(\bar{y}|\bar{x})$, $\bar{x} \in X, \bar{y} \in Y$, is a known blurring kernel, and $c(\bar{x})$, $\bar{x} \in X$, is a function to be recovered. SNYDER et al. (1992) established an iterative deblurring method that can be used for solving (1.28) subject to non-

negativity constraint so as to minimize Csiszàr's I-divergence monotonically. Mathematically,

$$c_{k+1}(\bar{x}) = c_k(\bar{x}) \frac{1}{H_0(\bar{x})}$$
$$\int_{\bar{y} \in Y} \left[\frac{h(\bar{y}|\bar{x})}{\int_{\bar{x}' \in X} h(\bar{y}|\bar{x}') c_k(\bar{x}') d\bar{x}'} \right] a(\bar{y}) d\bar{y}, \tag{1.29}$$

where $H_0(\bar{x}) = \int_{\bar{y} \in Y} h(\bar{y}|\bar{x}) d\bar{y}$, $c_k(\bar{x})$ and $c_{k+1}(\bar{x})$ are current and updated guesses to $c(\bar{x})$, respectively.

CT can be viewed as a deblurring problem. For the sake of clarity, we first formulate CT into this format with complete one-dimensional parallel-beam projection data, then repeat the procedures with incomplete projection data.

Following KAK and SLANEY (1987), a complete one-dimensional parallel-beam projection is a blurred two-dimensional object function:

$$P(\theta, t) = \int_{-R}^{R} \int_{-R}^{R} f(x, y) \delta(x \cos\theta$$
$$+ y\sin\theta - t) dx\, dy,$$
$$\theta \in [0, \pi] \text{ and } t \in [-R, R], \tag{1.30}$$

where θ and t denote respectively the projection orientation and detection position, and $f(x, y)$ is an object to be reconstructed with a supporting disk: $x^2 + y^2 \le R^2$. Since:

$$\bar{x} \Leftrightarrow (x, y)^t,$$
$$\bar{y} \Leftrightarrow (\theta, t)^t,$$
$$a(\bar{y}) \Leftrightarrow P(\theta, t),$$
$$c(\bar{x}) \Leftrightarrow f(x, y),$$
$$h(\bar{y}|\bar{x}) \Leftrightarrow \delta(x\cos\theta + y\sin\theta - t),$$
$$H_0(\bar{x}) \Leftrightarrow \int_0^\pi \int_{-R}^{R'} \delta(x\cos\theta$$
$$+ y\sin\theta - t) dt\, d\theta = \pi, \tag{1.31}$$

it follows from Eq. (1.29) immediately that:

$$f_{k+1}(x, y) = \frac{f_k(x, y)}{\pi} \int_0^\pi \int_{-R}^{R} \delta(x\cos\theta$$
$$+ y\sin\theta - t) \frac{P(\theta, t)}{P_k(\theta, t)} d\theta\, dt$$
$$= \frac{f_k(x, y)}{\pi} \int_0^\pi \frac{P(\theta, x\cos\theta + y\sin\theta)}{P_k(\theta, x\cos\theta + y\sin\theta)} d\theta$$
$$= f_k(x, y) g_k(x, y), \tag{1.32}$$

where:

$$g_k(x, y) = \frac{1}{\pi} \int_0^\pi \frac{P(\theta, x\cos\theta + y\sin\theta)}{P_k(\theta, x\cos\theta + y\sin\theta)} d\theta.$$

If a metallic object exists in the field of view, it is assumed that the cross-section of the metal is contained in a convex set, C, which is a subset of the circular reconstruction region. The characteristic function of C is expressed as:

$$M(x, y) = \begin{cases} 1, & (x, y) \in C; \\ 0, & \text{otherwise.} \end{cases} \qquad (1.33)$$

Denoting the projection profile of $M(x, y)$ as $P_M(\theta, t)$, an incomplete parallel-beam projection can be written as:

$$P(\theta, t) = \int_{-R}^{R} \int_{-R}^{R} f(x, y)\delta(x\cos\theta \\ + y\sin\theta - t)dxdy, \quad (\theta, t) \in Z, \qquad (1.34)$$

where $Z = \theta, t: \theta \in [0, \pi], t \in [-R, R]$ and $P_M(\theta, t) = 0$. In this case,

$$h(\vec{y}|\vec{x}) \Leftrightarrow \delta(x\cos\theta + y\sin\theta - t), \quad (\theta, t) \in Z,$$

$$H_0(\vec{x}) \Leftrightarrow n(x, y) = \int\int_Z \delta(x\cos\theta + y\sin\theta - t) \\ dt d\theta. \qquad (1.35)$$

Therefore, we have:

$$f_{k+1}(x, y) = \frac{f_k(x, y)}{n(x, y)} \int\int_Z \delta(x\cos\theta + y\sin\theta - t)$$

$$\times \frac{P(\theta, t)}{P_k(\theta, t)} d\theta dt$$

$$= \frac{f_k(x, y)}{n(x, y)} \int_{P_M(\theta, x\cos\theta + y\sin\theta)=0}$$

$$\frac{P(\theta, x\cos\theta + y\sin\theta)}{P_k(\theta, x\cos\theta + y\sin\theta)} d\theta$$

$$= f_k(x, y)g_k(x, y), \qquad (1.36)$$

where:

$$g_k(x, y) = \frac{1}{n(x, y)} \int_{P_M(\theta, x\cos\theta + y\sin\theta)=0}$$

$$\frac{P(\theta, x\cos\theta + y\sin\theta)}{P_k(\theta, x\cos\theta + y\sin\theta)} d\theta.$$

Geometrically, $P_k(\theta, x\cos\theta + y\sin\theta)$ is a synthesized projection based on the current guess $f_k(x, y)$, and

$g_k(x, y)$ is an overall correction factor computed by backprojecting ratios of measured and estimated projections.

To demonstrate the feasibility of metal artifact reduction using iterative deblurring, a software simulator was developed, and numerical tests were done. A representative study is described as follows. A simplified two-dimensional dental phantom was designed that consists of a low-density background disk modeling the soft tissue and a high-density half-ring representing the teeth. A metal denture was assumed to be a small disk opaque to x-rays. Both the dental phantom image and the metal denture mask image were generated separately, and then combined to form an input image. In the numerical implementation, projection and backprojection operations are needed. In both processes, linear interpolation was found to be sufficient. The normalization factor $n(x, y)$ was computed in a backprojection manner. First, projection masks were produced from the image mask by projecting it in various directions and binarizing the projection value to zero and one with a sufficiently small positive number. Then, projection masks were backprojected over all pixels. An element content of the normalization array was increased by one for each projection orientation if the projection ray passing through the element was associated with a zero value. The initial guess was selected to be a constant image. In each iteration, projection and backprojection were performed if and only if the required interpolation involved neither pixels in the metal region in the image mask nor detectors blocked by the projection mask. The constraint of the circular spatial support was enforced in all backprojection operations. For comparison, the method of filtered backprojection after linearly fitting missing projection portions was also implemented. The projection gaps can be directly identified using the projection masks, and linearly filled using the two nearest neighboring projection values.

Figure 1.27 presents typical simulation results on metal artifact reduction. All images are 128 by 128 matrices, one byte per pixel. Reconstruction was done using 128 parallel-beam projections, 128 detectors per projection, and 180° scanning. A point source and point detectors were assumed. The radius of the field of view was set to 1. The input image used in the simulation is shown in Fig. 1.27a, the direct filtered backprojection image in Fig. 1.27b treating all the missing projection data as zeros, the reconstructed image using filtered backprojection after linearly estimating missing data in Fig. 1.27c, and images recovered using the iterative deblurring

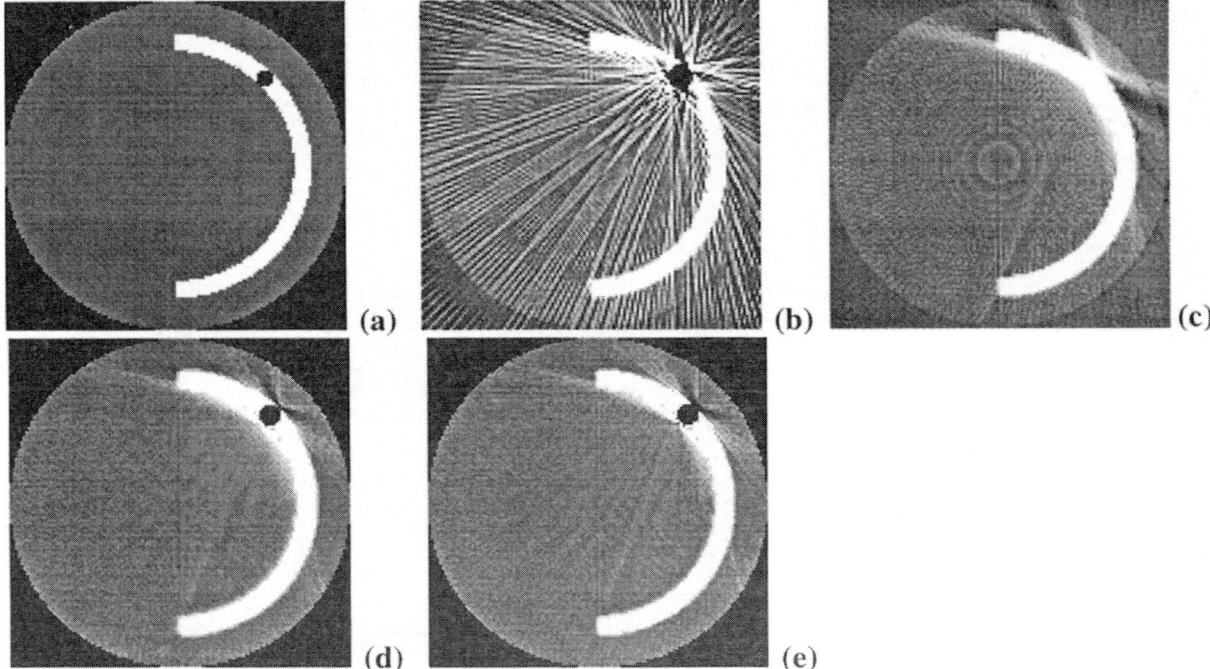

Fig. 1.27a–e. Simulation for metal artifact reduction. **a** Dental phantom with a metal denture; **b** image reconstructed using the filtered backprojection method; **c** image reconstructed using the method of filtered backprojection after linearly fitting missing gaps in projections; **d** image reconstructed using the iterative deblurring (ID) method with 50 iterations; **e** image reconstructed using the ID method with 100 iterations

method with 50, 100, and 150 iterations in Figs. 1.27d, 1.27e, and 1.27f, respectively.

It is reasonable to assume that the shape and position of metal objects are known because in practice the boundary will be clearly shown in a *directly* backprojected image. It is possible to develop a fully or semiautomatic image segmentation algorithm, such as a "snake" segmentation algorithm (KASS et al. 1987), to produce a metal mask image in practice. The snake algorithm performs well in many applications. In this approach, a contour is treated as a deformable curve that seeks to minimize its energy in internal and external force fields. The internal energy is specified by the resistance to the boundary stretching and bending. The external energy can be defined differently in various applications and may involve image intensities, their derivatives, prior knowledge, and user guidance. The contour is a minimizer of the total energy functional.

1.6.4 Motion Artifacts

In current CT, a patient is assumed to be rigid and motionless. This is unrealistic in many cases. In fact, anatomical structures move periodically due to respiration or cardiac pulsation during scanning. Severely injured and young patients frequently move while being scanned. It is often difficult for some adult patients to remain in a fixed position during scanning. In skull base and especially temporal bone imaging, high image resolution is critical, and even minimal patient movement could prevent accurate diagnosis. Since the commercial CT software does not take patient motion into consideration, motion artifacts may be produced in reconstructed CT images that blur structures of interest.

CRAWFORD (1993) and RITCHIE et al. (1992) developed a pixel-specific filtered backprojection approach for motion artifact reduction. In their algorithm, in-plane motion is corrected by performing pixel-specific reconstruction with the coordinate system moving according to the in-plane motion in the section, assuming the patient motion can be locally approximated as magnification and offset. Recently, WILLIS and BRESLER (1995a,b) reported their work on tomographic reconstruction of objects with temporal variation. They formulated the problem as signal recovery from time-sequential samples of a spatially and temporally band-limited signal, where one angular-independent view can be taken at a time. This requirement cannot be met with current spiral CT technology.

Rigid patient motion estimation and compensation in spiral CT was studied (WANG and VANNIER 1995b). To the first order approximation, rigid patient motion was modeled as being in-plane, translational, and uniform. A mismatch between adjacent fan-beam projections of the same orientation was determined via classical correlation, which is approximately proportional to the patient motion vector, defined as the patient displacement per gantry rotation, projected onto an axis orthogonal to the central ray of the involved fan-beam. The patient motion vector was estimated from its projections using a least-square-root method. To suppress motion artifacts, adaptive interpolation algorithms were developed that synthesize full-scan and half-scan planar projection data sets, respectively. In the adaptive scheme, the interpolation is performed along inclined paths dependent upon the patient motion vector. The simulation results demonstrated that the patient motion vector can be accurately estimated using our correlation and least-square-root method, patient motion artifacts can be effectively suppressed via adaptive interpolation, and adaptive half-scan interpolation is advantageous compared with its full-scan counterpart in terms of high contrast image resolution. The full-scan method is computationally simpler and statistically better for reduced image noise and improved low contrast resolution. Particularly if the table increment is relatively small and low contrast resolution is more important, the adaptive full-scan interpolation algorithm should be applied.

Nonlinear and nonrigid organ motion artifacts are more difficult to detect, characterize, and compensate. Therefore, the divide-and-conquer strategy was adopted, and motion artifact reduction in this case decomposed into two steps: motion estimation and motion compensation. Assuming the motion transform of an object function is known, a motion iterative deblurring (MID) approach was developed for nonlinear and nonrigid motion artifact reduction (WANG and VANNIER 1995a).

A time-varying object function is modeled in this context as $f(\tilde{x}, \tilde{y})$, where:

$$\begin{cases} \tilde{x} = m_1(x, y, \theta), \\ \tilde{y} = m_2(x, y, \theta), \end{cases} \quad (1.37)$$

and $m_1(x, y, \theta)$ and $m_2(x, y, \theta)$ define a regular nonlinear transform that can be visualized as an elastic mapping. In this case, a parallel-beam projection is a blurred time-varying object function:

$$\tilde{P}(\theta, t) = \int_{-R}^{R} \int_{-R}^{R} f(\tilde{x}, \tilde{y}) \delta(\tilde{x}\cos\theta + \tilde{y}\sin\theta - t) d\tilde{x} d\tilde{y}, \quad (1.38)$$

where the same supporting disk $(x^2 + y^2 \leq R^2)$ is assumed. Clearly, a family of straight lines $S: \{\tilde{x}\cos\theta + \tilde{y}\sin\theta - t, \theta \in [0, \pi]$ and $t \in [-R, R]\}$ corresponds to a family of curves $C: \{m_1(x, y, \theta)\cos\theta + m_2(x, y, \theta)\sin\theta - t, \theta \in [0, \pi]$ and $t \in [-R, R]\}$. In other words, the projection paths in the time varying case are bundles of curves. Following similar procedures as described in the preceding subsection for suppressing metal artifacts, an MID algorithm can be established as follows:

$$f_{k+1}(x, y) = f_k(x, y)\tilde{g}_k(\tilde{x}, \tilde{y}), \quad (1.39)$$

where

$$\tilde{g}_k(\tilde{x}, \tilde{y}) = \frac{1}{\pi} \int_0^{\pi} \frac{\tilde{P}(\theta, \tilde{x}\cos\theta + \tilde{y}\sin\theta)}{\tilde{P}_k(\theta, \tilde{x}\cos\theta + \tilde{y}\sin\theta)} d\theta.$$

Note that projection and backprojection are performed along curves in C.

To test our MID algorithm for motion artifact reduction, numerical simulation was performed with a time-varying Chinese Yin-Yang phantom. The Yin-Yang phantom was originally an ancient Chinese philosophical symbol consisting of asymmetric structures of continuously varying dimensions. In the numerical implementation, projection and backprojection operations are needed. In both processes, linear interpolation was found to be sufficient. The simulation results are given in Fig. 1.28. All images are 128 by 128. The pixel values for the light and dark colors in the actual Yin-Yang phantom are 1 and 2, respectively. For better visualization, the image gray-level was linearly transformed from [0.5, 2.5] into 256 gray levels. The synthetic time-varying phantom is shown in Fig. 1.28a at various scanning angles; reconstructed slices using filtered backprojection and motion iterative deblurring methods with 100 iterations are given in Figs. 1.28b and 1.28c, respectively.

If the patient motion cannot be characterized as global magnification and offset, no exact reconstruction algorithms have been available. The MID algorithm will produce the exact solution in this case as long as the problem is uniquely solvable. This is the major advantage of the MID method.

It was assumed that the motion transform can be

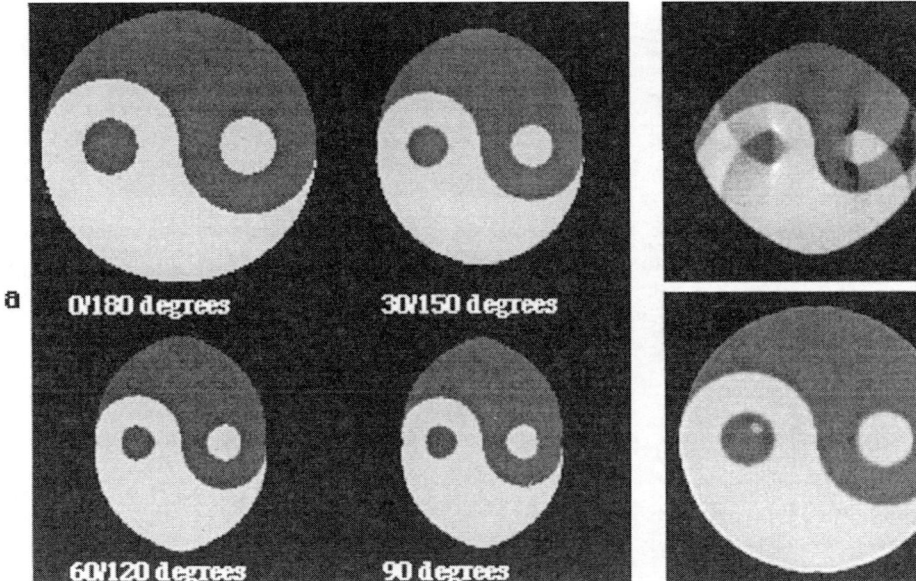

Fig. 1.28a–c. Nonrigid motion artifact reduction using the motion iterative deblurring (MID) method. **a** Synthesized time-varying Yin-Yang phantom images for projection direction $\theta = 0°$, 30°, 60°, 90°, 120°, 150°, and 180°; respectively; **b** reconstructed image using the filtered backprojection method; **c** reconstructed image using the MID method for $\theta = 0°$

estimated. This is actually also a difficult problem deserving more research effort. There are some preliminary results on patient motion estimation. As demonstrated previously, the patient motion vector can be reliably and accurately estimated directly from projection data under some conditions (WANG and VANNIER 1995b). Independent direct physical measurement may also play a role in motion estimation. It is hypothesized that superior motion estimation will be obtained by combining analysis in the projection and image domains with the shape modeling techniques.

Acknowledgements. The authors are grateful to Drs. D.L. Snyder, W.A. Kalender, C.R. Crawford, Y. Bresler, and J.A. Brink for helpful discussions, B. Brunsden, R. Knapp, R. Walkup, and N. Hente for technical assistance, and K. Smith and P. Commean for editorial help. This work was supported in part by grants from the Whitaker Foundation (The Biomedical Engineering Program) and the National Institutes of Health (1 R03 DC 02798, NIDCD R01-DC00581). The ANALYZE system was provided by Dr. R. ROBB of the Mayo Clinic. The research spiral CT software package was provided by Drs. W.A. Kalender, A. Polacin, and E. Klotz of the Siemens Medical Systems, Erlangen, Germany.

Glossary

Computed tomography (CT): Imaging modality in which projection data are collected by means of scanning x-rays across an object (a patient) from different orientations, and an image is mathematically reconstructed from the projections using computing technology.

Reconstruction: Term in CT; formation of an object image from its projections.

Filtered backprojection: Most popular CT reconstruction method, in which each projection profile is specially high-pass filtered, then backprojected over the field of view to recover a cross-sectional image.

Spiral CT: Also referred to as helical CT. Recent advance in CT which is achieved by continuous and simultaneous gantry rotation and patient translation.

Linear system: Any system whose output due to linearly combined input signals is equal to the same linear combination of output signals due to individual input signals.

Spatially invariant linear system: A special class of linear systems. If an input signal to such a system is shifted by a displacement, the output signal will also be shifted by the same amount.

High-contrast resolution: Imaging capability for resolving object details with high attenuation value differences.

Low-contrast resolution: Imaging capability for resolving object shading differences.

Slice sensitivity profile: The slice sensitivity profile (SSP) is currently used to quantify the slice thickness. An SSP can be defined as the longitudinal central profile of a CT scanner point spread function and is commonly measured along the longitudinal axis that passes through the geometric center of the gantry aperture.

FWHM/FWTM: Full-width at the half/tenth-maximum, which is defined as the distance between the two horizontal coordinates corresponding to the proximal and distal half/tenth maximum values of an SSP.

Interpolation: Process of determining an unknown value of a function from known values of the function. The most popular interpolation method is linear interpolation, in which it is assumed that the behavior of the function may be linearly approximated through adjacent known points.

Point spread function (PSF): Response of a linear system to an ideal impulse (point object) input.

Resolution: Quantified capability of an imaging system for resolving structural details and/or shading differences.

Deconvolution: Recovery of an input signal from the output response assuming that the relationship between the input and output can be modeled as a spatially invariant linear system.

Deblurring/restoration: Recovery of an input signal from the output response of a linear/nonlinear system.

Nyquist rate: The minimum sampling rate which determines how closely together the sampling points must be at least taken in order for this digital representation to be unique.

Aliasing effect: Errors produced due to sampling at less than the Nyquist rate.

Fourier transform: Fourier transform is a mathematical tool that is used to analyze periodic functions. A periodic function can be represented in terms of summation of a series of simpler trigonometric functions. If a function is not periodic, it can still be expanded as an integral of infinitely many weak trigonometric functions. Fourier transform was developed in the 1820s and has since been highly elaborated. An analogous method making use of localized mathematical fluctuations called wavelet transform was developed in the late 1980s. Wavelet analysis offers more flexibility.

Artifacts: Structured or patterned interference in reconstructed images due to limitations in data acquisition and image reconstruction.

References

Boyd DP, Lipton MJ (1983) Cardiac computed tomography. Proc IEEE 71:198-307

Bresler Y, Skrabacz CJ (1989) Optimal interpolation in helical scan computed tomography. Proc ICASSP 3:1472-1475

Brink JA (1995) Technical aspects of helical (spiral) CT. Radiol Clin North Am 33:834

Brink JA, Heiken JP, Balfe DM, Sagel SS, DiCroce J, Vannier MW (1992) Spiral CT: decreased spatial resolution in vivo due to broadening of section-sensitivity profile. Radiology 185:469-474

Brink JA, Heiken JP, Wang G, McEnery KW, Schlueter FJ, Vannier MW (1994) Spiral (helical) CT: principles and technical considerations. Radiographics 14:887-893

Crawford CR (1993) Motion artifact reduction in projection imaging. Patent Specification 5,251,128

Crawford CR, King KF (1990) Computed tomography scanning with simultaneous patient translation. Med Phys 17:967-982

Crawford CR, King KF, Hu H (1994) Helical CT noise reduction with optimized starting angles. Radiology 193(P): 170

Csiszàr I (1991) Why least squares and maximum entropy? An axiomatic approach to inference for linear inverse problems. Ann Stat 19:2032-2066

Dennis MJ (1989) Industrial computed tomography. In: Nondestructive evaluation and quality control, vol. 17. ASM International, Metals Park, Ohio

Elscint (1992) CT-twin double performance: the dream is now a reality. Elscint, Canada

Feldkamp LA, Davis LC, Kress JW (1984) Practical cone-beam algorithm. J Opt Soc Am [A] 1:612-619

Gerchberg RW (1974) Super-resolution through error energy reduction. Optica Acta 21:709-720

Grangeat P (1991) Mathematical framework of cone beam 3D reconstruction via the first derivative of the Radon transform. In: Herman GT, Louis AK, Natterer F (eds) Mathematical methods in tomography, lecture notes in mathematics. Springer, Berlin Heidelberg New York, pp 66-97

Gullberg GT, Zeng GL (1992) A cone-beam filtered backprojection reconstruction algorithm for cardiac single photon emission computed tomography. IEEE Trans Med Imaging 11:91-101

Hinderling T, Ruegsegger P, Anliker M, Dietschi C (1979) Computed tomography reconstruction from hollow projections: an application to in vivo evaluation of artificial hip joints. J Comput Assist Tomogr 3:52-57

Holmes TJ (1989) Expectation-maximization restoration of band-limited truncated point-process intensities with application in microscopy. J Opt Soc Am [A] 6:1006-1014

Hu H, Fox SH (1993) Effect of helical pitch and collimation on tumor contrast: a clinical model. Radiology 189(P):218

Hu H, Fox SH (1995) Effect of helical pitch and collimation on tumor contrast and slice profile in helical CT imaging. SPIE 2432:308-318

Ida Y, Sawada T, Tsujioka K et al. (1990) Basic studies of helical scan by a high-speed CT scanner. Jpn J Radiol Technol 46:1064

Jaszczak RJ, Greer KL, Coleman RE (1988) SPECT using a specially designed cone beam collimator. J Nucl Med 29:1398-1405

Kaiser G, Streater RF (1992) Windowed radon transforms, analytic signals, and the wave equation. In: Chui CK (ed) Wavelets: a tutorial in theory and applications. Academic Press, New York, pp 399-441

Kak AC, Slaney M (1987) Principles of computerized tomographic imaging. IEEE Press, New York

Kalender WA (1995) Principles of spiral CT. In: Goldman LW, Fowlkes JB (eds) Medical CT and ultrasound: current technologies and applications. American Medical Publ, Madison, Wisc.

Kalender WA, Polacin A (1991) Physical performance characteristics of spiral CT scanning. Med Phys 18:910-915

Kalender WA, Hebel R, Ebersberger J (1987) Reduction of CT artifacts caused by metallic implants. Radiology 164:576-577

Kalender WA, Seissler W, Vock P (1989) Single-breath-hold spiral volumetric CT by continuous patient translation and scanner rotation. Radiology 173(P):414

Kalender WA, Vock P, Seissler W (1990). Spiral CT scanning for fast and continuous volume data acquisition. In: Fuchs WA (ed) Advances in CT. Springer, Berlin Heidelberg, New York

Kalender WA, Polacin A, Marchal G, Baert AL (1992) Status and new perspectives in spiral CT. In: Langer N (ed) Advances in CT, vol. Springer, Berlin Heidelberg New York

Kalender WA, Polacin A, Süss C (1994) A comparison of conventional and spiral CT: an experimental study on detection of spherical lesions. J Comput Assis Tomogr 18:167-176

Kass M, Witkin A, Terzopoulos D (1987) Snakes: active contour models. Int J Comput Vision 1:321–331

Katada K (1993) Clinical usefulness of helical scan. In: Kimura K, Koga S (eds) Basic principles and clinical applications of helical scan: applications of continuous-rotation CT. Iryokagakusha Co, Tokyo, chapter 2

Katakura T, Kimura K Suzuki K et al. (1989) Basic studies of CT trial of helical scan. Jpn J Tomogr 16:247–250 (in Japanese)

Lewitt RM, Bates RHT (1978) Image reconstruction from projections. Projection completion methods. Optik 50:189–204

Lonn AHR, Crawford CR (1988) Reduction of artifacts caused by metallic objects in CT. Radiology 169(P):116

Medoff BP, Brody WR, Nassi M, Macovski A (1983). Iterative convolution backprojection algorithms for image reconstruction from limited data. J Opt Soc Am [A] 73:1493–1500

Mori I (1987) Computerized tomographic apparatus utilizing a radiation source. Patent Specification 4,630,202

Natterer F (1986) The mathematics of computerized tomography. John Wiley, New York

Papoulis A (1975) A new algorithm in spectral analysis and band-limited extrapolation. IEEE Trans Circuits Systems 22:735–742

Polacin A, Kalender WA, Marchal G (1992) Evaluation of section sensitivity profiles and image noise in spiral CT. Radiology 185:29–35

Rémy-Jardin M, Remy J, Giraud F, Marquette C (1993) Pulmonary nodules: detection with thick-section spiral CT versus conventional CT. Radiology 187:513–520

Rigauts H, Marchal G, Baert AL, Hupke R (1990) Scanning: phantom studies in patient material. In: Fuchs WA (ed) Advances in CT. Springer, Bderlin Heidelberg New York

Ritchie CJ, Crawford CR, Godwin JD, Kim Y (1992) Correction of respiratory motion artifacts in CT with pixel-specific backprojection. Radiology 185(P):271

Robb RA (1995) ANALYZE™ Reference Manual, 7.5 edn. Biomedical Imaging Resource, Mayo Foundation, Rochester, Minn.

Saint-Félix D, Trousset Y, Picard C, Ponchut C, Roméas R, Rougée A (1994) In vivo evaluation of a new system for 3D computerized angiography. Phys Med Biol 39:583–595

Schlueter FJ, Wang G, Hsieh P, Brink JA, Vannier MW (1994) Longitudinal image deblurring in spiral CT. Radiology 193:413–418

Sezan MI, Stark H (1984) Tomographic image reconstruction from incomplete view data by convex projections and direct fourier inversion. IEEE Trans Med Imaging 3:91–98

Skinner MW, Ketten DR, Vannier MW, Gates GA, Yoffie RL, Kalender WA (1994) Determination of the position of nucleus cochlear implant electrodes in the inner ear. Am J Otol 15:644–651

Skrabacz CJ (1988) Helical scan computerized tomography. Master's thesis, Dept of Elec & Computer Eng, University of Illinois at Urbana-Campaign

Smith BD (1985) Image reconstruction from cone-beam projections: necessary and sufficient conditions and reconstruction methods. IEEE Trans Med Imaging 4:14–28

Snyder DL, Schulz TJ, O'Sullivan JA (1992) Deblurring subject to nonnegativity constraints. IEEE Trans Signal Processing 40:1143–1150

Tohki Y (1991) The helical scanning technique. Toshiba Med Rev 38:1–5

Tohki Y (1993) Physical characteristics – principles of helical scan. In: Kimura K, Koga S (eds) Basic principles and clinical applications of helical scan: applications of continuous-rotation CT. Iryokagakusha Co, Tokyo, chapter 1

Tuy HK (1983) An inversion formula for cone-beam reconstruction. SIAM J Appl Math 43:546–552

Vannier MW, Wang G (1993) Spiral CT refines temporal bone imaging. Diagn Imaging 15:116–121

Vock P, Jung H, Kalender WA (1989a) Single-breathhold spiral volumetric CT of the lung. Radiology 173(P): 400

Vock P, Jung H, Kalender WA (1989b) Single-breathhold volumetric CT of the hepatobiliary system. Radiology 173(P):377

Wang G, Vannier MW (1993) Helical CT image noise – analytical results. Med Phys 20:1635–1640

Wang G, Vannier MW (1994a) Longitudinal resolution in volumetric x-ray CT – analytical comparison between conventional and helical CT. Med Phys 21:429–433

Wang G, Vannier MW (1994b) Spatial variation of section sensitivity profile in helical CT. Med Phys 21:1491–1497

Wang G, Vannier MW (1994c) Stair-step artifacts in three-dimensional helical CT – an experimental study. Radiology 191:79–83

Wang G, Vannier MW (1995a) Motion iterative deblurring in CT. Radiology 197(P):292

Wang G, Vannier MW (1995b) Preliminary study on helical CT algorithms for patient motion estimation and compensation. IEEE Trans Med Imaging 14:205–211

Wang G, Vannier MW (1996a) Maximum volume coverage in spiral CT. Acad Radiol 3:423–428

Wang G, Vannier MW (1996b) Optimal pitch in spiral CT. Submitted for publication.

Wang G, Lin TH, Cheng PC, Shinozaki DM, Kim H (1991) Scanning cone-beam reconstruction algorithms for X-ray microtomography. In Proc SPIE 1556:99–113

Wang G, Lin TH, Cheng PC, Shinozaki DM (1993) A general cone-beam reconstruction algorithm. IEEE Trans Med Imaging 12:486–496

Wang G, Brink JA, Vannier MW (1994) Theoretical FWTM values in helical CT. Med Phys 21:753–754

Wang G, Skinner MW, Vannier MW (1995a) Temporal bone volumetric image deblurring in spiral CT. Acad Radiol 2:888–895

Wang G, Snyder DL, Vannier MW (1995b) Iterative deblurring of CT image restoration, metal artifact reduction, and local reconstruction. Radiology 197(P):291

Wang G, Snyder DL, O'Sullivan JA, Vannier MW (1996) Iterative deblurring for CT metal artifact reduction. To appear in IEEE Trans. on Medical Imaging.

Willis NP, Bresler Y (1995a) Optimal scan for time-varying tomography. I. Theoretical analysis and fundamental limitations. IEEE Trans Image Processing 5:642–653

Willis NP, Bresler Y (1995b) Optimal scan for time-varying tomography. II. Efficient design and experimental validation. IEEE Trans Image Processing 5:654–666

Zeman RK, Brink JA, Costello P, Davros WJ, Richmond BJ, Silverman PM, Vieco PT (1994) Helical/spiral CT: a practical approach. McGraw-Hill, New York

2 Radiation Exposure

J.R. MAYO and J.E. ALDRICH

2.1 Introduction

Although computerized tomography (CT) represents only 2% of radiographic examinations, it results in 20% of the effective radiation dose from medical procedures (NRPB 1992). Radiation dose should nowadays be taken to mean the *effective dose* (ICRP 60 1991), which in radiology is the sum of the calculated absorbed doses to individual organs weighted for their radiation sensitivity. The surface dose obviously has a bearing on this effective dose but cannot directly be used to derive risk factors for radiological procedures. Effective dose can take into account partial irradiation of organs from noncontiguous CT slices and can be related to other forms of radiation exposure such as natural background or other radiological procedures. The risk of fatal cancer is 50 per million exposed to 1 mSv.

In comparison to plain film studies, the relatively high CT radiation dose results from two unique characteristics of this technique (SPRAWLS 1993). First, the ability to window or map the entire gray scale onto selected segments of the CT number scale enhances visualization of image noise. As a result, image degradation due to quantum noise is easily recognized with narrow window settings. Second, since CT is a digital technique, image acquisition and display are independent processes. Therefore, when CT dose is excessive, the image does not become too dark but merely improves because of decreased image noise (ROTHENBERG and PENTLOW 1992). As a result of these two effects, desired CT image quality often results in high patient radiation exposure which may not be recognized by the radiologist. Concern has been raised about radiation doses in chest CT (DiMARCO and BRIONES 1993; NAIDICH et al. 1994; DiMARCO and RENSTON 1994), and radiation dose surveys (NISHIZAWA et al. 1991) have documented wide variations in radiation exposure between different sites and equipment. Therefore, serious consideration needs to be given to the optimization of radiological exposures (ICRP 60 1991). As with all other radiological imaging modalities, optimal CT exposure requires an appropriate balance between diagnostic image quality and radiation dose.

This review is concerned with (a) the overall relationship between image quality and patient radiation dose, with reference to scanner dose efficiency and user-specified scan parameters, (b) the advantages of spiral over conventional data acquisition, and (c) current advances in dose reduction in chest CT. A review of radiation dosimetry and bioeffects is beyond the scope of this review and interested readers are referred to more complete works in these areas (METTLER and UPTON 1995; HUDA and ATHERTON 1995; JONES et al. 1992; METZ et al. 1995).

2.2 Scanner Radiation Efficiency

Optimally, the primary x-ray beam incident on the patient should exactly correspond to the sensitive regions of the CT detector array. Practically, this is not achieved because of imperfect collimation of the x-ray beam and physical gaps in the detector array due to its construction. Physical separation of individual detector elements creates gaps or dead

J.R. MAYO, MD, Department of Radiology, University of British Columbia and Vancouver Hospital and Health Sciences Centre, 855 West 12th Avenue, Vancouver, BC, Canada V5Z 1M9
J.E. ALDRICH, PhD, Department of Radiology, University of British Columbia and Vancouver Hospital and Health Sciences Centre, 855 West 12th Avenue, Vancouver, BC, Canada V5Z 1M9

space resulting in small zones of undetected primary beam. In some equipment this detector dead space effect can be exacerbated when detector apertures are partially masked to increase spatial resolution. The ratio of detected to incident primary beam is known as the geometric efficiency and ranges from 30% to 90% (ROTHENBERG and PENTLOW 1992).

In all radiology studies, scattered radiation is formed by the interaction of the primary beam with the patient. Scattered radiation exits in all directions and if detected, only contributes to noise in the image. In plain chest radiography, 90% of film darkening is due to scattered radiation, accounting for the low soft tissue contrast of this technique (CURRY et al. 1984). The extensive pre- and postpatient collimation in CT reverses this ratio, with 90% of detected x-rays being primary image photons. This partially accounts for the improved soft tissue contrast of CT. Compromises in CT scanner design can result in an increased scatter fraction, decreasing both image quality and CT number accuracy. Increased radiation dose may be used to compensate partially for these scanner limitations.

Scatter and imperfect collimation increase radiation dose outside of the image section. This effect is increased by contiguous or overlapping sections. Thus, with contiguous sections there is an increase in peak radiation dose by approximately 50% (Fig. 2.1) over that of a single section. Overlapping sections can give even higher doses. This dose build-up effect is accounted for mathematically in both the Multiple Slice Average Dose (MSAD) index and the Computerized Tomographic Dose Index (CTDI) (SHOPE et al. 1981). This effect can be minimized or eliminated through the use of wide intersection gaps (EVANS et al. 1989; MAYO et al. 1993). However, diagnostic information can be lost with this approach since only a portion of the chest is imaged. Intersection gaps are only practical when imaging diffuse processes such as interstitial lung disease (LEE et al. 1994).

Computerized tomography detectors vary in their efficiency. Ideally, a detector should identify all incident primary beam x-ray photons. However, depending on the technology used, detectors will record only from 60% (high-pressure xenon) to 95% (solid state) of the incident x-ray photons. The ratio of counted to incident x-ray photons is known as the quantum detection efficiency (QDE). The accuracy of conversion of the absorbed x-ray signal into an electrical signal is known as the conversion efficiency.

The product of the geometric efficiency, the quantum detection efficiency, and the conversion efficiency is the overall dose efficiency of the scanner (CUNNINGHAM 1995). This can vary significantly between scanners. Noise is also introduced by the electronics of the scanner data acquisition system. The sum of quantum noise and electronic noise results in differences in image quality between scanners. Again, increased radiation dose may be employed to

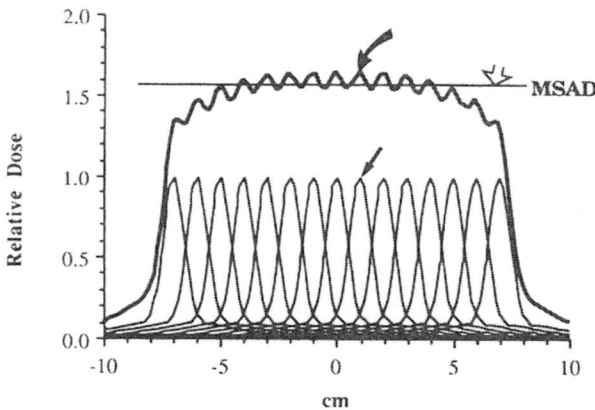

Fig. 2.1. Graph showing dose profiles for each of 15 contiguous single CT sections (*straight arrow*). The overall dose profile (*curved arrow*) is increased by approximately 50% secondary to scattered radiation and imperfect slice collimation. The calculated multiple slice average dose (*MSAD*) level is shown by the straight line (*open arrow*). (From ROTHENBERG and PENTLOW 1992)

improve image quality to compensate for increased image noise levels. Overall scanner dose efficiency can be assessed by measurement of image noise with standard phantoms. This is commonly performed by imaging physicists during the process of scanner purchase and installation.

Similar to all other radiological techniques, the primary x-ray beam in CT is filtered to eliminate low-energy photons which would be completely absorbed by the patient and only contribute to radiation dose. In CT additional spatially varying filtration is often placed in the primary beam. These filters reduce both the necessary dynamic range of the detector system in the periphery of the detector array and the radiation dose for larger fields of view (FOV). They are often referred to as "bow tie" filters due to their shape, and they create variations in entrance radiation exposure depending on both the size of the object and its position in the FOV. In some scanners these filters are moved into place depending on the specified scan FOV. In other scanners these filters are permanently positioned. Therefore, using identical technical parameters (kVp, mAs), the entrance exposure during head CT scan may be twice that during a body CT scan (MAYO et al. 1987, 1993).

2.3 User-Specified Scan Parameters

Computerized tomographic image quality can be reduced by patient motion, low subject contrast, and inadequate radiation exposure. In chest CT patient motion is minimized by use of rapid scan times and data acquisition in suspended respiration. However, the current conventional scan times of 0.7–1.0 s are still too slow to eliminate the effects of cardiac motion (RITCHIE et al. 1992). Thus, cardiac motion commonly degrades images of the lower chest region. Blurring due to motion may be reduced with electron beam CT scanners, but other compromises arise (BOYD and FARMER 1986). A full discussion of electron beam CT is beyond the scope of this review. Low subject contrast may be enhanced by the administration of intravenous contrast materials. When subject contrast remains inadequate, different imaging techniques such as magnetic resonance imaging or ultrasonography may be used.

The impact of radiation exposure on image quality occurs through its effect on image noise. Since all radiological images are derived from spatial maps of transmitted x-ray photons, counting or Poisson statistics govern the accuracy of the information on the image. As a result image noise decreases by the square root of increasing radiation exposure, giving more accurate estimates of tissue density and lower noise images. The appropriate radiation exposure for adequate image quality is determined by the radiologist based on the diagnostic question, previous experience, review of the literature, and consideration of the patient size. Patient radiation exposure or dose is linearly related to the product of tube current (mA) and scan time (s), otherwise known as mAs. In general, mAs is adjusted to create different levels of radiation exposure. Tube current (mA) is usually adjustable in steps, from 20 mA to approximately 400 mA. Scan time is related to both the gantry rotational speed and the angle over which the scan is obtained (e.g., 180° or 360°). Although the CT reconstruction technique only requires projections through a 180° arc, improved signal to noise and increased spatial resolution result from scans of 360–400°. Thus, a typical chest CT is obtained with a 360° rotation and a scan time of 1–2 s. Half scans are utilized when faster image acquisition is required, usually in dynamic bolus studies. The half scan technique results in a markedly asymmetric dose distribution which can be used to advantage, especially around the orbits. However, the introduction of newer spiral scanners with scan times of 1 s or lower has substantially limited the indications for half scan techniques. Since scan time is infrequently adjusted, the radiologist most commonly determines the trade-off between radiation exposure and image noise by setting the tube current.

Image noise represents the uncertainty or random variation in CT number determination and affects image quality. Image noise is easily measured by scanning with a phantom of uniform density such as a plastic cylinder or water bath (SPRAWLS 1992). The region of interest function on the scanner display console can be used to measure the mean and standard deviation from a large area (>100 pixels) of uniform attenuation in the phantom. Any variation in CT number as measured by the standard deviation represents image noise. Image noise in CT is primarily quantum noise related to the mAs or radiation exposure. Noise in CT is modified by the reconstruction process and has a different appearance to that on plain films. CT image noise is affected by the amount of smoothing or blurring produced by the reconstruction algorithm. As a result, image noise is higher with high spatial frequency reconstructions than with soft tissue reconstructions. Due to image reconstruction effects, low exposure CT images show more prominent streaks or lines arising from regions of high attenuation such as the vertebral bodies. On narrow collimation sections, an unrelated phenomenon, the aliasing artifact, has a similar appearance (BROOKS et al. 1979; MAYO 1991). The aliasing artifact results from incomplete data sampling and creates radiating streaks from regions of rapidly changing attenuation such as the cortex of vertebral bodies. Due to the volume averaging effect of the slice collimation, aliasing artifact is less visible on thick sections (10 mm) than on thin sections (1 mm). Aliasing artifact and correlated noise are often superimposed in the paravertebral regions of high-resolution chest images, where they form a basket-weave pattern of linear streaks. Only the correlated noise component of these streaks can be decreased by increasing tube current.

The relationship between CT image quality and radiation exposure has been previously studies (HAAGA et al. 1991; MAYO et al. 1995). In one study (MAYO et al. 1995), experienced chest radiologists showed consistently higher subjective image quality scores with higher tube current and resultant increased radiation exposure (Fig. 2.2). A linear relationship ($r^2 = 0.99$) was found between subjective image quality and square root of tube current from 20 to 200 mAs on both mediastinal and lung windows (Fig. 2.3). The inverse linear correlation between image noise and the square root of radiation exposure supports the concept that image noise is a major determinant of subjective image quality for this range of mAs. Of note, a much smaller increase in subjective image quality was seen between 200 and 400 mAs. This suggests that for these milliamperage levels, image noise reduction caused an insignificant improvement in subjective image quality.

Image noise is affected by other scan parameters including kVp, section thickness, FOV, reconstruction algorithm, and display window. In the following paragraphs trade-offs between these parameters will be described.

Along with mAs, kVp can alter the x-ray flux or entrance radiation exposure of the examination. Higher kVp values increase the radiation exposure while minimally decreasing subject contrast. Since subject contrast is high in the chest and beam hardening artifact is a problem at lower kVp values, 120 or 140 kVp is routinely used in chest CT.

Allowing for several approximations and assumptions, the relationship between CT image noise (σ) and the scan parameters of radiation dose (D), reconstruction algorithm unsharpness (ω), section thickness (h) and patient attenuation (B) has been derived by several authors (BROOKS and DICHIRO 1976; CHESLER et al. 1977; PENTLOW et al. 1977):

$$\sigma \alpha \left[1 \Big/ \sqrt{\left(B D h \omega^3 \right)} \right].$$

This equation allows us to explore the effects on image noise of alterations in scan spatial resolution (reconstruction algorithm, FOV, and slice thickness).

Due to the inverse relationship in the above equation, as the spatial resolution of the image improves by decreasing ω (e.g., decreased FOV, high spatial frequency algorithm), image noise increases. In high-resolution CT (HRCT) there is a twofold improvement of in-plane or xy spatial resolution (ω) and a tenfold improvement in slice thickness or z-axis (h) spatial resolution compared to conventional 10 mm CT. To generate an equivalent noise level on the two techniques, an increase in HRCT exposure of 80 times would be necessary. In practice, kVp and mAs levels are not changed in HRCT. The effect of increased noise in HRCT is minimized by primarily utilizing lung window settings. Patient attenuation or size (B) affects image noise, with higher exposures necessary for large patients.

The image display parameters also affect visualization, with narrow image windows enhancing both low contrast structures and image noise (WARREN and PANDYA 1982). Thus image noise is better perceived on narrow mediastinal windows (450 HU) than on the wide lung windows (1500 HU).

Finally, multiple scans of the same region increase the radiation dose in a linear fashion. Therefore, if a noncontrast acquisition is routinely performed before contrast, the radiation dose is doubled. This effect can be minimized if the noncontrast scan is a high-resolution study (e.g., 1 mm collimation at 10 mm spacing), for which the radiation dose is approximately 10% of that of a conventional or spiral scan.

2.4 Spiral CT

Spiral CT represents a different technique of acquisition of the raw scan data, which has implications with respect to image noise and radiation dose. In conventional CT, all scan data are acquired with the table stationary. The table is moved between sections. In spiral scanning, the table is continuously moved while data are acquired. Transverse sections are then created by interpolation of the spiral data set. The relative noise and section sensitivity profiles obtained with spiral CT depend on the angular interval (360° or 180°) of the interpolation algorithm (KALENDER and POLACIN 1991; POLACIN et al. 1992).

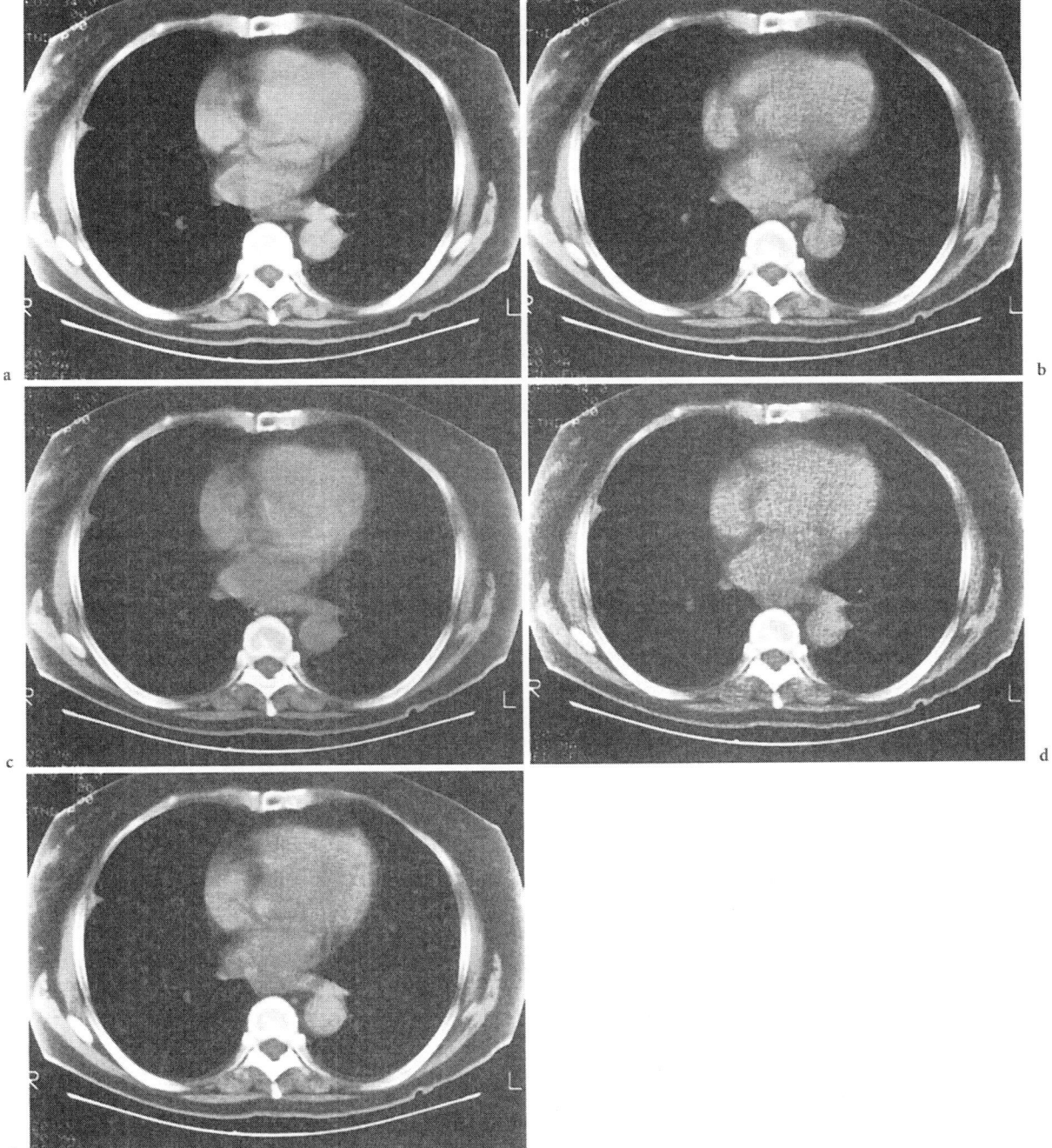

Fig. 2.2a–e. CT scans at mediastinal windows reconstructed using the standard algorithm at various mAs levels. **a** 400 mAs; **b** 200 mAs; **c** 140 mAs; **d** 80 mAs; **e** 20 mAs. Focal region of pleural thickening is identified laterally in the right major fissure. (From MAYO et al. 1995)

Compared to noise in a nonspiral acquisition, there is a 17% decrease in noise with a 360° interpolation algorithm and a 12% increase in noise with a 180° interpolation algorithm. The effect on the slice sensitivity profile is opposite, with greater broadening of the slice profile with 360° interpolation compared with 180° interpolation. Practically, the narrower slice profile of the 180° interpolation makes it the

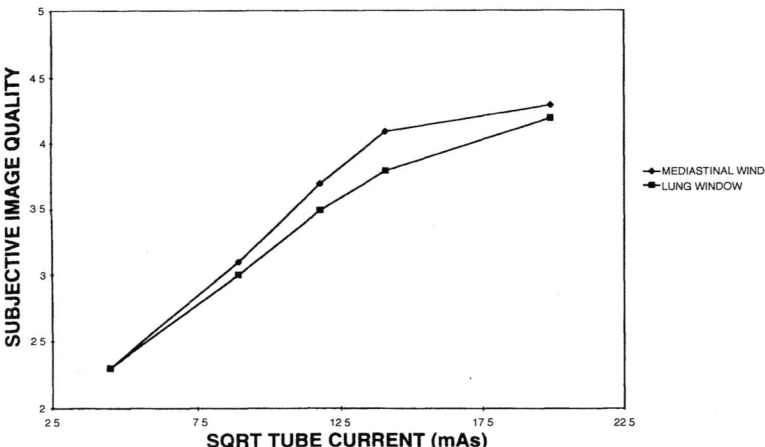

Fig. 2.3. Graph of subjective image quality versus square root of tube current for mediastinal and lung windows (high-spatial-frequency algorithm). For both windows a linear relationship ($r^2 = 0.999$) is present between subjective image quality and the square root (*SQRT*) of tube current from 20 to 200 mAs. However, a smaller increase in subjective image quality is seen between 200 and 400 mAs

commonly utilized technique. The use of either 360° or 180° interpolation does not affect the radiation exposure of the scan.

A further unique feature of spiral CT is the ability to vary the pitch of the scan (POLACIN et al. 1992). Pitch is defined as the table feed distance per 360° rotation divided by the section thickness. In many cases the table feed (e.g., 10 mm) and section thickness (e.g., 10 mm) are identical, with a resultant pitch of 1. This yields one spiral turn per section thickness and a radiation exposure essentially equal to a contiguous conventional CT scan. However, in spiral CT the table can be made to feed more rapidly (e.g., 20 mm) without changing the section thickness (10 mm). This results in a pitch of 2. This technique yields lower image quality due to broadening of the slice profile and reduction in the signal to noise ratio. However, the radiation exposure of the scan is decreased by the value of the pitch (e.g., one-half the radiation exposure for a pitch of 2) since the irradiated region of the patient now resembles the stripe on a barber pole.

Another significant advantage of spiral data acquisition is the capacity to produce multiple overlapping sections by reconstructing the data at rotational increments of less than 360°. Calculations indicate significant improvements in z-axis spatial resolution when five reconstructions per 360° rotation (WANG and VANNIER 1994) are performed. In comparison, a similar approach on conventional CT would require multiple overlapping sections with markedly increased radiation exposure. With further research

into z-axis deconvolution (SCHLUETER et al. 1994), it may be possible to produce isometric voxels with spiral CT. The very rapid data acquisition of the spiral technique leads to enhanced vascular opacification as all of the chest can be imaged during the bolus phase. The increased vascular contrast may allow reduction in radiation dose with no loss in diagnostic accuracy. However, this will require further research before clinical recommendations can be made. Finally, the rapid data acquisition of spiral CT creates very high x-ray tube loading, which often reduces the available mA, forcing the acquisition of a lower dose examination. Unfortunately, from a radiation dose viewpoint, this limitation is being obviated by the introduction of larger, more powerful x-ray tubes or modification of CT scanner gantry geometry to increase the entrance exposure.

2.5 Dose Reduction in Chest CT

The concept of reduced tube current for conventional 10 mm collimation chest CT was introduced by NAIDICH et al. in 1990 with demonstration of acceptable image quality for assessment of lung parenchyma with low tube current settings (20 mAs). While these images were adequate for assessing lung parenchyma, they had a considerable increase in noise, which resulted in marked degradation of image quality on mediastinal windows. For this reason the authors noted that such low-dose techniques were most suited for assessment of children and possibly for screening patients at high risk for lung cancer. The increased image noise present with the 20 mAs technique has precluded its routine use.

Similar findings were reported with chest HRCT, where no significant difference in lung parenchymal structures was seen between low-dose (40 mAs) and high-dose (400 mAs) HRCT images (ZWIREWICH et al. 1991). However, although not statistically significant, ground-glass changes were difficult to assess on low-mA images due to increased image noise. Therefore we recommend 200 mAs for routine HRCT images. Lower doses (i.e., 40–100 mAs) can be used for follow-up examination.

The radiation dose associated with HRCT has been controversial, with DiMarco quoting the high figure of 120–140 mGy (DIMARCO and BRIONES 1993) which was reported in an early HRCT paper (MAYO et al. 1987). This dose estimate was measured using contiguous 1.5-mm sections, 510 mAs, and CTDI methodology in a head-sized (16 cm) CT quality control phantom. The CTDI measurement was designed to facilitate dose comparisons between CT scanners and was not appropriate to describe the relative dose of HRCT. The effective dose (Table 2.1) is a better measure as it takes into account the significant reduction in radiation risk associated with the noncontiguous nature of HRCT. With 10-mm intersection gaps the effective dose of HRCT is 10% that of either conventional contiguous CT sections or spiral CT with a pitch of 1. The effective dose of HRCT is reduced to approximately 5% with the use of 20 mm intersection gaps. As noted previously, low-dose

HRCT can also be utilized in selected patients. It has been shown that three low-dose HRCT sections provide an effective dose comparable to that of a posteroanterior chest radiograph, with no significant loss of diagnostic accuracy in interstitial lung disease (LEE et al. 1994).

In conventional 10 mm collimation chest CT the relationship between radiation exposure and image quality on both mediastinal and lung windows has been evaluated between 20 and 400 mAs (MAYO et al. 1995). Although this study showed a consistent increase in mean image quality with higher radiation exposure, no significant difference in the detection of mediastinal or lung parenchymal abnormalities was seen from 20 to 400 mAs. As a result of this research we believe adequate image quality can be consistently obtained in average-sized patients with a radiation exposure of 100–200 mAs. This study was limited by a small number of patients (30) and an experimental design which limited low-dose sections to two levels, which in many cases were not the levels with clinically relevant findings. Comparison of complete chest CT studies at a variety of radiation exposures in a large number of patients will be required to evaluate further the effect of reduced radiation dose on diagnostic accuracy in chest CT.

The absorbed dose to the breast has been raised as a concern in chest CT, but this dose needs to be considered in terms of the risk from such a dose. In the paper by NISHIZAWA et al. (1991) the breast dose ranged from 8.72 to 39.6 mGy for chest CT. However, the contribution to total effective dose (which ranged from 5.67 to 14.05 mSv) from the absorbed dose to the breast was of the order of 10% (range 0.43–1.98 mSv), about the same as the annual effective dose from natural background.

Finally, although CT is a relatively high radiation dose modality, in selected instances it may replace studies with higher radiation exposures such as pulmonary angiography or bronchography (Table 2.1). In addition, its noninvasive nature and cross-sectional imaging perspective can result in a better tolerated and diagnostically more accurate examination.

Table 2.1. Comparison of effective doses

Procedure	Effective dose (mSv)
PA chest radiograph	0.05[a]
Conventional CT	7.0[b]
Spiral CT pitch 1	7.0[b]
Spiral CT pitch 2	3.5[b]
HRCT 10 mm intersection gap	0.7[b]
HRCT 20 mm intersection gap	0.35[b]
Thin-section low-dose HRCT	0.02[c]
Conventional pulmonary angiography	9.0[d]
Digital pulmonary angiography	6.0[d]
Conventional bronchography	3.0[e]
Natural background radiation	2.5[a]

[a] UNSCEAR (1993)
[b] NRPB (1992)
[c] LEE et al. (1994)
[d] Calculated using data from NRPB (1994) Report R262 assuming pulmonary angiography with 5 min of fluoroscopy and the equivalent of 30 PA and 30 lateral views
[e] Bronchography performed with the assumption of 2 min of fluoroscopy and six PA and six lateral views

2.6 Summary

The level of radiation exposure provided by CT is high relative to other radiological examinations. This is partially intrinsic to the technique but is also a result of the technical factors utilized. Currently, there is large variation in the technical factors employed, with resultant large variation in the radiation dose to the patients. Further research into the relationship between diagnostic accuracy and radiation exposure is necessary to ensure that the techniques utilized in chest CT are optimal.

References

Boyd DP, Farmer DW (1986) Cardiac computed tomography. In: Collin SM, Skorton DJ (eds) Cardiac imaging and imaging processing. McGraw-Hill, New York, pp 68–87

Brooks PA, DiChiro G (1976) Statistical limitations in X-ray reconstructive tomography. Med Phys 3:237–240

Brooks RA, Glover GH, Talbert AJ, Eisner RL, DiBianca FA (1979) Aliasing: a source of streaks in computed tomograms. J Comput Assist Tomogr 3:511–518

Chesler DA, Riederer SJ, Pelc NJ (1977) Noise due to photon counting statistics in computed X-ray tomography. J Comput Assist Tomogr 1:64–74

Cunningham IA (1995) Computed tomography: instrumentation. In: Bronzino JE (ed) The biomedical engineering handbook. CRC Press, Boca Raton, Fl., pp 990–1002

Curry TS III, Dowdey JE, Murray RC Jr (1984) Christensen's introduction to the physics of diagnostic radiology, 3rd edn. Lea & Febiger, Philadelphia, p 73

DiMarco AF, Briones B (1993) Is chest CT performed too often? Chest 103:985–986

DiMarco AF, Renston JP (1994) In search of the appropriate use of chest computed tomography. Chest 106:332–333

Evans SH, Davis R, Anderson W (1989) A comparison of radiation doses to the breast in computed tomographic chest examinations for two scanning protocols. Clin Radiol 40:45–46

Haaga JR, Miraldi F, MacIntyre W, LiPuma JP, Bryan PJ, Wiesen E (1991) The effect of mAs variation upon computed tomography image quality as evaluated in in vivo and in vitro studies. Radiology 138:449–454

Huda W, Atherton JV (1995) Energy imparted in computed tomography. Med Phys 22:1263–1269

ICRP 60 (1991) 1990 Recommendations of the International Commission on Radiological Protection. Pergamon Press, Oxford

Jones AP, Mott DJ, Parkinson L (1992) Experience with a new simple method for the determination of doses in computed tomography. Radiat Protection Dosimetry 43:139–142

Kalender WA, Polacin A (1991) Physical performance characteristics of spiral CT scanning. Med Phys 18:910–915

Lee KS, Primack SL, Staples CA, Mayo JR, Aldrich JE, Müller NL (1994) Chronic infiltrative lung disease: comparison of diagnostic accuracies of radiography and low- and conventional-dose thin-section CT. Radiology 191:669–673

Mayo JR (1991) High resolution computed tomography: technical aspects. Radiol Clin North Am 29:1043–1049

Mayo JR, Webb WR, Gould R, Stein MG, Bass I, Gamsu G, Goldberg HI (1987) High-resolution CT of the lungs: an optimal approach. Radiology 163:507–510

Mayo JR, Jackson SA, Müller NL (1993) High-resolution CT of the chest: radiation dose. AJR 160:479–481

Mayo JR, Hartman TE, Lee KS, Primack SL, Vedal S, Müller NL (1995) CT of the chest: minimal tube current required for good image quality with the least radiation dose. AJR 164:603–607

Mettler FA Jr, Upton AC (1995) Medical effects of ionizing radiation, 2nd edn. Saunders, Philadelphia

Metz CE, Wagner RF, Doi K, Brown DG, Nishikawa RM, Myers KJ (1995) Toward consensus on quantitative assessment of medical imaging systems. Med Phys 22:1057–1061

Naidich DP, Marshall CH, Gribbin C, Arams RS, McCauley DI (1990) Low-dose CT of the lungs: preliminary observations. Radiology 175:729–731

Naidich DP, Pizzarello D, Garay SM, Müller NL (1994) Is thoracic CT performed often enough? Chest 106:331–332

NRPB (1992) Documents of the NRPB 3;4:1–16 National Radiological Protection Board, Chilton, Didcot, Oxon., UK

NRPB (1994) Report R262: Estimation of effective dose in diagnostic radiology from entrance surface dose and dose-area product measurements. In: Hart D, Jones DG, Wall BF (eds) National Radiological Protection Board, Chilton, Didcot, Oxon., UK

Nishizawa K, Maruyama T, Takayama M, Okada M, Hachiya J, Furuya Y (1991) Determinations of organ doses and effective dose equivalents from computed tomographic examination. Br J Radiol 64:20–28

Pentlow KS, Beattie JW, Laughlin JS (1977) Parameters and design considerations for tomographic transmission scanners. In: Ter-Pogossian MM, Phelps ME et al. (eds) Reconstructive tomography in diagnostic radiology and nuclear medicine. University Park Press, Baltimore, pp 267–279

Polacin A, Kalender WA, Marchal G (1992) Evaluation of section sensitivity profiles and image noise in spiral CT. Radiology 185:29–35

Ritchie CJ, Godwin JD, Crawford CR, Stanford W, Anno H, Kim Y (1992) Minimum scan speeds for suppression of motion artifacts in CT. Radiology 185:37–42

Rothenberg LN, Pentlow KS (1992) Radiation dose in CT. Radiographics 12:1225–1243

Schlueter FJ, Wang G, Hsieh PS, Brink JA, Balfe DM, Vannier MW (1994) Longitudinal image deblurring in spiral CT. Radiology 193:413–418

Shope TB, Gagne RM, Johnson GC (1981) A method for describing the doses delivered by transmission X-ray computed tomography. Med Phys 8:488–495

Sprawls P Jr (1992) CT image detail and noise. Radiographics 12:1041–1046

Sprawls P Jr (1993) Physical principles of medical imaging, 2nd edn. Aspen, Maryland, pp 361–369

UNSCEAR (1993) Report to the General Assembly, with Scientific Annexes. United Nations, New York

Wang G, Vannier MW (1994) Longitudinal resolution in volumetric X-ray computerized tomography – analytical comparison between conventional and helical computerized tomography. Med Phys 21:429–433

Warren RC, Pandya YV (1982) Effect of window width and viewing distance in CT display. Br J Radiol 55:72–74

Zwirewich CV, Mayo JR, Müller NL (1991) Low-dose high-resolution CT of lung parenchyma. Radiology 180:413–417

3 Techniques of Acquisition

P. Vock

CONTENTS

3.1 Introduction

Having been introduced only half a decade ago (KALENDER et al. 1990), spiral CT is a technically young acquisition technique undergoing continuous development. New hardware performance characteristics are still being developed and there has been insufficient time for clinical experience to define consensus protocols even for frequent clinical indications (VERSCHAKELEN and VAN HOE 1995). This chapter will cover the current status of spiral CT application and, in view of the trends, suggest ranges for parameter selection or even cite two basically different approaches to the same problem.

Around 15 parameters can be controlled when spiral CT is performed (Table 3.1). Most of them are identical in conventional CT and spiral CT; some will hardly ever be changed when specific protocols are selected, and only for a few of the parameters is adaptation critical when spiral instead of conventional CT of the chest is performed.

Among the 15 parameters listed in Table 3.1, nearly all have to be chosen prospectively and, therefore, are true acquisition parameters. "Table feed per rotation (d)" and "reconstruction increment (RI)" are unique to spiral CT. It is a major advantage of spiral CT that the "reconstruction increment" can be selected and modified during postprocessing without keeping the patient in the gantry, whereas "interscan table motion," its analogue in conventional CT, must be selected in advance. Of course, reconstruction algorithm, reconstruction center, and field of view, as well as two-dimensional (2-D) reformations and three-dimensional (3-D) representations, are postprocessing options in both conventional CT and spiral CT; they may influence the acquisition protocol and will therefore be mentioned briefly although they are covered in detail in Chap. 5. Similarly, the details of intravenous contrast injection for vascular and parenchymal enhancement, although they are chosen prospectively, will be discussed in Chap. 4.

The influence of each parameter will be discussed first; then a practical approach to acquisition of spiral CT examinations of the chest will be suggested. Some frequent or important clinical indications will be covered, and the advantages spiral CT may offer and how it may be used best to resolve patient problems will be discussed.

3.2 Control of Acquisition Parameters

3.2.1 Rotation Time

The time needed for one tube rotation (t) is one of the major differences between scanner types, in both third- and fourth-generation CT. It usually corre-

P. VOCK, MD, Department of Diagnostic Radiology, University Hospital, 3010 Berne, Switzerland

Table 3.1. Acquisition parameters in spiral CT of the chest

Acquisition parameter	Available range	Selection criteria
1. Rotation time = t (s)	0.75 s, 1 s, 1.5 s, 2 s	Minimum available on scanner/ patient cooperation/dose needed
2. Scan collimation = section width = slice thickness = s (mm)	1–10 mm	Depending on indication
3. Table feed per rotation = d (mm)[a] $\rightarrow$ pitch = p = d/s	1–25 mm 1–2 (2.5)	Depending on indication
4. Voltage (kVp)	(80) 120–140 kVp	Usually 120–140 kV
5. mAs per rotation	(50–) 150–400 mAs	Depending on patient habitus
6. Gantry angulation	(−30°−) 0° (−+30°)[c]	Depending on indication
7. Scanning direction	Superoinferior, inferosuperior	Depending on indication
8. Scan duration (s)	24–60 s	Patient cooperation/scanner type
9. Multiple spiral scans	Modification of parameters 1–8	Patient/scanner/indication
10. Reconstruction increment = RI[a,b]	20%–50%–100% of scan collimation	See Chap. 5
11. Reconstruction center/size (targeting)	Any	See Chap. 5
12. Image reconstruction algorithm	a) Type of z-axis interpolation b) Soft/standard/high spatial resolution	See Chap. 5
13. Patient respiration	Inspiratory apnea, apnea, continuous respiration, expiration	Depending on indication and cooperation
14. Patient position	Supine (prone, lateral, oblique)	Prone scans to expand post. lung, lateral/oblique scans for intervention
15. Contrast	No/i.v. bolus/esophageal	See Chap. 4

[a] Unique to spiral CT $\rightarrow$ pitch = table feed per rotation/scan collimation
[b] Corresponds to interscan table motion in conventional CT but is independently selected in retrospect
[c] +(−), Anteroinferior (anterosuperior) to posterosuperior (posteroinferior) scanning plane

sponds to the standard scanning time for the conventional acquisition mode and varies between 0.75 and 2 s (Table 3.1); even in spiral CT, the number of projections used for reconstructing an image and the scanning time of one image are directly related to this parameter. In the chest, whether with or without respiratory cooperation of the patient, cardiovascular motion artifacts are critical, and the rotation time should be minimized to the duration compatible with the availability of sufficient photons to guarantee adequate image quality. Since the lung has a low physical density and offers high natural contrast, the shortest rotation time available for pulmonary and general chest examinations is usually selected, i.e., 0.75 or 1 s (Fig. 3.1). First, this will reduce cardiorespiratory motion artifacts and provide images of excellent quality even in uncooperative patients; second, based on a given maximal duration of apnea it will help one either to cover a larger volume with one scan or to choose a thinner slice without losing volume. Examinations of the spine and the shoulder region require higher mAs and more projections and, therefore, usually a longer rotation time of 1.5– 2 s.

3.2.2 Scan Collimation (Slice Thickness, Section Width, s)

Scan collimation can usually be selected in the range between 1 and 10 mm. If attention is paid to the potential degradation of the slice sensitivity profile (POLACIN et al. 1992) depending on the pitch and the reconstruction algorithm (see below), scan collimation can be selected according to the criteria used for conventional CT. Often, 10 mm is adequate for chest screening, for trauma studies, and for excluding major mass lesions and, specifically, metastases. As soon as resolution in the z-axis becomes critical, partial volume effects must be avoided, and the slice thickness has to be reduced. Volumetric coverage is an inherent advantage of spiral CT; with a fixed rotation time and an acceptable pitch (see Sect. 3.2.3) and scan duration, however, the volume covered by one spiral scan is limited by the slice thickness. The need to measure a maximum volume during one breathhold will sometimes require a compromise in scan collimation or pitch: A thicker slice or a higher pitch – both of which increase partial volume effects – can be partially compensated for by lowering the recon-

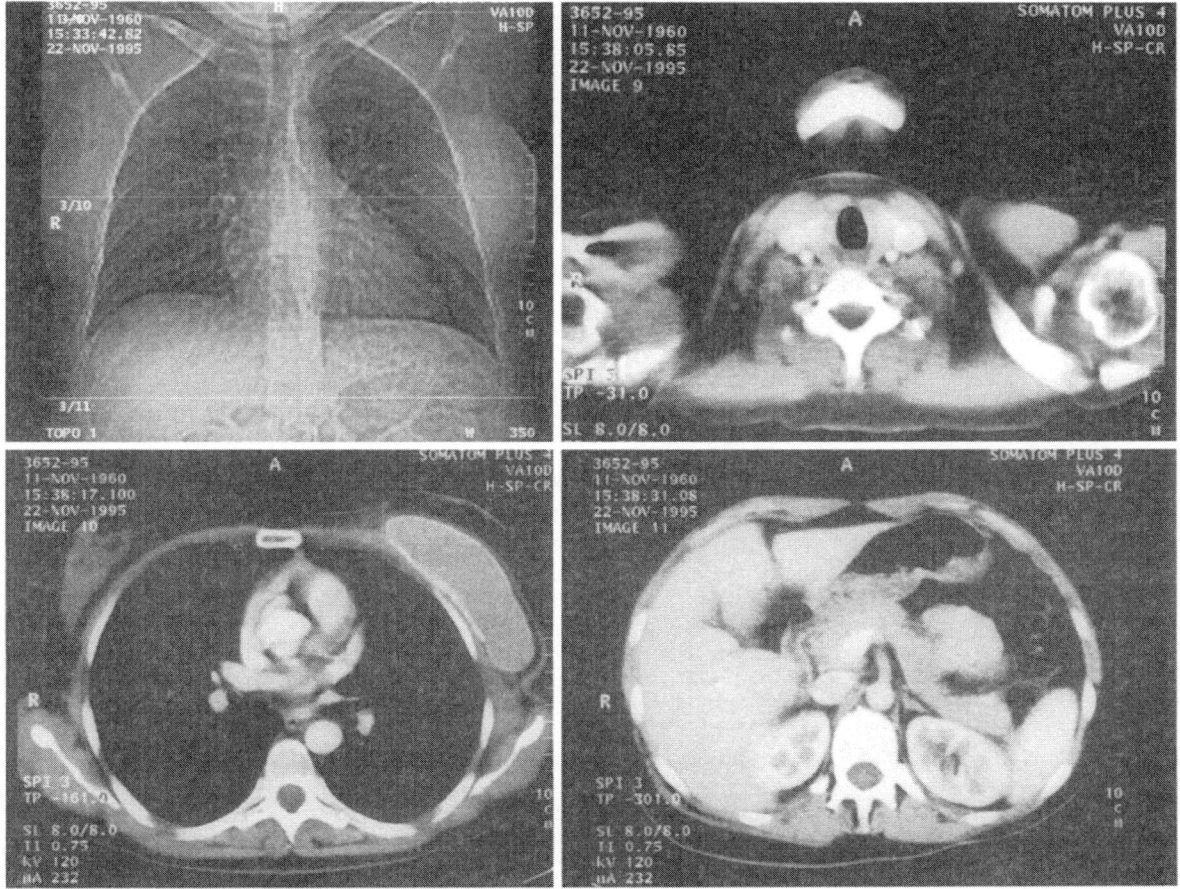

Fig. 3.1. Chest wall screening protocol in a 35-year-old patient after breast implant. Using a rotation time of 0.75 s, a collimation of 8 mm with a table feed of 8 mm per rotation (pitch = 1), and a scan duration of 26 s, a volume of 27 cm is covered

struction increment and, thus, calculating a higher number of overlapping, closely spaced images (BUCKLEY et al. 1995; FOLEY et al. 1994); this holds true especially for 2-D reconstructions and 3-D representations.

High-resolution computed tomography (HRCT), the modification introduced in the late 1980s and indicated for detailed analysis of pulmonary morphology, combines thin collimation (1–2 mm) with targeting and a high-resolution reconstruction algorithm. In our experience, the need to perform spiral HRCT is limited since complete volumetric coverage is usually unnecessary, and separate single sections spaced at 10–20 mm may provide all the information required at a lower radiation exposure. Spiral HRCT, however, is useful in analyzing topographical relations of a selected subvolume of the lung in chronic obstructive and infiltrative disease (see Chap. 7).

3.2.3 Table Feed per Rotation (*d*)

Instead of using the table transportation speed (mm/s), we prefer to look at the distance the table moves while the tube rotates 360° around the patient. This parameter is unique to spiral CT, and the greater the value chosen, the larger the volume that will be covered in a given amount of time. There is, of course, a trade-off in increasing table feed per rotation. First, the slice sensitivity profile will be degraded; the effective slice thickness, as measured by the full width at half maximum or at tenth area, will increase and therefore cause partial volume effects. For example, POLACIN et al. (1992) showed an increase in effective as compared to nominal thickness of 30% and more than 100% with a table feed per rotation of once and twice the slice thickness, respectively, using the old 360° linear interpolation algorithm (see Sect. 3.2.12). Besides partial volume effects (z-axis resolution), the resolution in the xy-plane is not significantly reduced by increasing the table feed per rotation.

For practical purposes, the selection of the table feed per rotation is determined by the *pitch factor, p*:

$$\text{pitch}\,(p) = \text{table feed per rotation}\,(\text{mm})\big/ \\ \text{slice collimation(mm)} = d/s \qquad (1)$$

Currently the useful range of pitch is between 1 and 2 (PARANJPE and BERGIN 1994); many authors will not go beyond 1.5. This means that acquisition protocols will use a table feed per rotation of 10–20 mm or 1–2 mm for slices of 10 and 1 mm respectively, with many possible values in between these two extremes, depending on the specific needs (Fig. 3.2). Table 3.2 demonstrates the influence of pitch selection on the volume (range in z-axis) covered by one spiral scan (Fig. 3.1).

3.2.4 Voltage

There is little discussion about the best voltage selection for CT; most manufacturers offer 120 kV with a filtration equivalent to around 5 mm of aluminum as a standard. Lowering the voltage from this standard base increases the relative contribution of photoabsorption and decreases that of Compton scattering. This may be a good option for quantitative densitometry of the spine by CT. In the chest, it might offer better recognition of calcification when characterizing solitary pulmonary nodules. However, dual-energy subtraction is not available with ordinary CT scanners, nor is low voltage (e.g., 80 kV) now widely used for densitometry of solitary pulmonary nodules. Lower voltage also means a higher exposure to ionizing radiation, since a smaller percentage of photons will penetrate the body unchanged and contribute to image formation. Conversely, increasing the voltage to 130–140 kV is advisable in high-contrast areas and when the number and penetration of photons are critical. Protocols

Table 3.2. Reconstructed volume [range in z-axis (cm)] in spiral CT of the chest depending on scanning time (scan duration), rotation time, and pitch. Nominal slice thickness = 10 mm [proportional correction for other collimations, based on 360° interpolation algorithm (slightly higher values with algorithm using 180° opposite projections)]

Pitch	Rotation time (s)	Spiral scan duration (s)									
		12	16	20	24	28	32	36	40	50	60
0.75	0.75	10.5	14.5	18.5	22.5	26.5	30.5	34.5	38.5	48.5	58.5
	1	7.5	10.5	13.5	16.5	19.5	22.5	25.5	28.5	36	43.5
	1.5	4.5	6.5	8.5	10.5	12.5	14.5	16.5	18.5	23.5	28.5
	2	3	4.5	6	7.5	9	10.5	12	13.5	17.3	21
1	0.75	14	19.3	24.7	30	35.3	40.7	46	51.3	64.7	78
	1	10	14	18	22	26	30	34	38	48	58
	1.5	6	8.7	11.3	14	16.7	19.3	22	24.7	31.3	38
	2	4	6	8	10	12	14	16	18	23	28
1.25	0.75	17.5	24.2	30.8	37.5	44.2	50.8	57.5	64.2	80.8	97.5
	1	12.5	17.5	22.5	27.5	32.5	37.5	42.5	47.5	60	72.5
	1.5	7.5	10.8	14.2	17.5	20.8	24.2	27.5	30.8	39.2	47.5
	2	5	7.5	10	12.5	15	17.5	20	22.5	28.8	35
1.5	0.75	21	29	37	45	53	61	69	77	97	117
	1	15	21	27	33	39	45	51	57	72	87
	1.5	9	13	17	21	25	29	33	37	47	57
	2	6	9	12	15	18	21	24	27	34.5	42
1.75	0.75	24.5	33.8	43.2	52.5	61.8	71.2	80.5	89.8	113.2	136.5
	1	17.5	24.5	31.5	38.5	45.5	52.5	59.5	66.5	84	101.5
	1.5	10.5	15.2	19.8	24.5	29.2	33.8	38.5	43.5	54.8	66.5
	2	7	10.5	14	17.5	21	24.5	28	31.5	40.3	49
2	0.75	28	38.7	49.3	60	70.7	81.3	92	102.7	129.3	156
	1	20	28	36	44	52	60	68	76	96	116
	1.5	12	17.3	22.7	28	33.3	38.7	44	49.3	62.7	76
	2	8	12	16	20	24	28	32	36	46	56

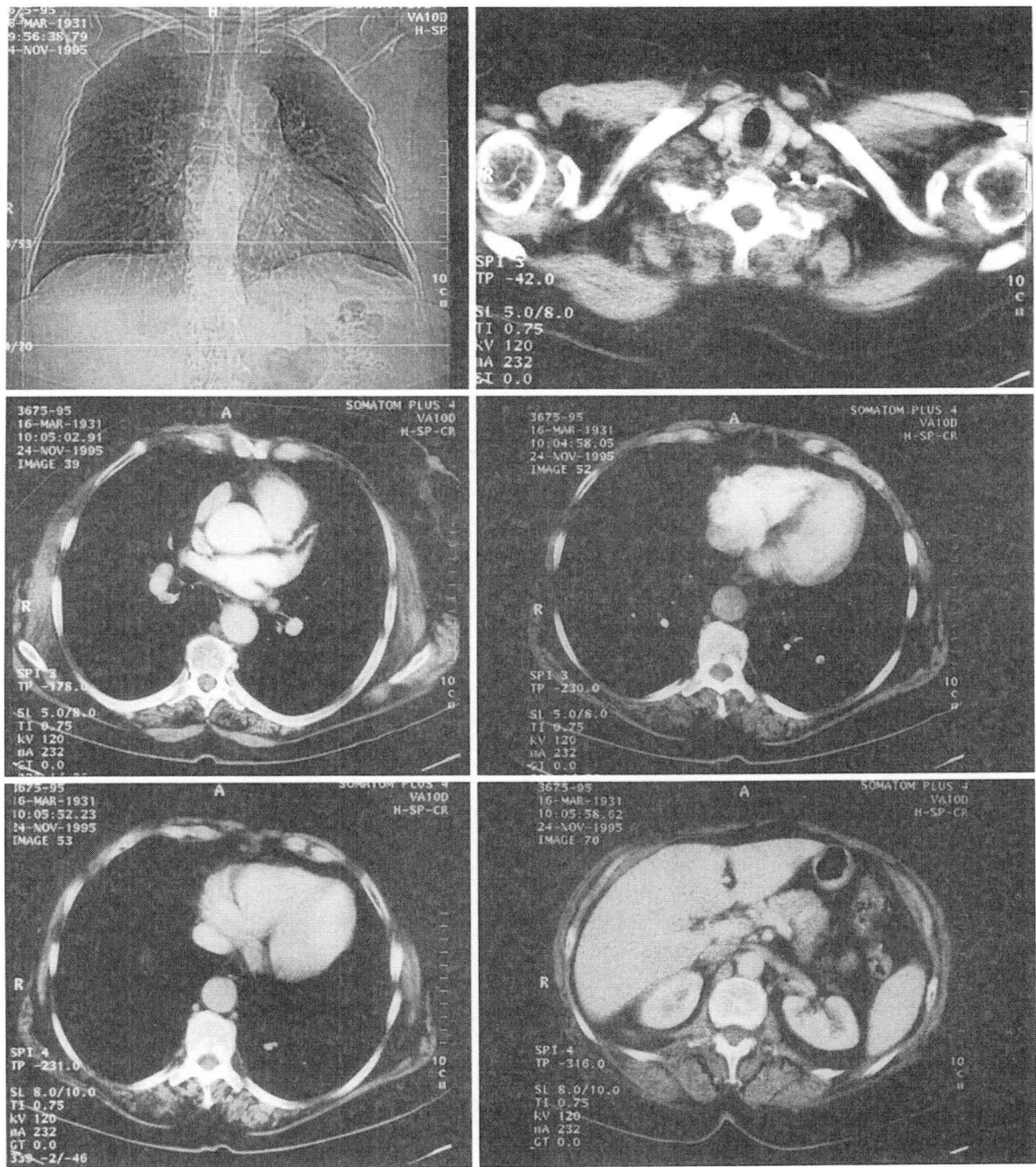

Fig. 3.2. Protocol as used for hilar pathology and lung cancer. This 64-year-old patient had nodal and pulmonary metastases from breast cancer. For the first inferosuperior spiral scan in inspiratory apnea (*upper right and middle left and right images*), the following parameters were selected: rotation time 0.75 s, collimation 5 mm, table feed 8 mm per rotation (pitch =

1.6), reconstruction increment 4 mm, and scan duration 18 s for a volume of 18.8 cm in the z-axis. The second superoinferior scan (*lower two images*) was added after an interval of 35 s, using a modified collimation of 8 mm (pitch = 1.25)

for the lung, the craniocervical and cervicothoracic junction, the shoulder area, and other parts of the spine often give preference to such higher voltage. Because of narrow collimation, increasing scatter is not critical in CT.

3.2.5 mAs per Rotation

The number of photons contributing to image formation is a limiting factor in image quality, and is best reflected by the product of current and time (mAs). Higher absorption in the body in heavy patients, the presence of many bony structures within the section level, and low voltage all require an elevated current or a longer measurement period to keep the signal-to-noise ratio constant. In spiral CT, noise is also increased by using 180° opposite views for interpolation instead of 360° (see Sect. 3.2.12); basically, both an elevated pitch factor and the use of 180° opposite views for interpolation reduce the effective measurement period per image, and the current has to be increased according to the specific clinical problem.

Since spiral CT requires long periods of continuous radiation, tube load was a critical limiting factor in its early application; reduced current (mA), as compared to conventional scans, was responsible for a generally noisier appearance of spiral CT studies. Even now, widespread use of spiral CT is limited by tube performance in some areas of the body, such as the skull and the spine (especially the petrous bone, the craniocervical junction, and the cervicothoracic junction). With some scanners the rotation time can be increased from 0.75–1 s to 1.5–2 s to resolve this problem. Otherwise, if the maximal current is not sufficient, the pitch can be reduced below 1 with 360° interpolation. Both measures increase the signal-to-noise ratio but, of course, have significant disadvantages and rarely make sense. For example, a pitch of 0.5 instead of 1 will roughly halve the volume covered and, thus, partly neutralize the strongest feature of spiral CT. Fortunately, most of the aforementioned very dense regions are easy to immobilize, and therefore several spiral scans can be added to cover the volume needed (see Sect. 3.2.9). In spiral examinations of the chest, due to the high contrast and low density available, current is usually sufficient and tube limitation minimal.

Besides pitch and voltage, the current-time product (mAs) is the main determinant of radiation exposure in spiral CT. Effective dose, the best global parameter of the biological risk, is higher in CT of the trunk than in most conventional radiographic examinations (COLLIE et al. 1994; MINI et al. 1995). Everything should be done to lower this value without causing a deterioration in information. Above all, mAs can be reduced in children; values around 100 mAs are sufficient for many indications, and 40–80 mAs can be used for the pediatric lung, even in HRCT (AMBROSINO et al. 1994). Similar dose reductions have been tried successfully in the adult lung, and in spiral CT lower mA can be combined with an increased pitch to further reduce exposure. Using

a pitch of 2 instead of 1 without changing other parameters means 50% less radiation exposure (CEDERLUND 1994; FOLEY et al. 1994; BLAKE et al. 1994; TAKAHASHI et al. 1994).

3.2.6 Gantry Angulation

Gantry angulation is most valuable for musculoskeletal and head studies. In the chest, two potential applications deserve mention. First, direct coronal or sagittal scanning has been proposed by some authors and requires flexible angulation of the gantry. Since even without table motion, positioning of the patient is difficult, this option is hardly ever used in spiral CT, except in pediatric or extremity studies. Second, the topographic course of segmental bronchi and arteries, e.g., in the middle lobe and lingula but also in the anterior upper lobe, corresponds to a plane inclined anteroinferiorly to posterosuperiorly. Direct visualization of bronchi is favored by a slight gantry angulation of around 20° (REMY-JARDIN and REMY 1988).

3.2.7 Scanning Direction

Historically, a majority of CT users preferred the superoinferior scanning direction but nonenhanced sequential single scans might equally well be obtained in the opposite direction. The introduction of bolus contrast enhancement and that of spiral CT were two important reasons to question this habit, since both offer arguments for an inferosuperior scanning direction.

Single-breathhold spiral CT requires longer periods of *apnea* than conventional sequential scans, and sick patients may start breathing before the end of the measurement. The superoinferior *respiratory displacement* of a voxel within the lung is much higher close to the diaphragm (up to 8 cm, YOUNG and SIMON 1972) than above the hilar level. In a volunteer study, from deep inspiration to expiration we found an upward motion of 7 cm for the right diaphragm and lung base, of 6.5 cm for the left diaphragm and lung base, and of around 2 cm for the upper lobar bronchi (unpublished MRI data with the volunteer in the supine position). It is likely that this displacement is smaller in sick and older people. Consequently, early continuation of breathing before the end of the spiral scan causes much more severe respiratory misregistrations and artifacts at the base with superoinferior scanning than it does at the apex with inferosuperior scanning.

Contrast enhancement requires an intravenous bolus of either highly concentrated or very rapidly injected iodinated contrast agent. Injection is usually performed using an antebrachial vein; therefore, the agent reaches the brachiocephalic vein essentially undiluted, and even in the superior vena cava it has a very high concentration that often causes severe *beam-hardening artifacts*. Major diagnostic problems may arise, especially when aortic dissection must be proven or excluded. To overcome these artifacts, injection into a leg vein has been proposed; however, this is combersome and not without risk of thrombophlebitis. Alternatively, with an inferosuperior scanning direction – ideally coupled with a small second bolus of saline –, the levels of the superior vena cava and brachiocephalic vein can be reached at or after the end of the bolus, when the iodine concentration has fallen to a value that no longer produces artifacts (RUBIN et al. 1995).

In conclusion, spiral CT protocols of the chest should *preferably* use an *inferosuperior scanning direction* (Fig. 3.2) unless more important reasons prevail, such as the need to continue the measurement to the liver. In this specific situation, the hardware and software configuration will strongly influence the decision as to the scanning direction.

3.2.8 Scan Duration

Scan duration is essentially limited by two technical and two patient-related factors: the heat capacity of the tube (requiring lower mA for prolonged scans), the data sampling capacity of the scanner, the degree of patient cooperation, and, sometimes, the pharmacokinetics of the contrast agent.

With new hardware, the data sampling capacity is no longer critical for most chest studies. Indeed, continuous spiral measurement during 60 s or even longer is available and allows large volumes of the body to be covered (more than 1 m in length, Table 3.2). However, using these long scan times, tube cooling again becomes a limiting factor and often results in a lower current. This applies for all studies that are independent of respiratory cooperation. However, many chest studies require apnea, and this usually entails a significantly shorter scan duration: usually below 30–40 s (see Sect. 3.2.13). Therefore, respiratory cooperation on the part of the patient

is the first factor to check when planning scan duration.

Pharmacokinetics are most critical for the liver when tumor staging requires a combined thoracoabdominal examination. Whether a single scan or, as is more likely, two sequential spiral measurements are employed, in order to maintain contrast between normal and neoplastic tissues the liver must be scanned before the equilibration phase of contrast distribution (i.e., within around 100 s; FOLEY and ONESON 1994).

3.2.9 Multiple Spiral Scans (Clusters)

Given the technical limitations of tube performance and the physiologic limitations of the period of apnea, it is logical that multiple segmental spiral scans came to be used to cover a larger volume of the body. Nowadays, this modification is also used to scan an organ twice (e.g., the liver during the arterial and the redistribution phase), to switch scanning parameters from one subvolume to the next, or to freely select the temporal sequence of subvolume scanning, with table transportation to any other level between scans and with a reversed scanning direction if necessary.

Of course, any interruption of the measurement will introduce anatomic misregistration between adjacent data sets since the lung volume will never reach exactly the same value with repeated apnea. This disadvantage is significant in the case of 2-D reformation and 3-D reconstruction, whereas a small overlap may avoid a potential scanning gap in mere cross-sectional diagnosis. In the chest, sequential examination of disease during two phases is much less important than in the abdomen. Respiratory cooperation, however, remains the single most important factor with newer high-capacity scanners, and it may be a good approach to divide the chest into three to four scans of around 10–15 s (FOLEY and ONESON 1994). This also allows one to adapt the slice thickness, e.g., to choose 10 mm above the hila, 5 mm through the hila, and 7–10 mm below them. In this "variable-mode helical CT technique," FOLEY and ONESON (1994) suggest intervals for respiration of 6–7 s, and of course, the protocol can be extended to include the liver, with the possibility also of modifying the current for sequential spiral scans (Fig. 3.3). We will discuss the need for multiple spiral scans further within the context of patient respiration. In summary, multiple spiral scans are a very powerful but also a complex tool. Their application depends

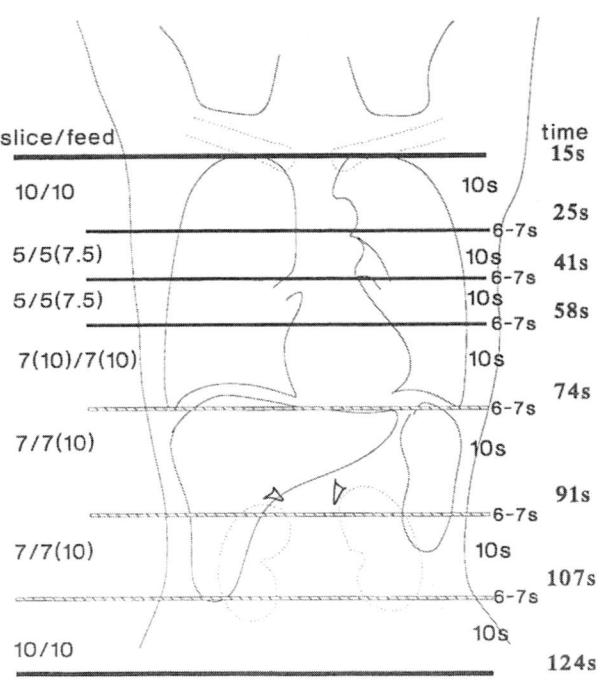

slice/feed

			time
			15s
10/10		10s	
			25s
		6-7s	
5/5(7.5)		10s	41s
		6-7s	
5/5(7.5)		10s	58s
		6-7s	
7(10)/7(10)		10s	
			74s
		6-7s	
7/7(10)		10s	
			91s
		6-7s	
7/7(10)		10s	
			107s
		6-7s	
		10s	
10/10			124s

Fig. 3.3. Lung cancer staging protocol by multiple spiral scans, adapted from the proposal of FOLEY and ONESON (1994). By using four sets of spiral scans one may adapt the slice thickness to 10 mm for the apex, 5 mm for the perihilar area, and 7–10 mm for the chest base; additional spiral scans with parameters appropriate for the upper abdomen can easily be added

Table 3.3. Factors to consider in selecting multiple spiral scans[a]

1. Need for absolute apnea
2. Individual patient cooperation
3. Scanner performance characteristics
4. Technical examination parameters
5. Need for modification of technical parameters for subvolumes
6. Need to include the liver in the chest study

[a] The first four factors determine the maximal volume covered by one spiral scan (Table 3.2). When this volume is not sufficient, when the parameters have to be modified for specific subvolumes, or when the upper abdomen has to be included, the decision is usually made to perform multiple scans

not only on the area of the body and the specific indication but also on the technical performance limits of the scanner and on the individual patient (Table 3.3). Due to the rapid developments in hardware and software since the introduction of spiral CT in 1989, no one has gathered enough experience in optimizing the protocols.

3.2.10 Reconstruction Increment (RI)

As mentioned in the introduction, the RI corresponds to interscan table motion in conventional CT but can be chosen retrospectively without respiratory misregistration. The center of a solitary pulmonary nodule can therefore be selected easily for morpho-

logic and densitometric analysis whereas in conventional CT it may be missed despite overlapping scans (KALENDER et al. 1990). Chapter 5 will cover all the details of how to select reconstruction increments. I shall therefore concentrate here on a few practical rules that help tailor acquisition protocols:

1. *Reduced reconstruction increments* (below one slice thickness) improve the information without increasing radiation exposure, at the cost only of a slightly longer reconstruction time and an increased number of images to analyse and archive (Fig. 3.2).

2. Practical reconstruction increments range between *20% and 100% of the slice thickness*. Values below 50% are mandatory for 2-D reformation, 3-D reconstruction, and maximal spatial resolution (KALENDER et al. 1994). Whether clinical diagnostic information is significantly improved below 40% (60% overlap, pitch = 1, 180° interpolation) or 60% (40% overlap, pitch = 2) remains to be determined (WANG and VANNIER 1994). Nonetheless, further development of spiral volumetric CT might lay the foundation for *isotropic* imaging, based on very thin collimation and reconstruction increments; isotropic data would compensate for several limitations of axial CT since multiplanar reconstructions would then allow any image plane to be obtained without loss of quality (KALENDER 1995).

At the other end of the sepctrum, with elevated reconstruction increments significantly above 100%, the need for spiral scanning is questionable; e.g., in diffuse infiltrative lung disease a good choice is to use conventional HRCT slices of 1–2 mm in width and an interscan table motion of 10–20 mm.

3. Practical experience seems to prove that *low reconstruction increments can compensate for higher pitch*. This means that protocols in the chest are much faster, allowing either larger volumes to be covered or thinner slices to be obtained.

3.2.11 Reconstruction Center and Field of View (FOV)

The selection of the center for image reconstruction and the FOV is exactly as in conventional CT and is entirely free during postprocessing. It will be discussed thoroughly in Chap. 5, and it is an important task of the radiologist to adapt these two parameters to the individual problem instead of losing geometric resolution by including a lot of air around the chest in the FOV. This usually means targeting to better show important tiny details, e.g., separate image reconstruction for lung analysis focused on the right and/or left lung (possibly helpful both in HRCT and with thick slices); however, it may also mean a greater FOV when pathology is expected in the subcutaneous soft tissues. In analogy, spiral CT of the shoulder or spine includes targeting and modifying the center of the FOV.

3.2.12 Reconstruction Algorithm

As the center and the FOV, the algorithm is a postprocessing parameter covered in detail in Chap. 5. Lung analysis is improved by high spatial resolution algorithms (PARANJPE and BERGIN 1994), and separate image reconstruction for pulmonary windows with targeting and adapted center of the FOV

(see Sect. 3.1.11) is routinely suggested. For the mediastinum and the soft tissues of the chest wall, a standard algorithm is used whereas bony structures are best visualized by a high-resolution algorithm. In contrast, densitometry is theoretically improved by low spatial resolution ("soft") algorithms.

Unlike in conventional CT, algorithm selection in spiral CT not only determines the mathematical procedure by which individual projection profiles (the raw data of one slice) are transformed into images. Before this step can be performed, interpolation is used to transform the spiral raw data into planar raw data. In brief, the initial 360° interpolation procedure using data from two consecutive tube rotations has largely been replaced by interpolating 180° opposite projections and, thus, data from not much more than one rotation (POLACIN et al. 1992). This means a slice profile close to the nominal value at the cost of signal-to-noise ratio, and it is compulsory with a pitch of more than 1 in order to avoid partial volume effects. In other words, reconstruction based on 180° opposite views allows spiral CT scanning at elevated pitch factors and therefore must be considered at the time of prospective planning of spiral CT of the chest.

3.2.13 Patient Respiration

Historically, CT of the chest was usually performed at maximal inspiratory apnea (close to total lung capacity). In parallel with the reduction of scanning time to around 1 s, respiratory artifacts have nearly disappeared. In spiral CT of the chest, respiration is again a critical parameter, with many options depending on the protocol, the patient, and the organ to be studied, but also on specific questions such as air trapping (Table 3.4).

The length of spiral CT acquisition is primarily limited by the *maximal duration of apnea*, which can be prolonged in critical cases by hyperventilation and nasal oxygen delivery prior to the scan. Most patients will be able to hold their breath for 32 s although in smokers, patients with chronic obstructive

Table 3.4. Patient respiration in spiral CT of the chest

Type of respiration	Chest wall	Lung	Mediastinum
Inspiratory apnea	+, diaphragm	++	++
Midtidal apnea	++	+ (child, biopsy)	+
Continuous superficial respiration	+ (spine, infants)	(+) (infants, above hilum)	+
During expiration	(+), (pleural shift)	+ (air trapping)	(+), (tracheal collapse)

++, First choice, preferred technique; +, alternative technique; (+), solution in specific situations

pulmonary disease, and those with congestive heart failure (mainly inpatients) the mean was found to be 25 s (GAY et al. 1994). Interestingly, it is often easier for patients with poor respiratory function to hold their breath once for an extended period than to perform 24–30 individual breathhold maneuvers (PADHANI and FISHMAN 1995). In routine investigations, 30 s can usually be achieved if patients are instructed correctly and supported by oxygen and hyperventilation before scanning. Predictive respiratory gating, as suggested recently (RITCHIE et al. 1994), is difficult to implement in spiral CT.

In the chest, *absolute apnea* is required for 2-D reformations and 3-D representations as well as for scanning the diaphragm and its neighborhood. Apnea is also needed for pulmonary parenchymal studies where maximal inflation decreases functional pseudo-lesions, such as tiny areas of atelectasis in dependent portions of the lung. If inspiratory apnea is not tolerated due to dyspnea or pain, midtidal apnea is a valuable alternative. Since superoinferior displacement of lung tissue is maximal at the base (YOUNG and SIMON 1972) and minimal at the apex, respiratory motion at the end of a scan is much less critical with an inferosuperior scanning direction. Indeed, respiratory artifacts are hardly ever seen in the apex. Similarly, apnea is not required for mediastinal evaluation; with severe chest pain and suspected aortic dissection, spiral CT can be done during *superficial continuous respiration* without loss in quality. For the chest wall, apnea is usually required to avoid motion artifacts caused by bone, except for the spine, which is sufficiently immobilized in the supine position. Specific functional changes are studied during expiration, such as air trapping in small airways disease or central bronchial obstruction, tracheal collapse in tracheomalacia, or the normal respiratory shift between lung tissue and the chest wall excluding infiltration by neoplasms. Finally, lung biopsy and other types of intervention are usually best done during midtidal apnea.

3.2.14 Patient Position

Patient position in spiral CT of the chest is basically identical to that in conventional CT. Absolute immobilization is more important than the specific position, and it can be improved by supporting cushions or analgesics when patients experience exquisite pain. The short duration of spiral CT is an advantage for patients with severe dyspnea or pain. Even orthopneic patients will usually tolerate around 1 min in a flat horizontal position, which is adequate for a spiral acquisition of the entire chest with bolus enhancement but without a localization scan. Chest spiral CT is usually done with the patient in the supine position with elevated arms except for the thoracic inlet and the shoulder region, where the arms are positioned parallel to the trunk. Axial scans can be obtained in any rotational position of the patient if this is more comfortable to the patient. If arm elevation is not possible unilaterally (due to osteoarthritis, trauma, or recent surgery), despite the lack of symmetry it is usually better to elevate the contralateral arm to decrease beam hardening artifacts. Spiral CT of the chest in different positions is rarely needed; as in conventional HRCT, the presence of linear subpleural densities in dependent portions of the lung is an indication for additional *prone* scans to differentiate morphologic interstitial lesions from meaningless functional findings (such as microatelectasis).

For biopsy and intervention, the best route of access determines patient position; again, immobilization is more important than an orthogonal biopsy direction. As mentioned above, *direct coronal, sagittal, or oblique nonaxial scanning* is rarely used. Whenever this technique is appropriate at all, the optimal position is a compromise between the requested scanning plane, patient habitus, and gantry diameter.

3.2.15 Contrast

Intravenous contrast enhancement is nearly compulsory in spiral CT of the chest except for pure pulmonary parenchymal and bone analysis. The details are covered by Chap. 4. In general terms, spiral CT is fast and allows better enhancement using the same amount of contrast, or enhancement equivalent to that of conventional CT using a lower amount of contrast agent. Other applications of contrast in the chest are less frequently used. However, for esophageal cancer intraluminal contrast is a requisite, as in conventional CT, and, of course, the same applies for intraarticular contrast in shoulder arthrography.

3.3 Examination Protocols for Specific Indications

With an awareness of the selection criteria in respect of the technical parameters, any radiologist will be able to adapt the protocols to the specific problems of individual patients. This section provides some hints on how to approach clinical spiral scanning and points out the most important parameters for specific indications. The ranges of parameter values will be rather broad, which is understandable given the great variety of hardware and software options currently available.

3.3.1 Chest Wall and Pleura (Table 3.5)

The *thoracic inlet,* a narrow space with many functional pathways between the trunk and the head as well as the upper extremities, requires thinner slices of 5 mm and targeting for optimal visualization of tiny structures. Several bony structures of high density, the scapulae, clavicles, spine, and sternum, will cause artifacts unless enough photons are used. Therefore, elevated voltage (140 kV), up to 400 mA, and longer than minimal rotation times are used; the pitch will hardly ever exceed 1. As long as examina-

tion of the complete chest is not required, arms are positioned parallel to the trunk rather than elevated. Gantry angulation (top towards the feet) to match the inlet at its narrowest plane is optional.

As for the thoracic inlet, sufficient dose is important to visualize *bony structures* of the chest wall (JURIK and ALBRECHTSEN 1994), and the same parameters will be adapted. For the spine, as soon as more than one vertebra is examined, even multiple shorter spiral scans can heat up the tube; in our experience the conventional nonspiral technique is preferable in most cases. Similar to the thoracic inlet, the spine can be scanned during shallow respiration whereas all other bony structures of the chest potentially move during breathing and therefore require scanning at apnea. Images are calculated with a high spatial resolution algorithm. Intravenous contrast enhancement is not required for pure studies of bone morphology. To characterize and stage inflammatory or neoplastic lesions, images during intravenous bolus injection of contrast are essential. The same is true for *soft tissue and pleural studies,* where avoid-

Table 3.5. Spiral CT acquisition protocols of the chest wall and pleura

Acquisition parameter (adult patients)	Region		
	Thoracic inlet	Bone + joints [diaphragm and neighborhood]	Soft tissues, pleura
1. Rotation time	1–2 s	≤2 s, [minimum]	Minimum
2. Scan collimation (slice thickness)	5 mm	2–5 mm (–8 mm)	5–10 mm
3. Table feed per rotation → pitch	5 mm 1	2–8 mm (spine: >1 segment → 0)[a] 1–1.6	5–16 mm 1–1.6
4. kVp	(120–) 140	(120–) 140 [120]	120 (–140)
5. mAs per rotation	200–400	150–400	150–250
6. Gantry angulation	0° (or 10°)	0°, spine +/–	0°
7. Scanning direction	si/is	si/is	is/si
8. Scan duration	≤30 s	≤30 s, spine: maximum	≤30 s
9. Multiple spiral scans	Usually not	spine +/–	Optional
10. Reconstruction increment	3–5 mm	1–5 (–8) mm	(3–) 5–10 mm
11. Reconstruction center/size (targeting)	As in conventional CT	As in conventional CT	As in conventional CT
12. Reconstruction algorithm	180 (360)° standard	180 (360)° interpolation, high resolution [standard resol.]	180 (360)° standard
13. Patient respiration	Apnea or continuous	(Inspiratory) apnea, (spine: continuous)	(Inspiratory) apnea (+ expir.: pleural shift)
14. Patient position	Supine, arms down	Supine, arms positioned according to indication [elevated]	Supine, arms elevated
15. Contrast	+	–, tumors + [–, +]	Usually +

si, Superoinferior; is, inferosuperior
[a] With more than one segment of the spinal column, tube heating is usually significant; instead of decreasing the current many people prefer conventional CT (table feed of 0 per rotation)

ance of motion artifacts and, thus, a short exposure time, is more critical than a high dose (Fig. 3.1). For the same reason, inspiratory or midtidal apnea is suggested; both inspiratory and expiratory scans are required to show the respiratory phase shift between middle and lower lobar pulmonary tissue and the chest wall that excludes parietal pleural infiltration by lung cancer (SHIRAKAWA et al. 1994).

Diaphragmatic studies (BRINK et al. 1994) deserve mention especially for two reasons: first, the central part of the diaphragm around the dome is oriented parallel to the section plane, a fact predisposing to partial volume effects and therefore requiring thin slices; second, the same area, due to its maximal respiratory excursions, needs to be imaged at apnea during minimal scan times.

3.3.2 Lung (Table 3.6)

The search for *lung metastases* of extrathoracic primary tumors is a fairly frequent clinical indication

for spiral CT, which has been reported to be superior to conventional CT for this purpose in many reports in the literature (COLLIE et al. 1994; COSTELLO et al. 1991; FRIESE et al. 1994; RÉMY-JARDIN et al. 1993; TURNBULL 1994). Most of these authors used a 10-mm slice thickness and a pitch of 1, based on scanning during one breathhold and on reduced reconstruction increments, a technique still adequate for screening. Recent modifications, above all for preoperative studies, included thinner slices to further increase sensitivity, elevated pitch factors of up to 2.5 without significant information loss (MORI et al. 1994), and a decreased dose of as low as 50–100 mAs per rotation, which is most important and appropriate in children. Where acquisition time is longer than 25 s, an inferosuperior scanning direction is suggested. Intravenous contrast enhancement is not needed.

Lung cancer staging, the other leading reason for chest CT, has to include the primary neoplasm, the entire lung, hilar and mediastinal lymph node stations, and adrenal glands. Often, abdominal staging

Table 3.6. Spiral CT acquisition protocols of the lung

Acquisition parameter (adult patients)	Problem						
	Search for metastases	Cancer staging	Solitary pulmonary nodule	Trauma, intensive care patient	Embolism/ vascular malformation	Bronchial disease (bronchiectasis)	Diffuse infiltrative lung disease
1. Rotation time	Minimum	Minimum	Minimum	Minimum	Minimum	Minimum	Minimum
2. Scan collimation (slice thickness)	4–10 mm	Hilum 4–5/ 8–10 mm	1–2 mm	7–10 mm	3–5–7/2–5 mm	1.5–3 mm	1–2 mm = HRCT
3. Table feed per rotation → pitch	4–25 mm 1–2	5–8/8–16 1–1.6	1–3 mm 1–1.5	7–16 mm 1–1.6	(3) 5–7 (10) mm 1–2	0 mm/2–7 mm[a] 1–2	0 mm/2–4 mm[a] 1–2
4. kVp	140 (120)	140 (120)	120	140 (120)	120 (140)	140 (120)	140 (120)
5. mAs per rotation	(50–) 150–250	180–250	150–250	150–250	150–250	150–250	(50–) 150–250
6. Gantry angulation	0°	0°	0°	0°	0°	−20°	0°
7. Scanning direction[b]	is/si	si/is	si/is	si/is	is/si	si/is	is/si
8. Scan duration	≤32 s	≤32 s	≤32 s	≤32 s	≤32 s	≤32 s	≤32 s
9. Multiple spiral scans[c]	(+)	−/+	−	(+)	−	(+)	(+)
10. Reconstruction increment	(2–) 4–10 mm	(2–) 4–10 mm	1–2 mm	(5–) 10 mm	3–7/2–5 mm	1–2–5 mm (cine)	1–3 mm
11. Reconstruction center/size (targeting)	Lung	Chest (targeting)	Lung area	Entire chest	Central/regional	Central bronchi	Lung (bilateral targeting)
12. Reconstruction algorithm	180 (360)° high	180 (360)° standard + high	180 (360)° standard	180 (360)° standard	180 (360)° standard	180 (360)° high	180 (360)° high
13. Patient respiration	(Inspiratory) apnea	(Inspiratory) apnea	(Inspiratory) apnea	Apnea/shallow respiration	(Inspiratory) apnea	(Inspiratory) apnea (+ expiration)	(Inspiratory) apnea (+ expiration)
14. Patient position	Supine	Supine	Supine	Supine	Supine	Supine	Supine (+ prone)
15. Contrast[c]	−	+	− (+)	+	+/− (+)	−/+	−

[a] Usually conventional scanning to screen for diffuse disease using 1.5 (1–2) mm slice thickness and 10-mm spacing between slices (less radiation exposure); spiral technique ideal for most suspicious subvolume of lung
[b] Inferosuperior when scan duration longer than 24 s; is, inferosuperior; si, superoinferior
[c] −, Not indicated; (+), possibly indicated; +, often indicated

is combined to include the entire liver. To fulfill these requirements, several protocols have been proposed, and optimization will continue during the next 2 years. As for conventional CT, historically 10-mm-thick slices have been the standard, and intravenous contrast enhancement has been used successfully during the past decade. Thinner slices have recently become standard for the hilum as well as to show exact relations of the neoplasm to the chest wall (KURIYAMA et al. 1994) and mediastinum; they are also suggested for the adrenals and the liver. Different approaches are currently being tested. One is to cover the apex down to the aortic arch or even the entire chest by a basic non-contrast-enhanced scan of 10-mm-thick slices; a second spiral scan with thin collimation for the hilum and the center of the mass is added during a contrast bolus injection to keep the breathhold below 20–30 s (PADHANI and FISHMAN 1995). Another approach uses multiple spiral scans and may include the abdomen; flexible modification of scan parameters, such as slice thickness, table feed, and mAs per rotation, as well as scan and interval duration, is the big advantage of this variable-mode technique. Whatever the selection, the liver has to be studied within 100 s, i.e., during the redistribution phase of contrast enhancement before equilibrium. One possible scheme is illustrated in Fig. 3.3 (FOLEY and ONESON 1994). We tend to prefer a third approach with just one thoracic measurement in the inferosuperior scanning direction that allows the patient to breathe at the end of the long scan, when the suprahilar level is investigated and respiratory motion is minimal (Fig. 3.2, 3.4); a second superoinferior spiral scan similarly extends the examination to include the upper abdomen. PARANJPE and BERGIN (1994) use a similar protocol. Individual patient factors as well as hardware and software limitations and new options preclude the use of one standard protocol for lung cancer screening in the near future. Furthermore, specific questions require specific modifications of the technique, e.g., when scanning under different lung volumes to ascertain whether there is parietal pleural infiltration by lung cancer (SHIRAKAWA et al. 1994, see Sect. 3.3.1).

Densitometry of the *solitary pulmonary nodule* by CT is usually intended to differentiate between calcified (or fatty hamartomatous) benign and non-calcified malignant subcentimeter lesions. Spiral CT helps in easily matching the center of the nodule without partial volume effects (CANN 1992; VOCK et al. 1990); it also shows 3D topographic relations to vessels and bronchi (NAIDICH 1994). Whether bolus contrast enhancement is a useful tool to further differentiate the two etiologic possibilities needs to be clarified in prospective studies.

Trauma and intensive care studies are both used to analyze pulmonary problems and at the same time to obtain important information on the pleura, chest wall, and mediastinum. Except for certain specific questions, 7- to 10-mm-thick slices are obtained at maximal speed to avoid motion artifacts and to shorten the examination.

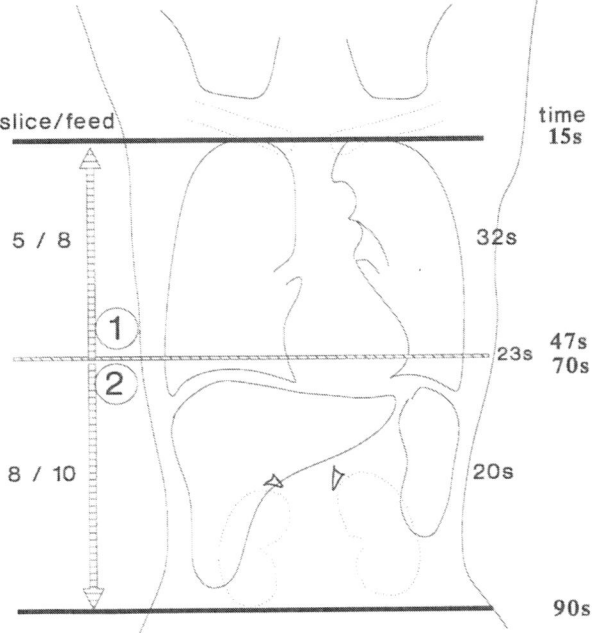

Fig. 3.4. Lung cancer staging protocol by two spiral scans using the inferosuperior scanning direction. The lung is covered nearly completely, and despite a relatively long scanning time (e.g., 32 s), respiratory artifacts are hardly ever visible at the apex. The second superoinferior scan for the upper abdomen starts with an overlap at the lung base within around 70 s of contrast injection; the liver is easily studied before the equilibrium phase

Central *pulmonary embolism*, a challenge despite a number of more or less noninvasive diagnostic methods, can be reliably shown by spiral CT (RÉMY-JARDIN et al. 1992). Thin slices centered on the pulmonary arteries coupled with optimal contrast enhancement help confirm or even detect unsuspected emboli. With improved CT hardware, subsegmental vessels are reproducibly visualized, and prospective studies in comparison with arteriography are likely to confirm the diagnostic equality or even superiority of CT in acute and chronic (KONTRUS et al. 1993) pulmonary embolism. Due to the natural contrast of the lung, the unique topography of *pulmonary arteriovenous malformations* shown without contrast injection is analyzed three-dimensionally (RÉMY et al. 1992, 1994); thin slices and an examination at breathhold are most essential. Using a collimation of 4 mm or less, targeting, and reduced reconstruction increments, it is even possible to visualize *bronchial arteries* (SCHWICKERT et al. 1994).

Bronchial disease similarly requires thin slices, and 20° of gantry angulation (top towards the patient's head) improves the demonstration of

bronchi (RÉMY-JARDIN and RÉMY 1988). CT has replaced bronchography in bronchiectasis. To screen for diffuse disease, 1.5- to 3-mm slices are scanned every 10–15 mm by the conventional technique. However, focal disease is better analyzed by spiral CT and cine display. Multiplanar reformations and/or 3-D reconstructions of spiral CT data are highly accurate (94%) in depicting stenosis of the central airways (QUINT et al. 1995; NEWMARK et al. 1994; PADHANI and FISHMAN 1995; COSTELLO 1995). Expiratory scanning may be helpful in obstructive disease of smaller aiways (NAIDICH 1994).

Similar to bronchiectasis, *diffuse infiltrative lung disease* is often studied by conventional HRCT. The spiral technique is appropriate when topographic relations and continuous information in a subvolume of the lung are of interest (VOCK and SOUCEK 1993; AMBROSINO et al. 1994). Narrow collimation and the high-resolution algorithm seem to be the most important factors in improving image resolution (PARANJPE and BERGIN 1994). As for conventional HRCT, prone scans differentiate between subpleural interstitial disease and dependent

Table 3.7. Spiral CT acquisition protocols of the mediastinum

Acquisition parameter (adult patients)	Problem			
	Screening	[Tracheal]/ esophageal disease	Aortic/arterial/venous/ [cardiac] disease	Adenopathy
1. Rotation time	Minimum	Minimum	Minimum	see screening and lung cancer staging
2. Scan collimation = slice thickness	5–10 mm	[3–] 5 (–10) mm	3–5–10 mm	
3. Table feed per rotation → pitch	8–20 mm 1–2	5–10 mm 1–1.6	5–15 mm 1–2	
4. kVp	120	120	120	
5. mAs per rotation	150–250	150–300	180–300	
6. Gantry angulation	0°	0°	0° / [0, −30°]	
7. Scanning direction	is/si	si/is	is (si)	
8. Scan duration	≤40 s	≤32 s	≤40 s	
9. Multiple spiral scans	(+)	(+)	−, +/[−]	
10. Reconstruction increment	4–10 mm	[3] 4–10 mm	[3–] 4–10 mm	
11. Reconstruction center/size (targeting)	Mediastinum or entire chest	Mediastinum/(chest)	Mediastinum/chest (collaterals)	
12. Reconstruction algorithm	180° (360°) standard	180° (360°) standard	180° (360°) standard	
13. Patient respiration	Inspiratory apnea/ shallow respiration	(Inspiratory) apnea/ [+ expiration]	Inspiratory apnea/ shallow respiration	
14. Patient position	Supine	Supine	Supine	
15. i.v. contrast	+	[−]/+, p.o.	+/[−, +]	

is, Inferosuperior; si, superoinferior; −, not indicated; (+), possibly indicated; +, often indicated

microatelectasis, and scanning at expiration is used to show air trapping.

3.3.3 Mediastinum (Table 3.7)

Mediastinal screening, e.g., in the search for mass lesions or lymphadenopathy, usually does not need thin slices; 8- to 10-mm sections with intravenous contrast enhancement are the standard (COSTELLO 1995), and apnea can be replaced by shallow respiration without major artifacts to include the entire chest or even larger volumes. Specific questions, such as *tracheal or esophageal disease*, require adapted solutions. For the trachea, expiration and thin collimation may be essential to show the functional cross-section, whereas contrast enhancement is optional (NEWMARK et al. 1994; NAIDICH 1994). For the esophagus, intraluminal contrast using a viscous preparation of CT barium sulfate is of great help.

Cardiovascular pathology can often be shown by spiral CT. The high degree of blood enhancement obtained with moderate amounts of contrast agents is ideal for visualizing the vessels of the entire chest, to detect intra- and extraluminal obstruction and collateral pathways. The scanning volume and slice thickness have to be adapted to the individual situation, and for the mediastinum, apnea and shallow respiration are nearly equivalent. Spiral CT has been shown to be superior to conventional CT in aortic dissection (COSTELLO et al. 1992; PROKOP et al. 1993), usually because additional levels between original images obtained during postprocessing clearly distinguish between artifacts and intimal flaps. Three-dimensional rendering for CT angiography is an advantage both for the aorta and for the smaller vessels (NAPEL et al. 1992; RUBIN et al. 1995).

Coronary calcifications have recently been identified by unenhanced electron beam CT and shown to correlate with coronary heart disease. Currently, there are not enough data to establish whether spiral CT can offer similar information. The patency of coronary artery bypass grafts potentially can be investigated by spiral CT (TELLO et al. 1993). The heart is usually imaged by echocardiography or magnetic resonance imaging. But CT, in most cases performed for other reasons, is excellent in demonstrating pericardial effusion and mass lesions of the heart.

In conclusion, spiral CT is an elegant tool that can usually replace conventional CT of the chest except for spinal studies and for the study of diffuse infiltrative lung disease. The selection of parameters has to be individualized and adapted to the specific scanner to achieve optimal results. Ongoing hardware innovations will further improve the results obtained with spiral CT of the chest.

References

Ambrosino MM, Genieser NB, Roche KJ, Kaul A, Lawrence RM (1994) Feasibility of high-resolution, low-dose chest CT in evaluation the pediatric chest. Pediatr Radiol 24:6–10

Blake S, Toma T, Flanagan FL, Breatnach E (1994) Comparison of thoracic helical CT protocols performed at 1:1 pitch and 2:1 pitch. Radiology 193(P):339

Brink JA, Heiken JP, Semenkovich J, Teefey SA, McClennan BL, Sagel SS (1994) Abnormalities of the diaphragm and adjacent structures: findings on multiplanar spiral CT scans. Am J Roentgenol 163:307–310

Buckley JA, Scott WW, Siegelmann SS, Kuhlman JE, Urban BA, Bluemke DA, Fishman EK (1995) Pulmonary nodules: effect of increased data sampling on detection with spiral CT and confidence in diagnosis. Radiology 196:395–400

Cann CE (1992) Quantitative accuracy of spiral CT versus discrete volume CT scanning. Radiology 185(P):126–127

Cederlund K (1994) Maintained image quality and dose reduction with spiral CT of the thorax and upper abdomen. In: Pokieser H, Lechner G (eds) Advances in CT, vol. III. Springer, Berlin Heidelberg New York, p 108

Collie DA, Wright AR, Williams JR et al. (1994) Comparison of spiral acquisition computed tomography and conventional computed tomography in the assessment of pulmonary metastatic disease. Br J Radiol 67:436–444

Costello P (1995) Thoracic imaging with spiral CT. In: Fishman EK, Jeffrey RB (eds) Spiral CT: principles, techniques and clinical applications. Raven Press, New York, p 109

Costello P, Anderson W, Blume D (1991) Pulmonary nodule: evaluation with spiral volumetric CT. Radiology 179:875–876

Costello P, Ecker CP, Tello R et al. (1992) Assessment of the thoracic aorta by spiral CT. Am J Roentgenol 158:1127–1130

Foley WD, Oneson SR (1994) Helical CT: clinical performance and imaging strategies. Radiographics 14:894–904

Foley WD, Jacobson DR, Tomiak MM (1994) Performance of new operating modes for CT. Radiology 193(P):127

Friese SA, Rieber A, Fleiter T, Brambs HJ, Claussen CD (1994) Pulmonary nodules in spiral volumetric and single slice computed tomography. Eur J Radiol 18:48–51

Gay SB, Sistrom CL, Holder CA, Suratt PM (1994) Breath-holding capability of adults; implications for spiral computed tomography, fast-acquisition magnetic resonance imaging, and angiography. Invest Radiol 29:848–851

Jurik AG, Albrechtsen J (1994) Spiral CT with three-dimensional and multiplanar reconstruction in the diagnosis of anterior chest wall joint and bone disorders. Acta Radiol 35:468–472

Kalender WA (1995) Thin-section three-dimensional spiral CT: is isotropic imaging possible? Radiology 197:578–580

Kalender WA, Seissler W, Klotz E, Vock P (1990) Spiral volumetric CT with single-breath-hold technique, continuous transport, and continuous scanner rotation. Radiology 176:181–183

Kalender WA, Polacin A, Süss C (1994) A comparison of conventional and spiral CT: an experimental study on the detection of spherical lesions. J Comput Assist Tomogr 18:167–176

Kontrus M, Zische R, Klapetko W, Thurnher S, Fleischmann D, Herold CJ (1993) Chronic thromboembolic pulmonary hypertension: pre- and post-operative evaluation with spiral CT angiography. Radiology 189(P):263

Kuriyama K, Tateishi R, Kumatani T et al. (1994) Pleural invasion by peripheral bronchogenic carcinoma: assessment with three-dimensional helical CT. Radiology 191:365–369

Mini RL, Vock P, Mury R, Schneeberger PP (1995) Radiation exposure of patients who undergo CT of the trunk. Radiology 195:557–562

Mori K, Sasagawa M, Moriyama N (1994) Detection of nodular lesions in the lung using helical computed tomography: comparison of fast couch speed technique with conventional computed tomography. Jpn J Clin Oncol 24:252–257

Naidich DP (1994) Helical computed tomography of the thorax, clinical applications. Radiol Clin North Am 32:759–774

Napel S, Marks MP, Rubin GD et al. (1992) CT angiography with spiral CT and maximum intensity projection. Radiology 185:607–610

Newmark GM, Conces DJ, Kopecky KK (1994) Spiral CT evaluation of the trachea and bronchi. J Comput Assist Tomogr 18:552–554

Padhani AR, Fishman EK (1995) Spiral CT evaluation of lung cancer. In: Fishman EK, Jeffrey RB (eds) Spiral CT: principles, techniques and clinical applications. Raven Press, New York, p 131

Paranjpe DV, Bergin CJ (1994) Spiral CT of the lungs: optimal technique and resolution compared with conventional CT. Am J Roentgenol 162:561–567

Polacin A, Kalender WA, Marchal G (1992) Evaluation of section sensitivity profiles and image noise in spiral CT. Radiology 185:29–35

Prokop M, Schaefer CM, Leppert AGA et al. (1993) Spiral CT angiography for diagnosis and follow-up of chronic aortic dissection. Radiology 189(P):112

Quint LE, Whyte RI, Kazerooni EA et al. (1995) Stenosis of the central airways: evaluation by using helical CT with multiplanar reconstructions. Radiology 194:871–877

Rémy J, Rémy-Jardin M, Wattinne L, Deffontaines C (1992) Pulmonary arteriovenous malformations: evaluation with CT of the chest before and after treatment. Radiology 182:809–816

Rémy J, Rémy-Jardin M, Giraud F, Wattinne L (1994) Angioarchitecture of pulmonary arteriovenous malformations: clinical utility of three-dimensional helical CT. Radiology 191:657–664

Rémy-Jardin M, Rémy J (1988) Comparison of vertical and oblique CT in evaluation of the bronchial tree. J Comput Assist Tomogr 12:956–962

Rémy-Jardin M, Rémy J, Wattinne L (1992) Central pulmonary thromboembolism: diagnosis with spiral volumetric CT with the single-breath-hold technique – comparison with pulmonary angiography. Radiology 185:381–387

Rémy-Jardin M, Rémy J, Giraud F, Marquette CH (1993) Pulmonary nodules: detection with thick-section spiral CT versus conventional CT. Radiology 187:513–520

Ritchie CJ, Hsieh J, Gard MF, Godwin JD, Kim Y, Crawford CR (1994) Predictive respiratory gating: a new method to reduce motion artifacts on CT scans. Radiology 190:847–852

Rubin GD, Dake MD, Semba CP (1995) Current status of three-dimensional spiral CT scanning for imaging the vasculature. Radiol Clin North Am 33:51–70

Schwickert HC, Kauczor HU, Schweden F, Schild HH (1994) Anatomie der Bronchialarterien – Darstellung mit der Spiral-CT. Fortschr Roentgenstr 160:506–512

Shirakawa T, Fukuda K, Miyamoto Y, Tanabe H, Tada S (1994) Parietal pleural invasion of lung masses: evaluation with CT performed during deep inspiration and expiration. Radiology 192:809–811

Takahashi M, Ashtari M, Papp Z, Khan A, Herman PG, Eacobacci T (1994) Low-dose spiral CT of the thorax: comparison with standard-dose technique. Radiology 193(P):338

Tello R, Costello P, Ecker C et al. (1993) Spiral CT evaluation of coronary artery bypass graft patency. J Comput Assist Tomogr 17:253–259

Turnbull CM (1994) Comparison of spiral acquisition computed tomography and conventional computed tomography in the assesment of pulmonary metastatic disease. Br J Radiol 67:436–444

Verschakelen JA, Van Hoe L (1995) Spiral CT of the chest: acquisition and injection techniques. Eur Radiol 5S:158

Vock P, Soucek M (1993) Spiral computed tomography in the assessment of focal and diffuse lung disease. J Thorac Imaging 8:283–290

Vock P, Soucek M, Daepp M, Kalender WA (1990) Lung: spiral volumetric CT with single-breathhold technique. Radiology 176:864–867

Wang G, Vannier MW (1994) Longitudinal resolution in X-ray CT: analytic comparison between conventional and helical CT. Med Phys 21:429–433

Young DA, Simon G (1972) Certain movements measured on inspiration-expiration chest radiographs correlated with pulmonary function studies. Clin Radiol 23:37–41

4 Injection Techniques

P. Schnyder, R. Meuli, and S. Wicky

CONTENTS

P. Schnyder, MD, Department of Radiology, University Hospital, CHUV Lausanne, 1011 Lausanne, Switzerland
R. Meuli, MD, Department of Radiology, University Hospital, CHUV Lausanne, 1011 Lausanne, Switzerland
S. Wicky, MD, Department of Radiology, University Hospital, CHUV Lausanne, 1011 Lausanne, Switzerland

4.1 Introduction

Computerized tomographic (CT) examination of the chest requires, for most clinical conditions, the acquisition of sections after intravenous injection of iodinated contrast material. The goal of the injection is to differentiate normal vascular, mediastinal, and hilar structures from pathological conditions, whether vascular or tumoral. In obese patients, whose mediastinal compartments are filled with large amounts of fat (an efficient natural contrast material), the role of intravenous contrast enhancement is probably less significant than in patients with sparse mediastinal fat. Indeed, in the latter subjects, nonenhanced CT sections will not afford identification of normal mediastinal structures such as upper pulmonary veins, esophageal walls, the azygos vein, and mediastinal and hilar lymph nodes. Reduction of slice thickness improves detection of these structures, but injection of intravenous contrast material remains essential in order to characterize pathological vascular conditions such as aneurysms or dissections, lymphadenopathy, tumors, and malformations.

In the mid-1970s, when CT was introduced into clinical use in selected patients with chest disease, iodinated contrast was intravenously injected with the use of drip perfusion. By the late 1970s, chest examinations were usually initiated with an injection of a bolus of 40–50 ml followed by rapid drip perfusion of 50–60 ml of contrast media (Naidich et al. 1991). The concentration of the iodinated material ranged between 300 and 360 mg/ml. Two to three 10-mm-thick sections per minute were obtained and the last sections of the chest examination were usually poorly enhanced.

In the late 1980s, third- and fourth-generation CT scanners allowed the number of sections obtained per minute to be increased, and there were calls for the use of power injectors and dynamic CT (Shepard et al. 1986; McCarthy and Moss 1984). This technique was rapidly adopted in most CT units dealing with chest and abdominal disease. Simultaneously, the volume of injected iodinated contrast material increased without diminution of its concentration (SHUMAN et al. 1986; MCCARTHY and Moss 1984). Currently, chest radiologists working with conventional incremental equipment use large amounts of iodinated contrast material (150 ml) at concentrations ranging between 320 and 360 mg/ml.

The introduction in the late 1980s of helical (or spiral) CT and its rapid incursion into the market has markedly changed injection techniques since: (a) chest examination now requires 20–30 s, according to the chosen x-ray beam collimation, the pitch value, and the length of the region of interest along the z-axis, (b) a reduced volume of contrast medium can be used, and (c) helical CT data acquisition within a single breath-hold affords more precise and uniform delivery of contrast medium and thus allows the acquisition of high-quality 2D and 3D images by eliminating respiratory inconstancies associated with incremental CT (DILLON et al. 1993; HEINKEN et al. 1993; COSTELLO 1994 a,b). Presently, no consensus has been reached regarding the optimal technique of injection for helical CT of the chest.

In this chapter we will consider the variable technical parameters of helical CT enhancement and propose protocols for the daily practice of chest radiologists.

4.2 Selection of Patients

Less than 10 years ago, almost all patients undergoing a CT examination of the chest had an injection of contrast material, unless they experienced an adverse reaction to iodinated media. Most of these patients had been referred for oncological reasons. With the tremendous improvement in the spatial and contrast resolution of CT devices and the simultaneous increase in interest by chest radiologists and pneumologists in the acquisition of high-resolution CT sections for the diagnosis of interstitial diseases, the total number of chest CT examinations has increased considerably, but the percentage of contrast-enhanced ones has decreased markedly, down to 15% in some institutions (COSTELLO et al. 1992; COSTELLO 1994a). Conditions requiring helical contrast-enhanced CT sections include neoplasms of the lung and mediastinum, vascular diseases and malformations, trauma, infectious diseases with possible extension to the hilum and mediastinum, and granulomatous and pleural space diseases. On the other hand, the majority of pathological conditions which involve the large and small airways and the

lung interstitial tissue, such as bronchiectasis, lung metastases, emphysema and pulmonary fibrosis, no longer require the injection of contrast medium.

4.3 Definition

A helical CT examination involving the injection of contrast medium should:

1. Be well tolerated
2. Increase the attenuation value of all systemic and pulmonary vessels and cardiac chambers by 150–200 Hounsfield units (HU), with respect to the attenuation value on the nonenhanced sections
3. Be reproducible
4. Induce few or no streak artifacts from the lumen of the thoracic veins ipsilateral to the injection sites (in particular from the subclavian and innominate veins and the superior vena cava)
5. Be applicable to most clinical conditions
6. Allow the dose of injected iodine to be optimized.

4.4 Iodine Concentration

Users are not yet in agreement on the iodine concentration of the contrast medium required by helical CT scanning. In a prospective study (SCHNYDER et al. 1995) in 200 patients divided into ten different groups, we tested iodinated contrast medium at different concentrations: 120, 150, and 300 mg iodine/ml. The amount of contrast injected was related to the body weight; the scan delay ranged from 10 to 20 s and the flow rate varied from 1.5 to 5 ml/s.

Chest CT examinations were analyzed in a double-blind manner by three radiologists who graded the importance of contrast medium-induced artifacts in the innominate veins, the subclavian veins, and the superior vena cava. They also scored the quality of the CT examinations with respect to the degree of enhancement of the vessels and cardiac chambers as compared with the other thoracic and mediastinal structures. HU values were measured in the following five areas: the ascending aorta, the descending aorta, the pulmonary artery, the left ventricle, and the distal thoracic aorta.

The incidence of chest examinations affected by venous artifacts was ascertained for each of the three tested iodine concentrations. Contrast medium-induced venous artifacts were observed in 31%, 47% and 86% of the chest CT examinations performed with 120, 150, and 300 mg iodine/ml, respectively

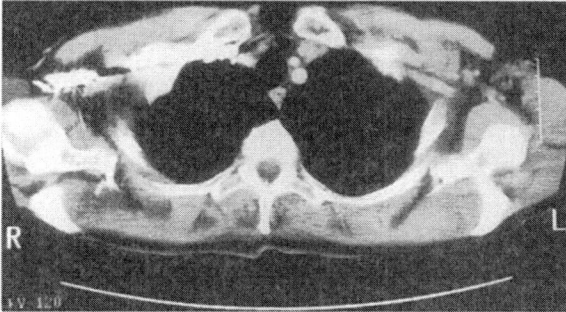

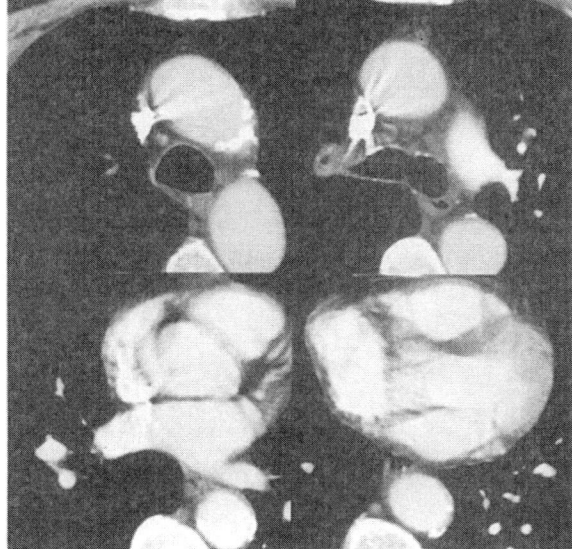

Fig. 4.1a,b. CT sections obtained with 300 mg iodine/ml ionic contrast medium injected at a flow rate of 3 ml/s and a delay of 20 s in the right antecubital vein. **a** Marked streak artifacts arising from the right subclavian vein do not permit adequate evaluation of axillary structures. **b** Similar streak artifacts arising from the superior vena cava spoil the image quality of the ascending aorta, the aortic arch, node station 4R, the right hilum and the right atrium

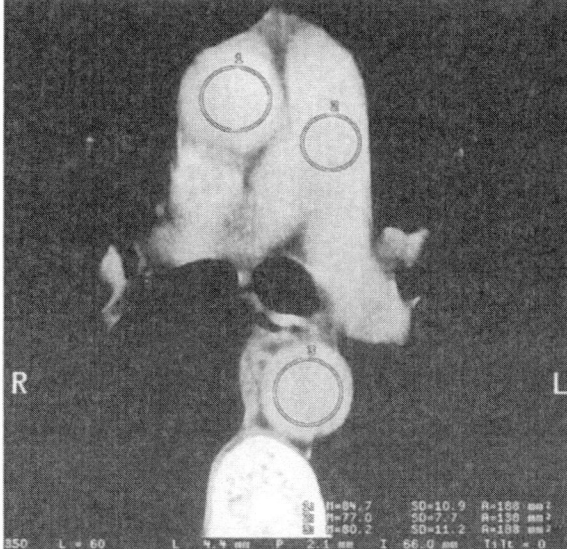

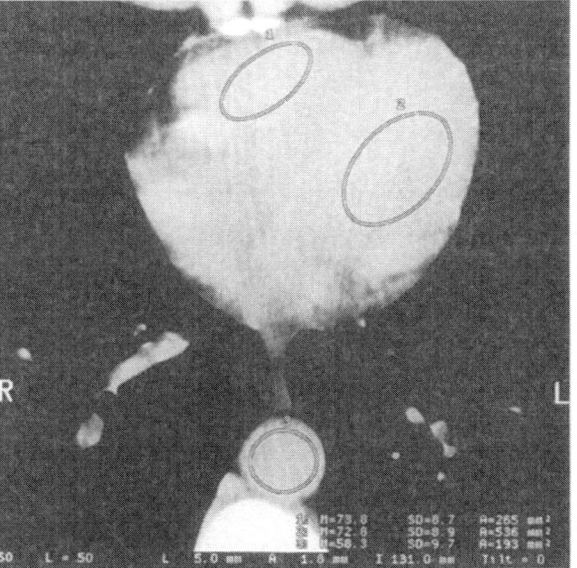

Fig. 4.2a,b. Enhanced helical CT of the chest was achieved with 200 ml of ionic contrast at a concentration of 120 mg iodine/ml, a flow rate of 4 ml/s, and a scan delay of 20 s. **a** The sections are free of streak artifacts arising from the superior vena cava, but afford mediocre enhancement of mediastinal vessels: 84, 77, and 80 HU for the ascending aorta, pulmonary trunk, and descending aorta, respectively. **b** The enhancement of cardiac cavities is also poor: 73 HU for the right ventricle, 72 HU for the left ventricle, and 58 HU for the descending aorta. Such mediocre enhancement does not allow identification of the ventricular walls and interventricular septum

(Fig. 4.1) Thus, the groups receiving 120 and 150 mg iodine/ml had approximately half as many artifacts as the group receiving 300 mg iodine/ml.

When the quality of the chest CT examinations and the degree of enhancement of the large mediastinal vessels and cardiac chambers were subjectively considered, most scans were assessed as excellent in patients who had received a concentration of 300 mg iodine/ml at a flow rate of 2 ml/s or a concentration of 150 mg iodine/ml at a flow rate of 3–5 ml/s. Patients examined with a concentration of 120 mg iodine/ml and flow rates ranging between 3 and 5 ml/s had poor enhancement of mediastinal vessels and cardiac cavities (Fig. 4.2).

Objective evaluation of the contrast enhancement of the five above-mentioned regions of interest af-

forded similar HU values for the groups of patients examined with concentration of 150 (Figs. 4.3, 4.4) and 300 mg iodine/ml (Fig. 4.5). HU values measured in patients examined with an iodine concentration of

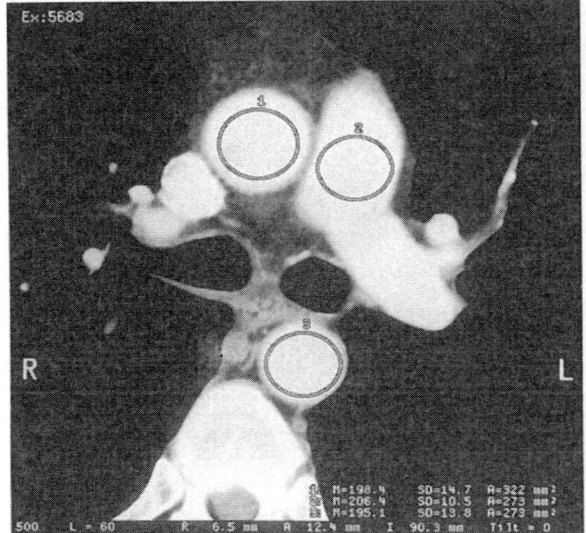

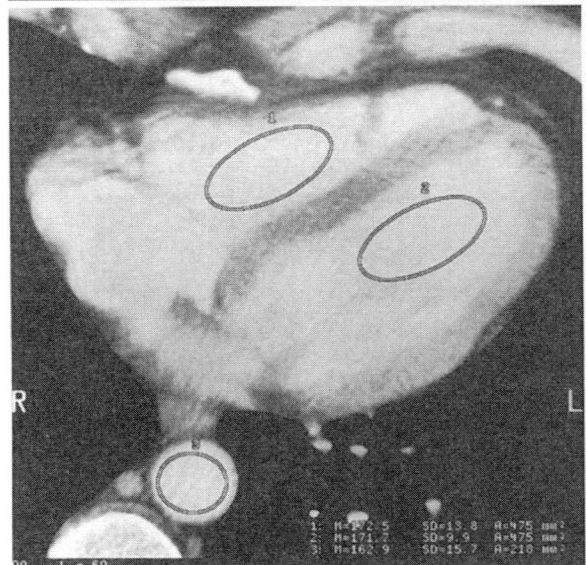

Fig. 4.3a,b. Enhanced helical CT examination obtained with 150 ml of ionic contrast material in a 75-kg, 39-year-old male patient. The concentration is 150 mg iodine/ml, the flow rate 3 ml/s, and the scan delay 20 s. **a** The section is free of streak artifacts and affords excellent enhancement of the ascending aorta, pulmonary trunk, and descending aorta, the respective values of which are 198, 206, and 195 HU. **b** The lumina of the right and left ventricles and descending aorta have enhanced up to 172, 171, and 162 HU, respectively

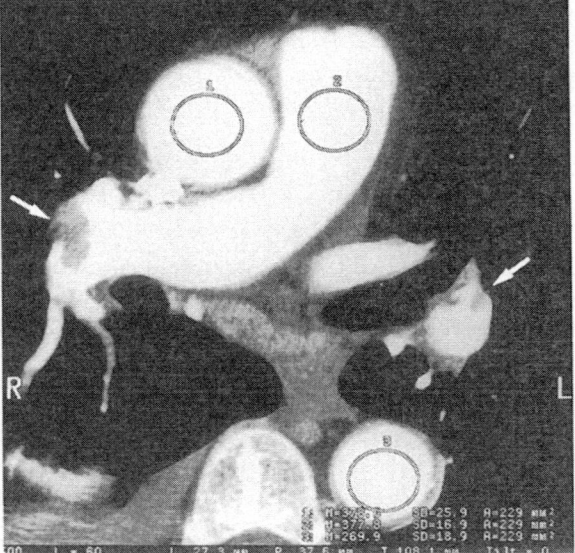

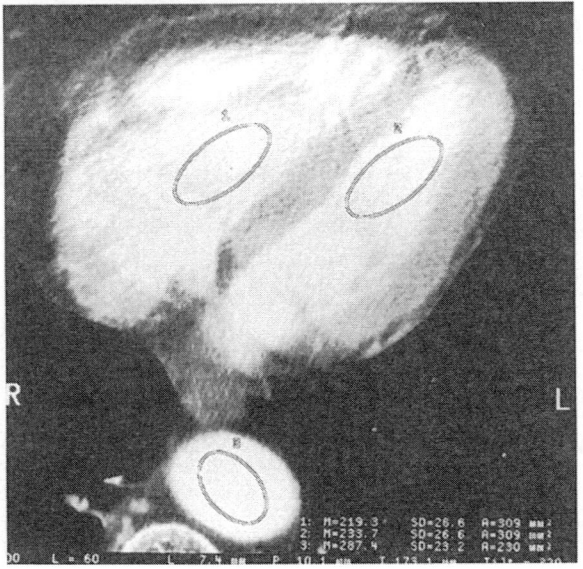

Fig. 4.4a,b. Enhanced helical CT of the chest performed with a concentration of 150 mg iodine/ml, a flow rate of 5 ml/s and a scan delay of 10 s in a patient suffering from bilateral pulmonary embolism (*arrows*). Measurements yielded the following values: **a** 378, 377, and 269 HU for the ascending aorta, pulmonary trunk, and descending aorta respectively; **b** 219, 233, and 287 HU for the right and left ventricles and descending aorta, respectively

120 mg/ml were 30–40 units lower than in patients examined with 150 and 300 mg/ml.

Based upon these data, we concluded that: (a) a 120 mg iodine/ml concentration induces few venous artifacts but provides poor or mediocre enhancement of mediastinal vessels and cardiac chambers; (b) a 300 mg iodine/ml concentration provokes numerous and marked venous artifacts but affords good enhancement; (c) a concentration of 150 mg iodine/ml is an excellent compromise (Fig. 4.6) which causes almost as few venous streak artifacts as 120 mg iodine/ml concentration and affords enhancement of mediastinal vessels identical in quality to that obtained with a concentration of 300 mg iodine/ml.

In a recent study, Storto et al. (1994), comparing

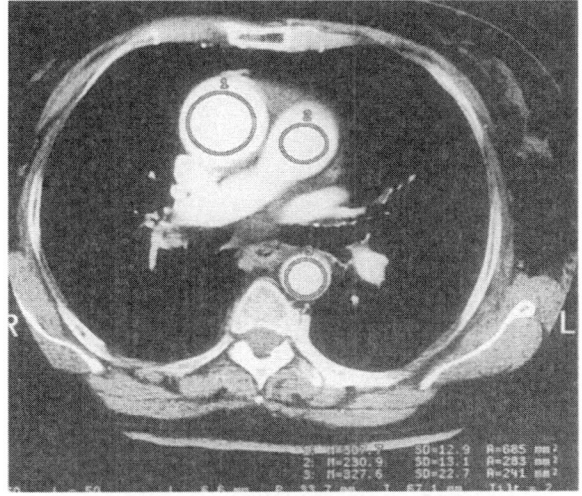

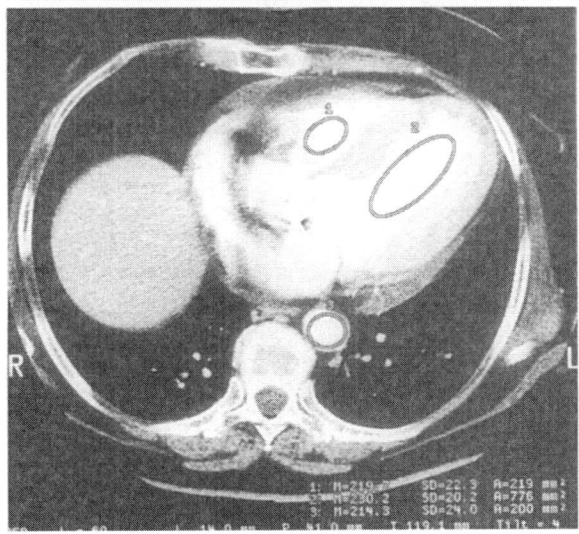

Fig. 4.5. a Enhanced helical CT obtained in a 75-kg woman with a concentration of 300 mg iodine/ml and a flow rate of 3 ml/s. On this section, streak artifacts arising from the superior vena cava are missing. The enhancement of mediastinal vessels is 307 HU for the ascending aorta, 230 HU for the pulmonary trunk, and 327 HU for the descending aorta. **b** More caudally, values of 219, 230, and 214 HU are obtained for the lumen of the right and left ventricles and the thoracic descending aorta, respectively. These values do not differ statistically from those obtained with a concentration of 150 mg iodine/ml and a flow rate of 3 ml/s

contrast medium concentrations of 200 and 300 mg iodine/ml injected at rates of 2 and 3 ml/s, found better overall enhancement of mediastinal vessels with the 300 mg iodine/ml concentration and a flow rate of 3 ml/s. These results differ greatly from ours and indicate that the higher the dose of iodine delivered per second, the greater the enhancement of mediastinal vessels. It should be noted that Storto et al.'s study did not deal with venous streak artifacts. Further evaluation is obviously required to clarify the aforementioned discrepancy.

4.5 Flow Rate

In the second part of our prospective study, six groups of 12 patients each were examined with a concentration of contrast material of 150 mg iodine/ml and flow rates of 3, 4, and 5 ml/s. Scan delays of 10 or 20 s were used.

Results (Table 4.1) indicate that a flow rate of 3 ml/s yields scans of excellent quality, almost as good as those obtained with a flow rate of 4 ml/s. Considering both flow rates together, mean measurements were: 200 ± 40 HU in the lumen of the ascending thoracic aorta, 190 ± 40 HU in the lumen of the proximal descending thoracic aorta, 220 ± 50 HU in the lumen of the main pulmonary artery, 170 ± 40 HU in the cardiac chambers, and 150 ± 50 HU in the distal thoracic aorta. Ten to fifteen percent higher values were obtained with a flow rate of 5 ml/s, a rate which delivers a dose of 750 mg iodine/s, which is close to the value of 900 mg iodine/s proposed by Storto et al. (1994). These data are not exactly in agreement with those of Reiser (1984), who, using a 300 mg iodine/ml contrast medium, showed with incremental CT scanners that the peak attenuation value of the lumen of the ascending aorta appears earlier and increases proportionally to the output of the power injector, with an upper threshold at 8 ml/s. We consider that iodine doses higher than 450–600 mg/s do not improve diagnostic performance,

Table 4.1. Measured HU values

Groups (flow rate, scan delay)	Ascending aorta	Descending aorta	Pulmonary trunk	Left ventricle	Septum	Distal aorta
3 ml/s, 10 s	188 ± 54	169 ± 64	197 ± 62	157 ± 28	80 ± 22	146 ± 34
3 ml/s, 20 s	201 ± 42	191 ± 36	206 ± 61	178 ± 49	99 ± 27	181 ± 56
4 ml/s, 10 s	215 ± 38	192 ± 39	234 ± 54	188 ± 30	108 ± 11	169 ± 46
4 ml/s, 20 s	238 ± 59	220 ± 50	254 ± 43	168 ± 31	109 ± 23	146 ± 49
5 ml/s, 10 s	240 ± 54	228 ± 51	260 ± 47	201 ± 32	121 ± 24	205 ± 37
5 ml/s, 20 s	255 ± 38	221 ± 42	255 ± 42	200 ± 43	118 ± 20	200 ± 41

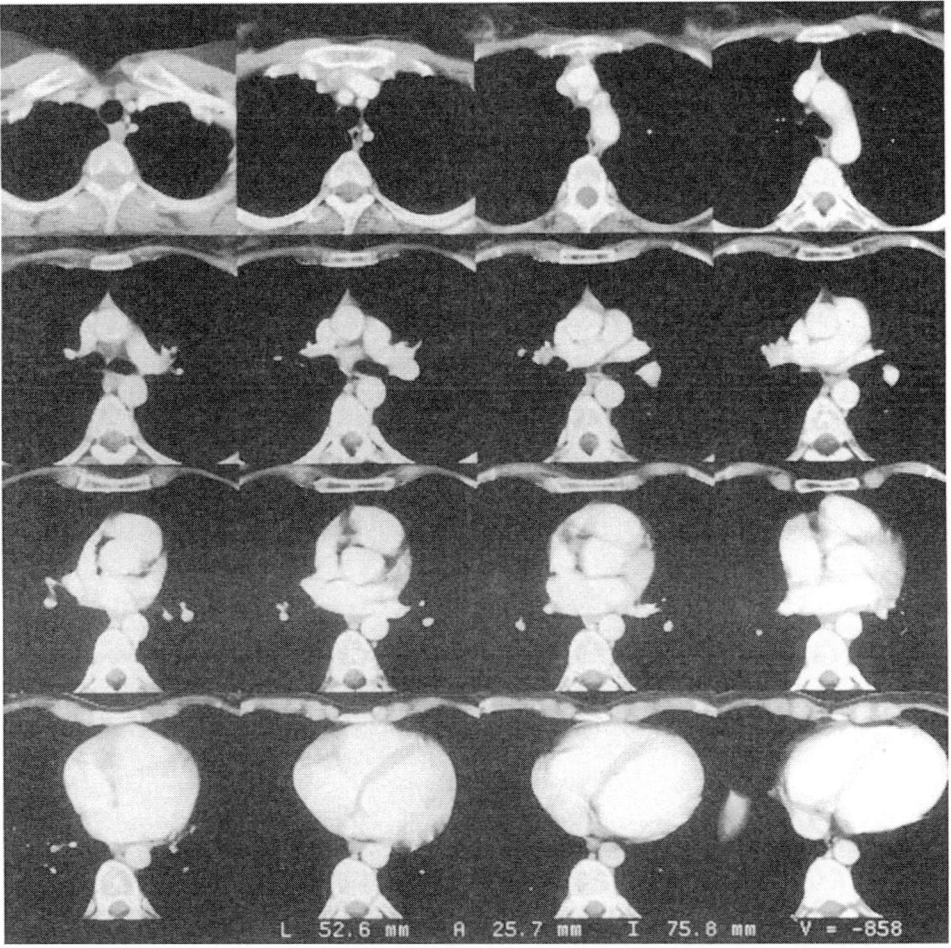

Fig. 4.6. Helical CT survey in a 31-year-old, 70-kg female patient with a cervical non-Hodgkins high-grade lymphoma. Helical CT of the chest was achieved with 140 ml of ionic contrast medium at a concentration of 150 mg iodine/ml and a flow rate of 3 ml/s. A 20-s scan delay afforded excellent enhancement of both innominate veins, of all mediastinal vessels and of the cardiac cavities without streak artifacts. This example is representative of the quality of imaging obtained with the aforementioned injection parameters

except when the radiologist is dealing with a patient suspected of having pulmonary embolism, a condition which requires high enhancement of segmental arteries. For this purpose, RÉMY-JARDIN et al. (1992) proposed the use of contrast material at a concentration of 120 mg iodine/ml and a flow rate of 7 ml/s, which delivers a dose of iodine of 840 mg/s. Presently, the same authors inject 1 g of iodine/s delivered by a 200 mg iodine/ml contrast solution and a flow rate of 5 ml/s for most helical CT examinations of the chest requiring contrast enhancement (PAUL 1994). We do not share this protocol, which markedly increases the doses of contrast and the related costs and prevents one from obtaining a complementary non-chest CT examination.

Surprisingly some authors, having tested our protocols (150 mg iodine/ml at 3 ml/s, are not as enthusiastic about them as we are. This may indicate that the quality of imaging obtained at a constant dose of iodine/s is related to the make and type of helical CT equipment, and possibly to the type and sensitivity of the detectors. Further evaluation on phantoms and patients is required.

4.6 Scan Delay

The preset delay between the initiation of contrast injection and the acquisition of helical CT data (the scan delay) is often determined by means of a test injection of 20 ml of contrast at the same flow rate (2–5 ml/s) as the planned chest CT examination (Morris 1988; Rubin et al. 1995). HU measurements at one or more regions of interest, usually the ascending and descending thoracic aorta, afford enhancement curves which allow determination of the peak enhancement and the appropriate scan delay (Morris 1988; Tello et al. 1993). This technique is not popular among many users, however, since it is time consuming and not cost-efficient and since it delivers an additional irradiation dose to the patient. The test injection is followed by the acquisition of sequential single-level scans at the anticipated time of initiation of the helical CT acquisition. Sequential scans are obtained every 2–5 s, starting 8 s after the beginning of the test injection. It should be noted that chest CT examinations are frequently performed in conjunction with an abdominal examination in oncological patients; this is important since a prior injection test with 20 ml decreases diagnostic performance in the detection of liver metastases and adversely affects the identification of pathological conditions involving the renal cortex.

In most instances a 12- to 15-s scan delay provides excellent opacification of pulmonary arteries and veins, and of systemic arteries including the aortic arch vessels. A 20-s scan delay affords additional opacification of the subclavian and jugular venous confluence, bilaterally. A 10-s scan delay offers good opacification of pulmonary arteries and veins but is insufficient for obtaining an adequate enhancement of the entire aorta and aortic arch vessels. These scan delays are in agreement with the values published by Naidich et al. (1991), who found that the average thoracic transit times from an antecubital vein are: 3.7 ± 1.5 s for the superior vena cava, 6.5 ± 2.5 s for pulmonary arteries, 10.5 ± 3.0 s for the ascending aorta, 12.3 ± 3.8 s for the descending aorta and neck vessels, and 17.8 ± 5.0 s for jugular veins. Such scan delays are approximations and must be adapted in accordance with the patient's estimated cardiac output and the suspected pathology.

In order to overcome variability in patient-related parameters, a new hardware/software system, called SmartPrep, was recently developed by General Electric Medical Systems (Milwaukee, USA); this allows the user to follow and monitor the enhancement curves during the injection of contrast material (Silverman et al.1995). For this purpose, low-dose scans (0.6 s, 40 mA) are obtained during quite superficial breathing at one level and at predetermined time intervals (usually every 3–5 s for a chest examination) (Fig. 4.7). Rapid reconstruction of sections

affords and almost real-time visualization of the enhancement of mediastinal vessels and other anatomical structures. HU measurements from one to three regions of interest are automatically subtracted from the baseline scan values abtained on the first unenhanced scan. The baseline values of each region of interest and the corresponding enhancement numbers are displayed on a graph on which the user has pre-established a desired threshold of enhancement. Once this threshold is reached by the ascending curve, the patient is automatically positioned in the gantry in 3–5 s at the desired level for acquisition of the helical CT data set (Tello et al. 1993). This program is now used routinely and we have applied it successfully in about 4000 spiral chest CT examinations performed in adults and children, with optimal mediastinal vessel and heart enhancement whatever the patient's age and cardiac output.

4.7 Scanning Direction

In order to decrease the importance of venous artifacts, which markedly detract from image quality, especially in the axillary and thoracic inlet areas and along the superior vena cava, some users choose a caudocranial direction when performing helical chest CT examinations. With an appropriate concentration of contrast material (150–200 mg iodine/ml), however, the cephalocaudal direction can be utilized, as for conventional incremental CT examinations. The advantage of the cephalocaudal direction is particularly obvious when an helical chest CT examination is performed in conjunction with a cervical and /or abdominal examination. Furthermore, when using a large volume of diluted contrast medium and a scan delay of 20 s, all upper and mid mediastinal vessels, including pulmonary arteries and veins, are opacified, with the exception in most instances of the innominate vein opposite to the injection site. At concentrations ranging between 150 and 200 mg iodine/ml and flow rates of 3–4 ml/s, no or few streak artifacts will arise from the superior vena cava and spoil imaging of the heart and mediastinum.

4.8 Injection Site and Catheter

Injection of contrast material in helical CT scanning must be performed in the largest available vein, usually in an antecubital vein – preferably the basilic one, which has collaterals with the humeral veins and which directs the contrast medium straight into

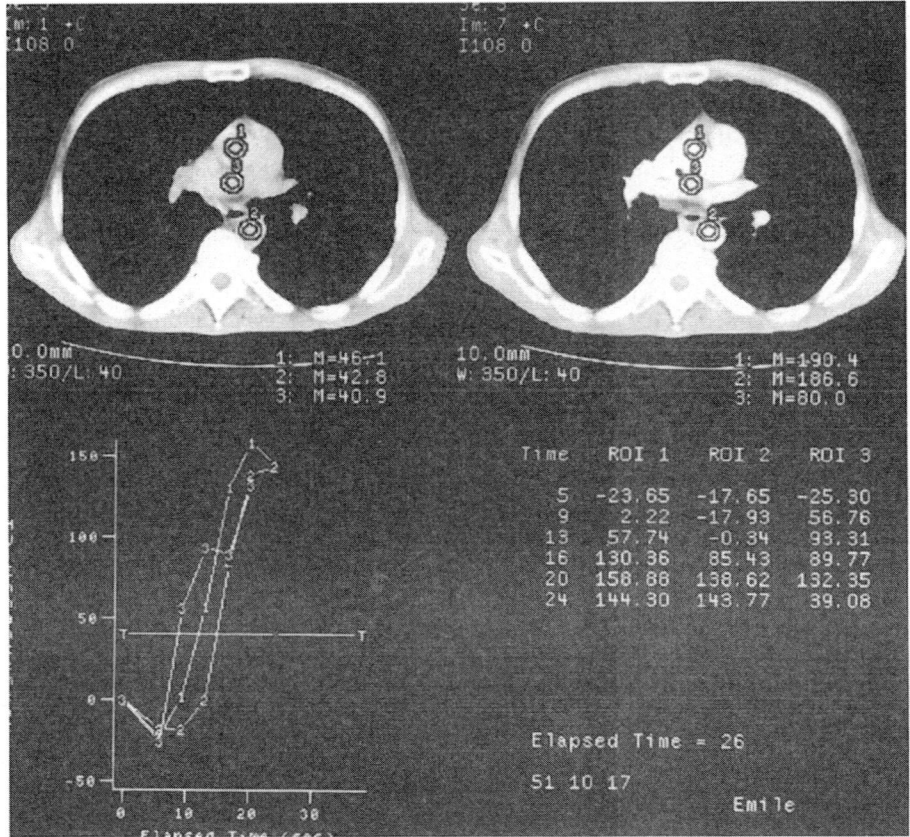

Fig. 4.7. SmartPrep display. The nonenhanced baseline scan (*upper left*), shows the three chosen regions of interest (ROIs) in the ascending aorta (*1*), descending aorta (*2*), and distal main pulmonary artery (*3*). The contrast-enhanced scan (*upper right*) shows that enhancement values three of the ROIs of 190.4, 186.6, and 80.0 HU. The *lower left graphic* displays en-hancement curves for each ROI. The *horizontal line* corresponds to the selected threshold (*T*), which has been fixed 45 HU over the baseline. In the *right lower quadrant* of the figure, time delays in seconds and enhancement over the baseline are presented for each ROI

the axillary and innominate veins. Injection in the cephalic vein directs the contrast material in a superficial, less straight route, since it has to flow through the arch of the cephalic vein before entering the axillary vein. Furthermore, when the upper limbs are placed above the head, the lumen of the arch of the cephalic vein is distorted and the blood flow is reduced. When antecubital veins are not available, the injection has to be done in the cubital vein or in a vein of the dorsal aspect of the wrist or hand. At this level, veins usually have a fragile wall and injections should be done with a 21- or 22- gauge Venflon (BOC Ohmeda AB, Helsingborg, Sweden) or needle at a maximum flow rate of 2 ml/s. Puncture of a lower limb superficial vein and catheterization of the common femoral vein with a 5F 15- to 20-cm-long catheter, using the Seldinger technique, represent two other options. The latter, which can be easily applied

on outpatients, is safe and efficient, but is rarely used in CT units.

The left upper limb is recommended for the injection (PAUL 1994; REMY et al. 1993). This choice is related to the direction of the left innominate vein, which axially and transversely crosses the retrosternal space and upper mediastinum. However, this venous segment is so easily recognized that a right-sided injection always affords equivalent diagnostic results. Obviously, if a bronchopulmonary or mediastinal or vascular mass is located on the course of an innominate vein, the opposite upper limb has to be chosen to achieve the injection (Fig. 4.8).

For many oncological patients, the only adequate site of injection may be an implanted infusion port, positioned in the subcutaneous tissues of the chest or at the root of the upper limb and linked to a catheter,

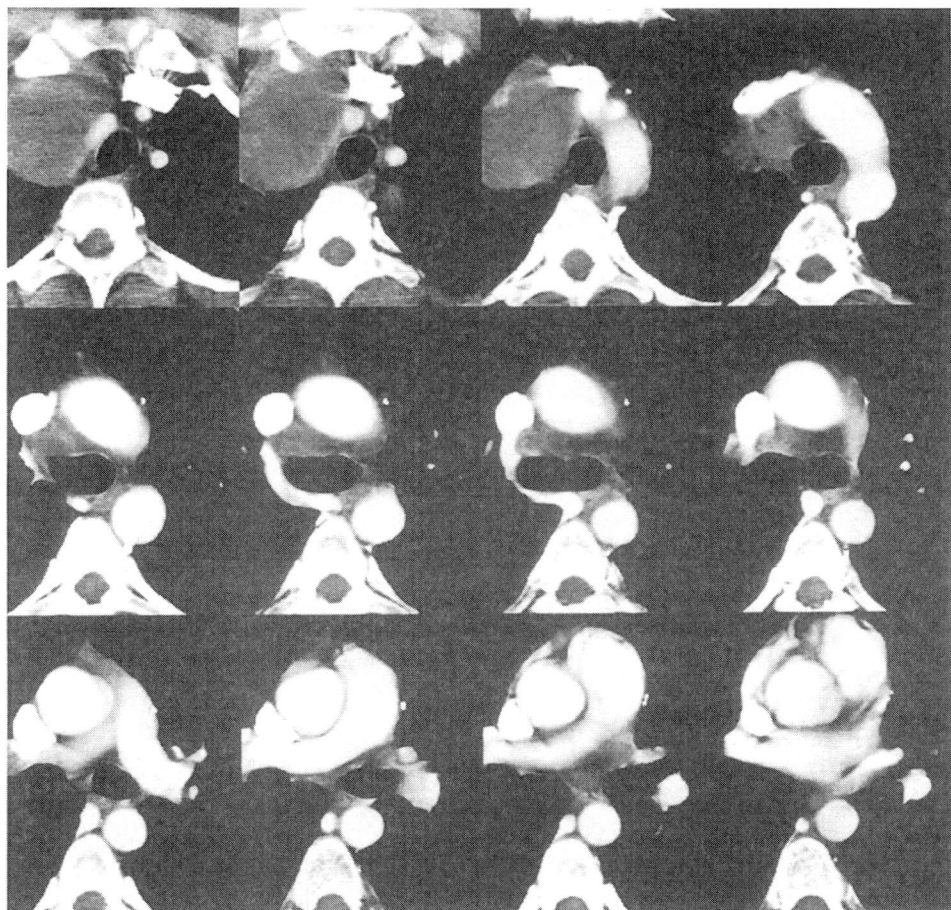

Fig. 4.8. Twenty-year-old female admitted with a 5-cm mass of the right pulmonary apex. Due to its position, the left antecubital vein was chosen for the injection of contrast material. Helical CT sections display a low-density lesion invading the lumen of the right innominate vein and the supra-aortic mediastinum. Lymphadenopathy is present in node station 4R. Biopsy revealed a primary leiomyosarcoma of the upper mediastinum. This helical CT examination, achieved with a concentration of 150 mg iodine/ml and a 3 ml/s flow rate, demonstrate marked reflux of contrast in the arch and vertical portion of the azygos vein. At this flow rate, such an important reflux is rarely encountered. It is certainly not related to the above-mentioned obstruction of the innominate vein

the distal end of which is located in the superior vena cava. Such infusion devices require a specially bent injection steel needle, the extremity of which does not damage the membrane of the port. The needle is fixed to an extension tube; the proximal end of this tube is adapted to the pump of the power injector. These ports should not be injected with a flow rate higher than 2 ml/s (CARLSON et al. 1992). Thus, the concentration of the contrast medium should be increased to 200 mg iodine/ml.

When the injection is made in the antecubital vein, an 18- to 20-gauge, 32- to 45-mm-long Venflon is used. It is firmly taped on the skin and connected to the power injector with an 83-cm-long extension tube with a Luer-Lock security system (Baxter Laboratory, Trieste, Italy). Injection rates of up to 3 ml/s are applied with a 20-gauge catheter. For higher flow rates, 19- or 18-gauge needles are preferred, even though 20-gauge ones have been demonstrated to withstand flow rates of 5 ml/s (McCARTHY and MOSS 1984). Before connecting the extension tube to the needle, it is checked that the Venflon is correctly positioned by obtaining a blood reflux followed by a bolus injection of 10 ml of sterile water in 2 or 3 s, with two fingers of the operator applied on the area of injection. In most patients this will allow early detection of a possible venous rupture.

Injection of contrast medium can also be achieved through central venous catheters; the latter were used mainly in patients referred from emergency or intensive care units. These 18-gauge catheters accept contrast medium flow rates of up to 5 ml/s (CARLSON 1992). Most central venous catheters contain in their wall a radioopaque marker, which can induce additional streak artifacts and spoil images. This is particularly true for patients referred for suspicion of pulmonary embolism, type A aortic dissection, or aortic rupture.

4.9 Patient Position

With few exceptions, spiral CT examinations of the chest, as well as incremental ones, are obtained with the patient supine. In adults, the upper limbs are positioned along the neck and above the head in order to reduce the body thickness at the level of the scapulohumeral joints and to minimize the related scan artifacts. However, this position, which somewhat mimics the Adson maneuver, is considered by some authors to obstruct the flow of the contrast medium through the axillary vein when it runs between the posterior aspect of the clavicle and the midcervical aponeurosis anteriorly and the anterior scalene muscle posteriorly (PAUL 1994; RÉMY et al. 1993). In fact, transit times of the contrast medium from the antecubital vein to the right heart and mediastinal vessels do not verify this supposition, and a complete obstruction or narrowing of the subclavian vein has never been observed in relation to the upper limb position. Achievement of the CT examination with only the injected upper limb lying along the body of the patient may represent a compromise, particularly in trauma patients. The prone position can be chosen for evaluation of posterior mediastinal lesions. Indeed, in this position the heart and mediastinum are anteriorly displaced (BALL 1980), a situation which affords good visualization of an esophageal tumor or provides an adequate route to perform a needle biopsy of a tumor located in a posterior segment of the lung (WESTCOTT 1988; COSTELLO et al. 1987). Radiologists are increasingly performing these minimally invasive procedures and must obtain contrast-enhanced helical CT examinations after having settled the patient in the optimal position for the maneuver, whether this be supine, prone, or lateral decubitus.

Although claustrophobia is less frequently encountered among patients than when performing magnetic resonance imaging, patients so affected (and particularly psychiatric ones) may generally benefit from the prone position, even if it renders the contrast injection and its control more hazardous.

4.10 Power Injector

The type of power injector does not play an important role in spiral CT scanning. However, the following conditions must be fulfilled: (a) the power injector computer program must be linked to that of the helical CT scanner, (b) the power injector must be easily moved from one side of the CT table or gantry to the other, (c) an emergency stop switch must be rapidly reachable on the power injector itself, (d) the syringe volume should be sufficient, i.e., not less than 200 ml, and (e) the injection pressure must be indicated on the remote control system with a maximal threshold at 150–200 PSI (11–14 kg/cm^2).

4.11 Precautions

Injection parameters (flow rate, volume) are chosen by the radiologist along with helical CT scanning parameters and are pre-established by the operator, The contrast injection is performed under the close supervision of the radiologist, who must stand next to the patient and carefully look for possible paravenous injection of contrast medium and be ready to immediately interrupt the injection manually. Extravasations of contrast material have occasionally been reported. They are certainly more frequent with the use of helical CT devices and power injectors. Despite strong recommendations and strict precautions, we have encountered three instances of extravasation of contrast material during the last 3 years, among 15 000 examinations (0.02%), an incidence similar to the 0.04% reported by COHAN et al. (1990). In one patient in whom a concentration of 300 mg iodine/ml of ionic contrast medium was used, extravasation of 40 ml occurred with subsequent necrosis of the skin, subcutaneous tissues, and muscles and transitory radial and cubital nerve palsy. The other two accidents occurred with ionic and nonionic contrast medium respectively, but at a concentration of 150 mg iodine/ml; The amounts of contrast were 100 and 50 ml respectively. The patients did not complain seriously and the injection was achieved through another vein. No short- or long-term complications occurred.

Necrosis of the skin and subcutaneous tissues as well as inflammatory local reactions are related to high-osmolality contrast medium only, with a maximum intensity of symptoms occurring during the first 3 days after the accident (SISTROM et al. 1991; ELAM et al. 1991). The recent literature dealing with the use of power injectors indicates that a much

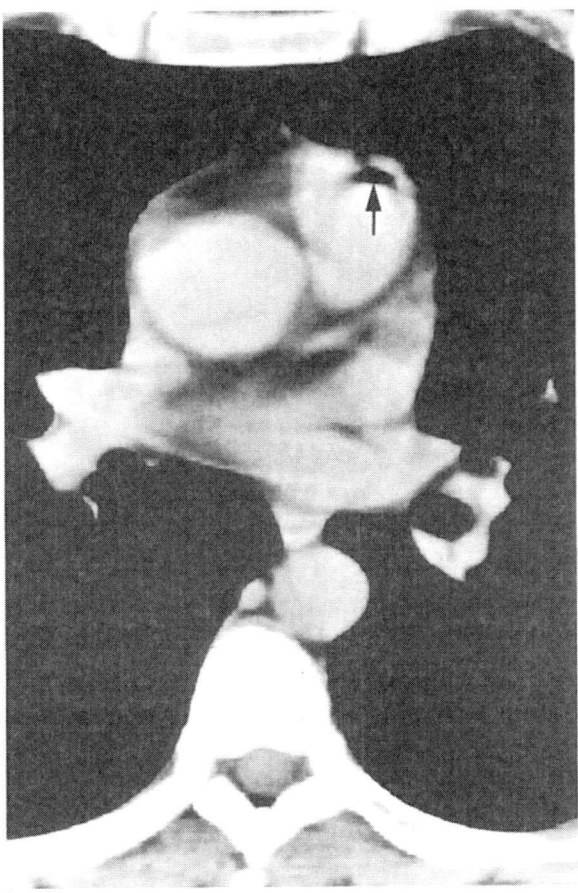

Fig. 4.9. Air bubble (*arrow*) anteriorly located in the lumen of the pulmonary trunk and related to a poorly flushed tubular extension or power injection syringe. Such findings are not uncommon and have been reported in up to 12% of CT examinations

higher incidence of massive extravasation occurs (50–150 ml) when a remote control injection is undertaken by the technician, without close supervision of the injection site (SHUMAN et al. 1986). In the various reported series, the incidence ranges from 0.1% to 2% (COSTELLO et al. 1992; PAUL 1994; SISTROM et al. 1991; SHUMAN et al. 1986; MILES et al. 1990).

Among other precautions, one has to verify that the syringe of the power injector has been carefully flushed, although small amounts of air, identified within the lumen of the innominate vein in up to 23% of patients in whom a manual injection has been performed (WOODRING and FRIED 1988), are totally asymptomatic. Air collections within the lumen of the pulmonary artery may be seen in up to 12% of CT examinations and are not related to the amount of the injected air volume (Fig. 4.9).

4.12 Choice of Contrast Medium Osmolality

At equal iodine concentrations, high osmolality contrast medium (HOCM: around 1500 mosmol/kg H$_2$O) and low osmolality contrast medium (LOCM: <600 mosmol/kg H$_2$O) have the same x-ray attenuation in vitro. In vivo, however, HOCM induces a dilution which leads to a decrease in the iodine concentration. This phenomenon is particularly obvious in the kidneys, and is less striking with LOCM (LLOYD 1991). It is not, however, apparent during the enhancement of chest blood vessels, and it is recognized that no gain in diagnostic efficiency is achieved by substitution of HOCM by LOCM (MCCLENNAN 1990; GRAINGER 1992). The choice of contrast medium is the sole responsibility of the radiologist and is determined by the patient's condition. All radiologists wish to replace conventional HOCM by the more physiological LOCM. This would result in a 3- to 15-fold increase in contrast-related costs, depending on the country (GRAINGER 1992). Thus, the choice of the osmolality is a constant dilemma for the radiologist, who has to face the decreasing resources devoted to medical care and yet must guarantee the comfort and security of patients (GRAINGER 1992; LEVIN et al. 1993; CARO et al. 1992; POWE 1992; POWE et al. 1993).

Large-scale prospective studies – both non-randomized (KATAYAMA et al. 1990; LASSER and Berry 1989; SCHROTT et al. 1986) and randomized (WOLF et al. 1989) – have investigated the safety of nonionic as compared with ionic contrast media. Although definitions of the severity of adverse reactions are not comparable, it appears in Katayama et al.'s series of 337 647 injections (KATAYAMA et al. 1990) that severe adverse reactions occurred in 0.22% and very severe ones in 0.04% of patients examined with HOCM. For patients examined with LOCM, the incidences dropped to 0.04% and 0.004% respectively. One death was reported in each group. Comparable results were obtained by WOLF et al. (1989) with a smaller series of 13 173 consecutive randomized patients and by SCHROTT et al. (1986), whose series comprised 24 756 patients. No death was reported in these two series. The same studies (KATAYAMA et al. 1990; WOLF et al. 1989) indicated that the incidences of nausea and vomiting are markedly reduced, from 4.6% and 1.8% to 1% and 0.4% when HOCM is replaced with LOCM. Fifty-two percent of patients with a history of allergy, asthma, urticaria, or another hypersensitivity reaction were found by KATAYAMA and TANAKA (1988) to show adverse reactions to HOCM. Patients having had prior mild or severe adverse reactions to HOCM have been shown to present a low incidence of adverse reactions during a second HOCM examination (KATAYAMA and TANAKA 1988). In such instances, the use of LOCM and steroid premedication have been recommended (LASSER et al. 1988; FISCHER and SPATARO 1988; LASSER and BERRY 1989; KATAYAMA et al. 1990), and the incidence of severe adverse reactions has been reported to be reduced by 40% by prescription of two doses of corticosteroids (LASSER et al. 1988; LASSER and BERRY 1989). The value of this premedication is, however, not widely recognized, and its use remains controversial (WOLF et al. 1989; GRAINGER 1992; POWE 1992).

We ourselves think that helical CT examinations, like all other radiological diagnostic procedures requiring an injection of iodinated contrast medium, must be achieved with a HOCM except in those patients presenting with cardiac failure, recent myocardial infarction, critical valvular diseases, coronary disease, unstable cardiac rhythm, or pulmonary hypertension. In such patients an LOCM should be used, this being less depressive for the myocardium. Other high-risk patients with diabetes, myeloma, a previous adverse reaction to iodinated injection, or renal insufficiency must also be examined with an LOCM, as must elderly patients and children.

The costs related to the use of contrast material in helical CT examinations of the chest are 30% lower as compared with the use of incremental CT (COSTELLO et al. 1992; COSTELLO 1994a,b; RÉMY-JARDIN et al. 1992). This is due to the reduced scan time, the improvement in scan delay, and the experience acquired by users who are constantly improving scanning protocols and adapting them to patient status and the pathology in question. Unfortunately, in some countries, such as Germany and Japan (and perhaps Switzerland in the near future) legislation now urges the use of nonionic contrast material only, which results in an unjustified and immediate threefold increase in the related costs.

4.13 Dilution of Contrast Medium

Concentrations of 150 and 200 mg iodine/ml are commercially available in Europe. Self-dilution is not recommended by companies, which claim that such a maneuver markedly increases the risk of infectious contamination. Surprisingly, 1 g of iodine at such a low concentration is significantly more expensive

than 1 g of iodine of contrast at a concentration of 300 or 360 mg/ml. Interestingly, the decrease in the initial osmolality of contrast media is not proportional to the dilution. Indeed, the osmolality of ioxithalamate 300 mg iodine/ml (Télébrix 30, Guerbet, Aulnay-sous-Bois, France), which is 1750 mosmol/kg H_2O, drops to 720 mosmol/kg H_2O when it is diluted with an equal volume of sterile water. Similarly, the 2300 mosmol/kg H_2O of ioxithalamate 380 mg iodine/ml (Télébrix 38, Guerbet, Aulnay-sous-Bois, France) is lowered to 950 mosmol/kg H_2O when it is similarly diluted (PAUL 1994). This reduction increases the patient's comfort and the quality of helical CT examination, since mild transitory adverse reactions such as nausea, vomiting, and warmth phenomena are markedly diminished at such osmolalities.

Furthermore, an experimental study in rats (DEAN et al. 1988) has demonstrated that dilution of contrast medium does not provoke lower iodine tissue concentrations, iodine distribution volumes, plasma volumes, or hematocrit, and concluded that lowering contrast medium osmolality by sterile water dilution should improve tolerance without affecting CT contrast enhancement.

In view of the above considerations, we do not follow commercial recommendations: we have routinely diluted contrast material for more than 3 years without any error arising. The concentration of 150 mg iodine/ml is obtained by diluting a 300 mg iodine/ml contrast medium with an equivalent volume of sterile water.

4.14 Volume

The volume of contrast required for a helical CT examination must be preset on the remote control system of the power injector and is estimated with the following formula:

$$\text{volume} = \text{flow rate } (\text{ml/s})$$
$$\times \left[\text{scan delay } (\text{s}) + \text{scan time } (\text{s}) - 7 \right],$$

where 7 s corresponds to the transit time to the pulmonary trunk. This formula has been adapted for a concentration of 300 mg iodine/ml injected at a flow rate of 2 ml/s. When using a concentration of 150 mg iodine/ml at a flow rate of 3–4 ml/s, the volume must be multiplied by 2. Another way of determining the volume (v) of contrast relates the amount of iodine to the body weight, such as:

$$V(300\,\mathrm{mgl/ml}) = \text{body weight}\,(\mathrm{kg})\ \text{or}$$
$$V(150\,\mathrm{mgl/ml}) = \text{body weight}\,(\mathrm{kg}) \times 2.$$

These formulae are more convenient for examination of children than the above-mentioned one. They are also easily applied to most adult patients. When helical CT examination of the chest is followed by an abdominal helical CT scan, an additional 30% of contrast volume is required.

4.15 Scan Time

The scan time is determined not only by the length of the chest along the z-axis, the x-ray beam collimation, and the pitch value, but also by the patient's aptitude for holding his breath. Most patients for whom an injection of contrast material is required are able to maintain a breath-hold for 30 s. This time is sufficient to achieve most helical CT chest examinations with an x-ray beam collimation of 7 mm and a pitch value of 1 : 1.5. When the planned apnea cannot be maintained, hyperventilation with 100% of oxygen for 2 min before the CT data acquisition will generally improve the patient's performances in holding his breath. Another possibility is to perform the examination with smaller volumes of data acquisition and to apply 5- to 7-s intergroup gaps. Examination of less cooperative patients (mainly chest trauma and intensive care patients or children) can be achieved with quite superficial breathing. Helical CT sections have been shown to be less sensitive to motion artifacts than incremental CT sections (KALENDER et al. 1990; VOCK et al. 1990).

4.16 Respiration and Physiologic Parameters

Even using a 150 mg iodine/ml concentration of contrast medium and a moderate flow rate of 3 ml/s, streak artifacts are still present in 47% of subjects. Furthermore, streak artifacts can arise from the subclavian vein and superior vena cava during one helical CT chest examination and yet be absent some weeks later in the same patient while using the same injection and CT parameters. Physiological parameters regarding cardiac output, respiratory position, lung volume, and lung vascular resistances are related to the flow of contrast material in the veins and right cardiac chambers of the patient. The pulmonary blood volume fluctuates not only during the cardiac cycle, due to the fact that inflow exceeds outflow during systole, but also, and more importantly, during the respiratory cycle. Indeed, the pulmonary blood volume decreases during positive pressure breathing (FENN et al. 1947) and, conversely, increases during negative pressure breathing (NUNN 1994).

The rise in intrathoracic pressure determined by the respiratory position is the main cause of the reduction of cardiac output in impairment of or obstruction to filling of the right atrium. Most helical CT examinations are performed at the full end-inspiratory position in order to permit maintenance of apnea for 20–30 s, and many patients can only sustain a full end-inspiratory position with the help of a closed glottis, thus achieving a Valsalva effect. The increase in intrathoracic and airway pressures related to this maneuver is important and reaches about 50–60 cmH$_2$O (5–6 kPa). This physiological response is complex and can be divided into four phases (NUNN 1994) (Fig. 4.10):

Phase 1 is characterized by an increase in the baseline pulmonary arterial pressure in accordance with the raised intrathoracic pressure. Simultaneously, the diastolic filling of the right cardiac cavities is markedly decreased by an unfavorable thoracoabdominal pressure gradient and by a striking reduction in the lumen caliber of the superior vena cava, directly related to the increased intrathoracic pressure. These two phenomena are well known and used in venous B-mode echo-Doppler imaging and upper and lower limb phlebograms. The decreased filling of right cardiac cavities results, in *phase 2,* in a reduction in the cardiac output and arterial pressure. Both reductions are rapidly stabilized and compensated in normal subjects by tachycardia, an increase in systemic vascular resistance, and an increase in peripheral venous pressure, the last-mentioned being the main mechanism of restoration of the blood input to the right heart. Thus, the decreased pressure will be followed by a plateau, at a level similar to the baseline pressure, which will last up to the end of the Valsalva maneuver. These systemic venous and pulmonary arterial complex variations occur during a 30-s Valsalve maneuver and certainly account for variations in the quality of contrast enhancement. *Phase 3* occurs immediately after the Valsalva maneuver, when the increased airway pressure returns to normal. At that time, an immediate decrease in pulmonary arterial pressure occurs due to a sudden improvement in cardiac output and in the resulting pulmonary capil-

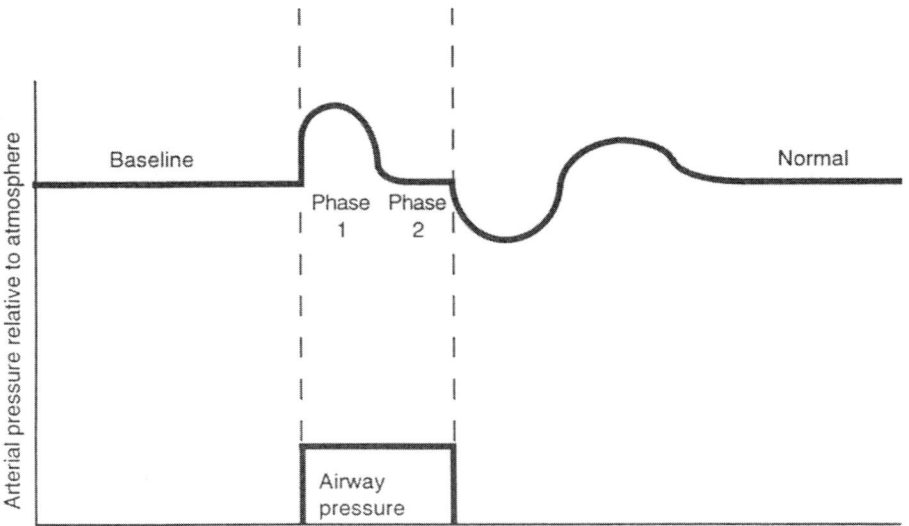

Fig. 4.10. Variation of the pulmonary arterial pressure during a Valsalva maneuver (adapted from NUNN 1994, with permission)

lary resistances (WEST 1990). During *phase 4*, a transient unclear arterial pressure overshoot or a rebound effect occurs.

These physiological variations have practical implications for the planning of helical CT examinations. First, patients must be trained to achieve and maintain apnea at the full end-inspiratory position and to avoid closing the glottis. Almost no pathological conditions examined by helical CT of the chest are better imaged as a result of the decreased heart filling, cardiac ouput, and flow within the systemic veins and pulmonary arteries induced by the Valsalva maneuver. A possible exception is the opacification of the venous pedicle of some complex pulmonary arteriovenous malformations, although some of the most experienced authors in this field recommend that such malformations be examined at the full end-inspiratory position and recommend the use of contrast material injection in selected cases only (RÉMY et al. 1994; WHITE and POLLAK 1994).

Low pulmonary vascular resistance is closely related to the lung volume. WEST (1990) has demonstrated that at the end of a normal expiration, when the functional residual capacity (FRC) is reached, the pulmonary vascular resistance will have dropped to its lowest value. When the lung volume linearly increases during inspiration, the pulmonary vascular resistance rises exponentially. This phenomenon is due to the intra-alveolar pressure, which increases relative to that of the capillary lumen, thereby stretching and constricting the lumen of the vessels and raising the pulmonary resistance. When the lung volume decreases, the smooth muscle and elastic tis-

sue tone of the vessels become very effective, leading to a collapse of the capillary lumen and an increase in the pulmonary artery pressure (WEST 1990).

The above-described physiological elements are to be taken into consideration when the radiologist is dealing with a superior vena cava syndrome or a bronchopulmonary tumor invading the hilum or mediastinum or is investigating the possible extension of a neoplastic mass to the wall of the superior vena cava. In all of these instances, the injection of contrast material should ideally be achieved with the lowest possible pulmonary vascular resistance, which means during quite superficial breathing. Examinations are, however, spoiled by breathing artifacts; therefore CT acquisition is preferably achieved at the full end-inspiratory position, though never during a Valsalva maneuver.

4.17 Cardiovascular Effects

Cardiovascular effects of HOCM are much more striking and must be considered in isolation from those induced by LOCM. Within a few milliseconds after entering the bloodstream, an HOCM induces (MORRIS 1988) transport of water from (a) the extravascular compartment and (b) the blood and endothelial cells to the intravascular compartment (MORRIS 1988; SUNNEGARDH et al. 1990; REES et al. 1988; BOCK et al 1990). This water shift is directly related to the high osmolality of the contrast medium, which provokes shrinkage of the cell cytoplasm and nucleus and widening of intercellular junctions (MORRIS 1988; THIESEN and MÜTZEL 1990; ALMEN et al. 1990; SCHNEIDER et al. 1988). These changes are markedly reduced with LOCM. Such cellular modifications lead to a dilution of the injected contrast medium in the veins of the injected upper limb, in the axillary and innominate veins, and in the superior vena cava. An additional dilution of the contrast medium occurs from the venous blood of the contralateral upper limb, the veins of the head and neck, and the azygos vein. This dilution is frequently observed as a low-attenuation filling defect within the lumen of the distal end of the homolateral innominate vein and proximal superior vena cava (Fig. 4.11). The HOCM then reaches the right cardiac cavities and has a depressive effect on the sinoatrial and atrioventricular nodes (negative chronotropic effect) (MORRIS 1988; HAGEGE 1994), as well as on the intraventricular bundle branches (negative dromotropic effect). Both negative chronotropic and dromotropic effects induce bradycardia, which is rapidly masked by tachycardia resulting from a collapse of both peripheral pulmonary and systemic resistances and from an increase in the pulmonary blood volume to the right heart (SUNNEGARDH et al. 1990. Furthermore HOCM have a depressive effect on the contractile power of the myocardium (negative inotropic effect), which decreases the aortic pressure, although LOCM have been shown to have a positive inotropic effect (SUNNEGARDH et al. 1990).

Once in the pulmonary artery, an HOCM increases the pulmonary artery pressure, although,

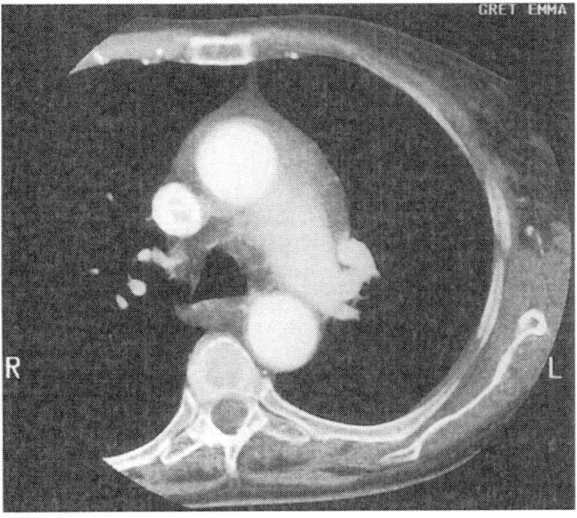

Fig. 4.11. Filling defect of the central part of the superior vena cava induced by the nonopacified blood arising from the left innominate vein. The injection of contrast was performed in the right antecubital vein

surprisingly, pulmonary vascular resistance decreases by about 20% in animals (SUNNEGARDH et al. 1990), just as in other vascular beds (MORRIS 1988; ALMEN et al. 1990; TAJIMA et al. 1991). This increase in pulmonary artery pressure, demonstrated in both animals (SUNNEGARDH et al. 1990; THIESEN and MÜTZEL 1990; ALMEN et al. 1990; BOCK et al. 1988) and humans (MORRIS 1988; BOCK et al. 1990; TAJIMA et al. 1991), is related (a) to the same water shift that occurs above the right cardiac chambers (MORRIS 1988; BOCK et al. 1990; TAJIMA et al. 1991) and also in the peripheric systemical circulation (MORRIS 1988; ALMEN et al. 1990) and (b) to an aggregation of red blood cells directly related to the osmolality of the contrast medium (MONNIER et al. 1991; MOREAU et al. 1988), which produces an increase in whole blood viscosity (MORRIS 1988; ALMEN et al. 1990). Such an increase in pulmonary artery pressure, which can reach 47% from the the baseline value in animals (SUNNEGARDH et al. 1990), occurs when contrast medium is injected intravenously, in the right cardiac cavities, or in the pulmonary arteries. It does not occur when the contrast is injected into peripheral arterial vessels (BOCK et al. 1990). First pass of contrast in the pulmonary capillaries is thus the main factor related to the increase in pulmonary arterial pressure.

Variations in aortic pressure during injection of contrast medium in the right atrium have been studied in animal models (SUNNEGARDH et al. 1990; ALMEN et al. 1990). In an early phase, 6–8 s after the start of injection, HOCM have a negative inotropic effect which leads to an immediate fall in the aortic pressure by about 20%. Soon 8–12 s after the start of the injection, the main aortic pressure increases again (by 20%–30%), simultaneously with the cardiac output. This increase is linked to the hyperosmolality of the contrast and the already mentioned water shift from the extravascular compartment to the intravascular one, and probably also to a positive inotropic effect of the contrast on the left ventricle (MORRIS 1988; SUNNEGARDH et al. 1990). Later, 15–25 s after initiation of injection, the aortic pressure drops again when the contrast medium reaches peripheral systemic arteries. Although pulmonary vascular resistances, pulmonary arterial and aortic pressures, and cardiac output are markedly influenced by intravenous injections of HOCM, the heart rate is only slightly modified. This is due to the antagonistic positive and negative chronotropic effects of HOCM (MORRIS 1988; BOCK et al. 1990).

Low osmolality contrast media have much lower endothelial and red blood cell toxicity. They induce no or few changes in the blood volume, and their effect on the contractility of the myocardium is much less than that of HOCM (MORRIS 1988). Although early changes in aortic pressure occur only with HOCM, the late reduction in systemic pressure occurs with both HOCM and LOCM; it is, however, more pronounced with HOCM (−40%) than with LOCM (−12%) (ALMEN et al. 1990).

Thus, most of the effects of intravenous injections of contrast medium are thought to be related to their osmolality. These effects have been shown to be significantly smaller with LOCM than with HOCM. This is of practical importance in helical CT sanning of patients with impaired cardiovascular function and/or pulmonary hypertension. There is now evidence that severe reactions to contrast media in these patients are reduced when using LOCM.

4.18 Causes of Opacification Failure

Failure to achieve adequate opacification is not uncommon in helical CT scanning even when the technique is performed by an experienced radiologist. Most instances of failure are related to the Valsalva maneuver performed by the patient in order to maintain a deep inspiratory position and to mild adverse reactions to the contrast medium (mainly nausea and vomiting, which warrant immediate interruption of the injection). Among other causes, cardiac insufficiency associated with bradycardia and arrhythmia is not uncommon. In these instances, the opacification quality is often unpredicable (Fig. 4.12), even with the help of injection tests or the SmartPrep program.

Right to left shunts, such as Eisenmenger complex and large arteriovenous malformations, can be responsible for opacification failure at the first helical CT examination. A second acquisition, with modified injection parameters, may be necessary, and close evaluation of the behavior of the contrast enhancement in both series affords much anatomical and physiological information.

Subjects with normal heart function and a patent superior vena cava usually do not present reflux into the arch of the azygos vein at an injection rate of 3 ml/s (see, however, Fig. 4.8). Such reflux is observed more frequently, i.e., in about 20% of cases, when the flow rate is increased to 4 ml/s and in about 50% of examinations performed at 5 ml/s or more. The reflux usually does not occur in the jugular veins, due to the presence in more than 80% of subjects (FISCHER et al. 1982) of valves which remain compe-

tent even when submitted to high gradient pressure (DRESSER and MCKINNEY 1987).

4.19 Injection Techniques in Children

Parameters of contrast medium injection in children vary according to the age of the patient. However, some of them are constant: The use of LOCM is required by the recommendations of many national societies and the European Society of Pediatric Radiology (MCALISTER and KISSANE 1990). The dose of iodine should be limited to a maximum of 1 g iodine per kilogram of body weight. Most helical CT examinations require a smaller amount of iodine since, as for adults, the optimal iodine concentration is around 150 mg/ml and the flow rate 2–4 ml/s. The total volume of contrast and consequently the dose of iodine will be determined by the slice thickness, the pitch value, and the length of the examined areas along the z-axis.

Newborn babies are generally examined asleep under mild chloral sedation or after a meal, during quite superficial breathing.

Young children under 4–5 years of age require deep sedation or brief general anesthesia. Tracheal intubation is usually not required and causes streak artifacts which considerably impair image quality, especially with respect to mediastinal structures. At the age of 6 years, most children are able to cooperate and even to maintain apnea at the full end-inspiratory position, without the Valsalva maneuver, or to breath superficially.

Most children enter the CT unit after the positioning of an efficient Venflon or other type of needle (e.g., butterfly); the needle should be of 20–22 gauge and firmly taped to the skin, allowing an injection flow rate of at least 2–3 ml/s. The positioning of the

---

Fig. 4.12a,b. Seventy-year-old patient with right heart failure and pulmonary hypertension following chronic pulmonary embolism disease. **a** Contrast injection was performed in the right antecubital vein with 200 ml of nonionic contrast at 150 mg iodine/ml concentration, a flow rate of 3 ml/s, and a scan delay of 20 s. A marked reflux of contrast opacifies the right enlarged jugular vein. The right innominate vein and superior vena cava are also enlarged. The aorta has barely enhanced, although **b** the pulmonary arteries display high attenuation values. Even by the end of the acquisition, 68 s after the initation of the injection, the lumen of the left atrium and ventricle remain poorly enhanced. This discrepancy between the right and left heart cavities results from high pulmonary resistance due to chronic pulmonary embolism. A 70-mgHg pressure was measured during a previous pulmonary catheterization

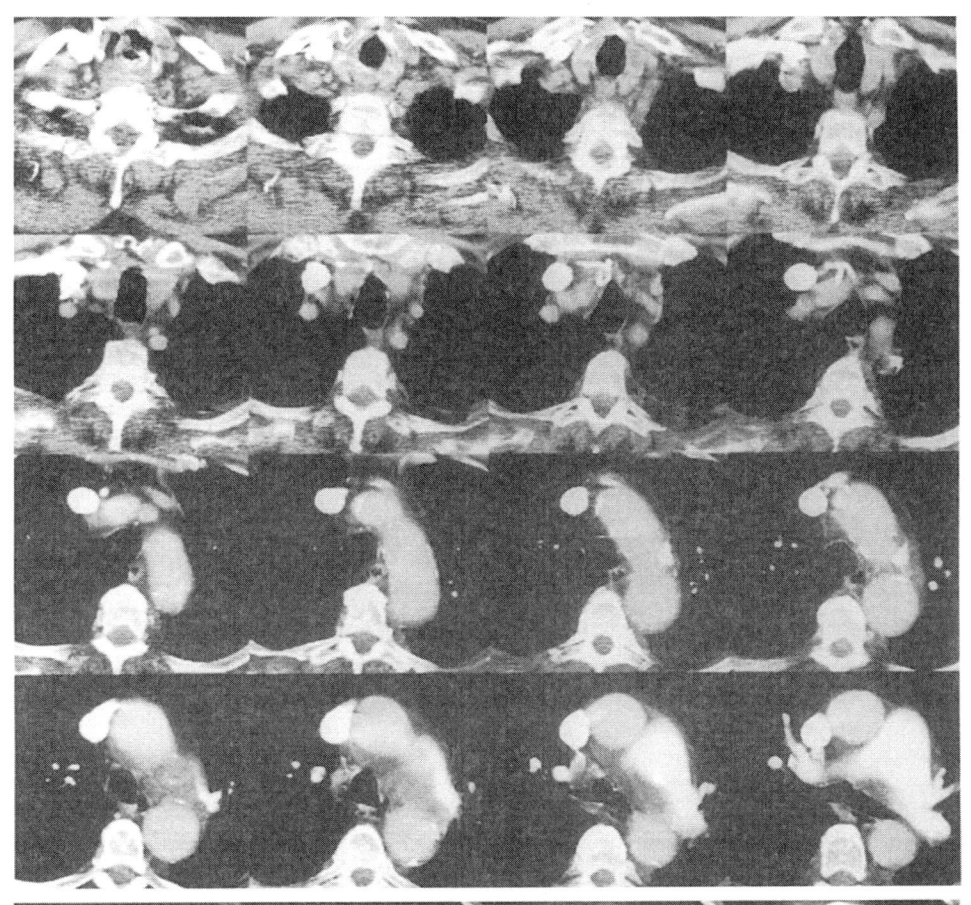

a

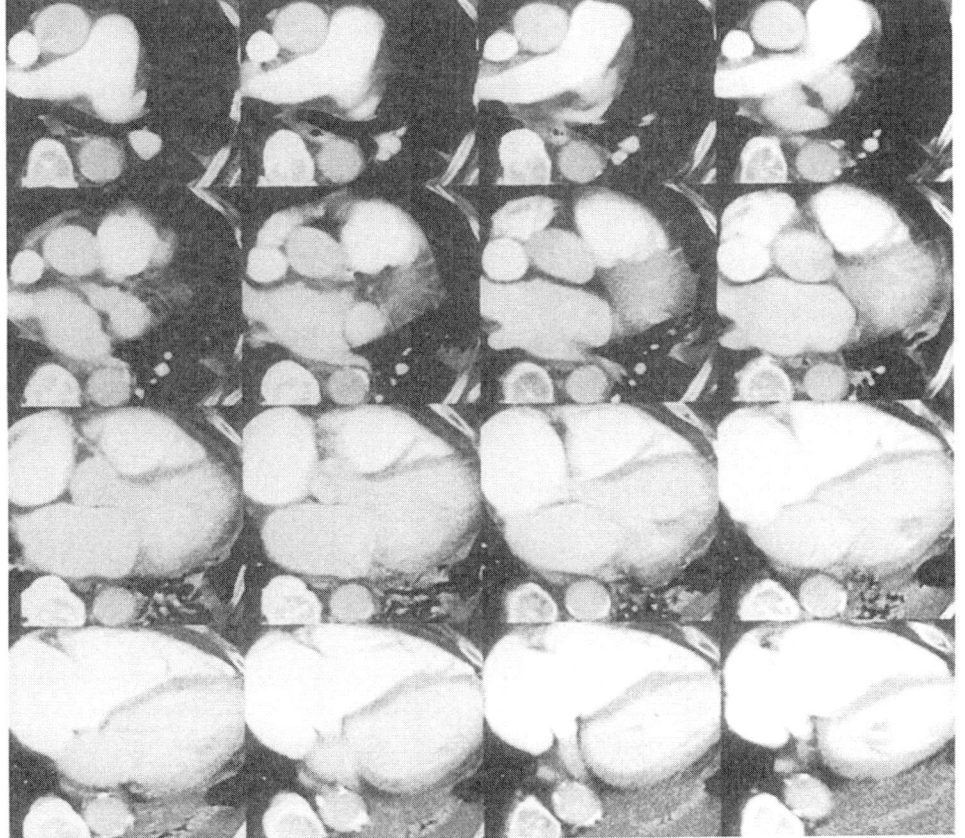

b

Venflon has to be done in the pediatrics department at least 1 h before the CT examination. Newborn babies and small children should be injected by hand rather than with the power injector in order to control the injection site. The use of 20-ml syringes and some experience allow one to inject the contrast medium very regularly, at the desired flow rate. As for adults, the scan delay is preferably determined with the SmartPrep program. It can also be accurately estimated by taking account of the short distance from the injection site to the heart and the cardiac rate. Transit times given for adults can be divided by 2 for children under the age of 4 or 5 years.

The appropriate position of children for helical CT scanning is supine. However, due to the small size of the chest and shoulders, the upper limbs can be easily placed along the body. Scan parameters such as kilovoltage, mA, slice thickness, and pitch value must be adapted in accordance with the patient's age, condition, and stoutness, and the suspected pathology.

4.20 Protocols

The protocols outlined below provide the radiologist with guidelines for daily helical CT practice. Comments and proposed examination parameters are based on the literature data (COSTELLO et al. 1994a,b; STORTO et al. 1994; PAUL 1994, RÉMY et al. 1993; BLUM and RÉGENT 1995) and on the experience we have acquired during the last 3 years with one helical CT unit and, over the past year, with an additional scanner installed within an emergency unit. The proposed protocols mostly concern examinations requiring the injection of contrast material. They must be adapted to (a) the patient's condition, (b) the type and make of helical CT scanner, and especially the x-ray tube characteristics, (c) the local conditions of work, and (d) financial (institutional or insurance) restrictions, such as costs related to the use of contrast media, x-ray tube wear, patient through put, etc.

4.20.1 Protocol for Helical CT Imaging of Bronchopulmonary Cancers

Bronchopulmonary cancer represents the most frequent indication for helical CT scanning of the chest, which is performed in order to determine the TNM staging. In most instances, helical CT scans following adequate injection of contrast material can dif-

ferentiate a central lung tumor from distal postobstructive lobar collapse (Fig. 4.13) or postobstructive pneumonitis (ONITSUKA et al. 1991). Identification of invasion of the chest wall or mediastinum by lung cancers, which distinguishes T3 from T2 lung cancers, remains a difficult task. Criteria of invasion (GLAZER et al. 1985, 1989; MCCAUGHAN et al. 1985) established with contrast-enhanced incremental CT scans, with their mediocre sensitivity and specificity, seem to remain unchanged with helical enhanced CT techniques. Contrast-enhanced spiral CT scanning using 3- to 5-mm x-ray beam collimation has been shown to be efficient, in a limited number of subjects, in demonstrating on 3D images the adhesion and retraction of both pleural sheaths by the lung cancer, the so-called puckering sign (KURIJAMA et al. 1994). The efficiency of this time-consuming technique, however, is not convincing when compared to the reliability of dynamic inspiratory and expiratory helical CT. Indeed, the latter method, which does not require the injection of contrast medium, has a sensitivity of 100% and a specificity of 70% for the evaluation of chest wall or mediastinal invasion (MURATA et al. 1994). The number of false-positive results recorded with the dynamic respiratory technique is similar to the number encountered with the technique combining chest CT with iatrogenic artificial pneumothorax (WATANABE et al. 1991; YOKOI et al. 1991) or with ultrasonography (SUZUKI et al. 1993).

Upper abdominal survey, including the adrenal glands and liver, is part of the helical CT examina-

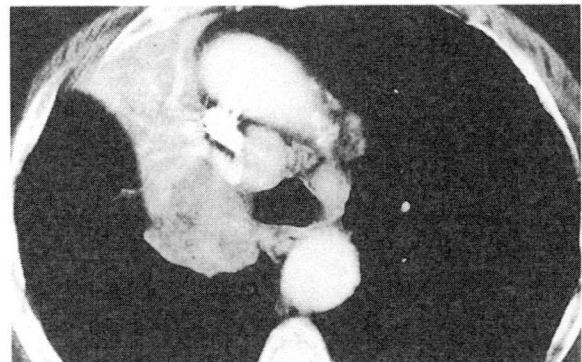

Fig. 4.13. T4N3 squamous cell carinoma of the right main bronchus extending to the posterior aspect of the carina, readily differentiated from the distally collapsed right upper lobe. Such a differentiation is possible on this contrast-enhanced helical CT scan, which enhances the collapsed lobe more than the tumor. Markedly enhanced segmental and subsegmental arteries and veins coursing within the collapsed lung parenchyma are well displayed

Fig. 4.14. a Poorly differentiated T3N3 central adenocarcinoma invading the mediastinal pleura and fat. Incremental 3-mm CT sections have been obtained before and during injection of contrast medium, at 10-s intervals during 90 s. **b** The graph displays the enhancement curve of the tumor, which increases from 25 HU before injection to a peak enhancement of 57 HU 60 s after the start of the injection

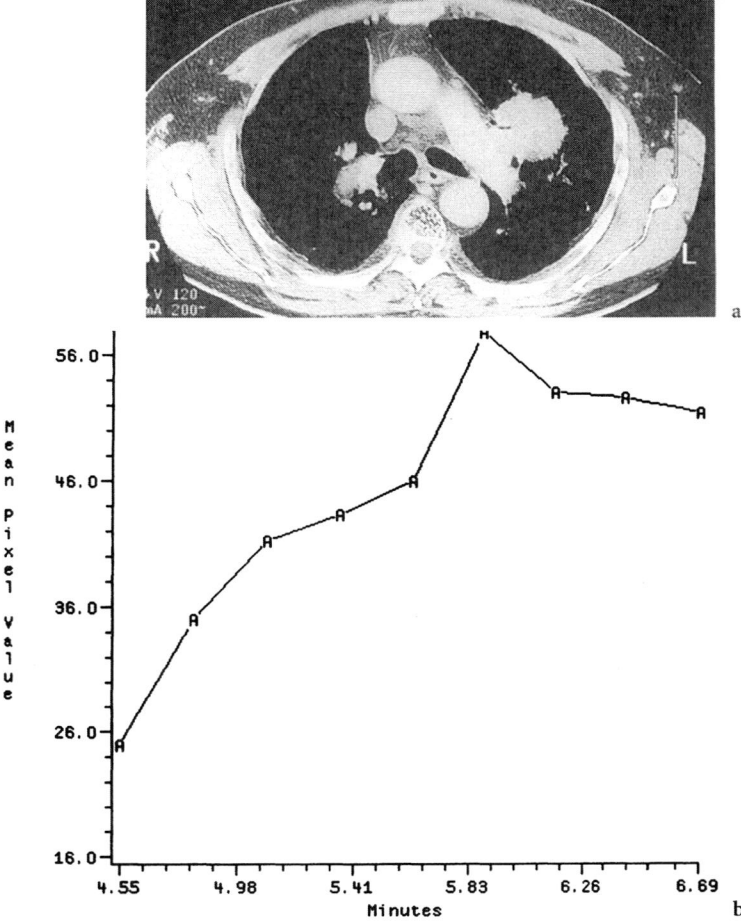

tion. When a brain CT examination is required for TNM assessment, it is achieved with incremental postcontrast sections only at the end of the session.

Most of the time, precontrast chest sections are not justified. However, they can be recommended to better focus the helical acquisition on the tumor and thus determine its upper and lower aspects and its relationships with the mediastinum or the chest wall. Precontrast sections can also be required for evaluation of the enhancement of a pulmonary nodule in order to statistically determine its benignity or malignancy, as recently proposed (SWENSEN et al. 1995; YAMASHITA et al. 1995) (Fig. 4.14). Scan parameters for precontrast helical CT acquisitions are identical to those used for postcontrast acquisitions.

Contrast-enhanced helical CT acquisition is pre-established on two front and lateral scout views required by an x-ray dose optimization program (SmartScan, General Electric, Milwaukee, USA). Upper sections include the thoracic inlets, and caudal sections include the diaphragm. Data acquisition is planned with a 7-mm x-ray beam collimation, a pitch of 1.5, and image reconstruction intervals of 5 mm (B/P/R: 7/1.5/5), with x-ray tube parameters of 125 kV and 140–200 mA according to the patient's stoutness, an FOV of 28–32 cm, and a craniocaudal acquisition direction (Table 4.2).

High- or low-osmolality contrast media are used at a concentration of 150 mg iodine/ml injected at a flow rate of 3 ml/s. The volume of contrast is determined by the scan parameters, and is usually 130–150 ml. This amount is increased by 30% when the upper abdomen is simultaneously examined, and does not exceed 200 ml, which corresponds to 30 g of iodine.

Table 4.2. Protocol for helical CT imaging of bronchopulmonary cancers

	Chest	Upper abdomen
Patient position	Upper limbes above the head or injected upper limb along the body	Same
Respiratory position	Full end-inspiratory position	Same
Nonenhanced survey	Optional	Optional
B/P/R	7/1.5/5	7/1.5/7
X-ray tube	125 kV, 140–200 mA	125 kV, 280–320 mA
FOV	Entire chest	30–35 cm
Algorithm	Standard + high frequency	Standard
Injection site	Antecubital vein	Same
Contrast concentration	150 mg iodine/mL	Same
Contrast volume	130–200 ml	+30%
Contrast flow rate	3 ml/s	Same
Scan delay	Smart Prep/15–25 s	45–75 s
Image display	350/50 and 1600/−600	350/50
Acquisition direction	Craniocaudal	Same

B/P/R: X-ray beam collimation/pitch value/reconstruction interval

The scan delay is determined with the SmartPrep program, if available. When it is not, a scan delay of 15 s affords optimal enhancement of mediastinal systemic and pulmonary vessels.

For elderly subjects or patients suffering from cardiac insufficiency and/or arrhythmia, the scan delay is greatly modified. Over the age of 70, a scan delay of 20–25 s can be applied. In these situations, however, the 20-ml injection test (STORTO et al. 1994; RUBIN et al. 1995) is a good alternative to the SmartPrep program.

Abdominal examination follows chest data acquisition in the helical mode during the portal phase in the full end-inspiratory position, usually 45–60 s after the beginning of injection. In most instances, a 15-s interval can be set between the two acquisitions and will allow the patient to breath.

Abdominal helical CT examination is obtained with parameters of 7/1.5/7 (see above), 125 kV, 280–320 mA, and a field of view (FOV) adapted to the patient's habitus.

Chest sections are reconstructed with standard and high-frequency algorithms and imaged with window settings of 350/50 and 1600/−600, respectively. Abdominal sections are reconstructed with a standard algorithm and imaged with a window setting of 350/50.

When a complementary chest acquisition is required with higher resolution on a smaller FOV, it is achieved with a second injection, rather than incorporating it into the initial examination planning. Indeed, any change in the scanning parameters will stop the helical acquisition for at least 5–7 s

and require more contrast and a longer period of apnea.

4.20.2 Helical CT Imaging of Mediastinal and Hilar Masses

Primary bronchopulmonary central cancers, lymphoma, metastatic lymphadenopathy, and, less frequently, inflammatory diseases, (mainly sarcoidosis and tuberculosis) represent the commonest indications for helical CT imaging in the mediastinum and hilum (COSTELLO 1994b; PUGATCH 1995; QUINT et al. 1995; WEBB et al. 1991; NAIDICH 1994). All these conditions are preferably imaged by CT rather than by MRI (PUGATCH 1995; WEBB et al. 1991), although large series have demonstrated mediocre sensitivity and specificity of both techniques (PUGATCH 1995; WEBB et al. 1991; GRENIER et al. 1989; McLOUD et al. 1992). Presently, no series has evaluated the accuracy of helical CT. However, one can expect no significant improvement as a result of its use, since the diagnosis of metastatic lymphadenopathy relies only on the smallest diameter of each lymph node, 10 mm in the smallest horizontal diameter usually being considered the maximal normal size (GLAZER et al. 1984). The quality of examination of the hilum and mediastinum is nevertheless better with spiral CT by virtue of the degree and homogeneity of opacification of vessels, the variable image reconstruction intervals and the instantaneously available 2D multiplanar reconstruction (Fig. 4.15).

In some instances, contrast-enhanced helical CT helps to establish the diagnosis, such as in patients carrying tuberculous lymphadenopathy. It has been shown (PASTORES et al. 1993) that contrast injection induces an early rim enhancement of tuberculous lymphadenopathy, which surrounds a low-attenuation necrotic centre (Fig. 4.16). This sign, which can be observed in other infectious diseases, such as cryptococcosis and AIDS, is not seen in lymphoma, metastatic cancer, or sarcoidosis (PASTORES et al. 1993).

Helical CT examination protocols in respect of mediastinal and hilar masses preferably include a precontrast helical CT survey, identical to that proposed for lung cancers. The patient maintains his upper limbs above the head (Table 4.3). The examination is preferably achieved in the full end-inspiratory position. Large tumors can, however, be examined during quiet breathing (Fig. 4.17); this is particularly true for tumors involving the upper and posterior aspects of the mid mediastinum (Fig. 4.18), which are less subject to breathing artifacts. The volume of enhanced data acquisition should include all lymphatics of the chest, including those of the diaphragm. For this purpose, a first enhanced helical CT examination is acquired with parameters identical to those proposed for bronchopulmonary cancers. The injected contrast volume, however, has to be limited to 100–120 ml so that another 100 ml can be used for a second enhanced acquisition, focused on the regions of interest, such as the hilum or a tumor–mediastinum interface, with narrower scan parameters (Fig. 4.19).

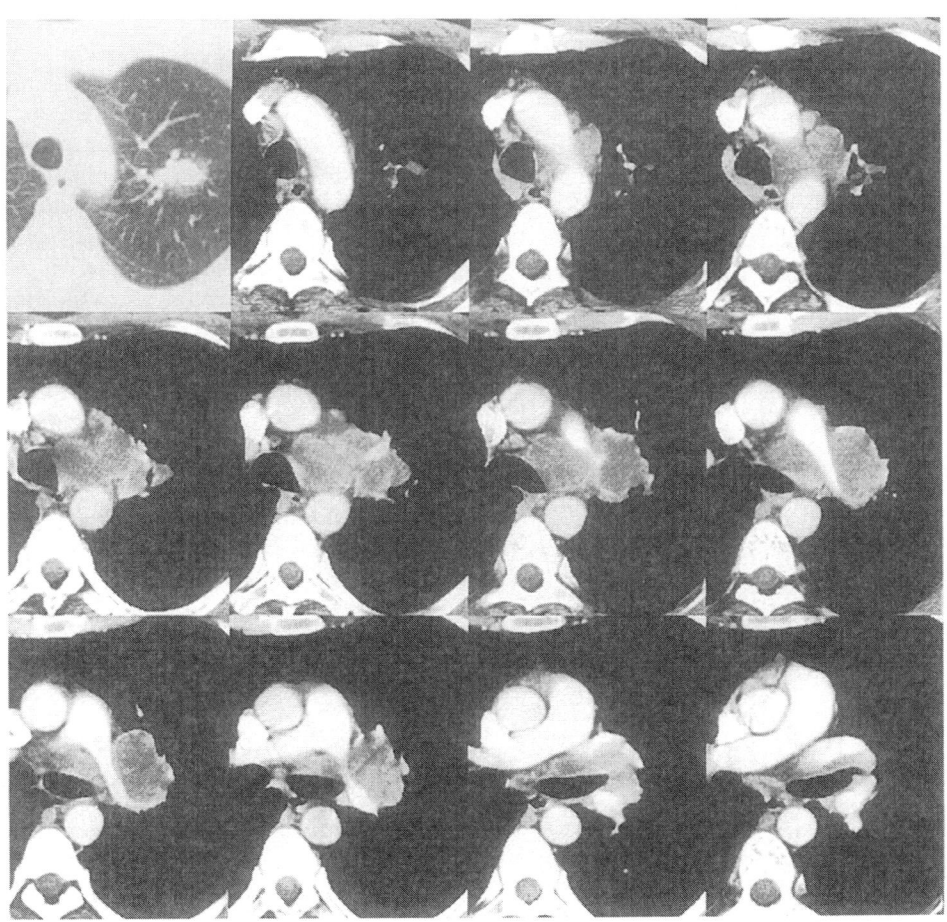

Fig. 4.15. a Forty-year-old HIV + male patient admitted with a left upper lobe 2.5 cm squamous cell carcinoma and extensive hilar and mediastinal lymphadenopsthy. Contrast injection affords homogeneous enhancement of mediastinal vessels but axial sections alone do not permit a precise evaluation of the degree of invasion of the left pulmonary artery. b,c 2D sagittal oblique and d coronal reconstructions demonstrate the extent of lymphadenopathy to the aorticopulmonary window, the marked stenosis of the distal left pulmonary artery (*arrow head*), the obstruction of the left upper lobe artery (arrow), and the patency of the left lower lobe artery (*circle*)

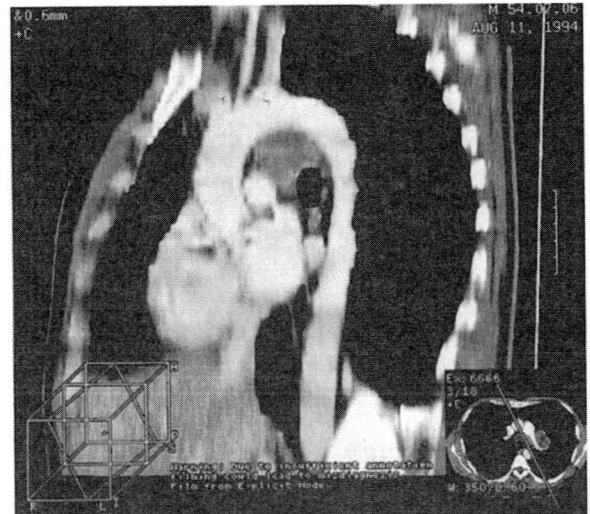

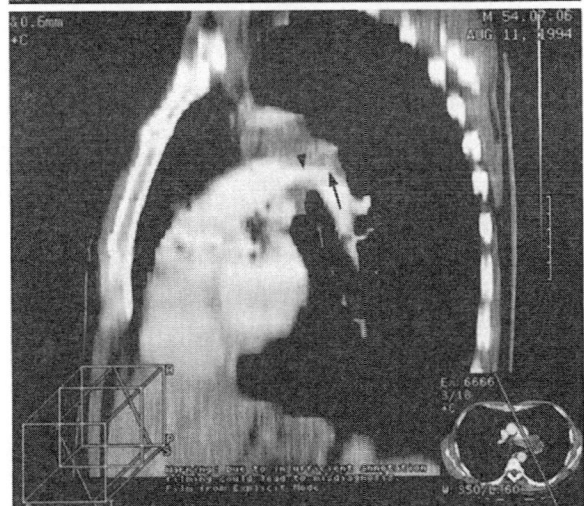

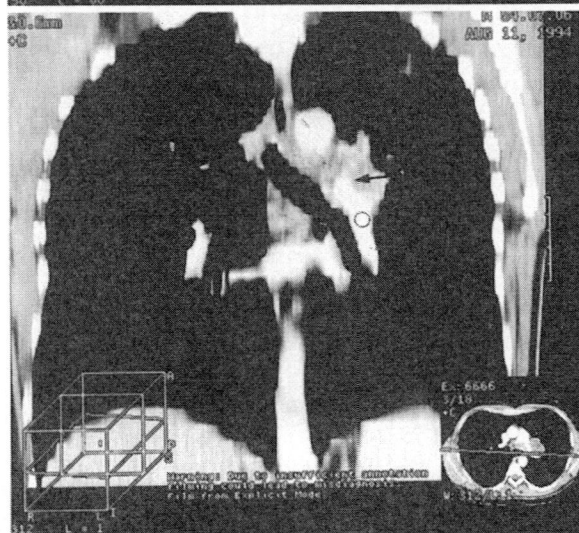

Fig. 4.15b–d

4.20.3 Protocol for Helical CT Imaging of Vascular Malformations

Vascular malformations of the lung include in particular pulmonary arteriovenous malformations (PAVMs) and partial anomalous pulmonary venous return (PAPVR). These conditions can be examined with an identical basic protocol which does, however, require some adaptation to the patient's condition, such as dyspnea due to right to left shunt or length of the malformation along the z-axis. This protocol is designed to demonstrate the precise extension of the malformation in the axial plane on 3D reconstructions, as well as to provide angiodynamic information by comparison of the kinetics of the lesion with those of cardiopulmonary vascular structures (RÉMY et al. 1994; WHITE and POLLAK 1994).

Following a front scout view, it is mandatory that nonenhanced helical CT sections are obtained over the whole chest. The examination is performed in the full-end inspiratory position, with B/P/R of 5–7/1.5/5 at 120 kV and as low an mA as possible (100–120 mA) in order to prevent a heat overload of the x-ray tube during the contrast-enhanced acquisition. The field of view must include both lungs and a standard reconstruction algorithm is suitable.

While non-enhanced spiral CT acquisitions permit reliable analysis of the angioarchitecture in 95% of PAVMs (RÉMY et al. 1994), selection of the threshold value for 3D reconstructions is sometimes problematic and must be done with care. Thus, helical CT contrast-enhanced acquisition should be considered; this will ensure inclusion of a maximal number of vascular voxels enhanced above the selected threshold and decrease the partial volume effects of horizontally oriented vessels. Injection of contrast material should be performed only for PAVMs larger than 10 mm (RÉMY et al. 1994).

The helical CT examination is achieved with the patient supine, with both upper limbs above the head, in the full end-inspiratory position, with a contrast medium concentration of 150 mg iodine/ml, an injection rate of 5 ml/s, and a maximal volume of 200 ml (30 g iodine) (Table 4.4). A scan delay of 7 s is adequate for the evaluation of the size, number, and origin of the arterial pedicles of the PAVM, and in most instance for the venous ones as well.

The helical CT acquisition is obtained in the craniocaudal direction with B/P/R of 1–3/1–1.5/1–1.5 at 125 kV and 140–200 mA, depending on the length of the malformation in the z-axis and on the orientation and length of the vascular pedicles. Indeed, pedicles mainly oriented in the horizontal plane and/

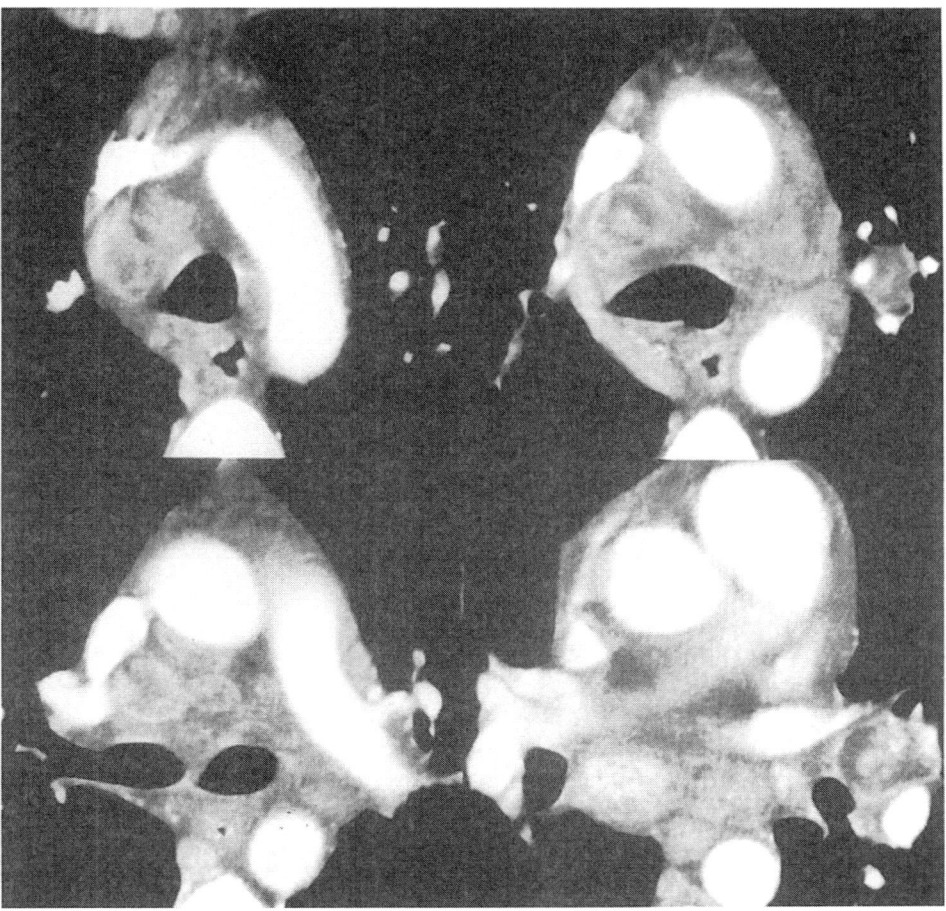

Fig. 4.16. Thirty-six-year-old HIV + female patient with a CD4 count level of 40 cells/ml and extensive mediastinal and hilar lymphadenopathy. Contrast-enhanced helical CT displays, for most of the diseased lymph nodes, a rim enhancement which circumscribes a low-attenuation necrotic center. This pattern is very suggestive of tuberculosis. Lymphadenopathy was removed by mediastinoscopy and the diagnosis was confirmed by histology and cultures. Injection parameters: 140 ml of ionic contrast material; flow rate 3 ml/s; scan delay 15 s concentration: 150 mg/ml. Technical parameters: B/P/R: 5/1/5

or with a short vertically oriented portion (z-axis) require a thinner x-ray beam collimation (1–2 mm), a smaller pitch value (1–1.2) and smaller image reconstruction intervals (1–1.5 mm) in order to minimize partial volume effects and improve 3D reconstructions (Fig. 4.20).

Like PAVMs, PAPVR is a dysgenesis in which the embryological pulmonary venous plexus does not anastomose to the primitive sinus venosus. This results in a left to right shunt due to abnormal communication between the portions of the pulmonary venous plexus and the cardiac cavities, or a persistent cardinal or omphalomesenteric venous system (FRIEDMAN 1992). The frequency of PAPVR ranges between 0.4% and 0.7% in autopsy series of patients with congenital heart disease, particularly an atrioseptal defect of the sinus venosus type

(FRIEDMAN 1992). The right lung is twice as often involved by PAPVR as the left one; 85%–90% of PAPVRs drain into the superior vena cava (Fig. 4.21) or the right atrium, while 10%–15% drain into the inferior vena cava, giving rise to the so-called scimitar syndrome on plain chest radiographs (OLSON and BECKER 1986).

Contrast-enhanced helical CT sections are particularly valuable in differentiating PAPVR of the left upper lobe from a duplicated left superior vena cava – two frequently confusing malformations. PAPVR of the left superior lobe is constituted by a vertically oriented vascular channel coursing along the left aspect of the aortic arch, into which drain the pulmonary veins of the left upper lobe. This abnormal vessel changes its orientation, and its cephalic, distal end is connected to the left subclavian vein (DILLON

Table 4.3. Protocol for helical CT imaging of mediastinal and hilar masses

	Chest	Upper abdomen
Patient position	Upper limbs above the head	
Respiratory position	Full end-inspiratory position	
Non-enhanced chest survey	Recommended	
	First enhanced acquisition	**Second enhanced acquisition**
B/P/R	7/1.5/5	3–5/1–1.5/3–5
X-ray tube	125 kV, 140–160 mA	125 kV, 160–200 mA
FOV	Entire chest	Region of interest: 15–18 cm
Algorithm	Standard + high frequency	Standard
Injection site	Antecubital vein	
Contrast concentration	150 mg iodine/ml	150 mg iodine/ml
Contrast volume	100 ml	100 ml
Contrast flow rate	3 ml/s	3 ml/s
Scan delay	Smart Prep/15–25 s	Smart Prep/15–25 s
Image display	350/50 and 1600/–600	350/50
Acquisition direction	Craniocaudal	Craniocaudal

B/P/R: X-ray beam collimation/pitch value/reconstruction interval

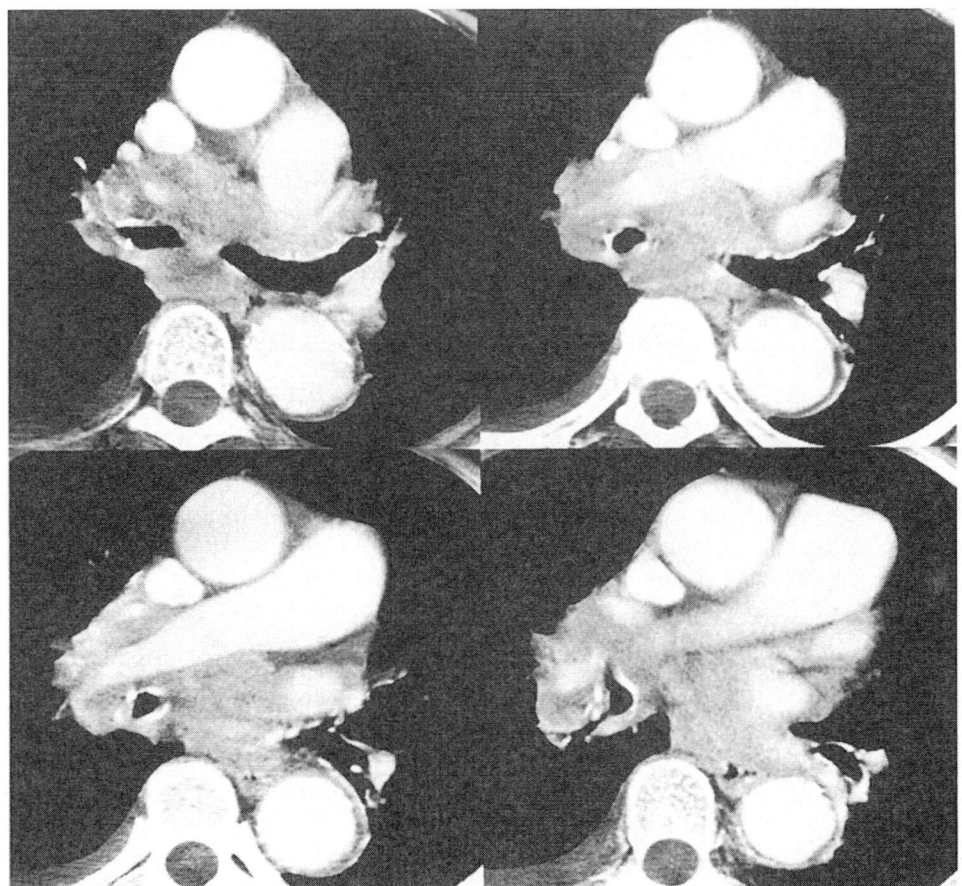

Fig. 4.17. Seventy-three-year-old female, 3 months after chemotherapy and partial remission of a poorly differentiated carcinoma of the intermediate bronchus. Enhanced helical CT sections show a large tumor recurrence involving the entire mid mediastinum with contralateral extension and an obvious stenosis of the right pulmonary artery. 2D reconstructions were not obtainable owing to the scanning parameters, which were chosen in accordance with the poor condition of the patient, and breating artifacts. Technical parameters: B/P/R: 7/1.5/5

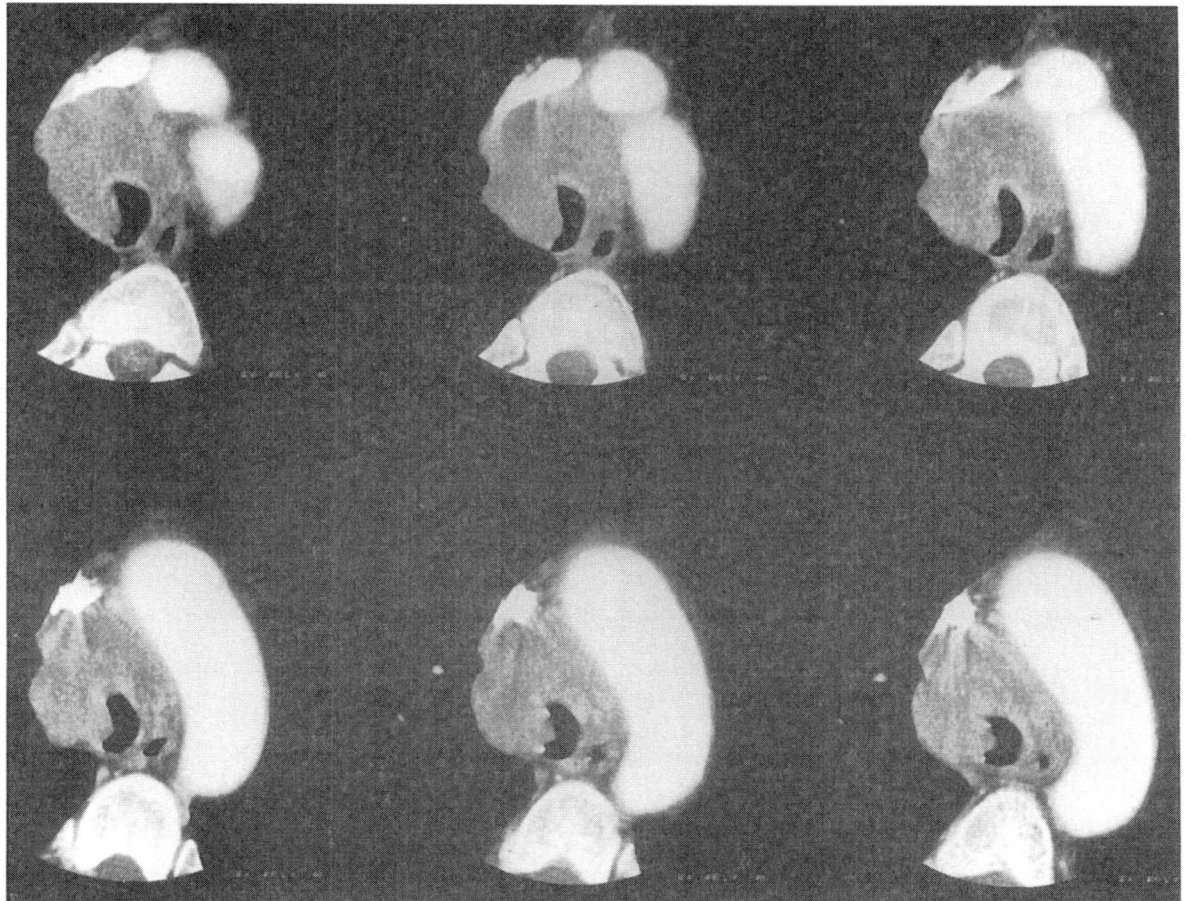

Fig. 4.18. Sixty-year-old patient with dyspnea, presenting with a large tracheal carcinoma invading and obstructing the right main bronchus. Contrast-enhanced helical CT examination, obtained during quite superficial breathing and focused on the region of interest, demonstrates the precise extension of the lesion and its relationships with the arterial and venous mediastinal structures. Injection parameters: 100 ml of nonionic contrast; flow rate 3 ml/s; scan delay 15 s. Technical parameters: B/P/R: 5/1/3

Table 4.4. Protocol for helical CT imaging of PAVMs and right PAPVR

Patient position	Arms above head	
Respiratory position	Full end-inspiratory position	
Nonenhanced survey	For all cases	
	Nonenhanced acquisition focused on the malformation	Contrast-enhanced acquisition focused on the malformation
B/P/R	1–3/1–1.5/1–1.5	Same
X-ray tube	125 kV, 140–200 mA	Same
FOV	ROI + heart and mediastinum	Same
Algorithm	Standard + high frequency	Same
Injection site	–	Antecubital vein
Contrast concentration	–	150 mg iodine/ml
Contrast volume	–	Max. 200 ml
Contrast flow rate	–	5 ml/s
Scan delay	–	7 s
Image display	350/50 and 1600/–600	350/50
Acquisition direction	Craniocaudal	Craniocaudal

B/P/R: x-ray beam collimation/pitch value/reconstruction interval

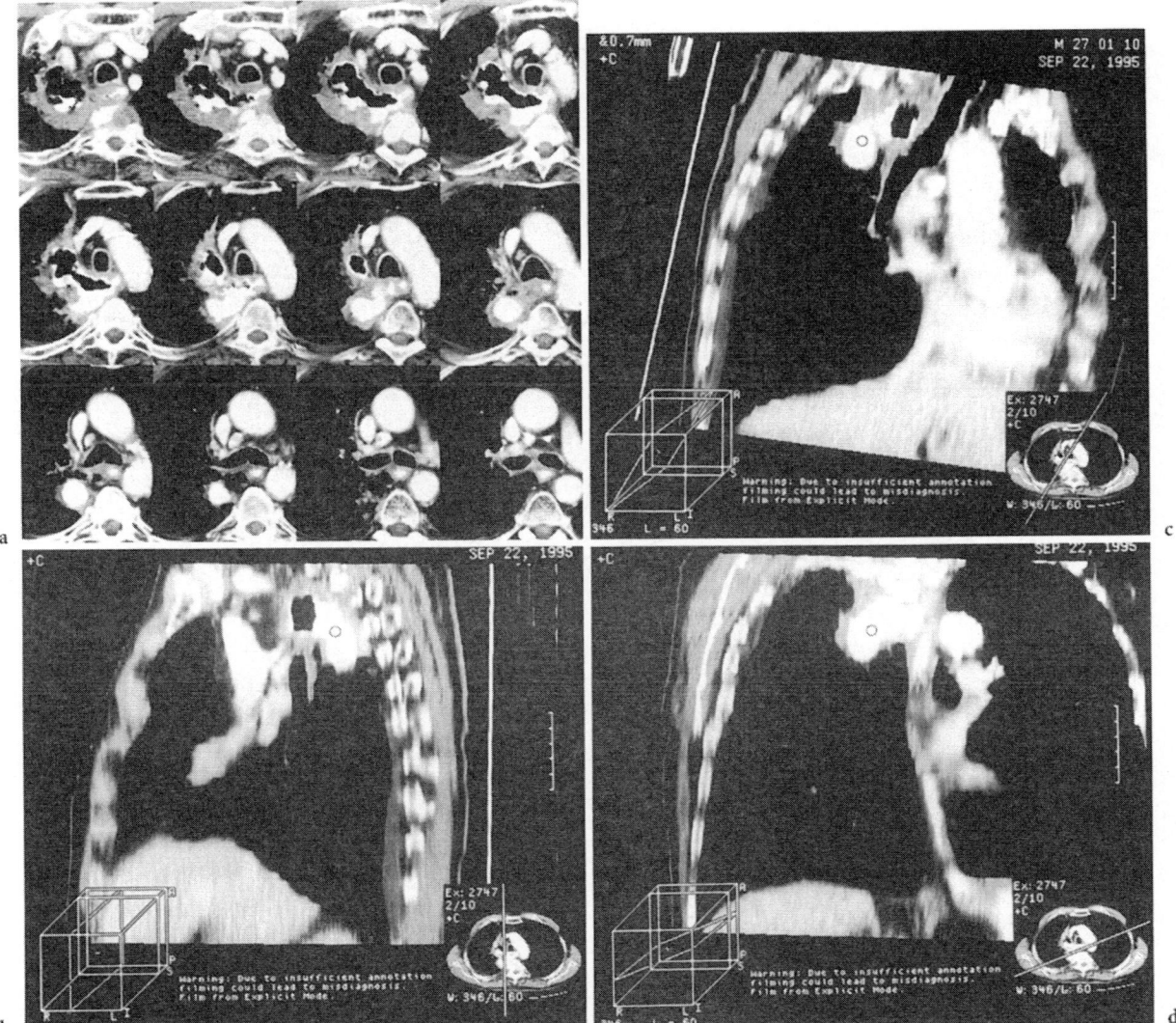

Fig. 4.19a–d. Sixty-eight-year-old patient operated on and irradiated 4 months previously for a bronchogenic carcinoma of the right upper lobe. **a** Helical CT sections display a large recurrent exavated tumor invading the esophagus, the posterior wall of the trachea, and the mediastinal fat. The excavation is filled with air and oral contrast material. A large communication between the esophagus and the recurrence is observed on four adjacent images. Delineation of the recurrence and its mediastinal invasion are improved by contrast enhancement. A cylindrical oral contrast-filled channel, which belongs to the necrotic excavted tumor, extends caudally in the right paravertebral sulcus on seven adjacent sections. The relationships of this recurrent necrotic tumor (*circle*), and its water-soluble contrast and air content, with the trachea and other mediastinal elements, are advantageously displayed by sagittal (**b**), oblique sagittal (**c**), and oblique coronal (**d**) 2D reconstructions. Technical parameters: B/P/R: 7/1.5/3

Fig. 4.20a–e. Helical CT examination in a 68-year-old male patient who had long suffered from an arteriovenous malformation of the middle lobe, provoking a major right to left shunt. **a** Helical CT acquisition was obtained 7 s after injection of 200 ml of 150 mg iodine/ml contrast medium at a flow rate of 5 ml/s. Scan parameters: B/P/R: 7/1.2/2. **a,b** Sections displaying delayed enhancement of the arteriovenous malformation, similar to that of the aorta, probably due to marked cardiac insufficiency. **c,d** Sections demonstrating that the venous pedicle enters the right atrium, with the inferior pulmonary vein. **e** 3D reconstruction displaying the arteriovenous malformation (*avm*) with one arterial (*ap*) and one venous (*vp*) pedicle

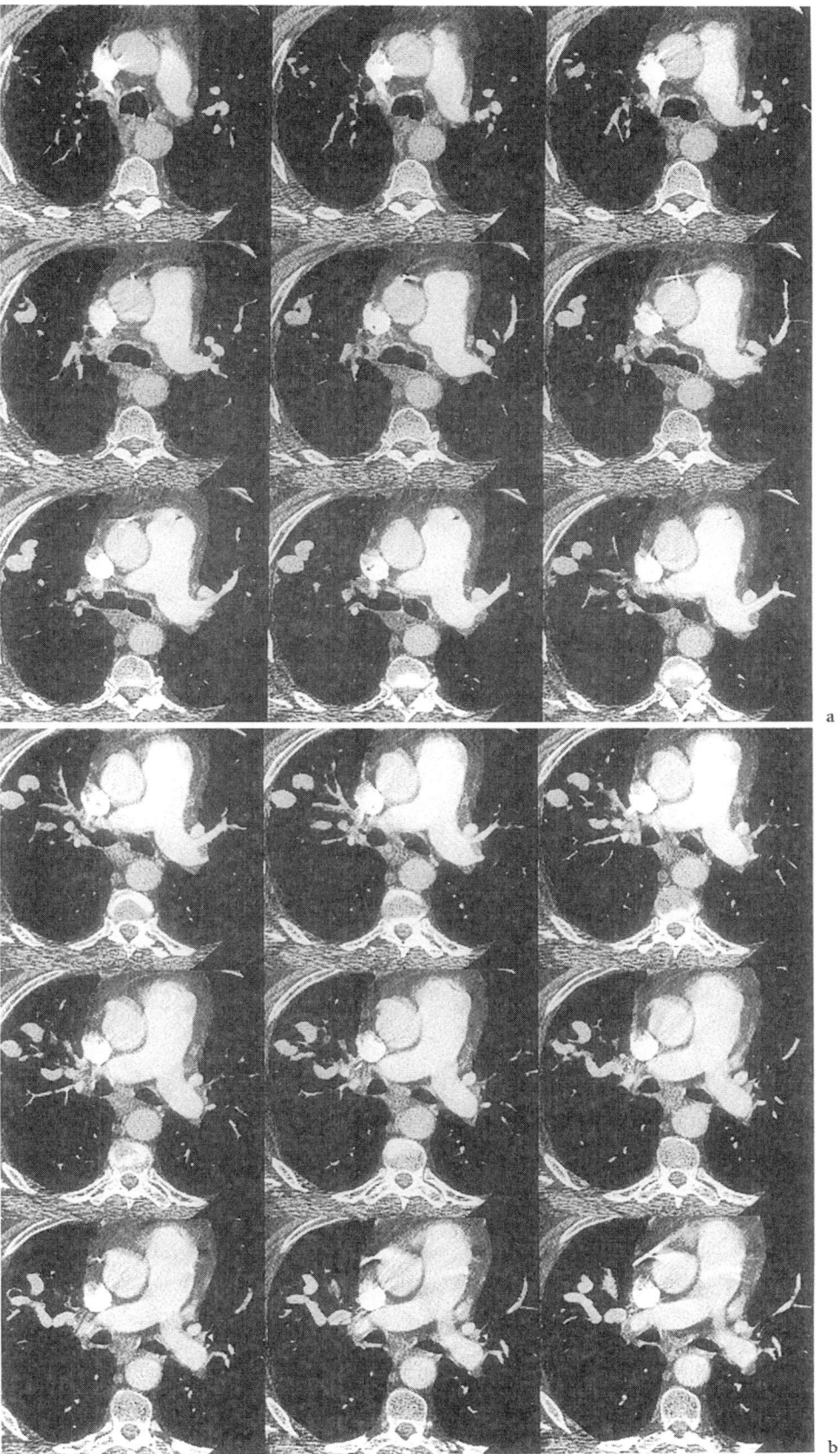

a

b

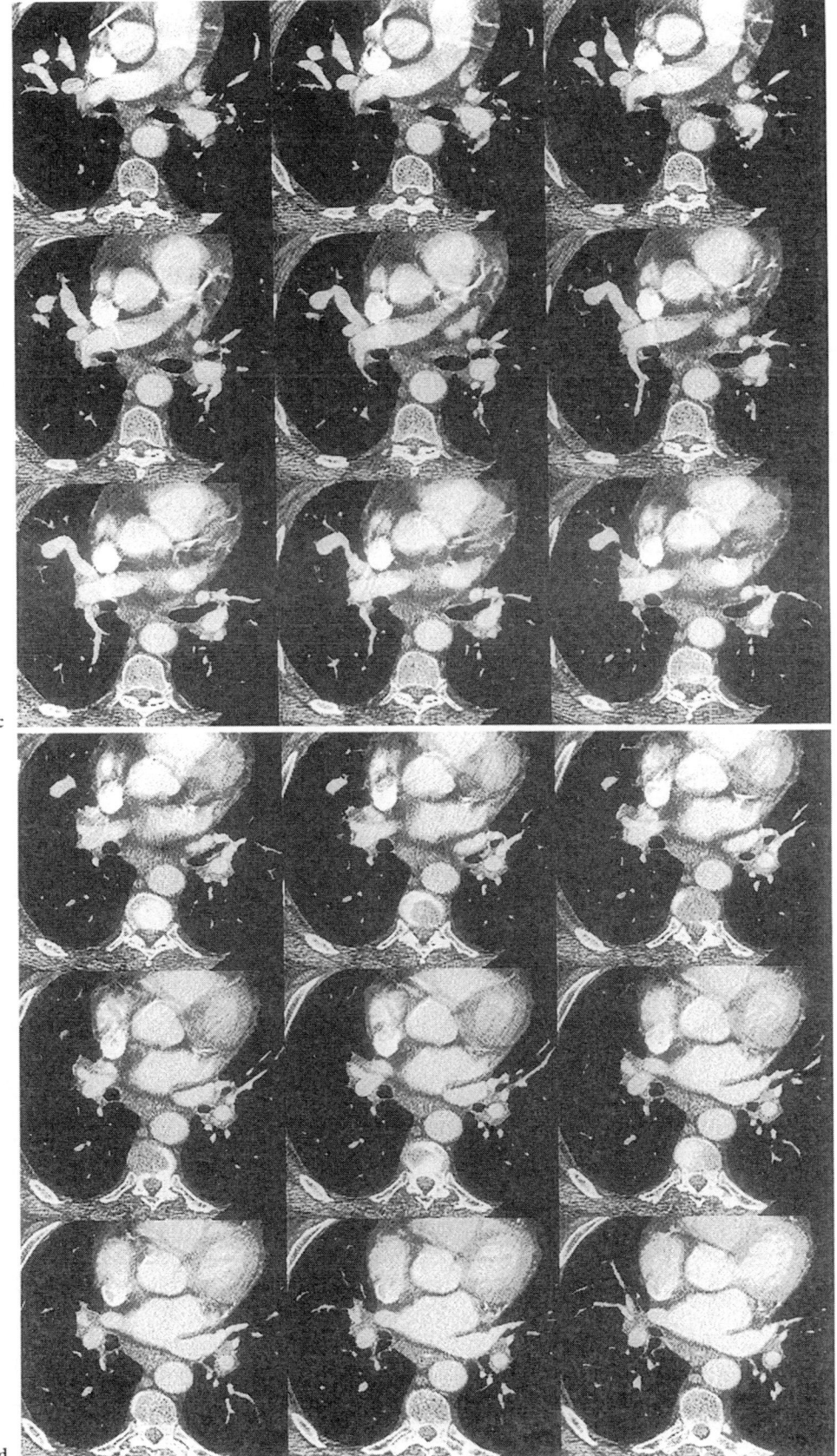

Fig. 4.20c,d

Fig. 4.20e

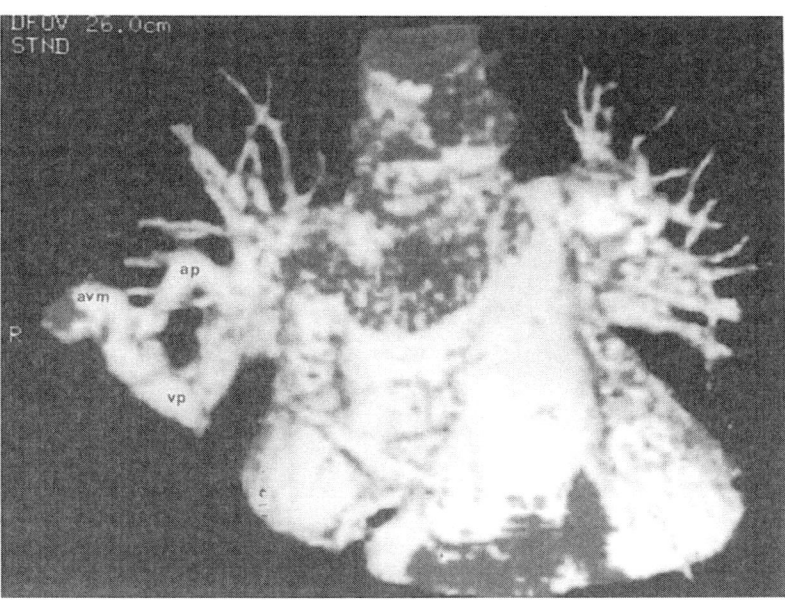

and Camputaro 1993; Kellmann et al. 1988; Godwin and Chen 1986). The superior pulmonary vein, anterior to the left main bronchus, is always missing and the coronary venous sinus has a normal size (Dillon and Camputaro 1993).

Duplication of the superior vena cava (Fig. 4.22), an abnormality easily identified by contrast-enhanced helical CT, includes the following features: (a) the right and left jugular and subclavian veins drain into the right and left superior vena cava, respectively; (b) as with left PAPVR, the left superior vena cava courses vertically along the lateral aspect of the aortic arch. The left innominate vein is, however, frequently missing or has a reduced diameter.

More caudally, the left superior vena cava passes posteriorly to the left superior pulmonary vein and anteriorly to the left main bronchus. Inferiorly, the left superior vena cava circumscribes the left atrium, acquires a horizontal course, and drains into an enlarged coronary venous sinus (Dillon and Camputaro 1993; Kellmann et al. 1988). As each subclavian vein drains into the homolateral vena cava, the injection is preferably achieved simultaneously in both antecubital veins.

If the evaluation of right PAPVR can be achieved by helical CT without enhancement (Table 4.4), left PAPVR and duplication of the superior vena cava are preferably examined with contrast-enhanced helical CT acquisitions (Table 4.5), which allow 3D reconstruction for a better comprehension of the abnor-malities (Falaschi et al. 1992; Rémy et al. 1994; Zwetsch et al. 1995).

4.20.4 Protocol for Helical CT Imaging of Pulmonary Embolism

Helical CT has been demonstrated to be of value for the identification of pulmonary embolisms within the lumen of the pulmonary trunk and segmental arteries, with an accuracy of 98% when compared to pulmonary angiography (Rémy-Jardin et al. 1992; Tardivon et al. 1993; Petasnick 1991). The relative performances of helical CT and ventilation-perfusion scans have not yet been established.

Patients with suspected pulmonary embolism undergo helical CT examination with the arms positioned above the head. A front scout view allows determination of the upper and lower limits of the region of interest, which correspond to the upper aspect of the aortic arch and the upper third of the right border of the right atrium, respectively. The acquisition is preferably obtained in the full end-inspiratory position, sometimes with oxygen assistance. Patients with dyspnea and tachypnea are examined with superficial breathing. Nonionic contrast medium must be used in these unstable patients, at a concentration of 150 mg iodine/ml (Table 4.6). A flow rate of 5 ml/s delivers 750 mg iodine/s and affords excellent pulmonary artery enhancement with only

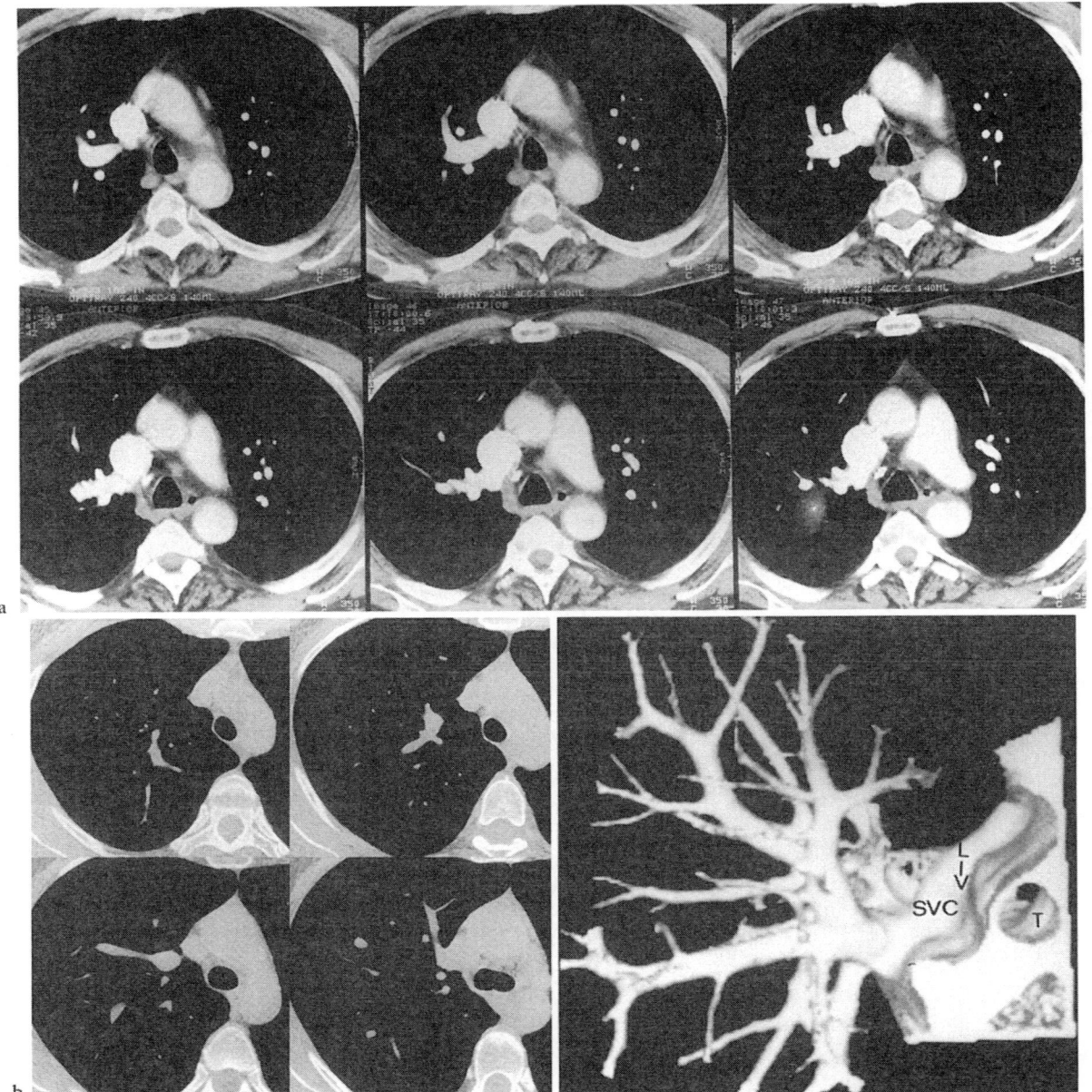

Fig. 4.21. a Right upper lobe PAPVR displayed by enhanced helical CT examination. The PAPVR drains into the posterior aspect of the superior vena cava, at the same level as the azygos vein. Injection parameters: 140 ml; concentration 240 mg iodine/ml; flow rate 4 ml/s; scan delay 10 s (courtesy of Dr J. Rémy, Lille, France). **b** A similar PAPVR of the right lung, adequately displayed by nonenhanced helical CT. In this patient, the malformation drains into the lateral aspect of the superior vena cava. **c** 3D surface reconstruction obtained from nonenhanced helical CT acquisition, showing the PAPVR draining into the superior vena cava (*SVC*). *LIV*, Left innominate vein; *T*, trachea

---

→

Fig. 4.22a,b. Helical CT scanning of a duplicated superior vena cava (SVC). Although the injection was performed in the left antecubital vein only, both left and right innominate veins are adequately enhanced due to a scan delay of 20 s. The right innominate vein courses posteriorly to an enlarged right lobe of the thyroid gland and laterally to the innominate artery. More caudally, it appears as a normal right-sided SVC. Some contrast reflux can be observed in the azygos arch. The left innominate vein does not course anteriorly to the innominate artery. As it courses vertically along the lateral aspect of the left subclavian artery and aortic arch, it becomes the left SVC (*arrows*). At this level, the superior left thoracic vein (*arrowheads*) drains into the left-sided vena cava, which more caudally lies anterior to the left pulmonary artery and medial to the left superior pulmonary vein (*lspv*). More distally, the left SVC courses anteriorly to the left inferior pulmonary vein, and runs along the left posterolateral aspect of the left atrium before entering an enlarged venous coronary sinus (*curved arrows*)

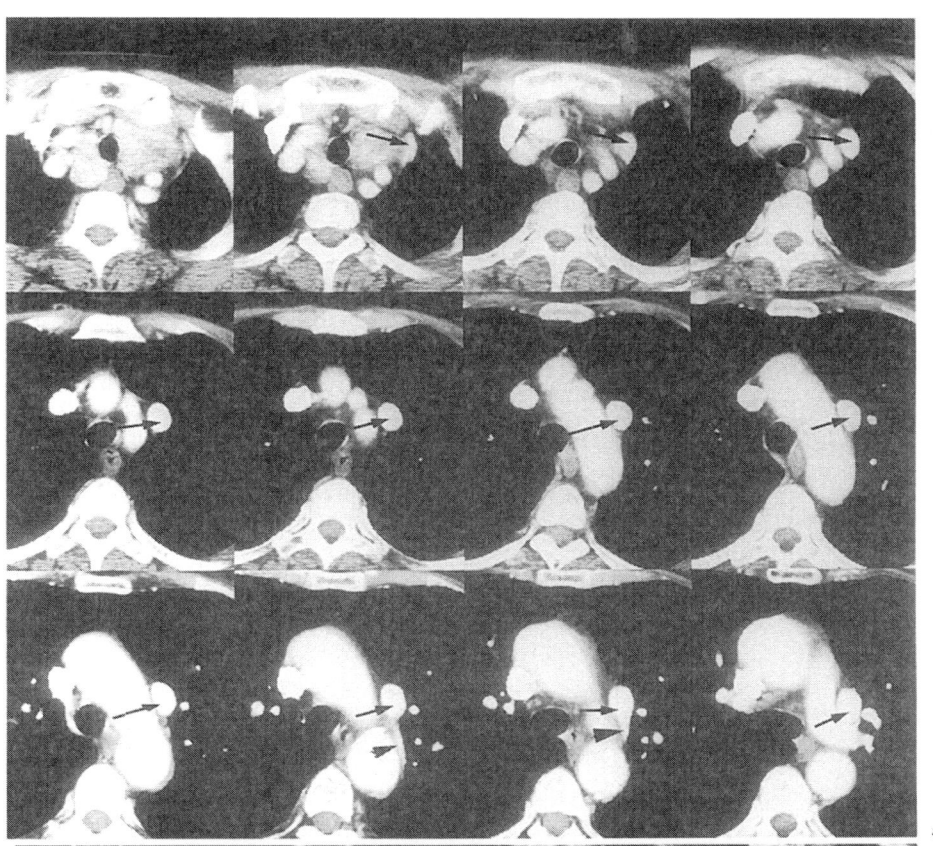

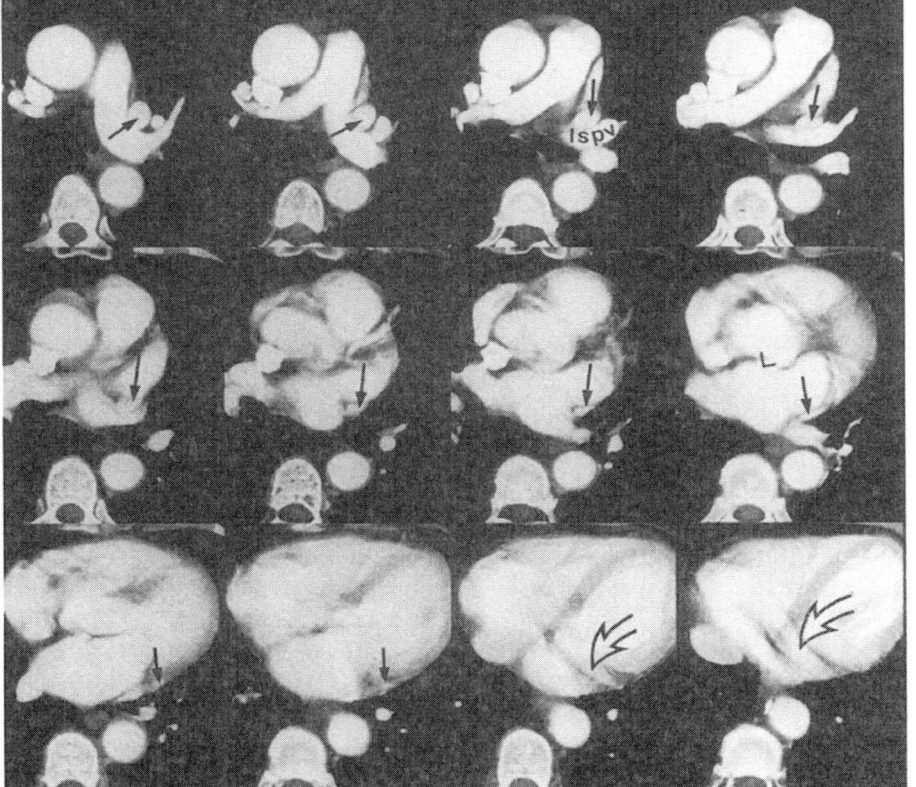

a

b

Table 4.5. Protocol for helical CT injection of left PAPVR and duplication of the superior vena cava (DSVC)

	Left PAPVR	DSVC
Patient position	Arms above the head	Arms above the head
Respiratory position	Full end-inspiratory position	Full end-inspiratory position
Nonenhanced survey	Yes	Yes
B/P/R	5/1/3	7/1.5/5
X-ray tube	125 kV, 140–200 mA	125 kV, 140–200 mA
FOV	Both lungs	Both lungs
Algorithm	Standard + high frequency	Standard
Injection site	Antecubital vein, bilaterally	Antecubital vein, bilaterally
Contrast concentration	150 mg iodine/ml	150 mg iodine/ml
Contrast volume	100–140 ml, max. 200	100–140 ml, max. 200
Contrast flow rate	5 ml/s	3 ml/s
Scan delay	7 s	5 s
Image display	350/50 and 1600/−600	350/50
Acquisition direction	Craniocaudal	Craniocaudal

B/P/R: X-ray beam collimation/pitch value/reconstruction interval

Table 4.6. Protocol for helical CT imaging of pulmonary embolism

Patient position	Arms above head
Respiratory position	Full end-inspiratory position. If not possible, quiet superficial breathing with oxygen assistance
B/P/R	5/1/3
X-ray tube	125 kV, 200 mA
FOV	Chest size (30–33 cm)
Algorithm	Standard
Injection site	Antecubital vein, or central catheter
Contrast concentration	150 mg iodine/ml, nonionic
Contrast volume	120–130 ml
Contrast flow rate	5 ml/s
Scan delay	10 s
Image display	350/50 and 1600/−600
Acquisition direction	Craniocaudal

B/P/R: X-ray beam collimation/pitch value/reconstruction interval

limited streak artifacts arising from the superior vena cava (Fig. 4.23). In this respect, one has to pay attention to the patient's apnea, which must be maintained for about 20 s without the Valsalva maneuver. X-ray beam collimation of 5 mm, a pitch value of 1, image reconstruction intervals of 3 mm, a standard algorithm, and a scan delay of 10 s yield optimal images. All images must be displayed with narrow and wide window settings (350/50 and 1600/−600) in order to clearly differentiate segmental arteries, running parallel to the corresponding bronchi, from veins, which may not be enhanced at the time of acquisition and thus may mimic an artery obstructed by an embolism (RÉMY-JARDIN et al. 1992).

4.20.5 Protocol for Helical CT Imaging of Obstruction of Innominate Veins and Superior Vena Cava Syndrome

Most innominate vein obstruction result from thrombosis induced by positioning of catheters. Superior vena cava (SVC) obstructions or compressions result mainly from direct invasion by primary lung cancers, mediastinal metastatic lymphadenopathy, or lymphoma.

Helical CT examination is preferably achieved using a bilateral injection of the arms, which are positioned along the body. The region of interest is determined by a scout view and must include both thoracic inlets. The examination can be achieved in the full end-inspiratory position, but this is rarely achievable by patients with a SVC syndrome and the acquisition has to be done with oxygen assistance during quiet breathing. A Valsalva maneuver must be avoided as it would narrow the lumen of the intrathoracic collateral veins. A large field of view allows the identification of subcutaneous, retrosternal, paravertebral, juxtadiaphragmatic, phrenic (Fig. 4.24), and mediastinal (Fig. 4.26) collateral veins (CHASEN 1994; TRIGAUX and VAN BEERS 1990). Nonionic contrast medium should be preferred to an ionic contrast medium, and should be administered at a concentration of 150 mg iodine/ml and a flow rate of 4 ml/s when bilaterally injected (Table 4.7). A scan delay of 5 s is sufficient for the acquisition, which is performed in the craniocaudal direction. Parameters such as 5/1.5/5 afford good-quality CT sections. A reduced image reconstruction interval of 2.5 or 3 mm is more suitable if a 3D reconstruction of

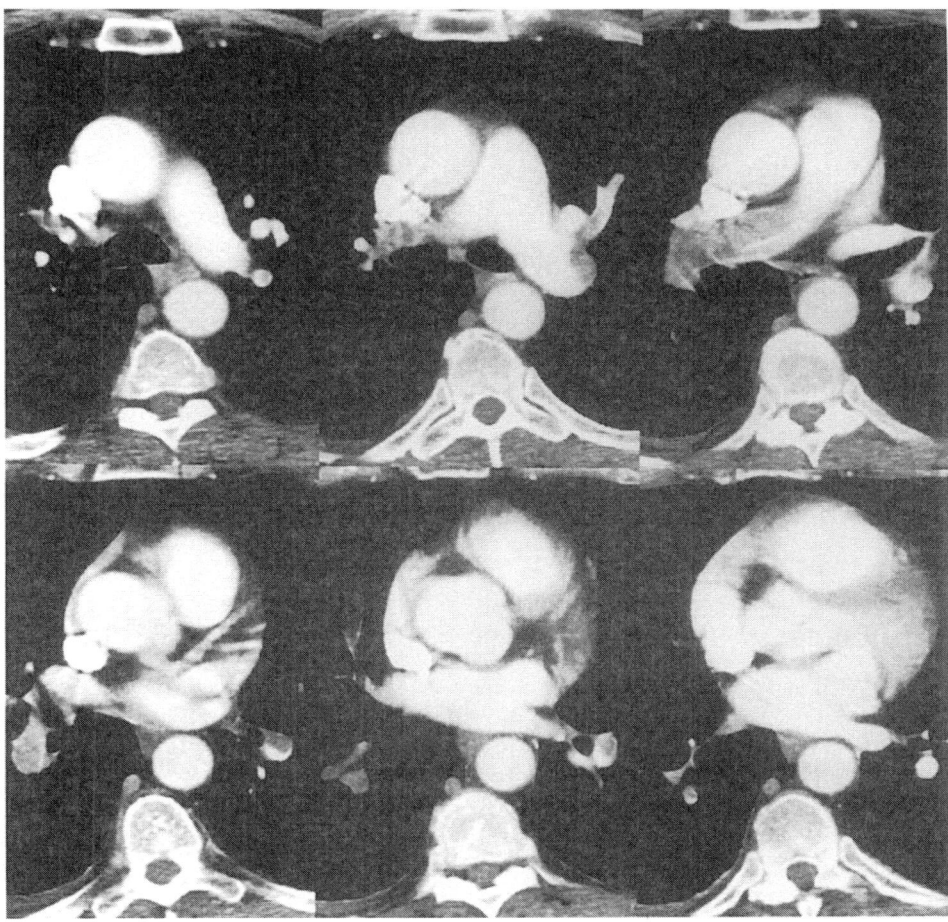

Fig. 4.23. Helical CT acquisition demonstrating bilateral central and segmental pulmonary embolisms. The examination was obtained with a contrast concentration of 150 mg iodine/ml, a flow rate of 5 ml/s, and a scan delay of 10 s

Table 4.7 Protocol for helical CT imaging of obstruction of innominate veins and SVC syndrome

Patient position	Arms down
Respiratory position	Full end-inspiratory position. If not possible, quiet superficial breathing with oxygen assistance
Nonenhanced survey	Not required
B/P/R	5/1/3–5 or 5/1/2.5–3 for 3D
X-ray tube	125 kV, 250 mA
FOV	Chest size including axillary veins
Algorithm	Standard
Injection site	Bilaterally, antecubital veins
Contrast concentration	150 mg iodine/ml
Contrast volume	120–140 ml, max. 200 ml
Contrast flow rate	4 ml/s
Scan delay	5 s
Image display	350/50
Acquisition direction	Craniocaudal

B/P/R: X-ray beam collimation/pitch value/reconstruction interval

the compressed or invaded superior vena cava is required.

4.20.6 Protocol for Helical CT Imaging of Aortic Dissection

Type A and B aortic dissections (Fig. 4.25) occur in arteriosclerotic patients and frequently mimic symptoms of a heart infarct. CT examination of these patients may require the acquisition of nonenhanced sections in order to detect displaced aortic calcifications and to determine the position of the aortic arch vessels, the origin of which must be included in the helical enhanced CT acquisition. The distal end of the acquisition has to include the entire thoracic and abdominal aorta down to the iliac vessels.

The patient is examined with the arms above the head. The injection is performed with nonionic con-

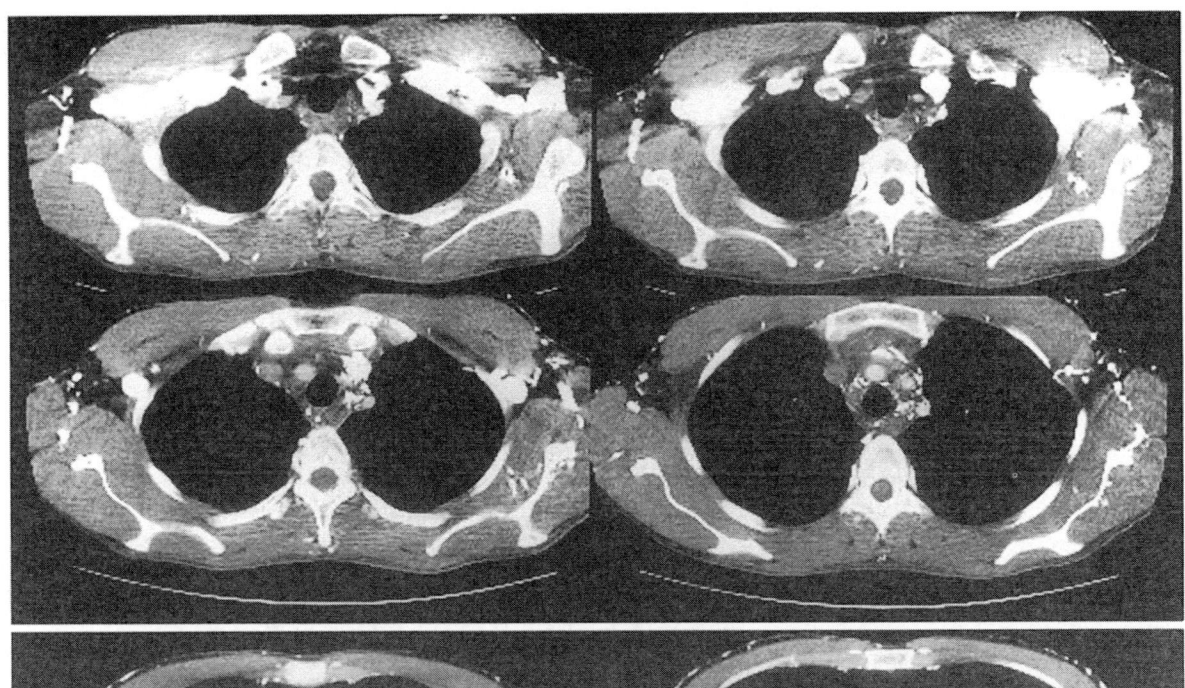

a

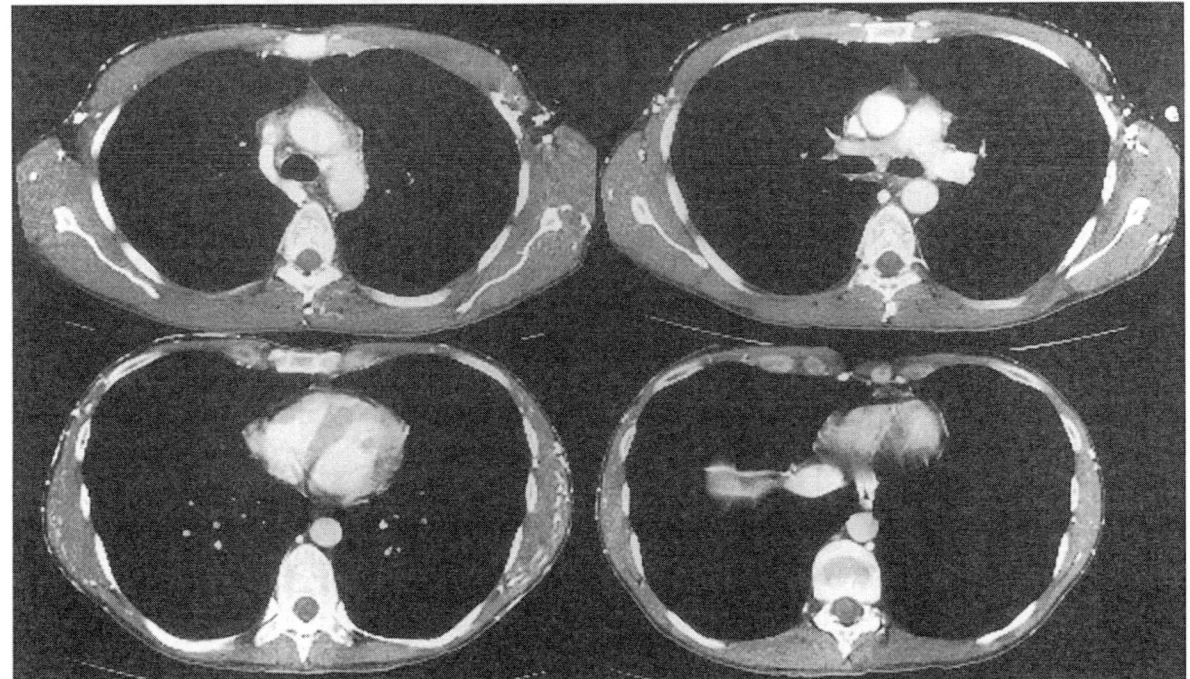

b

Fig. 4.24a, b. Thirty-year-old female with a superior vena cava syndrome, induced by an infusion port positioned in the lumen of the proximal end of the superior vena cava for treatment of high-grade lymphoma. **a** Helical CT acquisition following bilateral antecubital injection of contrast medium demonstrates the thrombosed right innominate vein and up-per segment of the superior vena cava and numerous collaterals of the chest wall and mediastinum. **b** The azygos vein is opacified in the retrograde direction. A right diaphragmatic vein is coursing towards the inferior vena cava. Injection parameters: contrast volume, 150 ml; concentration, 150 mg iodine/ml; flow rate, 4 ml/s. Technical parameters: B/P/R: 5.1.3

→

Fig. 4.25a,b. Helical CT in a 58-year-old male, demonstrating a 7.5-cm aneurysm of the ascending aorta, associated with a type A dissection arising from the posterior wall of the mid ascending aorta (*open arrows*) and extending to the aortic arch and to the three aortic arch vessels (*arrowheads*). The root of the ascending aorta is so dilated that it induces a clinically silent marked compression of the superior vena cava (*curved arrows*). This narrowing is responsible for the important re-flux of contrast in the azygos vein, which can be followed down to the level of the left ventricle. Injection parameters: 140 ml nonionic contrast medium; concentration, 150 mg iodine/ml; flow rate, 4 ml/s. Technical parameters: B/P/R: 7/1.5/5

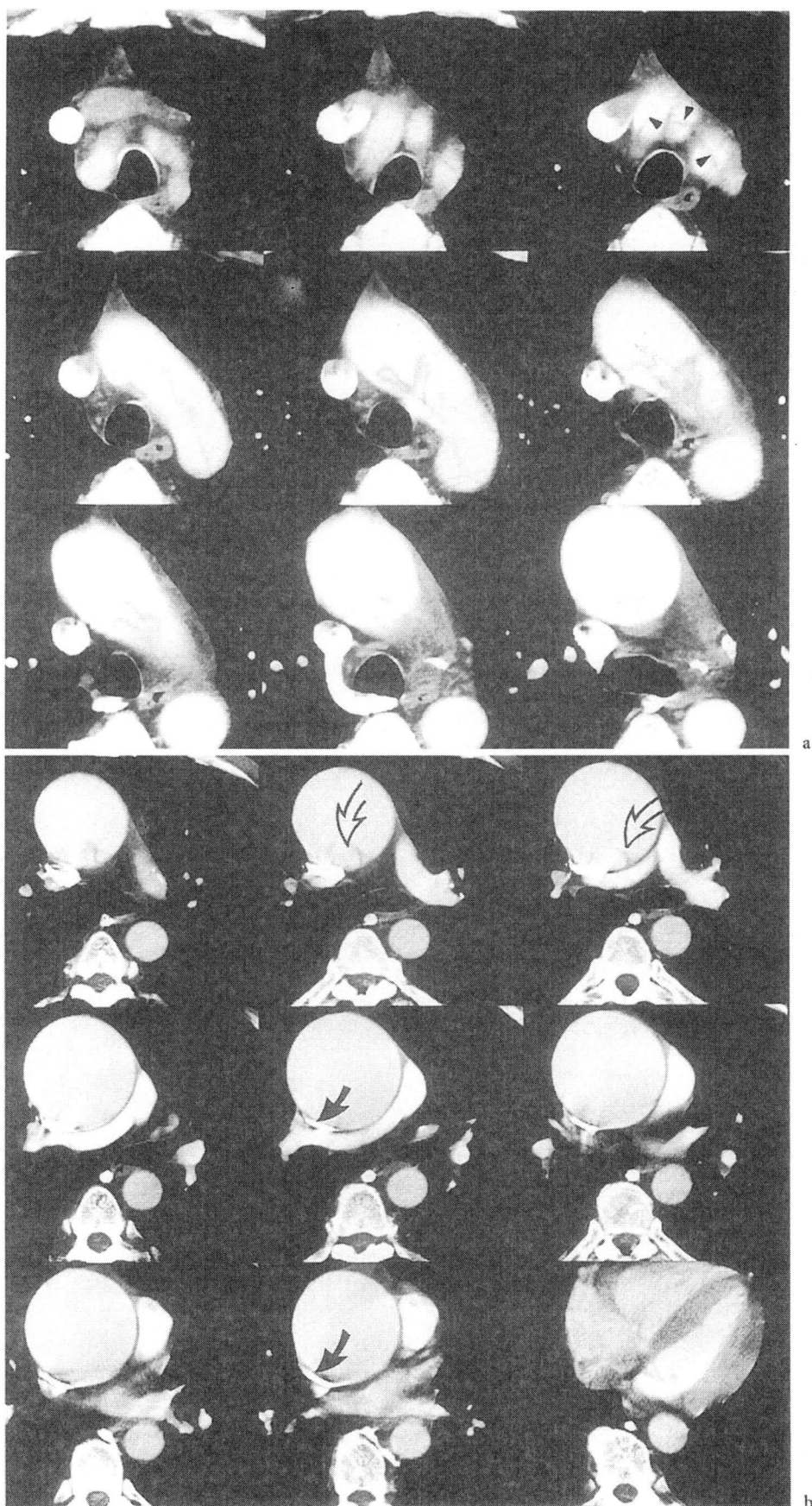

trast medium, with a 150 mg iodine/ml concentration and a flow rate of 4 ml/s. Type A and B dissections require 200 ml of contrast medium in order to maintain a high concentration level in the abdominal aorta.

The SmartPrep program is ideal for obtaining a highly enhanced true lumen. When this program is not available, a scan delay of 12 s affords excellent opacification of the aorta and aortic arch vessels. The remarkable length of the aorta in the z-axis favors an x-ray beam collimation of 7 mm, a pitch of 1.5, and image reconstruction intervals of 5 mm for the thoracic aorta. Below the diaphragm, the second helical acquisition can be obtained with a 10-mm x-ray beam collimation, a pitch of 2, and reconstruction intervals of 10 mm (Table 4.8). This acquisition has to include the origin of both iliac arteries.

The full end-inspiratory position cannot be sustained for such a long acquisition. Examinations of quality can be easily obtained during superficial quiet breathing, occasionally with oxygen assistance.

Surface rendering or MIP 3D reconstructions of type A or B aortic dissections do not facilitate the diagnosis. Multiplanar 2D reconstructions can display the dissecting membrane and both true and false aortic lumina. However, axial sections alone depict more precisely the origin and the extent of the dissection. The diagnosis of dissection no longer requires angiography (PESTANICK 1991; NIENABER et al. 1993), an exception being symptomatic dissections extending into the lumen of the aortic arch vessels. Transesophageal echocardiography (LAISSY et al. 1995) and magnetic resonance imaging are

recognized equivalent optional diagnostic modalities (NIENABER et al. 1993; CIGARROA et al. 1993; SOMMER et al. 1993; NAIDICH 1994).

Pseudo images of dissections occur in about 30% of patients examined by helical CT, at the root of the ascending aorta (STANFORD 1992; MUKHERJI et al. 1992; POSNIAK et al. 1993). They can fool radiologists inexperienced in helical CT. These so-called ring artifacts are related to the acquisition time of 1 s or less and to the motion of the aorta, rather than to the geometry of the equipment.

4.20.7 Protocol for Helical CT Imaging of the Chest Trauma Patient

Trauma of the chest includes many conditions, among which fractures of the ribs and spine, tears of the pleura and pericardium, myocardial contusions, and aortic ruptures are the most frequent.

Aortic ruptures occur during high-speed abrupt deceleration. This disastrous condition is associated with an immediate fatality rate of 85% at the site of the accident. A mortality of 1% per hour affects the remaining 15%. Less than 1% of untreated patients are alive 6 months after the trauma (PARMLEY et al. 1958). Conventional supine chest x-rays have been shown inaccurate for screening of patients; rather, patients must undergo aortography, which is the gold standard modality in this condition (MORGAN et al. 1992; RAPTOPOULOS et al. 1992). Large series dealing with incremental CT examinations as a screening modality have shown that patients with an

Table 4.8. Protocol for helical CT imaging of aortic dissection

Patient position	Arms above the head	
Respiratory position	Quiet breathing with oxygen assistance	
Nonenhanced survey	Mandatory	
Injection site	Antecubital vein or central catheter	

	Chest	Abdomen
B/P/R	7/1.5/5	10/2/10
X-ray tube	125 kV, 160 mA	250 mA
FOV	Includes heart, ascending and descending aorta	25 cm
Algorithm	Standard	Same
Contrast concentration	150 mg iodine/ml	Same
Contrast volume	200 ml	No additional contrast
Contrast flow rate	4 ml/s	–
Scan delay	12 s	–
Image display	350/50	350/50
Acquisition direction	Craniocaudal	Same

B/P/R: X-ray beam collimation/pitch value/reconstruction interval

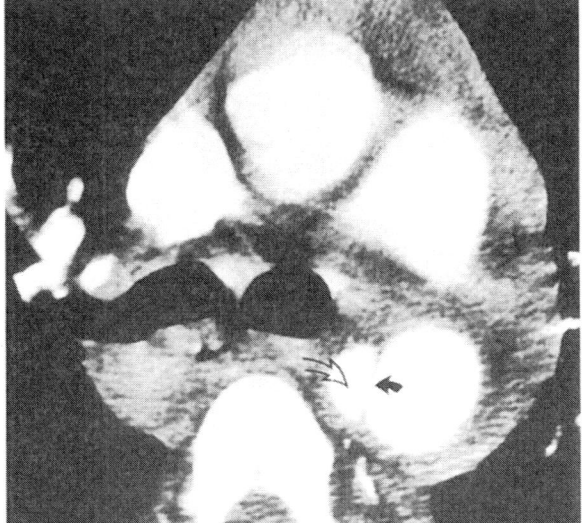

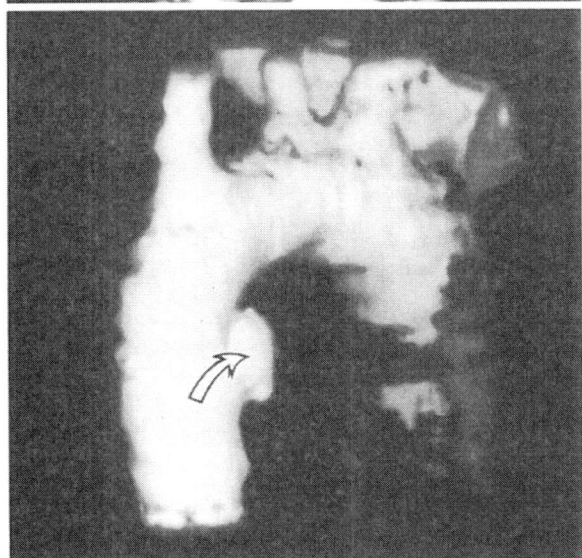

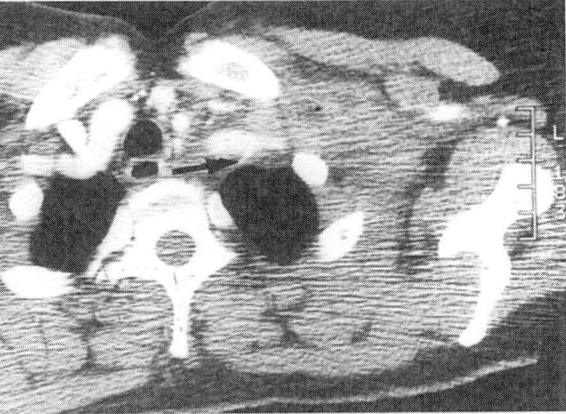

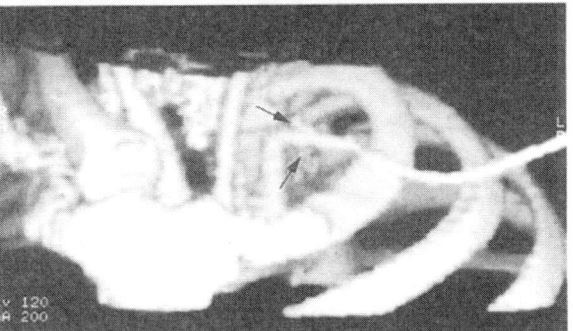

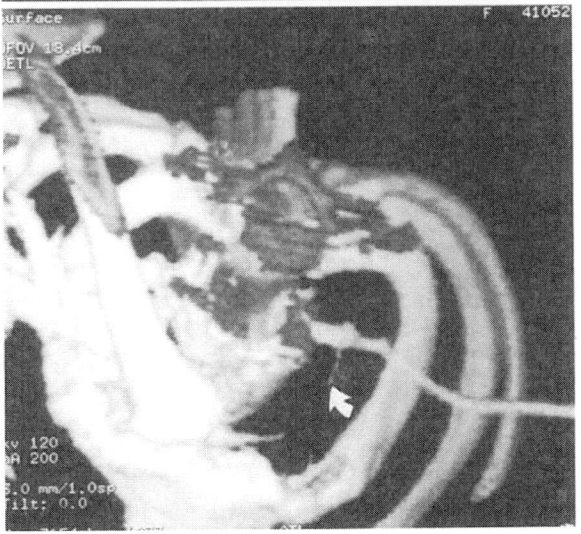

Fig. 4.26a,b. Traumatic aortic rupture in a 45-year-old patient involved in a motor vehicle accident with marked deceleration. **a** The rupture appears as an additional pouch (*open arrow*) of the medial border of the isthmus, associated with an intimal dissection (*arrow*). This section displays an unequivocal hemomediastinum. **b** Posterior oblique view of a 3D reconstruction obtained immediately after the helical CT acquisition, displaying the striking isthmic rupture (*open arrow*). The patient was immediately operated upon on the basis of this sole examination without having had an angiogram. CT findings were confirmed at surgery

Fig. 4.27a–c. Iatrogenic trauma of the left subclavian artery which occurred during an attempt at catheterization of the left subclavian vein in a 48-year-old obese patient. **a** Helical CT scanning performed during injection of the right antecubital vein with 180 ml of 150 mg l/ml contrast medium, at 4 ml/s, with a scan delay of 20 s. The posterior aspect of the horizontal segment of the subclavian artery displays the bleeding point (*arrow*) responsible for a large left subclavian hematoma. **b** Front and **c** craniocaudal oblique views of a 3D surface reconstruction showing a posterior and an anterior leak of contrast (*arrows*). Later, this was barely identifiable on axial sections

unequivocally blood-free mediastinum have only a 0.7% likelihood of having an aortic rupture (RAPTOPOULOS et al. 1992; MILLER et al. 1989). CT has also been shown to be a cost-effective means of triage of patients by angiography for the detection of blunt aortic ruptures (HUNINK and BOS 1995).

Table 4.9. Protocol for helical CT imaging of the chest trauma patient

	CT survey	Aortic rupture	Rupture of Aortic arch vessels
Patient position	Arms down	Arms above the head when feasible	Arms above the head when feasible
Respiratory position	Quiet breathing with oxygen assistance, sometimes mechanical ventilation	Same	Same
B/P/R	7/1.5/7	3/1.3/2	3/1.3/2
X-ray tube	125 kV, 200 mA	125 kV, 200–220 mA	125 kV, 200–250 mA
FOV	Entire chest	Includes ascending and descending aorta	Includes both subclavian arteries
Algorithm	Standard	Standard	Standard
Injection site	Antecubital vein or central catheter	Antecubital vein or central catheter	Antecubital vein opposite to trauma or central catheter
Contrast concentration mg iodine/ml	150	150	150
Contrast volume		200 ml	200 ml
Contrast flow rate	3 ml/s	5 ml/s	5 ml/s
Scan delay	15 s	12 s	12 s
Image display	350/50 and 1600/−600	350/50	350/50
Acquisition direction	Craniocaudal	Craniocaudal	Craniocaudal

B/P/R: X-ray beam collimation/pitch value/reconstruction interval

Sixty-six per cent of chest trauma patients have associated severe lesions (DOUGALL et al. 1977) of the head (22%), abdomen (14%), and/or extremities (56%). Therefore enhanced helical CT examinations of the chest and abdomen are frequently obtained as a survey with 10-mm x-ray beam collimation, a pitch of 1.5–2, and image intervals of 10 mm. If a hemomediastinum is displayed by this CT survey, patients must undergo an aortogram. Four cases of aortic rupture displayed by helical CT were recently reported (SCHNYDER et al. 1996) (Fig. 4.26). Examinations are carried out with the patient supine and with the arms above the head when possible, usually during quiet superficial breathing or mechanical assistance. A scout view determines the level of the aortic arch vessels, the origin of which must be included in the acquisition. A 3-mm x-ray beam collimation, a pitch value of 1.3, and image reconstruction intervals of 2 mm afford optimal 3D surface rendering and MIP reconstructions. The examination is achieved at 125 kV and 200–220 mA (Table 4.9). The helical acquisition must include the entire thoracic aorta and the origin of the aortic arch vessels.

For most patients, this examination requires 200 ml of nonionic contrast material at a concentration of 150 mg iodine/ml. The flow rate of the power injector is 5 ml/s. The acquisition has to be achieved in a craniocaudal direction, starting 2 cm above the level of the aortic arch, with a scan delay of 10–12 s. The field of view must encompass the ascending and descending aorta. Images are calculated with a standard algorithm and displayed with a 350/50 window setting. Immediate 3D surface rendering and MIP reconstructions are obtained. Further evaluation is needed to assess the statistical value of this method.

Presently, aortography, using two or three different incidences, remains the modality of choice to rule out an aortic rupture (FISCHER et al. 1994; PAUL 1994). In one of our reported patients (SCHNYDER et al. 1996), the diagnosis of aortic rupture was so obvious on 3D surface rendering and MIP reconstructions that the patient entered the operating room immediately after the helical CT procedure.

Trauma of the aortic arch vessels and subclavian arteries (Fig. 4.27) can also be imaged by means of the helical CT mode (MEIER et al. 1993; STEHLING et al. 1984). Due to the horizontal direction of subclavian arteries, a 3-mm x-ray beam collimation, a pitch value of 1–1.3, and image reconstruction intervals of 1.5 mm must be used for adequate 3D reconstructions (WANG and VANNIER 1994). Injection and x-ray beam parameters and scan delay are identical to those used to rule out an aortic rupture.

4.20.8 Protocol for Helical CT Imaging of Aneurysms of the Thoracic Aorta

Arteriosclerotic aneurysms of the thoracic aorta, whether saccular or spindle-shaped, are associated with a high mortality when their diameter exceeds 5 cm (DINSMORE et al. 1986). They involve, in decreasing frequency, the descending aorta, the aortic arch, and the ascending aorta.

Helical CT scanning of aortic aneurysms represents a minimally invasive modality when compared to aortography. It provides diagnostic information regarding the size of the aneurysm and reveals the presence and extent of a partially calcified or noncalcified thrombus, an associated intimal dissection, a compression of the superior vena cava (Fig. 4.25), or vertebral erosion. Ruptures are usually clinically suspected when the patient is referred for a CT examination. Helical CT is able in most instances to precisely display the site of the rupture, which is frequently related to a hemothorax or hemomediastinum or hemopericardium.

Spindle-shaped aneurysms involving the thoracoabdominal aorta also have an arteriosclerotic origin and are defined as aortic ectasia exceeding 4 cm in diameter, extending above and below the diaphragm. They have been classified into four types (CRAWFORD et al. 1986): type 1 (Fig. 4.28), which involves the descending aorta from the aortic isthmus and the abdominal aorta down to the origin of renal arteries; type 2, which involves the entire thoracic descending and abdominal aorta; type 3, which

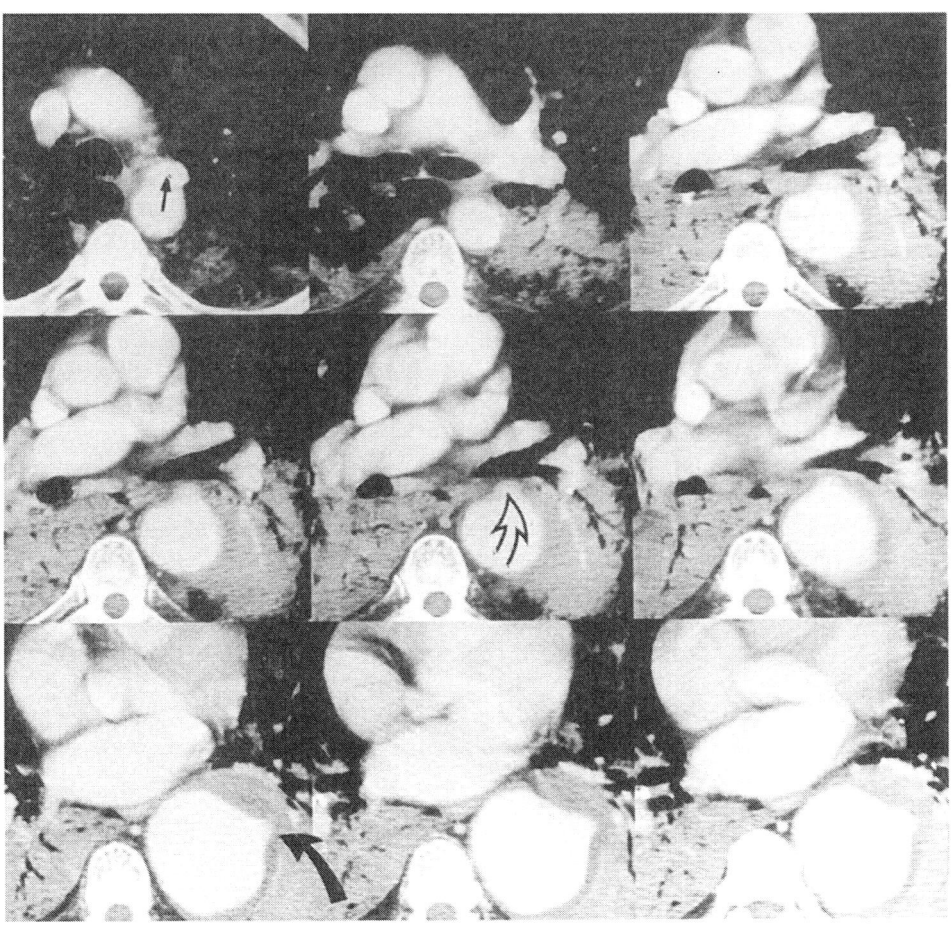

Fig. 4.28. Seventy-three-year-old patient admitted for massive hemoptysis which was shown to arise from the left lung at bronchoscopy. Enhanced spiral CT examination displays a saccular aneurysm at the isthmus (*arrow*) and a type 1 spindle-shaped aneurysm, which presents a double rupture: a superior one (*open arrow*), responsible for the massive hemoptysis, located on the posterior aspect of the left main bronchus, and an inferior one (*curved arrow*), located on the anterolateral aspect of the distal thoracic aorta

Table 4.10. Protocol for helical CT imaging of aneurysms of the thoracic aorta

	Thoraclc aneurysm	Thoracoabdominal aneurysm
Patient position	Arms above head	Same
Respiratory position	Quiet superficial breathing	Same
Nonenhanced survey	Chest	Chest and abdomen
B/P/R	5/1.3/3	7/1.5/3
X-ray tube	125 kV, 200 mA	125 kV, 160 mA (chest), 250 mA (abdomen)
FOV	Chest	Chest and abdomen
Algorithm	Standard	Standard
Injection site	Antecubital vein	Antecubital vein
Contrast concentration	150 mg iodine/ml	150 mg iodine/ml
Contrast volume	120–140 ml	200 ml
Contrast flow rate	4 ml/s	4 ml/s
Scan delay	15 s/test/SmartPrep	15 s/test/SmartPrep
Image display	350/50	350/50
Acquisition direction	Craniocaudal	Craniocaudal

B/P/R: X-ray beam collimation/pitch value/reconstruction interval

involves the distal end of the descending thoracic aorta and the entire abdominal aorta; and type 4, which involves the abdominal and preserves the thoracic aorta.

With respect to the considerable extent of thoracic aneurysms, obtainment of a nonenhanced CT acquisition is recommended, in either the helical or the incremental mode. This chest survey can reasonably be obtained with a 10-cm x-ray beam collimation and a pitch value of 2, with image reconstruction intervals of 10 mm. The contrast-enhanced helical acquisition is obtained with nonionic contrast at a concentration of 150 mg iodine/ml and a flow rate of 4 ml/s (Table 4.10). Scan parameters must be adapted to the length of the aneurysm and an x-ray tube heat evacuation characteristics. Parameters such as 5/1.3/3 are suitable for evaluation of aneurysms with a length exceeding 10 cm. The acquisition can be obtained during quite superficial breathing. The arms of the patient are positioned above the head. The scan direction is preferably craniocaudal and a scan delay of 15 s should suit most examinations. However, the use of an injection test or the SmartPrep program is recommended since patients frequently suffer from associated cardiac insufficiency and present slow-moving blood in their ectatic aortic lumen.

4.21 Conclusion

The use of iodinated contrast material at a concentration of 150 mg/ml, of a power injector, and of the SmartPrep program have greatly contributed to the achievement of very high quality imaging by means of enhanced helical CT examination. The above-described protocols and parameters must, however, be adapted to the patient's condition and the suspected disease. A flow rate of 3 ml/s will be appropriate for most pathological conditions. The flow rate is increased to 4 ml/s when an aortic dissection, aneurysm, or traumatic rupture is suspected and to 5 ml/s when the radiologist is looking for a pulmonary embolism.

In most clinical situations, the patient's arms are positioned above the head. Optimal conditions require apnea in the full-end-inspiratory position, without a Valsalva maneuver. However, helical CT acquisitions obtained during quite superficial breathing afford excellent 2D and 3D reconstructions as well. Finally, scan parameters must be adapted to the patient, to the region of the interest and to the x-ray tube characteristics.

References

Almen T, Aspelin P, Lewin B (1990) Effect of ionic and nonionic contrast medium on aortic and pulmonary arterial pressure: an angiocardiographic study in rabbits. Invest Radiol 25:437–443

Ball WS, Wicks JD, Mettler FA Jr (1980) Prone-supine change in organ position: CT demonstration. AJR 135:185–189

Blum A, Regent D (1995) Scanner hélicoïdal – Principes et modalités pratiques d'utilisation. Masson, Paris, pp 72–85

Bock J, Heilbron DC, Hoeft A et al. (1988) No pulmonary edema or congestion after central venous injection of conventional and newer contrast media in dogs. Invest Radiol 23:836–841

Bock J, Barker BC, Federle MP, Lewis FR (1990) Iodinated contrast media effects on cardiovascular lung water, central blood volume, and cardiac output in humans. Invest Radiol 25:938–941

Carlson JE, Heldlund LJ, Trenkner SW, Ritenour R, Halvorsen RA (1992) Safety considerations in the power injection of contrast media via central venous catheters during computed tomographic examinations. Invest Radiol 27:337–340

Caro JJ, Trinidade E, McGregor M (1992) The cost-effectiveness of replacing high-osmolality with low-osmolality contrast media. AJR 159:869–874

Chasen MH (1994) Arteries and veins of the thorax: anatomy, pathology and imaging – thoracic venous anatomy. Radiology 193(Suppl):57

Cigarroa JE, Isselbacher EM, Dessanctis W, Eagle KA (1993) Medical progress. Diagnostic imaging of suspected aortic dissection: old standards and new directions. AJR 161:485–493

Cohan RH, Dunninck NR, Leder RA, Baker ME (1990) Extravasation of nonionic radiologic contrast media: efficacy of conservative treatment. Radiology 176:65–67

Costello P (1994a) Spiral CT of the thorax. Semin Ultrasound CT MR 15:90–106

Costello P (1994b) Thoracic helical CT. Radiographics 14:913–918

Costello P, Onik G, Cosman E (1987) Computed tomographic-guided stereotaxic biopsy of thoracic lesions. J Thorac Imaging 2:27–32

Costello P, Dupuy DE, Ecker CP, Tello R (1992) Spiral CT of the thorax with reduced volume of contrast material: a comparative study. Radiology 183:663–666

Crawford ES, Crawford JL, Safi HJ et al. (1986) Thoracoabdominal aortic aneurysms: preoperative and intraoperative factors determining immediate and long-term results of operations in 605 patients. J Vasc Surg 3:389–404

Dean P, Kivisaari L, Kormano M (1988) Does dilution of contrast media affect contrast enhancement? An experimental study in rats. Invest Radiol 23(Suppl):S118–S121

Dillon EH, Camputaro C (1993) Partial anomalous pulmonary venous drainage of the left upper lobe vs duplication of the superior vena cava: distinction based on CT findings. AJR 160:375–379

Dillon EH, van Leeuwen MS, Fernandez MA et al. (1993) Spiral CT angiography: pictorial essay. AJR 160:1273–1278

Dinsmore E, Liberthson R, Wismer L et al. (1986) Magnetic resonance imaging of thoracic aortic aneurysms: comparison with other imaging methods. AJR 146:309–314

Dougall AM, Paul ME, Finley RJ, Holliday RL, Coles JC, Duff JH (1977) Chest trauma – current morbidity and mortality. J Trauma 17:547–553

Dresser L, McKinney W (1987) Anatomic and pathophysiologic studies of the human internal jugular valva. Am J Surg 154:220–224

Elam EA, Dorr RT, Lagel KE, Pond GD (1991) Cutaneous ulceration due to contrast extravasation. Experimental assessment of injury and potential antidotes. Invest Radiol 26:13–16

Falaschi F, Palla A, Formichi B et al. (1992) CT evaluation of chronic thromboembolic pulmonary hypertension. J Comput Assist Tomogr 16:897–903

Fenn WO, Otis AB, Rahn H, Chadwick LE, Hegnauer AH (1947) Displacement of blood from the lungs by pressure breathing. Am J Physiol 151:258–269

Fischer HW, Spataro RF (1988) Use of low-osmolality contrast media in patients with previous reactions. Invest Radiol 23(Suppl):S186–S188

Fischer J, Vaghaiwalla F, Tsitlik J, Levin H, Brinker J (1982) Determinants and clinical significance of jugular venous competence. Circulation 65:188–196

Fisher RG, Chasen MH, Lamki N (1994) Diagnosis of injuries of the aorta and brachiocephalic arteries called by blunt chest trauma: CT vs aortography. AJR 162:1047–1052

Friedman WF (1992) Partial anomalous pulmonary venous connection. In: Brownwald E (ed) Heart disease: a textbook of cardiovascular medicine. Saunders, Philadelphia, p 951

Glazer GM, Orringer MB, Gross BH, Quint LF (1984) The mediastinum in non-small cell lung cancer: CT surgical correlation. AJR 142:1101–1105

Glazer HS, Ducan-Meyer J, Aronberg DJ, Moran JF, Levitt RG, Sagel SS (1985) Pleural and chest wall invasion in bronchogenic carcinoma. CT evaluation. Radiology 157:191–194

Glazer HS, Kaiser LR, Anderson DJ, Molina PL, Emami B, Roger CL, Sagel SS (1989) Indeterminate mediastinal invasion in bronchogenic carcinoma: CT evaluation. Radiology 173:37–42

Godwin JD, Chen JTT (1986) Thoracic venous anatomy. AJR 147:674–684

Grainger RG (1992) Optimum utilisation of intravascular radiological contrast media. Eur Radiol 2:121–123

Grenier P, Dubray B, Carette MF, Frija G, Musset D, Chastang C (1989) Preoperative thoracic staging of lung cancer: CT and MR evaluation. Diagn Intervent Radiol 1:23–28

Hagege A (1994) Influence des teneurs en sodium et en iode des produits de contraste iodés sur la fonction myocardique: étude sur coeur isolé. (Résumés des mémoires de DEA d'imagerie médicale 1993). Rev Im Méd 6:425–434

Heinken JP, Brink JA, Vannier MW (1993) Spiral (helical) CT. Radiology 189:647–656

Hunink MGM, Bos JJ (1995) Triage of patients by angiography for detection of aortic ruptura after blunt chest trauma: cost-effectiveness analysis of using CT. AJR 165:27–36

Kalender W, Seissler W, Klotz E, Vock P (1990) Spiral volumetric CT with single-breath-hold technique, continuous transport, and continuous scanner rotation. Radiology 176:181–183

Katayama H, Tanaka T (1988) Clinical survey of adverse reactions to contrast media. Invest Radiol 23(Suppl):S88–S89

Katayama H, Yamaguchi K, Kozuka T, Takashima T, See ZP, Matsuura K (1990) Adverse reactions to ionic and non ionic contrast media. A report from the Japanese Committee on the safety of contrast media. Radiology 175:621–628

Kellman GM, Alpern MB, Sandler MA, Craig BM (1988) Computed tomography of vena caval anomalies with embryologic correlation. Radiographics 8:533–556

Kurijama K, Tateishi R, Kumatani T et al. (1994) Pleural invasion by peripheral bronchogenic carcinoma: assessment with three-dimensional helical CT. Radiology 191:363–369

Laissy JP, Blanc J, Soyer P et al. (1995) Thoracic aortic dissection: diagnosis with transoesophageal echocardiography versus MR imaging. Radiology 194:331–336

Lasser EC, Berry CC (1989) Nonionic vs ionic contrast media: what do the data tell us? AJR 152:945–946

Lasser EC, Berry CC, Talner LB, Sautin LC, Lang EK, Gerber FH, Stolberg HO (1988) Protective effects of corticosteroids in contrast material anaphylaxis. Invest Radiol 23(Suppl):S93–S94

Levin DC, Gardiner GA, Karasick S et al. (1993) Cost containment in the use of low-osmolar contrast agents: effect of guidelines, monitoring and feedback mechanisms. Radiology 189:753–757

Lloyd DA, Stein JS, Rowe MI (1991) The effects of a hyperosmolar intravenous contrast medium on blood viscosity. Invest Radiol 26:220–223

McAlister WH, Kissane JM (1990) Comparison of soft tissue effects of conventional ionic, low osmolar ionic and nonionic iodine containing contrast material in experimental animals. Pediatr Radiol 20:170–174

McCarthy S, Moss AA (1984) The use of a flow rate injector for contrast-enhanced computed tomography. Radiology 151:800

McCaughan BC, Martinin N, Bains MS, McCormack PM (1985) Chest wall invasion of carcinoma of the lung: therapeutic and prognostic implications. J Thorac Cardiovasc Surg 89:836–841

McClennan BL (1990) Ionic and nonionic iodinated contrast media: evolution and strategies for use. AJR 155:225–233

McLoud TC, Bourgouin PM, Greenberg RV et al. (1992) Bronchogenic carcinoma: analysis of staging in the mediastinum with CT by correlative lymphnode mapping and sampling. Radiology 182:319–323

Meier RA, Marianacci EB, Costello P, Fitzpatrick PJ, Hartnell GG (1993) 3D image reconstruction of right subclavian artery aneurysms. J Comput Assist Tomogr 17:187–190

Miles SG, Rasmusen JF, Litwiller T, Osik A (1990) Safe use of intravenous power for CT: experience and protocol. Radiology 176:69–70

Miller FB, Richardson JD, Thomas HA, Cryer HM, Whiding SJ (1989) Role of CT in diagnosis of major arterial injury after blunt thoracic trauma. Surgery 106:596–603

Monnier L, Laurent A, Othmane A, Dufaux J, Mills P, Moyse D, Merland JJ (1991) Produits de contraste et microcirculation: étude de l'agrégation de la déformation érythrocytaire. Rev Im Med 3:237–242

Moreau JF, Lesavre P, de Luca H, Hennessen U, Fischer AM, Giwerc M (1988) General toxicity of water-soluble iodinated contrast media. Pathologic concepts. Invest Radiol 23(Suppl):S75–S78

Morgan PW, Goodman LR, Aprahamian C, Foley WD, Lipchick EO (1992) Evaluation of traumatic aorta injury: does dynamic contrast-enhanced CT play a role? Radiology 182:661–666

Morris TW (1988) The cardiovascular effects of iodinated contrast media injections. Invest Radiol 23:S133–S136

Mukherji SK, Varma P, Stark P (1992) Motion artifact simulating aortic dissection on CT. AJR 159:674

Murata K, Takahashi M, Mori M, Shimoyama K, Mishina A, Fujino S, Itoh H, Morita R (1994) Chest wall and mediastinal invasion by lung cancer: evaluation with multisection expiratory dynamic CT. Radiology 191:251–255

Naidich DP (1994) Helical computed tomography of the thorax. Radiol Clin North Am 32:759–774

Naidich DP, Zerhouni EA, Siegelman SS (1991) Principles and techniques of thoracic CT and MR. In: Naidich DP, Zerhouni EA, Siegelman SS (eds) Computed tomography and magnetic resonance of the thorax, 2nd edn. Raven Press, New York, pp 13–18

Nienaber CA, von Kodolitsch J, Nicolas V et al. (1993) The diagnosis of thoracic aortic dissection by noninvasive imaging procedures. N Engl J Med 328:1–9

Numm JF (1994) Nunn's applied respiratory physiology, 4th edn. Butterworth/Heinemann, Oxford, pp 138–139 and pp 457–459

Olson MA, Becker GJ (1986) The scinitar syndrome: CT findings in partial anomalous pulmonary venous return. Radiology 159:25–26

Onitsuka H, Tsukuda M, Araki A, Murakami J, Torii Y, Masuda K (1991) Differentiation of central lung tumor

from postobstructive lobar collapse by rapid sequence computed tomography. J Thorac Imaging 6:28–31

Parmley LR, Thomas WM, Marion WC, Jahuke EJ (1958) Nonpenetrating traumatic injury of the aorta. Circulation 15:405–410

Pastores SM, Naidich DP, Aranda CP, McGuinnes G, Rom WN (1993) Intrathoracic adenopathy associated with pulmonary tuberculosis in patients with human immunodeficiency virus infection. Chest 103:1433–1437

Patz EF, Lowe VJ, Hoffman JM, Paine SS, Harris L, Goodman PC (1994) Persistant or recurrent bronchogenic carcinoma: detection with PET and 2 (F18)-2-deoxy-D-glucose. Radiology 191:379–382

Paul JL (1994) Techniques d'injection en tomodensitométrie thoracique par balayage spiralé volumique. PhD thesis, University of Lille, France

Pestanick JP (1991) Radiologic evaluation of aortic dissection. Radiology 180:297–305

Posniak H, Olson MC, Demos TC (1993) Aortic motion artifact simulating dissection on CT scans: elimination with reconstructive segmented images. AJR 161:557–558

Powe NR (1992) Low versus high osmolality contrast media for intravenous use: a health care luxury or necessity? Radiology 183:21–22

Powe NR, Moore RD, Steinbeg EP (1993) Adverse reactions to contrast media: factors that determine the cost of treatment. AJR 161:1089–1095

Pugatch RD (1995) Radiologic evaluation in chest malignancies. A review of imaging modalities. Chest 107:294S–297S

Quint LE, Francis IR, Wahl RL, Gross BH, Glazer GM (1995) Preoperative staging of non-small-cell carcinoma of the lung: imaging method. AJR 164:1349–1359

Raptopoulos V, Steinman RG, Philips DA, Davidoff A, Silva WE (1992) Traumatic aortic tear: screening with chest CT. Radiology 182:667–673

Rees CR, Palmaz JC, Garcia O et al. (1988) Hemodynamic effects of the administration of ionic and nonionic contrast materials into the pulmonary arteries of a canine model of acute pulmonary hypertension. Invest Radiol 23:184–189

Reiser UJ (1984) Study of bolus geometry after intravenous contrast medium injection: dynamic and quantitative measurements (chronogram) using an X-ray CT device. J Comput Assist Tomogr 8:251–262

Rémy J, Rémy-Jardin M, Wattine L, Giraud L (1993) Le balayage spiralé volumique en tomodensitométrie thoracique. Feuillets de Radiologie 33:239–256

Rémy J, Rémy-Jardin M, Giraud F, Wattine L (1994) Angioarchitecture of pulmonary arteriovenous malformations: clinical utility of three-dimensional helical CT. Radiology 191:657–664

Rémy-Jardin M, Rémy J, Wattine L, Giraud F (1992) Central pulmonary thromboembolism: diagnosis with spiral volumetric CT with the single-breath-hold technique – comparison with pulmonary angiography. Radiology 185:381–387

Rubin GD, Dake MD, Semba CP (1995) Current status of three-dimensional spiral CT scanning for imaging the visculature. Radiol Clin North Am 33:51–70

Schneider KM, Ham KN, Friedhuber A, Rand MJ (1988) Functional and morphologic effects of ioxilan, iohexol and diatrizoate on endothelial cells. Invest Radiol 23 (Suppl):S147–S149

Schnyder P, Meuli RA, Mayor B, Wicky S (1994) Injection techniques in helical CT of the chest. Annual Meeting of the European Society of Thoracic Imaging. 13–15 June 1994. Paris, France

Schnyder P, Meuli RA, Wicky S, Mayor B (1995) Injection techniques in helical CT of the chest (abstract). Eur Radiol (Suppl) 5:126

Schnyder P, Chapuis L, Mayor B, Meuli R, Wicky S, Lepori D, Essinger A (1996) Helical CT aortography in correlation with angiography and surgery for traumatic aortic rupture, J Thorac Imaging 11; 39–45

Schrott KM, Behrends B, Klauss W, Kaufman J, Lehnert J (1986) Iohexol in der Ausscheidungsurographie: Ergebnisse des Drug-monitoring. Fortschr Med 104:153–156

Seely J, Mayo JR, Miller RR, NL Müller (1993) T1 lung cancer: prevalence of mediastinal nodal metastases and diagnostic accuracy of CT. Radiology 186:129–132

Shepard JAO, Dedrick CG, Spizarni DL, Mcloud TC (1986) Dynamic incremental computed tomography of the pulmonary hila using flow-rate injector. J Comput Assist Tomogr 10:369–371

Shuman WP, Adam JL, Schoenecker SA, Taziolo PR, Moss AA (1986) Use of a power injector during dynamic computed tomography. J Comput Rssist Tomogr 10:1000–1002

Silverman PM, Brown B, Wray H, Fox SH, Cooper C, Roberts S, Zeman PK (1995) Optimal contrast enhancement of the liver using helical (spiral) CT: value of SmartPrep. AJR 164:1169–1171

Sistrom CL, Gay SB, Peffley L (1991) Extravasation of iopamidol and iohexol during contrast-enhanced CT: report of 28 cases. Radiology 180:707–710

Sommer T, Holzknecht N, Smekal J (1993) Thin-section spiral CT in the evaluation of aortic dissection: comparison with MR and transoesophageal echocardiography (abstract). Radiology 189:112

Stanford W (1992) Motion artifact simulating aortic dissection. AJR 158:1048

Stehling MK, Lawrence JA, Weintraub JL, Raptopoulos V (1994) CT angiography: expanded clinical applications. AJR 163:947–955

Storto ML, Ciccotosto C, Patea RL, Spinazzi A, Bonomo L (1994) Spiral CT of the mediastinum: optimization of contrast medium use. Eur J Radiol 18:S83–S87

Sunnegardh O, Hietala SO, Wirell S, Reiz S, Haggmark S (1990) Systemic, pulmonary and renal haemodynamic effects of large intravenous doses of high and low-osmolar contrast media. An investigation in the pig of ratio 1,5 and ratio 3 media. Acta Radiol 33:297–302

Suzuki N, Saitoh T, Kitamura S (1993) Tumor invasion of the chest wall in lung cancer: diagnosis with US. Radiology 187:39–42

Swensen SJ, Brown LR, Colby TV, Weaver AL (1995) Pulmonary nodule: CT evaluation of enhancement with iodinated contrast material. Radiology 194:393–398

Tajima H, Kumazaki T, Ito K et al. (1991) Effects of an iso-osmolar contrast medium on pulmonary arterial pressure at pulmonary angiography. Acta Radiol 32:134–136

Tardivon AA, Musset D, Maitre S, et al. (1993) Role of CT in chronic pulmonary embolism: comparison with pulmonary angiography. J Comput Assist Tomogr 17:345–351

Tello R, Costello P, Ecker C, Hartnell G (1993) Spiral CT evaluation of coronary bypass graft patency. J Cmput Assist Tomogr 17:253–259

Thiesen B, Mützel W (1990) Effects of angiographic contrast media on venous endothelium of rabbits. Invest Radiol 25:21–126

Trigaux JP, van Beers B (1990) Thoracic collateral venous channels: normal and Pathologic CT findings. J Comput Assist Tomogr 14:769–773

Vock P, Soucek M, Daepp M, Kalender W (1990) Lung: spiral volumetric CT with single-breath-hold technique. Radiology 176:864–867

Wang G, Vannier MN (1994) Stair-step artifacts in three-dimensional helical CT: an experimental study. Radiology 191:79–83

Watanabe A, Shimokata K, Saka H, Nomura F, Sakai S (1991) Chest CT combined with artifical pneumothorax: value in determining origin and extent of tumor. AJR 156:707–710

Webb WR, Gatsonis C, Zerhouni EA, Heelan RT, Glazer GM, Francis IR, McNeil BJ (1991) CT and MR imaging in staging non-small cell bronchenic carcinoma: report of the radiologic diagnostic oncology group. Radiology 178:705–713

West JB (1990) Respiratory physiology – the essentials. Willians and Wilkins, pp 35–40

Westcott JL (1988) CT percutaneous transthoracic needle biopsy. Radiology 169:593–601

White RI, Pollak JS (1994) Pulmonary arteriovenous malformations: diagnosis with three-dimensional helical CT – a breakthrough without contrast media. Radiology 191:613–614

Wolf GL, Arenson L, Cross AP (1989) A prospective trial of ionic vs nonionic contrast agents in routine clinical practice: comparison of adverse effects. AJR 152:939–944

Woodring JH, Fried AM (1988) Nonfatal venous air embolism after contrast-enhanced CT. Radiology 167:405–407

Yamashita K, Matsunobe S, Takahashi R et al. (1995) Small peripheral lung carcinoma evaluated with incremental dynamic CT: radiologic-pathologic correlation. Radiology 196:401–408

Yokoi K, Mori K, Miyazawa N, Saito Y, Okuyama A, Sasagawa M (1991) Tumor invasion of the chest wall and mediastinum in lung cancer: evaluation with pneumothorax CT. Radiology 181:147–152

Zwetsch B, Wicky S, Meuli R, Schnyder P (1995) Three-dimensional image reconstruction of partical anomalous pulmonary venous return to the superior vena cava. Chest 108:1743–1745

5 Techniques of Reconstruction

G.D. Rubin

CONTENTS

5.1 Introduction

Compared with conventional CT, spiral CT data offer greater flexibility for image reconstruction and are uniquely suited for multiplanar reformation and three-dimensional rendering. The goal of this chapter is to provide an explanation of spiral CT reconstruction and rendering techniques with an emphasis on practical considerations to maximize image quality and the extraction of diagnostic information.

5.2 Spiral Reconstruction

Once the spiral scanning has been completed, there are four fundamental choices to be made prior to reconstructing transverse sections. Two of these, the section derivation algorithm and the reconstruction

G.D. Rubin, MD, Assistant Professor, Department of Radiology, S 072B, Stanford University Hospital Medical Centre, 300 Pasteur Drive, Stanford, CA 94305-5105, USA

interval, are unique to spiral CT, while the selection of reconstruction kernel and display field of view are similar to conventional CT. All four variables strongly influence the quality of the reconstructed CT section.

5.2.1 Section Derivation

The section derivation algorithm, using either interpolation or extrapolation, determines how the continuous volumetric data are used to create axial sections. If projection data were reconstructed with equal weighting over a 360° segment of the spiral acquisition, as is performed with conventional CT, considerable motion artifacts would result due to the patient's translation through the CT gantry. The section derivation algorithm is a mathematical process that attempts to compensate for these motion effects.

The simplest method termed 360° linear interpolation or "wide" interpolation uses 720° or two full gantry rotations to reconstruct a single axial section (Kalender et al. 1990). 360° linear interpolation uses two projections obtained with the same angle of rotation at table locations z' and $z' + d$, where d denotes the table travel for 360° rotation, to estimate a projection in planar geometry (Napel 1995; Polacin et al. 1992). 360° linear interpolation offers a small advantage relative to conventional CT in that image noise is reduced by approximately 30%; however, there are significant limitations. Most importantly, the section sensitivity profile, which defines the thickness of the reconstructed section, is considerably broadened relative to conventional CT, which results in image blurring (Brink et al. 1992; Wang and Vannier 1994a). The full width at half maximum is broadened approximately 30% as compared to conventional CT while the full width at tenth area is broadened 66% when 5-mm collimation is used. The profile is further degraded when pitch is increased. With a pitch of 2 and 5-mm collimation, the full width at half maximum is broadened 116% while the full width at tenth area is broadened 182% relative to conventional CT (POLACIN et al. 1992). Therefore pitch values greater than 1.0 should never be used with 360° interpolation. Because two full gantry rotations are required to reconstruct a single axial section with 360° linear interpolation, 2 s of spiral data are required, resulting in a 50% diminution in temporal resolution relative to conventional CT. Finally, positions scanned during the first and last rotation of the spiral path cannot be reconstructed with this technique; therefore in order to acquire 30 s of spiral images, a 32-s exposure is required.

An alternative approach introduced by Polacin and colleagues interpolates between projections separated by 180° (POLACIN et al. 1992). This approach, termed 180° linear interpolation or "slim reconstruction," requires [2 × (180° plus fan angle)] or approximately 440° of projection data to reconstruct an axial section. It overcomes several significant limitations of 360° linear interpolation. Most importantly, the section sensitivity profile is degraded considerably less relative to conventional CT. With a pitch of 1 and 5-mm collimation, the full width at half maximum is not measurably broadened and the full width at tenth area is broadened only 18%. At a pitch of 2, the full width at half maximum is broadened 30%, and the full width at tenth area is broadened 68%. This significant improvement in spatial resolution as compared to 360° linear interpolation makes scanning with pitch values up to 2.0 practical. In fact, the use of increased scan pitch is a valuable method for improving the spatial resolution of a scan as the collimator width can be reduced while the same volume of tissue is imaged within the required scan duration (RUBIN and NAPEL 1995).

There is a price for using 180° linear interpolation, however, and that is a 12% increase in noise over conventional CT and a 29% increase in noise over 360° linear interpolation. While it is tempting to consider that 360° linear interpolation might be a useful technique for diminishing image noise, the loss of spatial resolution is unacceptable and alternative methods for diminishing image noise (increased exposure or lower spatial frequency reconstruction kernels) are advised.

CRAWFORD and KING (1990) have described a similar approach to that of Polacin, called "half scan with extrapolation," which is used on some scanners. Although other section derivation techniques have been proposed for spiral CT data, currently these are the most widely applicable approaches. The reader is referred to additional resources for more detailed information on this subject (CRAWFORD and KING 1990; NAPEL 1995).

5.2.2 Reconstruction Kernel

Parallel to spiral interpolation, a reconstruction kernel is employed which determines the in-plane resolution and noise of the CT section (PELC and COLSHER 1987). Higher spatial frequency reconstruction kernels termed "bone" or "high" provide the highest spatial resolution and highest image noise. Within the lung, where contrast differences between air and surrounding pulmonary interstitium and bronchovascular structures are high, high spatial frequency reconstruction kernels facilitate visualization of fine structure without significant interference from the increased noise. Within the mediastinum, where intrinsic contrast differences between mediastinal fat, fluid collections, and soft tissue are less, the increased noise of high spatial frequency reconstruction kernels can limit assessment of the mediastinum, particularly in large patients with scanners that cannot achieve adequate exposure rates. While some users prefer to minimize image noise by reconstructing the images of the mediastinum with a lower spatial frequency reconstruction kernel, images reconstructed with a high spatial frequency kernel are typically diagnostic for evaluating pulmonary parenchyma, mediastinum, and chest wall. Conversely, use of a low spatial frequency reconstruction kernel may limit evaluation of pulmonary parenchymal lesions.

Although the increased noise of a high spatial frequency algorithm typically does not present problems in the interpretation of transverse CT sections, it can degrade the quality of three-dimensional (3-D) renderings considerably. If 3-D rendering is contemplated, then a low spatial frequency reconstruction kernel or "soft reconstruction" is advised to minimize noise (Fig. 5.1). While this diminishes in-plane resolution, the overall voxel dimensions are usually such that the voxel length along the z-axis is considerably greater than its in-plane (x, y) dimensions. Therefore, a small diminution in in-plane resolution does not impact greatly on the 3-D rendering. However, the diminished noise has a significant impact on creating high-quality 3-D images.

5.2.3 Reconstruction Interval

The contiguity of the spiral data enables sections to be reconstructed at arbitrary intervals along the axis of table travel (KALENDER et al. 1990; VOCK et al. 1990). The capability for overlapping sections to be reconstructed has two significant effects on

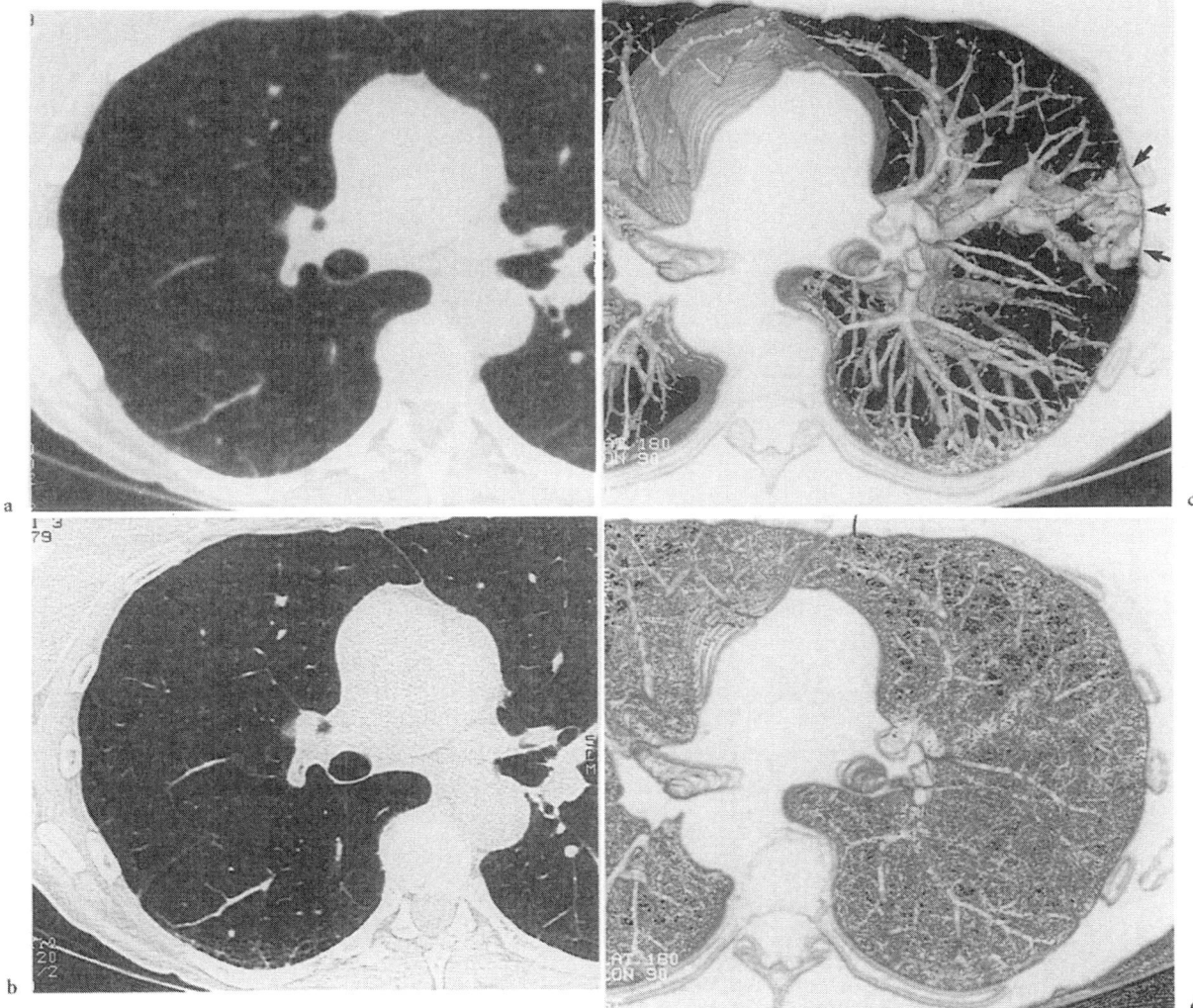

Fig. 5.1. a,b One-millimeter collimation, pitch 2.0 spiral CT section reconstructed with "soft" reconstruction kernel (**a**) and "high" or "bone" reconstruction kernel (**b**). Detail within the pulmonary parenchyma is much more distinctly visualized with the higher resolution kernel; however, noise, best visualized within the mediastinum and chest wall, is greater than with the soft reconstruction kernel. **c** Shaded surface display (SSD) of a 3-cm-thick slab, viewed from above, using the images reconstructed with the soft kernel and a threshold of −600 HU demonstrates a right upper lobe pulmonary arteriovenous malformation (*arrows*). **d** SSD of a 3-cm-thick slab using the images reconstructed with the high kernel and a threshold of −600 HU is dominated by noise within the lung which masks the arteriovenous malformation. **e,f** SSDs viewed from below and created from the images reconstructed with soft (**e**) and high (**f**) kernels with a threshold of −200 HU en-able better separation of the complex arteriovenous malformation from adjacent vasculature. While the lesion is unmasked on the image reconstructed with bone kernel (**f**), the surfaces are highly irregular and many small holes appear within the anatomy due to the higher degree of noise within this image. **g** Maximum intensity projection, viewed from below, created using the images reconstructed with the soft kernel demonstrates the embolic metallic coils within the arterial branches of this complex arteriovenous malformation. **h** Maximum intensity projection created using the images reconstructed with the high kernel. The high degree of image noise and edge enhancement inherent in the bone reconstruction kernel results in a poorer quality maximum intensity projection than with the soft reconstruction kernel and makes visualization of the metallic emboli more difficult

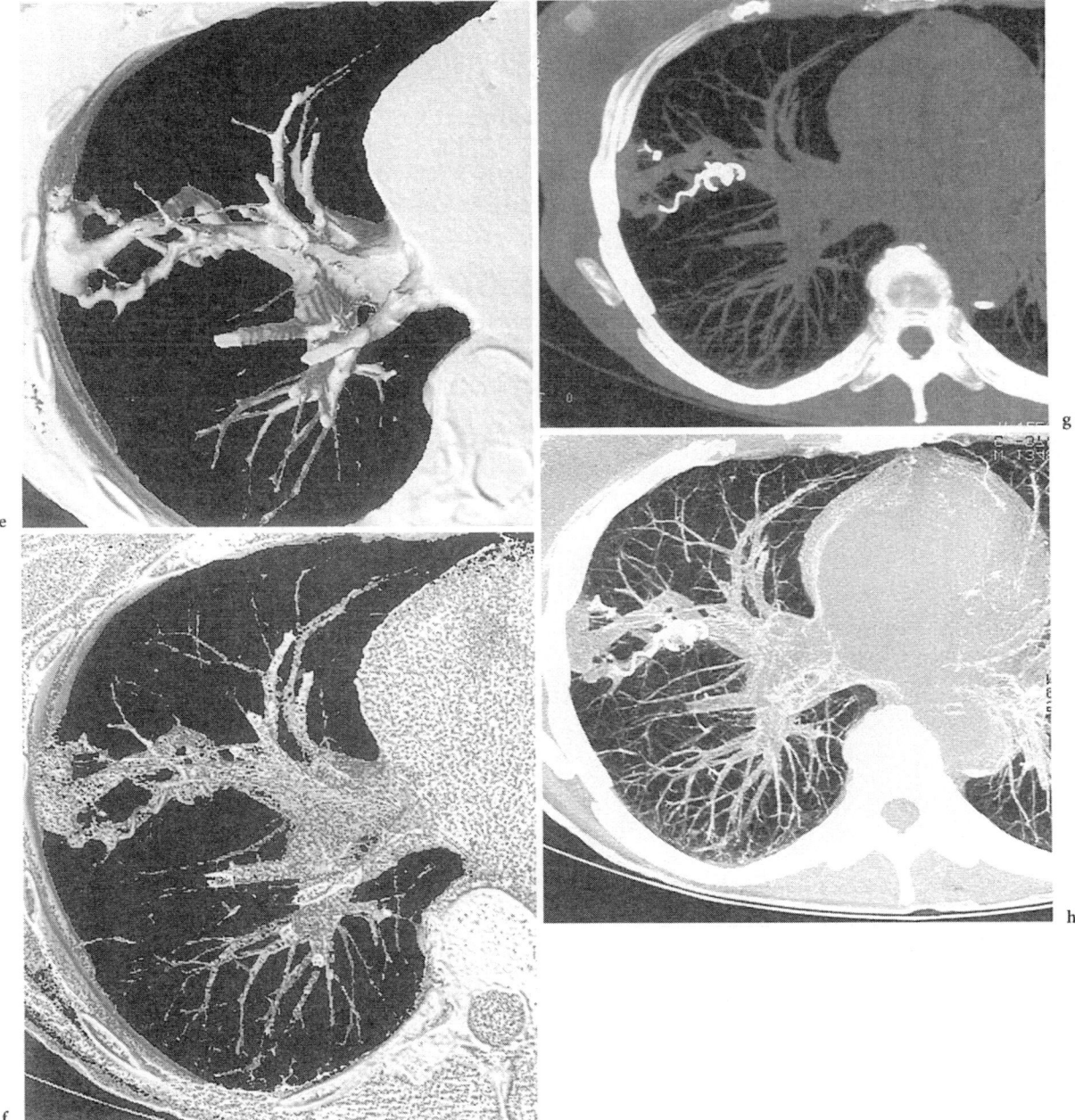

Fig. 5.1e–h

multiplanar reformations and 3-D reconstructions. Firstly, the creation of overlapping sections improves longitudinal resolution (KALENDER et al. 1994) and minimizes volume averaging, which can cause structures, particularly those with edges parallel to the acquisition plane, to have lower attenuation due to averaging with adjacent mediastinal fat or pulmonary gas. Reconstruction with overlapping sections minimizes the probability that small pulmonary nodules or vessels such as intercostal or bronchial arteries will be lost. Further, sections reconstructed with at least 50% overlap increase the likelihood that a pulmonary nodule will be centered within a section and improve densitometry (Fig. 5.2). A recent investigation of the utility of overlapping reconstructions for the detection of pulmonary nodules was performed. Thoracic CT scans obtained with 8-mm collimation were reviewed independently with 8-mm

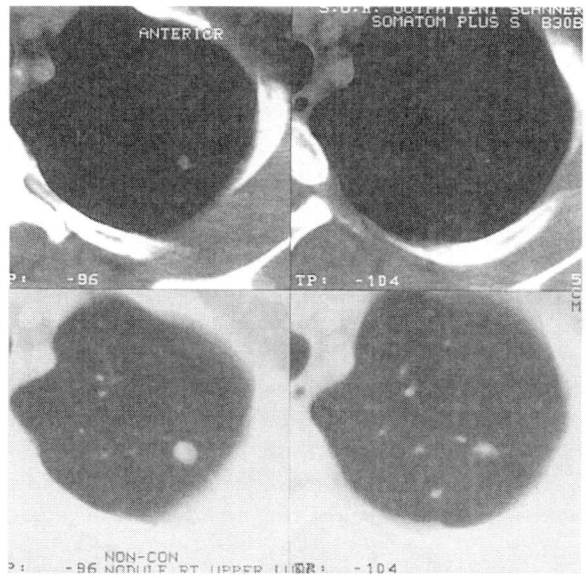

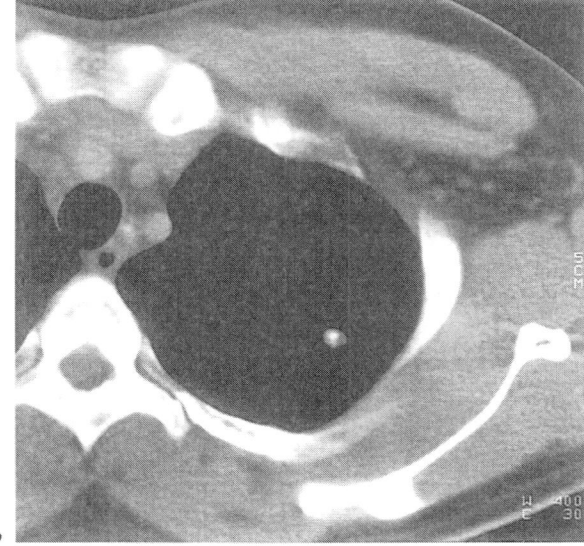

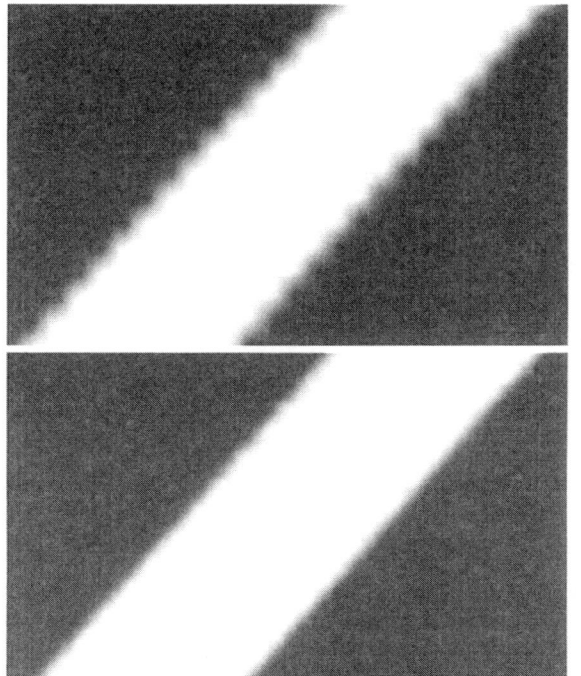

Fig. 5.3. a Coronal reformation of a tilted plastic rod scanned with 5-mm collimation, 1.0 pitch, and 5-mm reconstruction interval. "Stair-step" artifact is prominent along the edges of the rod. b Same scan data reconstructed at 1-mm intervals demonstrate how overlapping reconstruction greatly reduces "stair-step" artifacts. (From NAPEL 1995)

Fig. 5.2. a Serial transverse spiral CT sections obtained with 8-mm collimation, pitch 1.3 and reconstructed at 8-mm intervals. A pulmonary nodule is demonstrated within the left upper lobe. Mediastinal windows fail to demonstrate calcification within the nodule. b Intermediate section retrospectively reconstructed between the two sections in a demonstrates that the pulmonary nodule is calcified. By creating this intervening section, volume averaging is minimized and the calcification is unmasked

when contiguous sections are reformatted is greatly reduced (WANG and VANNIER 1994b) (Fig. 5.3). High-quality multiplanar reformations or 3-D renderings require high-resolution (3-mm or lesser collimation) data free of respiratory misregistration reconstructed with overlapping sections. The overlap should be at least 50% of the collimator width. Although a higher degree of overlap may result in further improvement in multiplanar reformations and 3-D renderings, a significant price is paid in reconstruction time and data storage for these additional images. Perhaps more importantly, a data set consisting of more than 120–150 images will unacceptably slow most rendering workstations.

5.2.4 Field of View

Current spiral CT scanners reconstruct images on a 512×512 display matrix. With a maximal scanning field of view of approximately 50 cm diameter, reconstruction of the entire scan field would result in pixel dimensions of approximately 1 mm. The maximum

(no overlap) and 4-mm (50% overlap) reconstruction intervals. Pulmonary nodules were detected with greater frequency and confidence when overlapping reconstructions were created (BUCKLEY et al. 1995).

The second advantage of the creation of overlapping sections is that the "stair-step" artifact observed

spatial resolution of the CT scanner is typically 0.5 mm or higher. As a result, selection of a smaller display field of view improves in-plane resolution to a maximum between 20 and 25 cm field of view. Although it is possible to reconstruct images with very small fields of view (5–10 cm) with pixel dimensions of 0.1 mm, scanner geometry (e.g., detector size, focal spot size) dictates the actual resolution of the scan. In fact, use of such extremely small fields of view can increase noise within the image without significantly improving spatial resolution. As a result, a field of view less than 20 cm is rarely indicated for reconstruction.

While a 20- to 25-cm field of view provides optimal in-plane spatial resolution, most patients are larger, and therefore only a subset of patient information is reconstructed. The periphery of the lungs and chest wall will likely be eliminated from a section obtained with a 20-cm field of view centered over the mediastinum. This may be satisfactory for CT angiography or dedicated airway evaluations but not for imaging patients with neoplasia or chest wall disease. Therefore, for routine scanning some in-plane spatial resolution is sacrificed in order to image the chest wall in its entirety and avoid missing lesions in the axilla and chest wall. It is better to limit spatial resolution with a larger field of view than potentially miss a peripheral lesion.

Regardless of the reconstruction technique used, as long as the original spiral data are reserved in memory, additional reconstructions can be created to optimize visualization of structures of interest. If a patient requires a large field of view to display all pertinent anatomy, selected sections can be retrospectively reconstructed through an area of interest with a smaller field of view, smaller reconstruction interval, different reconstruction kernel, and, if necessary, different section derivation algorithm to optimize visualization of this structure.

5.3 Methods of Rendering

There are two main alternatives to viewing axial CT sections – multiplanar reformation and 3-D rendering. Multiplanar reformation creates images along arbitrary straight or curved planes that are one voxel thick. Multiplanar reformation ignores all data except those which are found along the single-voxel-thick path defining the plane of reformation. True 3-D rendering techniques consider the entire data set or an edited subset of data to generate an image.

5.3.1 Multiplanar Reformation

Multiplanar reformations can be created through any arbitrary plane intersecting the CT volume (FISHMAN et al. 1991). They can be selected from transverse sections, other multiplanar reformations, or 3-D renderings. In general, selections using transverse sections or multiplanar reformations are adequate; however, when complex branching needs to be presented in a multiplanar reformation, 3-D views can be particularly useful for aligning the anatomy to define the plane of reformation. The routine creation of 3-D views for the purpose of selecting planes of reformation tends to be impractical because of the additional time required to create the 3-D views. Ultimately, the design of the software package dictates the ease and methods of creating multiplanar reformations and 3-D rendering. While sagittal and coronal reformations can be very helpful for displaying anatomic features which course perpendicular to the plane of acquisition, most pertinent anatomic features are not perfectly perpendicular to the plane of acquisition and therefore reformation of oblique planes is frequently more valuable than sagittal or coronal sections (QUINT et al. 1995). Of even greater utility is the curved planar reformation which is created when a curved path is drawn on any multiplanar reformation or 3-D view and then extruded through the volume perpendicular to the plane on which it was drawn (RUBIN et al. 1995). The advantage of this technique is that it enables structures that do not traverse a single plane to be displayed with a two-dimensional (2-D) view (Fig. 5.4). A limitation of this technique is that considerable anatomic distortion results from the curved drawing and relationships between structures as well as distances are inaccurately displayed (Fig. 5.5). A further disadvantage of curved planar reformations is that inaccurate curved drawing can spuriously imply lesions. In particular, vascular stenoses can be simulated when the curve is not well centered over the vessel of interest. It is additionally possible to underestimate eccentric lesions by drawing curves only perpendicular to the axis of least disease. A prudent practice when creating curved planar reformations is always to create two curved reformations using orthogonal views to better delineate eccentric lesions.

5.3.2 Three-Dimensional Rendering

Two strategies exist for creating 3-D renderings of spiral CT data – shaded surface display and volume

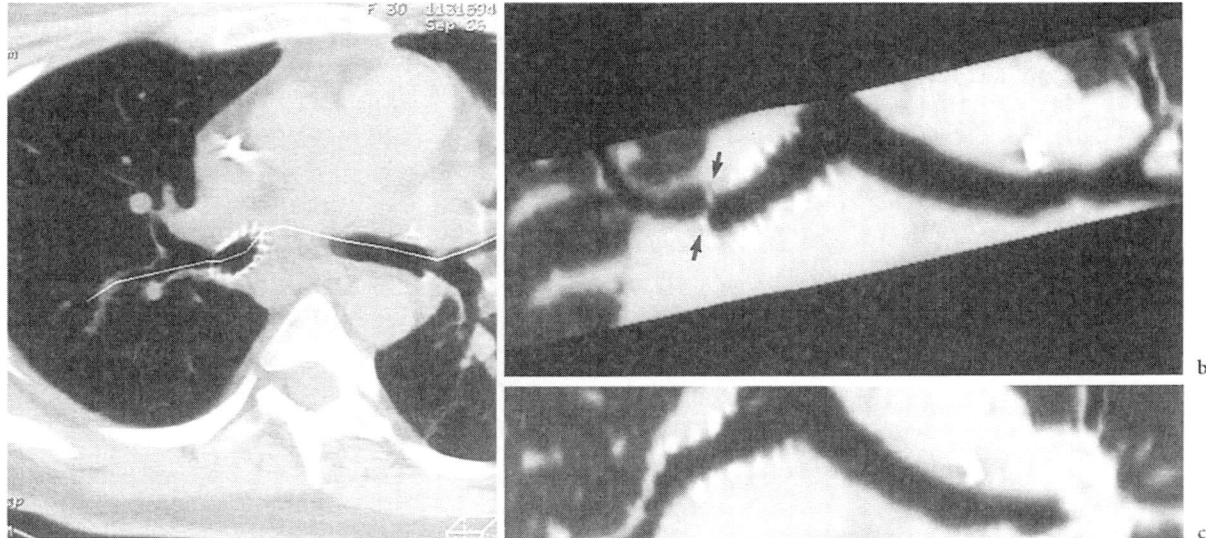

Fig. 5.4. a Transverse CT section through a stent placed in the right main stem bronchus. A curved path has been defined to demonstrate the relationship of the stent relative to the right upper lobe bronchus. **b** Corresponding curved planar reformation demonstrates that the stent covers the origin of this bronchus (*arrows*). Atelectasis is not seen within the corresponding pulmonary segment because the interstices of the stent are open. **c** Alternative curved planar reformation demonstrates that the stent does not encroach upon the right lower lobe bronchial ostium

rendering. Both 3-D rendering techniques result in 2-D images which portray 3-D relationships by depth cues created with surface shading, shadowing, perspective, or motion around an axis of rotation presented as a cine loop of multiple images.

5.3.2.1 Shaded Surface Display

Shaded surface displays (SSDs) require a threshold to be applied to the CT data such that all values within a threshold range are retained for rendering and the remainder are removed from the data set (CLINE et al. 1991; MAGNUSSON et al. 1991). This effectively reduces the bit depth from 12 to 1 and as a result removes 99.97% of the information content of the volume data. The remaining data are used to create isosurfaces using polygonal patches at the boundaries of structures. One or more imaginary sources of illumination are applied and calculated reflections provide depth cueing through surface shading. SSDs can provide an exquisite view of anatomic relationships particularly in regions of vessel or bronchial overlap and become particularly important when viewing aortic branches to be sure that the origins of the branches are visualized (RUBIN et al. 1995).

Shaded surface displays come at a high price. The loss of information resulting from the thresholding process establishes arbitrary boundaries for structures. The perceived size of a structure is dependent upon the threshold chosen. This has particular importance when evaluating strictured segments of the bronchial tree or arterial stenoses, where luminal narrowing can be depicted as a complete discontinuity or a mild stenosis depending on the threshold selection (RUBIN et al. 1994; RUBIN and SILVERMAN 1995). Multiple surfaces that have been derived with different thresholds can be displayed simultaneously. The surfaces are distinguished by color coding (DILLON et al. 1993). While this can be helpful for differentiating bone from blood vessels and even some calcium deposits in the walls of blood vessels, each additional surface increases the computational time of the display, and the fundamental limitations of arbitrary boundary selection are not overcome.

5.3.2.2 Volume Rendering

Volume rendering uses mathematical rays cast through the reconstructed volume to create a projectional image based upon some function applied to each ray. The simplest form of volume rendering is an "average" or "ray sum" projection where each pixel in the output image corresponds to the average or sum of all voxel values found along the corresponding ray. In general, these projections are of

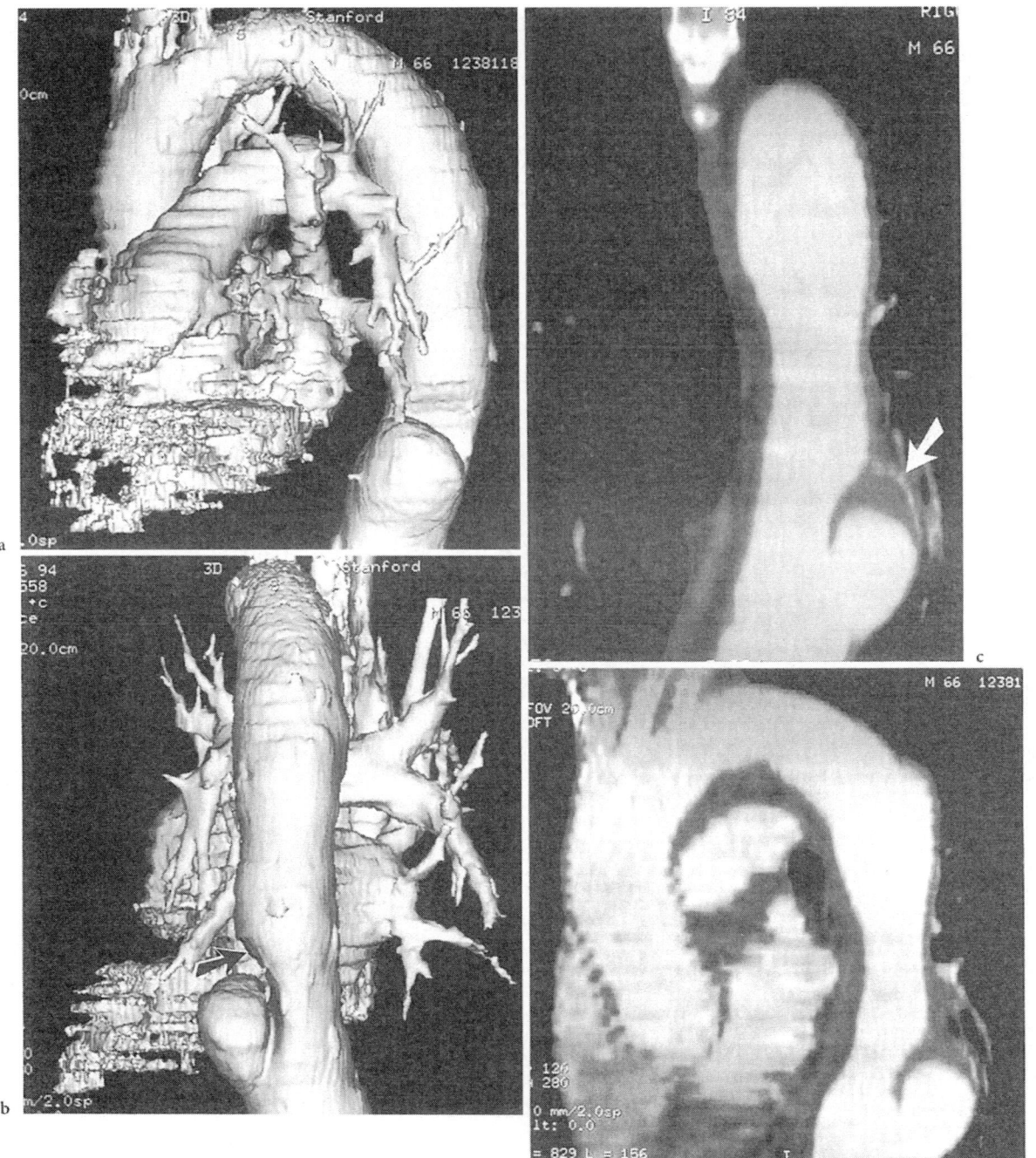

Fig. 5.5. a Left lateral and **b** posterior SSDs of a spiral CT angiogram, obtained with 3-mm collimation, 2.0 pitch, and 2-mm reconstruction interval, demonstrate a penetrating ulcer on the left lateral wall of the descending thoracic aorta. Mass effect (*arrow*), suggestive of thrombus, is observed on the aorta just proximal to the ulceration. **c** Oblique coronal reformation enables delineation of both the patent portion of the intramural ulceration and the superior thrombosed portion (*arrow*). **d** Curved planar reformation delineates the thoracic aorta along its entire course; however, considerable distortion results from curved drawing, which erroneously gives the impression that the ulceration is on the posterior wall. Curved planar reformations must always be reviewed in association with transverse sections, maximum intensity projections, or SSDs to clarify where regions of anatomic distortion might exist

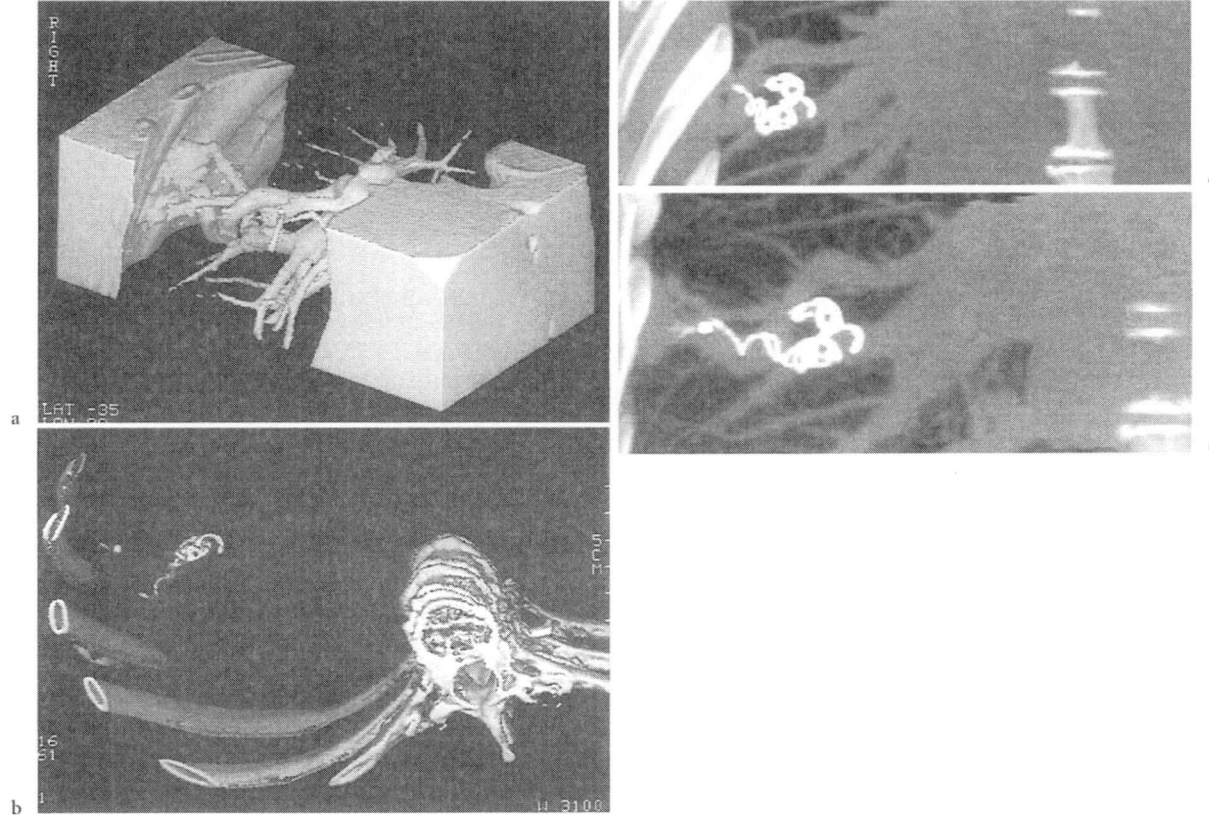

Fig. 5.6. **a** Spiral CT of an arteriovenous malformation following coil embolization. The angioarchitecture of this complex arteriovenous malformation is clearly demonstrated on an SSD created with a threshold of −200 HU. The embolic material, however, cannot be visualized because of the single threshold surface display technique. **b** In order to identify the embolic material with the SSD, a higher threshold (500 HU) is applied. While the embolic material is clearly delineated, the arteriovenous malformation is lost in the thresholding process. **c** Corresponding maximum intensity projection demonstrates the embolic material relative to the arteriovenous malformation; however, the peripheral nidus of the lesion is obscured by overlying chest wall. Extensive editing would be required to remove the chest wall yet maintain visualization of the nidus. **d** Alternatively the anatomy can be viewed from an angle perpendicular to the chest wall in order to delineate the feeding vessels and nidus of the arteriovenous malformation. While this is an easy solution, view angles that demonstrate the entire AVW are limited without removal of the chest wall. Additionally, note the difficulty with which the feeding arteries and draining vein are separated. Portions of the embolic material erroneously appear to be within the vein

little value in processing CT data because the high degree of contrast resolution inherent in CT is reduced due to the volume averaging. Small structures are lost and the edges of structures become indistinct. Ray sum projections may be useful when a thin slab (2–10 mm) is selected as a subvolume for the ray sum projection. The diminished number of voxels that each ray encounters results in an image where fine structures are not completely lost and may be a useful technique for visualizing intimal flaps within the aorta or regions of mural thrombus (ZEMAN et al. 1995).

The most widely implemented volume rendering technique is the maximum intensity projection (KELLER et al. 1989; NAPEL et al. 1992b; RUBIN et al. 1994), which is used when structures of interest are brighter (bones or iodine-enhanced blood vessels) than adjacent structures. Each pixel in the output image corresponds to the maximum voxel value encountered by each ray. Unlike SSDs, this technique preserves the relative density information present in the CT data. However, there are no depth cues in a maximum intensity projection. Multiple maximum intensity projections rendered about an axis of rotation can be displayed as a cine loop with recovery of some depth information. Because only one voxel per ray contributes to the corresponding output pixel, 98%–99.8% of the information contained within the volume information is lost. Fine structures can be visualized, and the edges of structures are well de

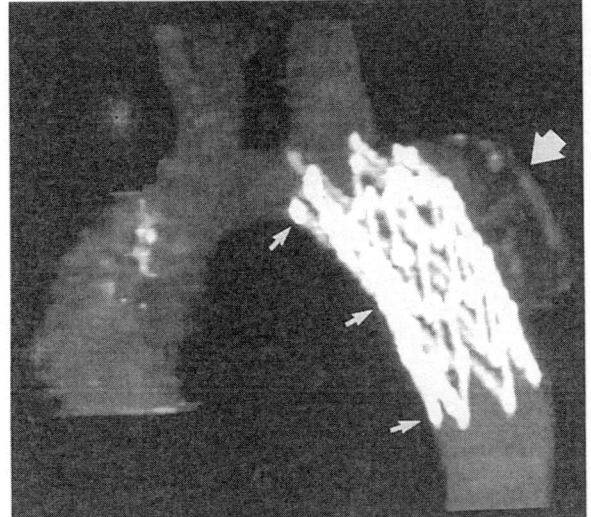

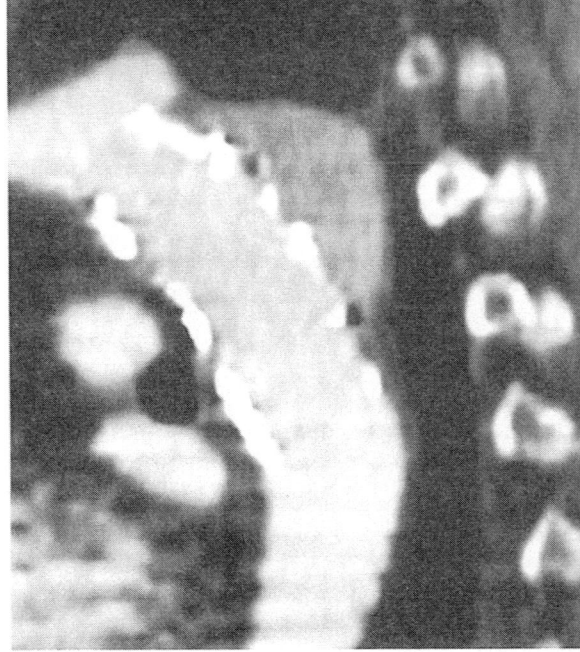

fined. An advantage of the maximum intensity projection, when compared to surface displays, is that differences in attenuation between mural calcium and luminal contrast (RUBIN et al. 1993b), varying contrast concentrations within true and false lumina (RUBIN 1994; RUBIN and COSTELLO 1994), and metal within blood vessels or airways (Fig. 5.6) are readily distinguished. Significant disadvantages of the use of the maximum intensity projection exist in the chest, however. Because only the brightest voxel along the ray is encoded, smaller overlapping vessels are not displayed. While this is less of a problem in the abdomen, vessel overlap is a significant problem in the mediastinum and pulmonary parenchyma due to the divergent course of the blood vessels. It can be particularly difficult to identify the origins or aortic branches. Additionally, the lumina of metallic stents or stent-grafts are obscured by the circumferential high-attenuation metal cage. Curved planar reformations overcome this limitation by slicing through the stent, revealing the interior (Fig. 5.7). A minor limi-

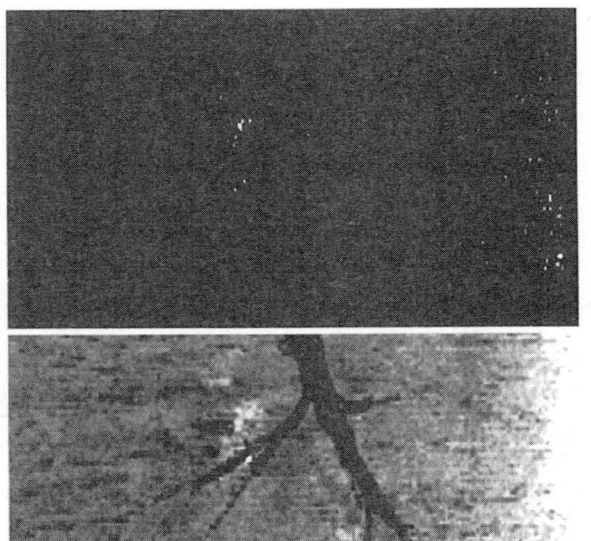

Fig. 5.7. a Maximum intensity projection of a CT angiogram performed with 3-mm collimation, 1.5 pitch, and 2-mm reconstruction interval demonstrates the highly attenuative metallic endoskeleton of a stent-graft (*small arrows*) within the proximal descending aorta. There is thrombosis of a pseudoaneurysm that had resulted from a failed coarctation repair (*wide arrow*). The struts of the stent graft are clearly visualized; however, the interior of the stent graft is obscured by the metallic struts. The arch is hypoplastic and the left subclavian artery is large. **b** Curved planar reformation allows clear visualization of the interior of the stent graft as well as delineation of both the thrombosed portion of the pseudoaneurysm and the patent enhancing aorta. Although differentiation of the pseudoaneurysm and the patent aorta can be appreciated from both views, the maximum intensity projection required slice-by-slice region of interest editing, taking 45 min to perform. The curved planar reformation required no editing and was created in less than 2 min

Fig. 5.8a,b. Lateral minimum intensity projection of images obtained through the right middle and lower lobes of spiral CT data with 1-mm collimation and reconstructed with "high" (**a**) and "soft" (**b**) kernels. Because the attenuation difference between the interior of airways and the surrounding lung is typically less than 100 HU, minimum intensity projections of he airways are degraded by background noise to a greater extent than are maximum intensity projections of the vasculature. The airways are completely lost when the "high" reconstruction kernel is used (**a**). The same data reconstructed with the "soft" kernel enable clear visualization of the medial an lateral segments of the right middle lobe, the superior segmental bronchus, the medial basilar bronchus, and the common trunk of the anterior lateral and posterior basal bronchi

tation of the maximum intensity projection is that there is an overall increase in background attenuation, which can result in small blood vessels being lost.

A rendering technique akin to the maximum intensity projection which has unique applicability in the thorax is the minimum intensity projection (NAPEL et al. 1992a). Pixels encode the minimum voxel value encountered by each ray. This can be useful for visualizing the airways because air contained within the tracheobronchial tree is lower in attenuation than surrounding pulmonary parenchyma. In general, however, the density difference between pulmonary parenchyma and airways is small (50–150 HU). In order to see small airways, narrow collimation is required to achieve thin sections. The increased spatial resolution resulting from narrow collimation is accompanied by an increase in noise. Successful minimum intensity projections require that the noise within the data is minimized, and therefore reconstruction with a low spatial frequency, low noise (soft) kernel is advised (Fig. 5.8). Minimum intensity projections can be particularly difficult to implement in patients with emphysema due to the diminished attenuation of the surrounding pulmonary parenchyma. In contrast, minimum intensity projections can be very effective through regions of consolidation or other causes of increased pulmonary parenchymal attenuation. Nevertheless, bronchial stenoses are accentuated using minimum intensity projections even when the volume is reduced to a thin slab (Fig. 5.9).

A more sophisticated and computationally intensive form of volume rendering can be used to preserve all voxel information in the output image (DREBIN et al. 1988; LEVOY 1988; NEY et al. 1992; RUSINEK et al. 1989). Voxel values are rendered with varying opacity and color, as defined by an opacity curve and color table applied to a histogram of voxel values. This allows different tissues to be visualized as different colors and opacities by virtue of their CT attenuation (Fig. 5.10). Spatial gradients are calculated and used to simulate gray-scale lighting effects which provide depth cues.

5.3.3 Alternative Transverse Rendering Techniques

Depending upon the reconstruction interval and imaging volume, hundreds of axial images can be generated from less than 1 min of scan time, and it is anticipated that future generations of spiral CT scanners will be capable of greater data acquisition rates.

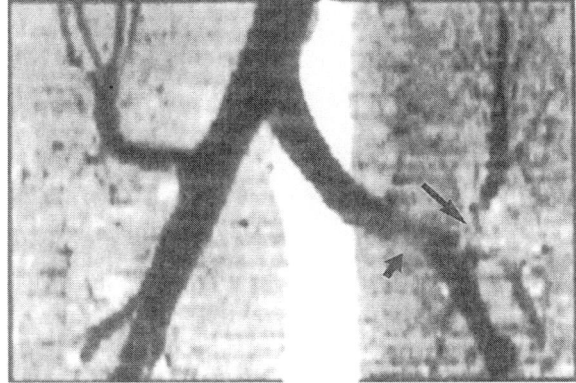

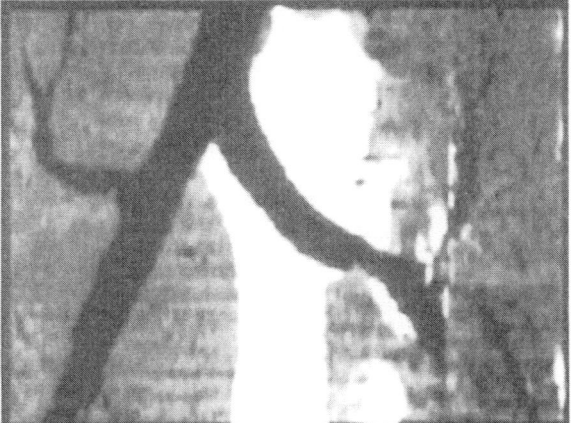

Fig. 5.9. a Minimum intensity projection obtained through the full thickness of the lung demonstrates an apparent discontinuity in the proximal aspect of the left upper lobe bronchus (*long arrow*) and what appears to be a high-grade stenosis of the horizontal portion of the left main stem bronchus (*short arrow*). **b** Minimum intensity projection created through a 2-cm-thick slab demonstrates that the apparent occlusion at the origin of the left upper lobe bronchus is patent yet highly stenotic and the distal horizontal left main stem bronchus is not as stenotic as is suggested on the thicker slab minimum intensity projection. Note that some bronchial branches, particularly in the right upper lobe, right lower lobe, and left lower lobe, are not visualized because they are excluded from the thinner slab. **c** Curved reformation demonstrates a moderate stenosis of the left upper lobe bronchial origin and localized granulation tissue on the inferior wall of the horizontal portion of the left main stem bronchus. Because stenoses are over-accentuated and intraluminal filling defects are not well visualized with minimum intensity projections, the curved and oblique planar reformations are preferable for visualizing airway stenoses

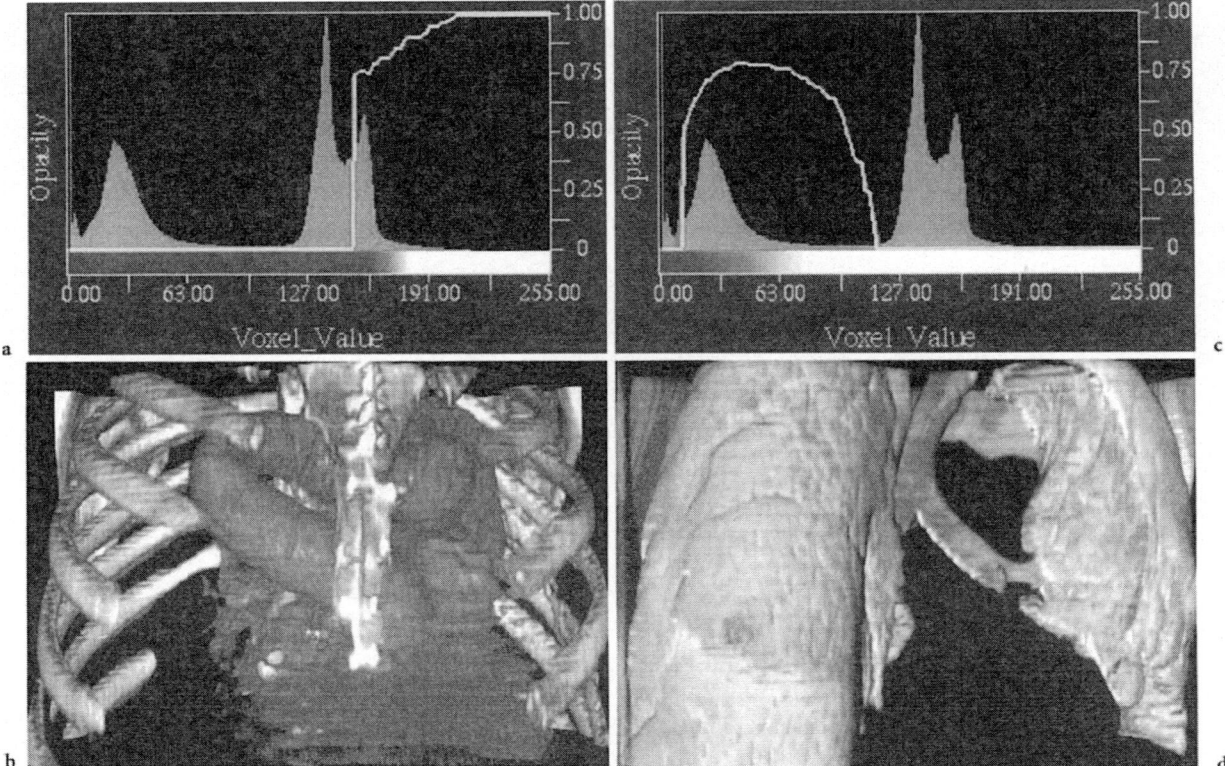

Fig 5.10. a Histogram of voxel values within a spiral CT data set of the thorax. The yellow line is the opacity curve which is drawn to demonstrate the vasculature and bones. Opacity of zero indicates complete transparency and opacity of 1.00 is completely opaque. Intermediate values are semiopaque. The color scale is indicated between the x-axis and the histogram plot. The color scale enables differentiation of the blood vessels from the bones. **b** Volume rendering corresponding to opacity and color values defined in **a**. **c** Same data as in **a** with opacity curve and color scale to demonstrate the pulmonary parenchyma and the central airways. **d** Volume rendering corresponding to opacity and color values defined in **c**. An advantage that volume rendering holds over shaded surface displays is that the opacity and color curves can be altered with immediate re-rendering to demonstrate different aspects of the anatomy. Surface displays may require 10–15 min to recalculate isosurfaces once the threshold level is changed (From Rubin et al. 1996)

There is considerable expense in printing these individual sections and time requirements to review them, so alternatives have been proposed for reviewing numerous axial sections. One such approach is to simply review the images sequentially on a display monitor in "cine" mode. A recent investigation suggests that cine mode review of transverse images improves the detection of pulmonary nodules over film-based presentation (SELTZER et al. 1995). For current routine applications, this approach represents a practical alternative to film-based review; however, for special high-resolution applications such as airway studies or CT angiography, hundreds of images may be available for sequential review, requiring that large amounts of random access memory be present.

An additional alternative is the use of sliding thin slab maximum intensity projection and/or sliding thin slab minimum intensity projection to review the data (NAPEL et al. 1993). The sliding thin slab maximum intensity projection is defined by two variables – the number of sections per slab and the interval between slab centers (Fig. 5.11). The sections are typically thin sections (1–2 mm) rendered into 5- to 20-mm slabs. Therefore the total number of images for review can be reduced by a factor of 10 or more. Further investigations are required to determine the optimal number of sections per slab and degree of overlap required for accurate interpretation. Thin slab maximum intensity projection permits smaller blood vessels to be visualized on a 1- to 1.5-cm rendered section that would be lost to partial volume averaging on a section acquired with 1- to 1.5-cm thickness. The advantage over a single thin section is

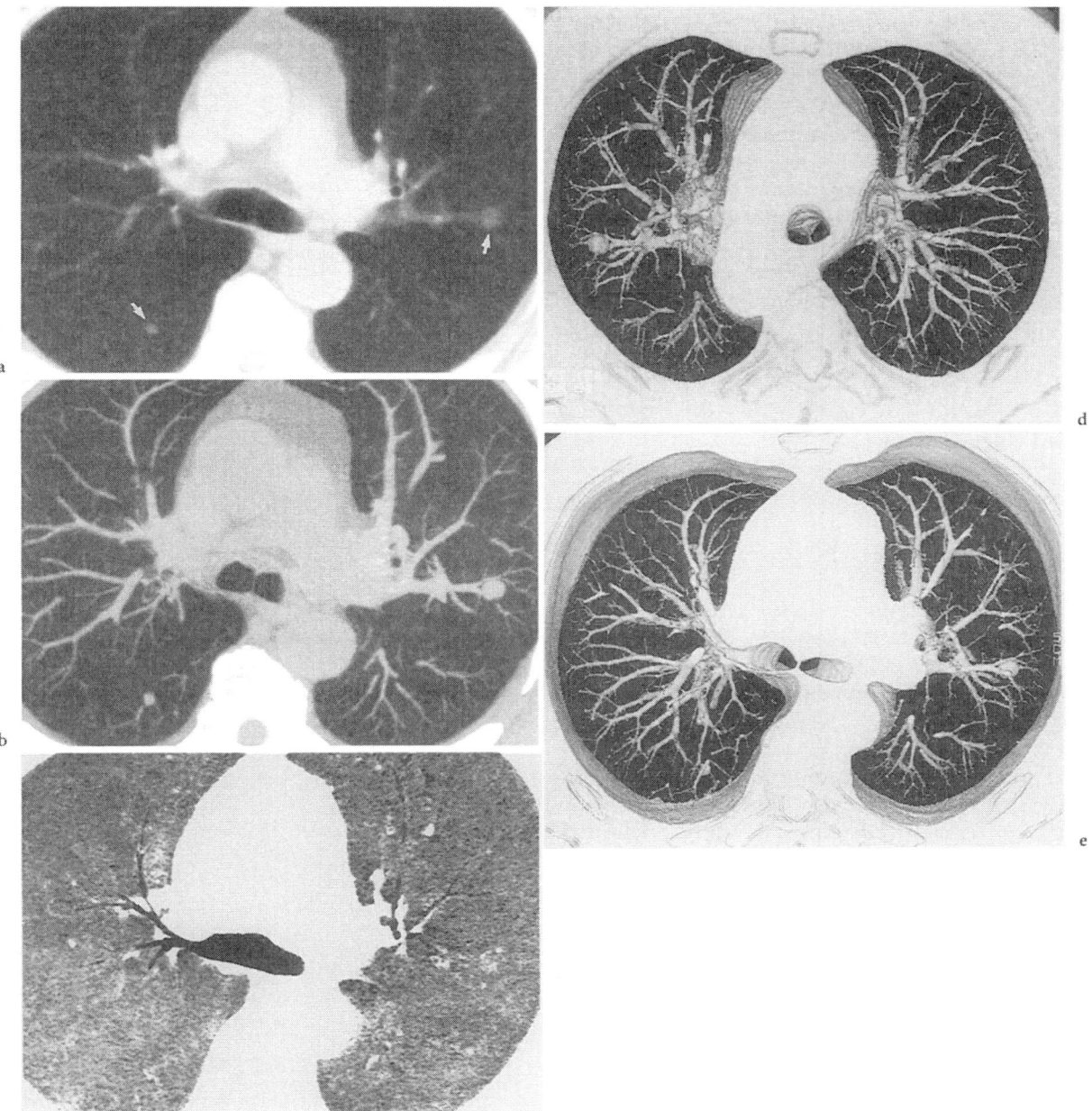

Fig. 5.11. a Spiral CT scan with 1-mm collimation, pitch 2.0 and reconstructed with a 1-mm interval and soft kernel. Ten contiguous sections were averaged (ray-sum) to create a 10-mm-thick slab. This view simulates the appearance of a 10-mm-thick CT section. Pulmonary nodules are demonstrated within the superior segment of the right lower lobe and the apical posterior segment of the left upper lobe (*arrows*). **b** Ten-millimeter-thick slab maximum intensity projection using the same sections as **a** demonstrates the pulmonary nodules and intrapulmonary vasculature more distinctly. Small peripheral arterial branches are better visualized; however, smaller central airways as well as the lateral aspect of the main stem bronchi are lost in the maximum intensity projection process. **c** Ten-millimeter-thick slab minimum intensity projection demonstrates the airways more clearly than in the averaged image or in the maximum intensity projection. The pulmonary nodules, however, are lost in the background. **d** Superior and **e** inferior 10-mm-thick slab SSDs providing unique visualization of the pulmonary nodules relative to the vasculature; however, the clinical utility of these images is limited

that vessels can be appreciated over a much longer segment of their course. This can facilitate localization of pulmonary parenchymal lesions. A limitation of the maximum intensity projection is that low attenuation structures such as the airways are lost. The sliding thin slab minimum intensity projection enables airway anatomy to be visualized; however, parenchymal and bronchial abnormalities associated with the airways may not be adequately rendered. It is possible that superimposition of thin slab maximum intensity projections and thin slab minimum intensity projections would be a preferred technique.

5.3.4 Perspective Rendering

Currently, the predominant application of 3-D rendering creates views from points external to the data set, generated using parallel rays cast through the volume or reflected off surfaces as if the model were viewed from an infinite distance with magnification. A more realistic technique is to render with slightly divergent rays to mimic the perspective provided by the human visual system, where similarly sized structures closer to the viewing point appear larger than those farther away (RUBIN et al. 1996). While perspective rendering is not critical when viewing CT data sets from external view points, it becomes critical when rendering occurs from within the data. Both SSDs (VINING et al. 1994) and volume rendering (RUBIN et al. 1996) can be used to render perspective images from within the CT data to simulate endoscopy (Fig. 5.12). This technique has only recently become available and to date has not been validated in a clinical series; however, preliminary images show considerable promise for uniquely visualizing endobronchial, endovascular, and intrathoracic anatomy and disease.

Currently a minimum of 10–20s is required to volume render a individual image with perspective, depending on the type of computer hardware. Multiple images must be generated along a flight path to perform "virtual endoscopy." Using currently available hardware (Silicon Graphics Onyx workstation with Reality Engine Two, costing approximately $250 000) a 2-min movie created with 30 frames per second requires up to 20h of rendering time. The computational speed of this hardware is expected to increase considerably over the next several years, while prices should fall. Perspective volume rendering is particularly attractive when compared to other 3-D rendering techniques because editing of the data

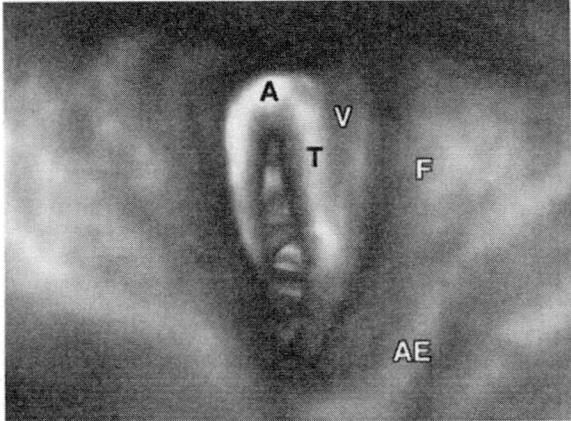

a

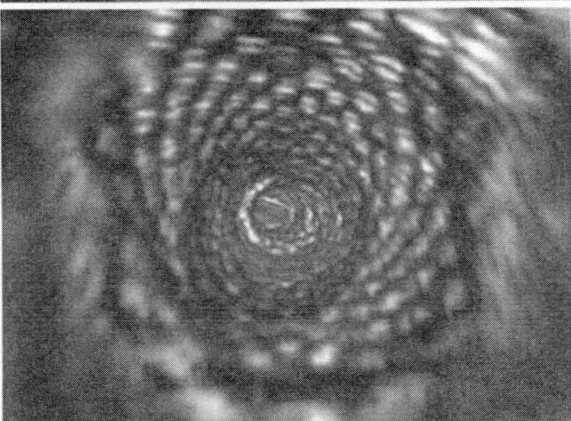

b

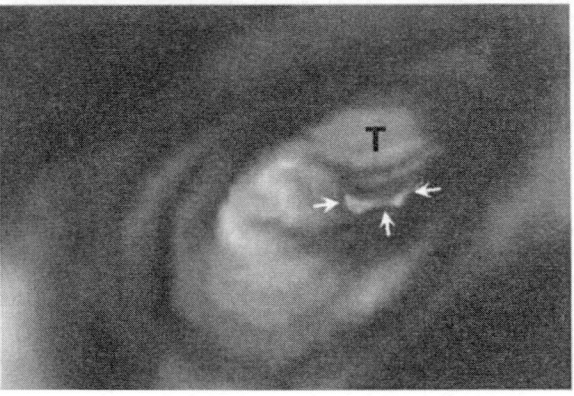

c

Fig. 5.12. a Perspective volume rendering of a spiral CT scan (1-mm collimation, 2.0 pitch, 0.5-mm reconstruction interval) viewed form the glottis looking inferiorly demonstrates the true vocal cord (*T*), false vocal cord (*F*), laryngeal ventricle (*V*), anterior commissure (*A*), and aryepiglottic fold (*AE*). **b** Perspective volume rendering within the proximal trachea looking inferiorly through a Wall stent placed to treat a high-grade tracheal stenosis. The tracheal lumen is widely patent. **c** Perspective volume rendering within the right main stem bronchus looking inferolaterally demonstrates an adenocarcinoma (*T*), which is markedly narrowing the bronchus intermedius (*arrows*). This region could not be passed with a fiberoptic bronchoscope; however, the CT bronchoscopy, performed with perspective volume rendering, allowed passage to demonstrate near-complete occlusion of the right middle lobe bronchus and provided views of the tumor from below looking superiorly – an impossibility with fiberoptic bronchoscopy

may not be required when views can be generated between structures that would overlap on external views.

Although SSDs, being less computationally intensive, allow near-interactive rendering rates, the sur-

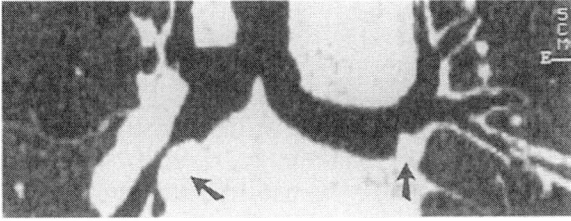

Fig. 5.13. Curved planar reformation in a patient 1 year following heart-lung transplant, demonstrating granulation tissue within the right lower lobe and horizontal portion of the left main stem bronchi (*arrows*). Curved planar reformations facilitate visualization of subtle intraluminal filling defects that may be missed on transverse sections

face extraction process with its inherent reduction in voxel information ultimately limits these renderings by creating surfaces at assumed boundaries. Discontinuities in the walls of airways or blood vessels can be artifactually created and structures typically appear irregular due to the polygonal modeling applied to the surfaces.

5.4 Editing

Two strategies for editing CT data are widely in use – region of interest selection and connectivity, or region growing. Region of interest editing is performed when a region is defined on either an axial image, multiplanar reformation, or 3-D rendering (RUBIN and JEFFREY 1994). Voxels within or those outside of the region of interest are then eliminated. The region of interest can be defined to extend through a single

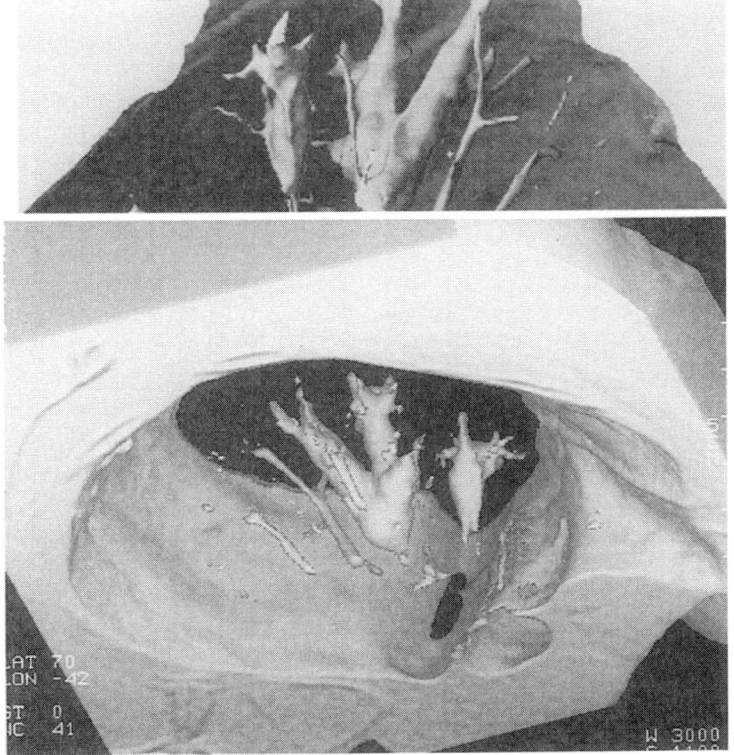

Fig. 5.14. a Lateral and **b** oblique SSDs created with a 20-HU threshold in a patient with allergic bronchopulmonary aspergillosis demonstrate the classic finger in glove appearance of the mucous-filled bronchi. Note, however, that parenchymal vessels are difficult to distinguish from the mucus-filled airways, because they have similar densities. The only clues to the differentiation are morphologic. This is a limitation of all currently used 3-D techniques. SSDs may be the best means of data display in this situation, because they provide the greatest morphologic detail. Other techniques capable of differentiating densities, e.g., maximum intensity projections, are not as useful when all structures of interest have the same density. Images were obtained using 1-mm collimation, 2.0 pitch, and 1-mm reconstruction interval. (From Rubin et al. 1996a)

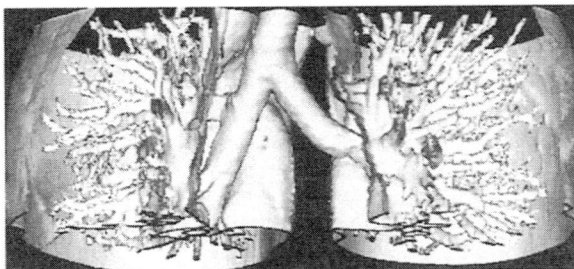

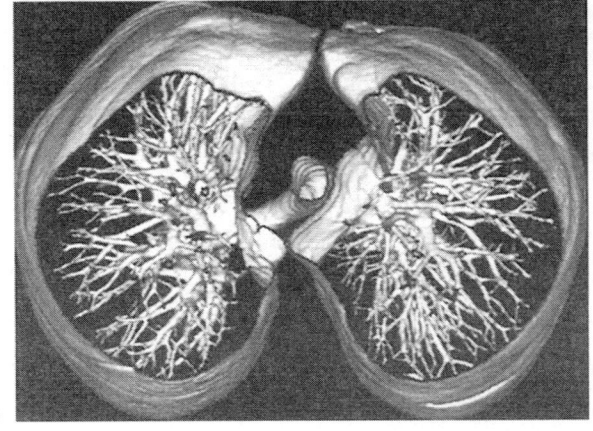

a

b

Fig. 5.15. a Anterior and **b** craniocaudal SSDs created with a upper threshold of −150 HU and a lower threshold of −600 HU clearly demonstrate the distal trachea, main stem bronchi, and proximal lobar bronchi. The selection of thresholds that render surfaces at the interface between air and soft tissue results in visualization of the central airways within the mediastinum, but within the lung only the vasculature and pleural surface are seen. Images were obtained using 1-mm collimation, 2.0 pitch, and 1-mm reconstruction interval

voxel thickness (2-D region of interest) or can be extruded through a slab of more than one voxel thickness to define a 3-D region. While 2-D region of interest editing offers the greatest degree of control, it is the most time intensive. As slab thickness increases, editing time decreases, but control diminishes.

Connectivity can be a useful technique for removing structures of sufficiently different density from the structure of interest or for removing structures of similar density that are not in continuity. A seed point is placed within a structure to be identified and that seed is allowed to grow in three dimensions within a range of voxel values defined by threshold levels (CLINE et al. 1987). The structure identified is either selectively retained or removed from the data. Connectivity can be an effective means of removing complex structures such as the thoracic cage; however, in practice, the proximity of the brachial-cephalic branches and high attenuation inflowing

venous contrast material makes region of interest editing necessary in the upper mediastinum and thoracic inlet.

Threshold selection for object removal or identification results in the edges of structures being excluded from the identification. This is remedied by applying a dilation process where voxels adjacent to the selected region are recruited to join the region selected with connectivity alone. Without this dilation step, maximum intensity projections will have artificially sharp edges, appearing to have been cut with scissors. By including the "edge voxels' with dilation, the maximum intensity projection is improved. Dilation is also important when removing structures identified with connectivity. Without dilation, the subtracted structure remains visible, because the edge pixels that fall below the threshold are not subtracted.

5.5 Current Applications

5.5.1 Airways

The majority of the tracheobronchial tree does not course in the transverse plane. As a result, only cross-sections of bronchi are visible on transverse sections. Although the sections can be very useful for assessing bronchial wall thickening and dilation, it can be difficult to identify the origin of a given bronchial generation. Further, regions of bronchial narrowing may be difficult to appreciate when not viewed adjacent to normal bronchial lumen. Minimum intensity projections and multiplanar reformations provide a means for visualizing bronchial branching and identifying regions of stenosis. While minimum intensity projections are effective in showing proximal tracheobronchial branching, subsegmental branches are typically lost in the background of lung parenchyma, and narrowing within regions of stenoses is artifactually increased. For these reasons, multiplanar and particularly curved planar reformation can be very useful for visualizing the airways (Fig. 5.13). Surface displays can be applied to the trachea and proximal main bronchi as well (SILVERMAN et al. 1995); however, threshold selection must be performed with care to accurately display lesions. Surface displays are particularly effective when airways are filled with mucus (Fig. 5.14), although air-filled intrapulmonary airways cannot be rendered with surface displays because of their similar attenuation to the parenchyma (Fig. 5.15). If a successful algorithm for airway

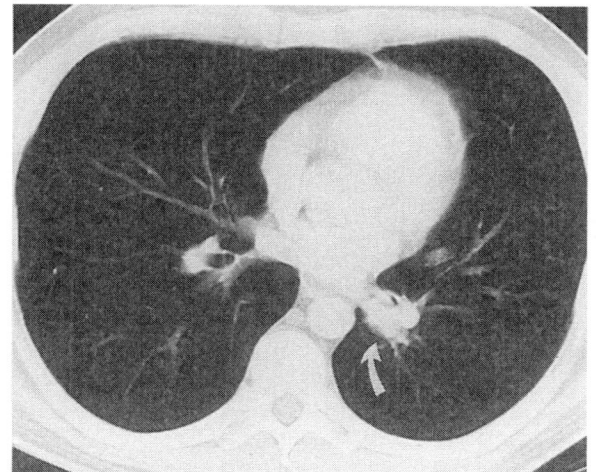

Fig. 5.16. a Eight-millimeter collimated transverse section demonstrates a 2.5-cm mass within the inferior aspect of the left pulmonary hilum (*arrow*). The relationship of this mass to the left lower lobe bronchus is difficult to ascertain on this thick section. **b** Contiguous 1-mm collimated spiral CT sections obtained with pitch 2.0 and 1-mm reconstruction interval demonstrate the considerable detail that can be shown when thin spiral sections are used to characterize a pulmonary nodule. Although the mass clearly has an intraluminal component, it is difficult to appreciate the relative intra- and extraluminal extent of the mass and its relationship to bronchial branches. **c** Sagittal oblique and **d** coronal oblique reformations clearly delineate the extraluminal component of this bronchial carcinoid (*arrows*) as well as the intraluminal component (*x*)

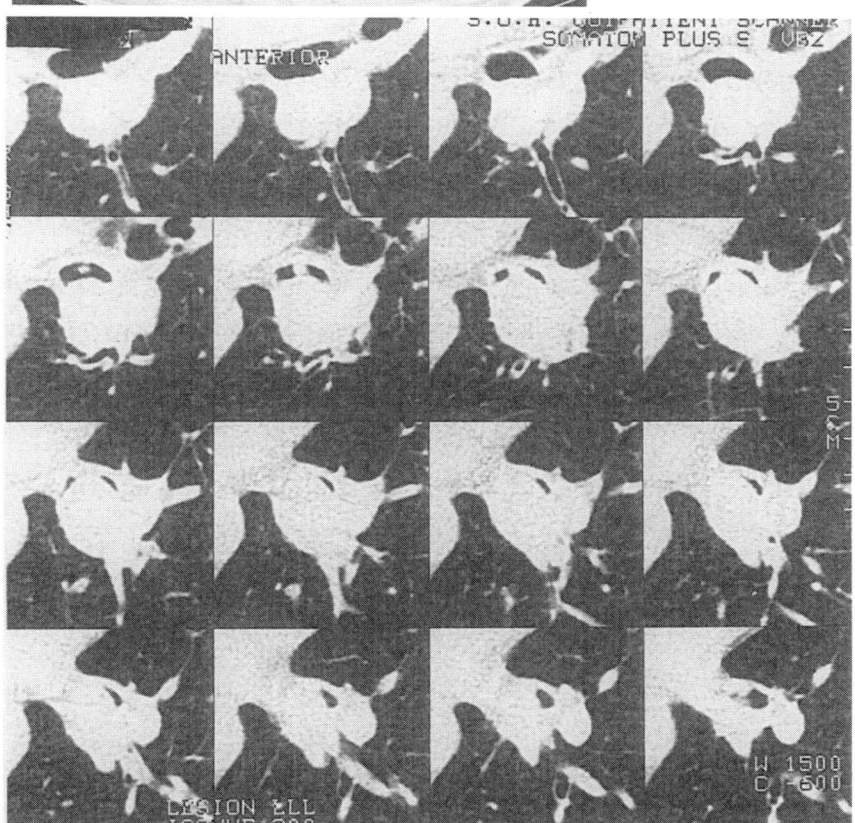

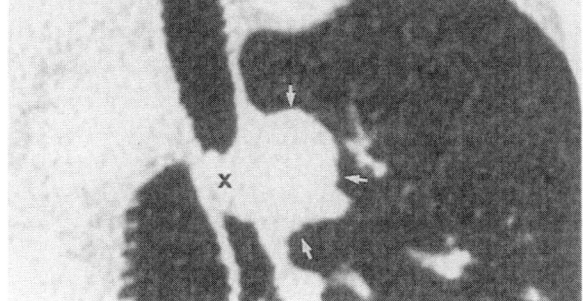

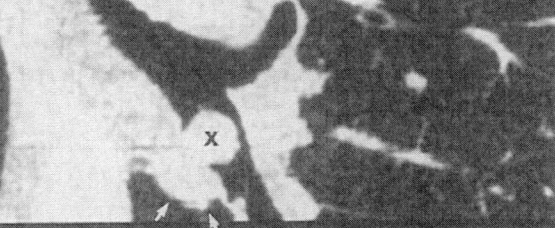

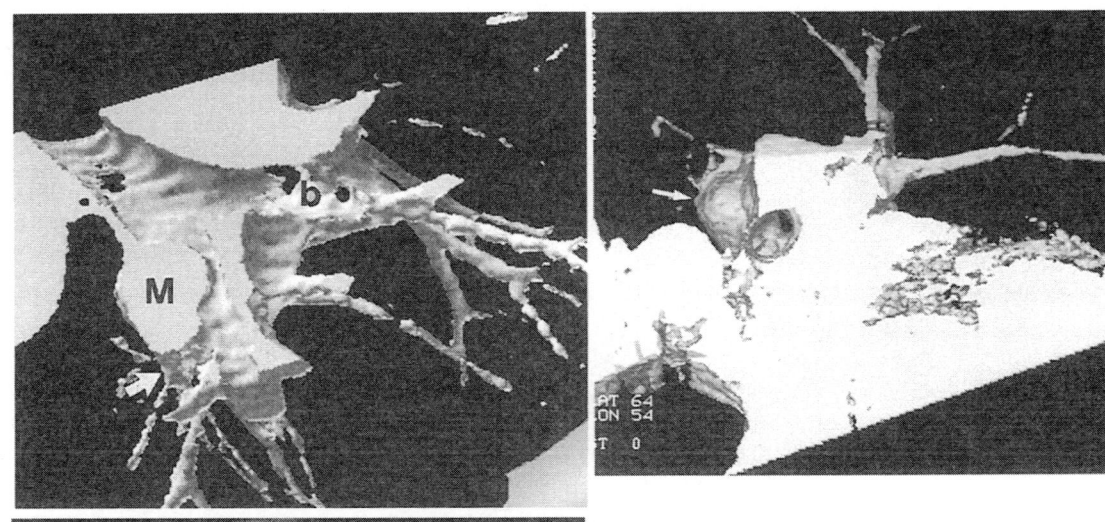

e

f

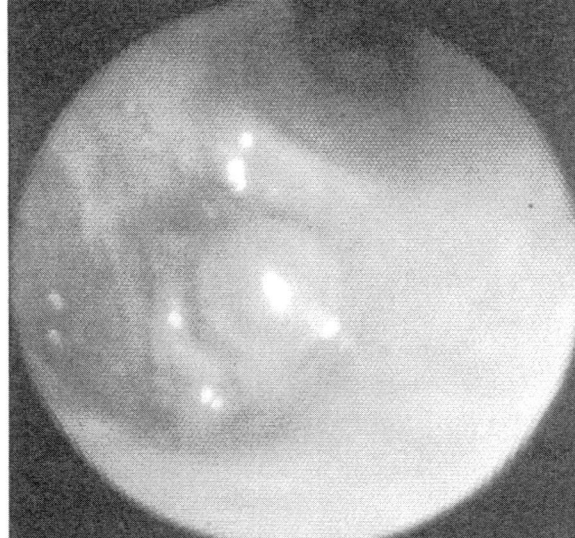

Fig. 5.16. e Sagittal oblique SSD demonstrates the relationship of the mass (*M*) to the left upper lobe bronchus (*b*) and the superior segmental bronchus of the left lower lobe (*arrow*). This image facilitated surgical planning, demonstrating that a left lower lobectomy was possible and a total pneumonectomy need not be performed. f Craniocaudal SSD demonstrates the intraluminal component of the lesion as might be viewed with a bronchoscope as well as the extraluminal component (*arrow*). g Correlative bronchoscopic image demonstrates the intraluminal component of this carcinoid tumor. (From Rubin et al. 1996a)

g

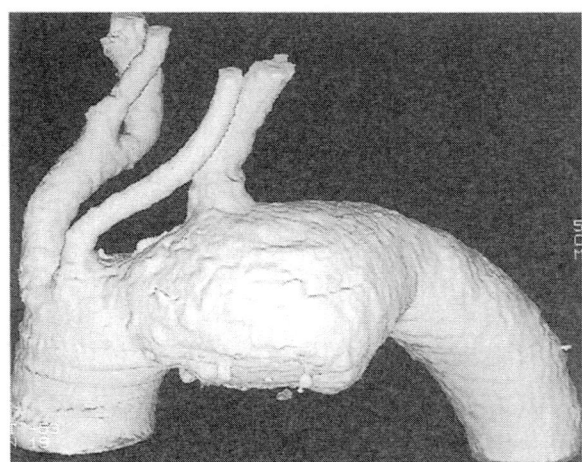

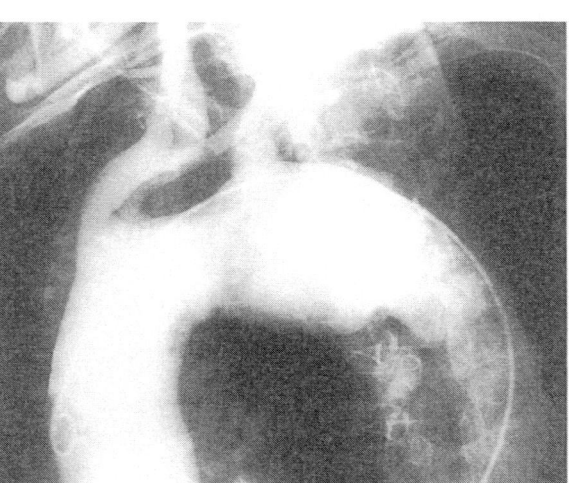

a

b

Fig. 5.17. a CT angiogram of a thoracic aortic aneurysm (3-mm collimation, 1.0 pitch, 2-mm reconstruction interval) demonstrates that the lateral extent of the aneurysm is better appreciated on the shaded surface display when compared to b the conventional angiogram. (From Rubin and Jeffrey 1995)

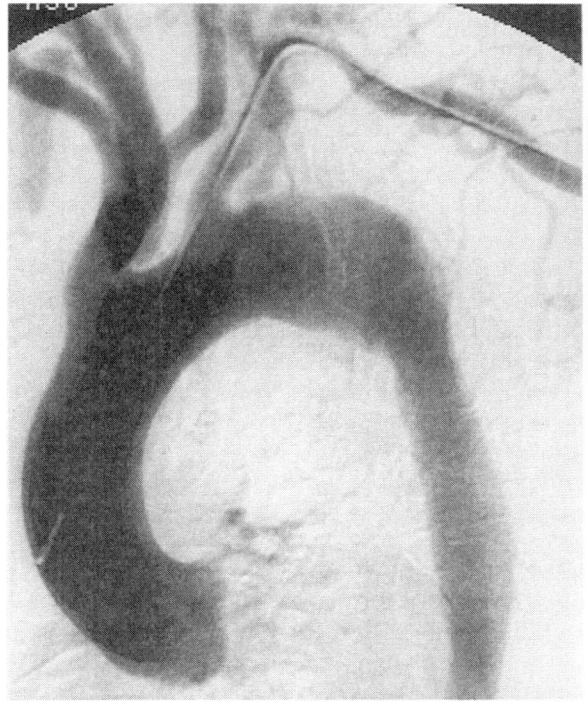

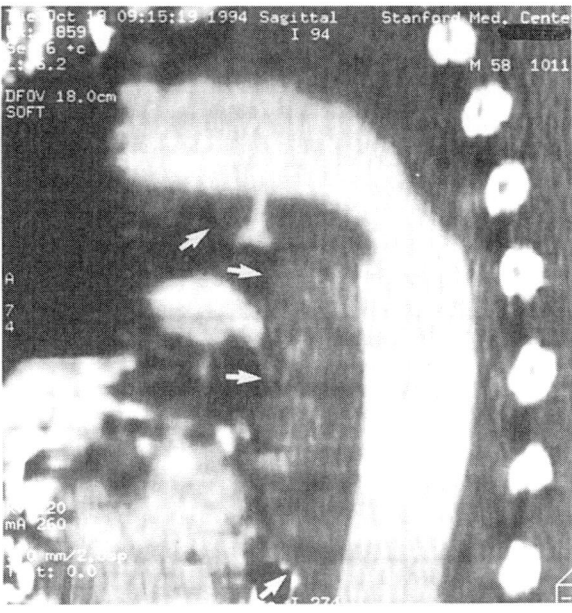

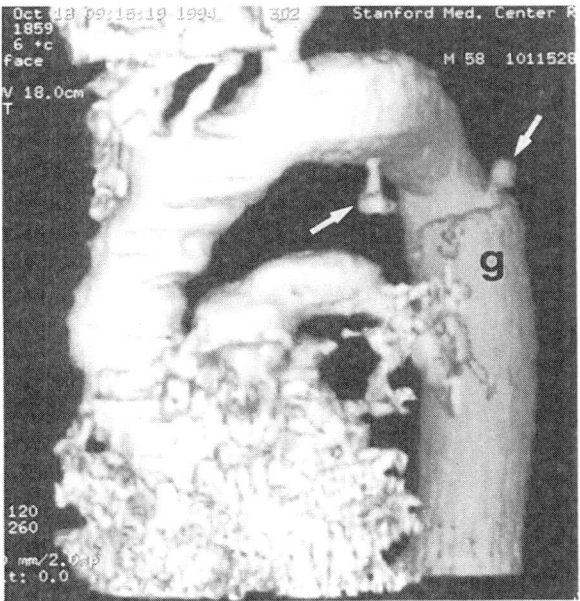

Fig. 5.18. a Digital subtraction arteriogram opacifies the true lumen of a type B aortic dissection. b Following placement of a descending aortic graft a spiral CT angiogram was performed (3-mm collimation, 2.0 pitch, 2-mm reconstruction interval). An SSD demonstrates two areas of contrast extravasation (*arrows*). The region adjacent to the descending aortic graft (*g*) may be due to an anastomotic leak; however, the leak on the underside of the aortic arch was likely present preoperatively, but unopacified on the arteriogram due to slow flow. c Curved planar reformation demonstrates associated thrombus on the underside of the aortic arch and around the descending aortic graft (*arrows*)

extraction were developed, then this limitation might be solve. Perhaps the best means of assessing the airways is with a combination of perspective volume rendering and multiplanar reformations. Neither technique requires airway extraction or thresholding. Seventh order bronchial branching has been visualized with perspective volume rendering (Rubin et al. 1996). Multiplanar and 3-D rendering of thin-section airway data can be useful for identify-

ing the extent of lesions and planning surgery (Fig. 5.16).

5.5.2 Vasculature

The use of multiplanar reformations and 3-D renderings has greatly facilitated the visualization of aortic disease with CT. Although a high-resolution acquisition is required for all multiplanar and 3-D rendering in the thorax, CT angiography additionally requires that a high-flow (3–5 ml/s) accurately timed iodinated bolus is delivered (RUBIN et al. 1993b, 1995). CT angiograms of the thoracic aorta allow aortic pathology to be presented to surgeons in a manner that is analogous to conventional arteriography or intraoperative views. As a result, spiral CT angiography has found greater acceptance as a single imaging modality for many aortic diseases where conventional CT was viewed with skepticism. Two main advantages of CT angiography exist relative to conventional angiography. Firstly, aortic anatomy can be viewed from arbitrary view angles providing views that are geometrically impossible with conventional angiography. Additionally, CT angiography enables vessels to be "sliced open" and their interior directly visualized. The two most common abnormalities of the thoracic aorta warranting CT angiography are aneurysms and dissections. Both have very different rendering requirements.

5.5.2.1 Aortic Aneurysms

Thoracic aortic aneurysms are best rendered using SSDs to visualize the aneurysm in its entirety and appreciate its relationship to aortic branches (Fig. 5.17). Mural thrombus is typically not rendered with SSDs unless a two-threshold, colorized technique is applied after extensive editing.

Because of the potential for considerable vessel overlap, particularly in the region of the aortic arch, maximum intensity projections may not clearly delineate the full extent of the aneurysm, although mural thrombus and calcium are distinguished from the patent lumen. If treatment with an aortic stent graft is contemplated, multiplanar reformation, particularly curved planar reformations, and SSDs provide a clearer depiction of the aneurysm neck than axial sections and facilitate planning of stent graft placement. The proximity of the left subclavian artery to the aneurysm must be accurately delineated lest the left subclavian artery is inadvertently occluded at the time of stent graft deployment. Accurate preoperative imaging that suggests that the left subclavian artery origin might be covered by a portion of the stent graft might indicate the need for an additional procedure to transplant the left subclavian artery onto the left common carotid artery prior to stent-graft deployment. An additional advantage of surface displays is that when rendered with the spine and ribs, they typically delineate intercostal

artery origins so that occlusions of these vessels can be avoided during graft placement.

CT angiography is equally or perhaps more valuable than conventional angiography for assessing postprocedural complications (RUBIN et al. 1993a). Because periaortic leaks both at traditional graft anastomoses and around stent grafts typically have slow flow, conventional angiography may not delineate these regions of extravasation. CT angiography has been found to be more sensitive than conventional angiography in delineating the degree of perigraft extravasation (Fig. 5.18). Further, 3-D renderings are often required to clearly understand the site of origin for the extravasation.

5.5.2.2 Aortic Dissection

Recent data suggest that multiplanar reformations and 3-D reconstructions facilitate the assessment of thoracic aortic dissection, particularly when establishing the extension of intimal flap into brachiocephalic branches (ZEMAN et al. 1995). The difficult differentiation of intramural hematoma and aortic dissection is also facilitated with spiral CT and multiplanar reformations (Fig. 5.19). Maximum intensity projections are typically the least helpful ren-

---

Fig. 5.19. a,b DSA images demonstrate flattening of the posterior wall of the descending aorta and a posterior collection of contrast material within the distal descending aorta suggestive of focal ulceration with intramural hematoma formation (*arrows*). Although the arteriogram suggests that there is thrombus within the posterior wall of the descending aorta proximal to the ulceration, the aortic arch and ascending aorta are normal. **c,d** Transverse spiral CT sections (3-mm collimnation; 2.0 pitch; 2-mm reconstruction interval) through the region of apparent ulceration demonstrate the communication between the aorta and intramural collection as well as band-like filling defect proximal to the ulceration (*arrows*). **e** Transverse spiral CT section 2 cm below the aortic arch demonstrates hematoma within the lateral aspect of the aorta. The wall of the aorta (*arrows*) can be delineated from pleural fluid and the intramural collection. **f** Transverse spiral CT section through the aortic arch demonstrates that the mural abnormality extends across the entire aortic arch to the ascending aorta, where a localized region of contrast extravasation (*arrow*) is observed. The demonstration of contiguity between this abnormality of the ascending aorta extending to the apparent ulceration in the distal descending aorta suggests that in fact this lesion represents a predominately thrombosed type A aortic dissection. The region of extravasation seen in the ascending aorta could not be visualized on a conventional arteriogram. **g** Curved planar reformation demonstrates the region of extravasation anteriorly on the ascending aorta (*large arrow*) as well as the extensive hematoma present throughout the descending aorta (*small arrows*)

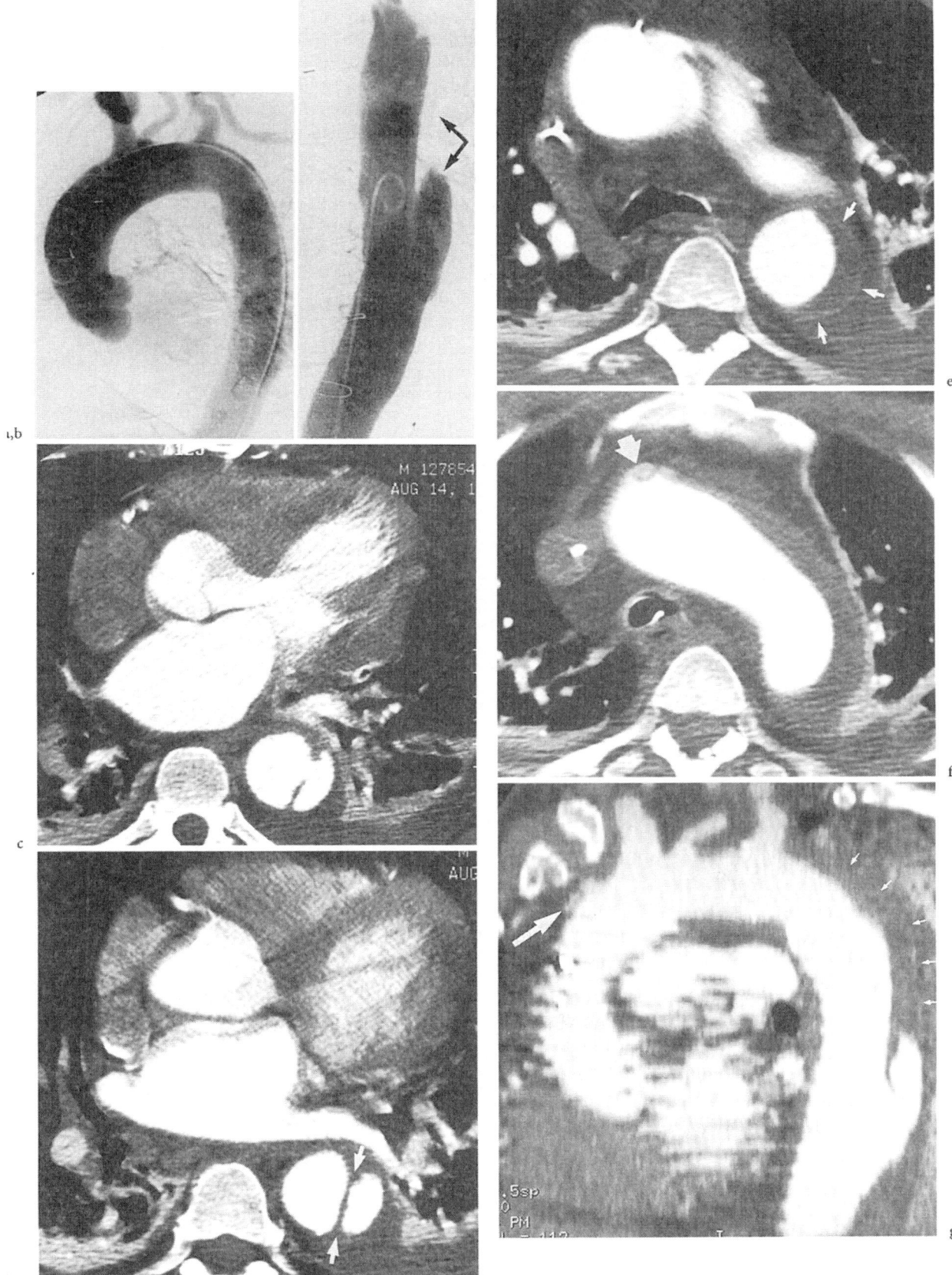

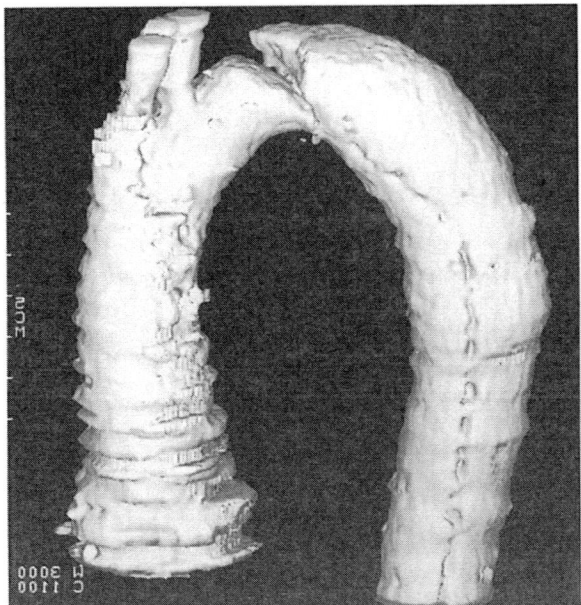

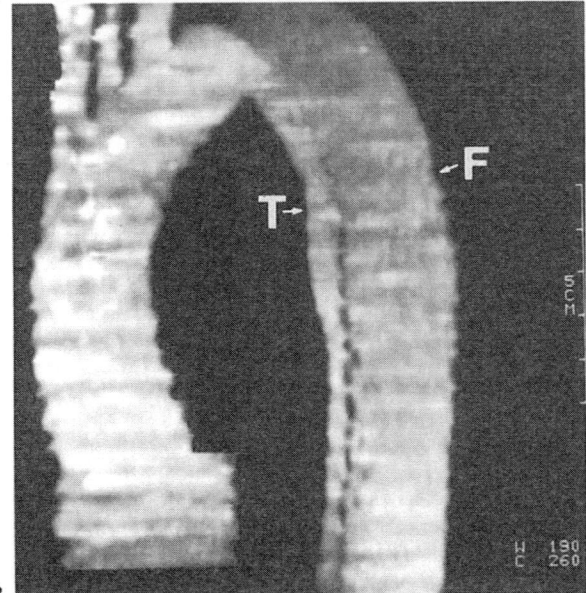

dering technique for delineating the intimal flap be-cause the flap is the lowest attenuation structure found within the blood vessel and therefore is lost in the maximum intensity projection process. The only clue available indicating the presence of a true and a false lumen is when differential enhancement between these two lumina occurs due to slower flow within the false lumen (TOULIOPOULOS and COSTELLO 1995). SSDs typically define the course of the intimal flap at its intersection with the vessel wall (Fig. 5.20). In order to visualize the intimal flap within the aorta using SSDs, a double threshold tech-nique is required so that only the wall and intimal flap of the aorta are rendered (ADACHI et al. 1994; KOBAYASHI 1995). The upper threshold is selected at approximately 100–150 HU, and the lower threshold is selected between 0 and 50 HU. Using this technique it is possible to visualize intimal flaps within the lu-mina of the blood vessel; however, considerable trial and error is required to identify the optimum thresh-old levels. Surface displays can be particularly help-ful in the presence of pseudoaneurysm formation.

Perhaps the easiest and frequently most helpful technique for evaluating aortic dissection is the curved planar reformation (Fig. 5.21). The single-

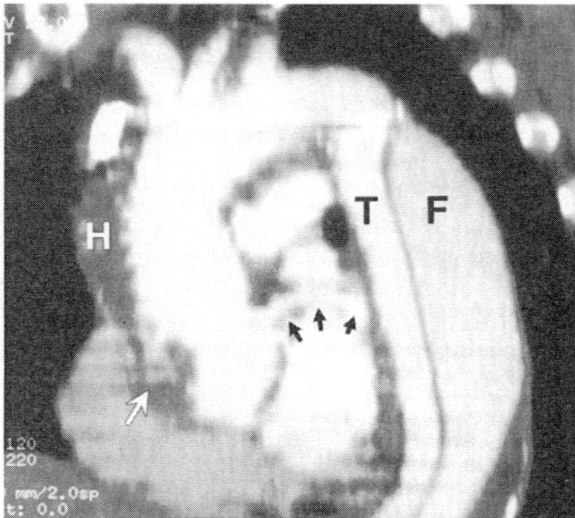

Fig. 5.20. a SSD of a CT angiogram (3-mm collimation, 2.0 pitch, 2-mm reconstruction interval) in a patient with a type B thoracic-aortic dissection demonstrates the intimal flap at its intersection with the wall of the aorta. b Maximum intensity projection demonstrates the intimal flap only in regions where the intimal flap is tangential with the maximum intensity pro-jection view. Superiorly the intimal flap cannot be directly visualized; however, its position is inferred because of the differential enhancement that can be seen between the lesser attenuating false lumen (F) and the greater attenuating true lumen (T). These variations in luminal enhancement cannot be appreciated on the SSD. (From RUBIN and COSTELLO 1994)

Fig. 5.21. Curved planar reformation CT angiogram (3-mm collimation, 2.0 pitch, 2-mm reconstruction interval) demon-strating a dissection flap originating 5-cm distal to the left subclavian artery. The false lumen (F) is differentiated from the true lumen (T) by its lesser attenuation due to delayed flow of contrast media into the false lumen. An extensive ascend-ing aortic mural hematoma (H) is present anteriorly with extravasation of contrast material (white arrow) from the true aortic lumen into this predominately thrombosed false lumen at the aortic root. The origin of the left main and course of the left circumflex coronary artery is demonstrated (black arrows)

voxel-thick view enables clear delineation of the intimal flap relative to aortic branches and is capable of delineating complex flap anatomy free of averaging. Ray sum projections have been described as being preferable to maximum intensity projections for demonstrating the intimal flap (ZEMAN et al. 1995). While it is true that the intimal flap is frequently delineated on a ray sum projection, it tends to suffer from significant blurring due to the averaging that occurs through the subvolume and in my experience is not as helpful as the curved planar reformation. The application of spiral CT to imaging the thoracic aorta is described in detail later within this volume.

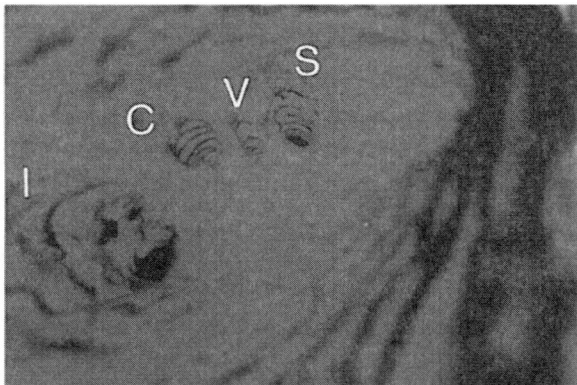

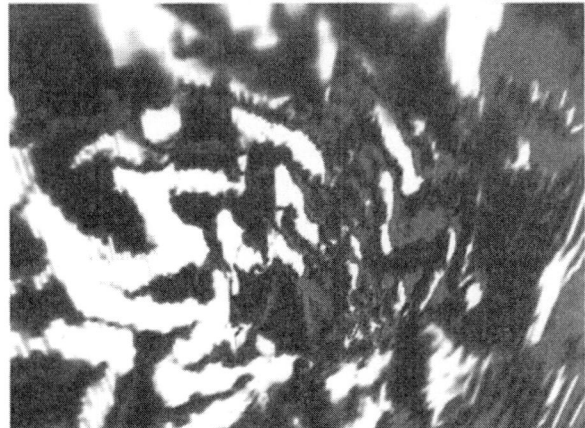

Fig. 5.22. a Perspective volume rendering of a CT angiogram (3-mm collimation, 2.0 pitch, 2-mm reconstruction interval) viewed from the ascending aorta looking into the aortic arch. The innominate artery (*I*), left common carotid artery (*C*), left vertebral artery (*V*), and left subclavian artery (*S*) are visualized. b Perspective volume rendering within the proximal descending aorta looking inferiorly. The metallic struts of a stent-graft are visualized as white, while the aortic wall is red. The Dacron covering the stent cannot be differentiated from the interior of the aortic wall. Perspective volume rendering may become a valuable technique for evaluating the vasculature with spiral CT without the need for time-consuming and artifact-producing editing

Perspective volume rendering may be useful in the future for assessing the thoracic aorta and its branches as editing of the data is not required prior to rendering and high-quality aortic editing is highly time consuming (Fig. 5.22).

5.5.2.3 Pulmonary Vasculature

Perhaps one of the most elegant applications of spiral CT for imaging the vasculature is in imaging arteriovenous malformations (REMY et al. 1992). Iodinated contrast material is not required. Once a high-resolution volumetric acquisition has been acquired, SSDs have been demonstrated to be very effective in demonstrating the angioarchitecture of arteriovenous malformations. These techniques are described in detail later within this volume. Although maximum intensity projections can be used to view arteriovenous malformations, the degree of vessel overlap associated with these lesions makes it very difficult to interpret the maximum intensity projections. One application for the maximum intensity projection is the visualization of embolic material, typically coils, within the feeding arteries (Fig. 5.6).

Shaded surface displays can additionally be of value in demonstrating anomalies of the pulmonary arteries (Fig. 5.23). For the evaluation of pulmonary embolus, multiplanar reformations can be helpful in delineating the extent of thrombus; however, there is little role for maximum intensity projections or SSDs.

5.5.3 Peridiaphragmatic Lesions and Chest Wall

Both thoracic and abdominal lesions found in contiguity with the diaphragm have traditionally been difficult to evaluate with transverse sections. Multiplanar reconstructions of thin-section spiral data sets can greatly facilitate characterization of these lesions (BRINK et al. 1994). Three-dimensional images tend to be less helpful in this region because of the importance of displaying relatively small variations in attenuation that may be found when assessing hepatic parenchyma, diaphragmatic muscle or fluid, pulmonary parenchymal consolidation, and tumor masses. In contrast, assessment of the bony structures of the chest wall, specifically the sternum and sternal clavicular joints, is well suited to SSDs (JURIK and ALBRECHTSEN 1994). Multiplanar, particularly curved planar reformations enable visualization of nonossified costal cartilage and soft tissue lesions.

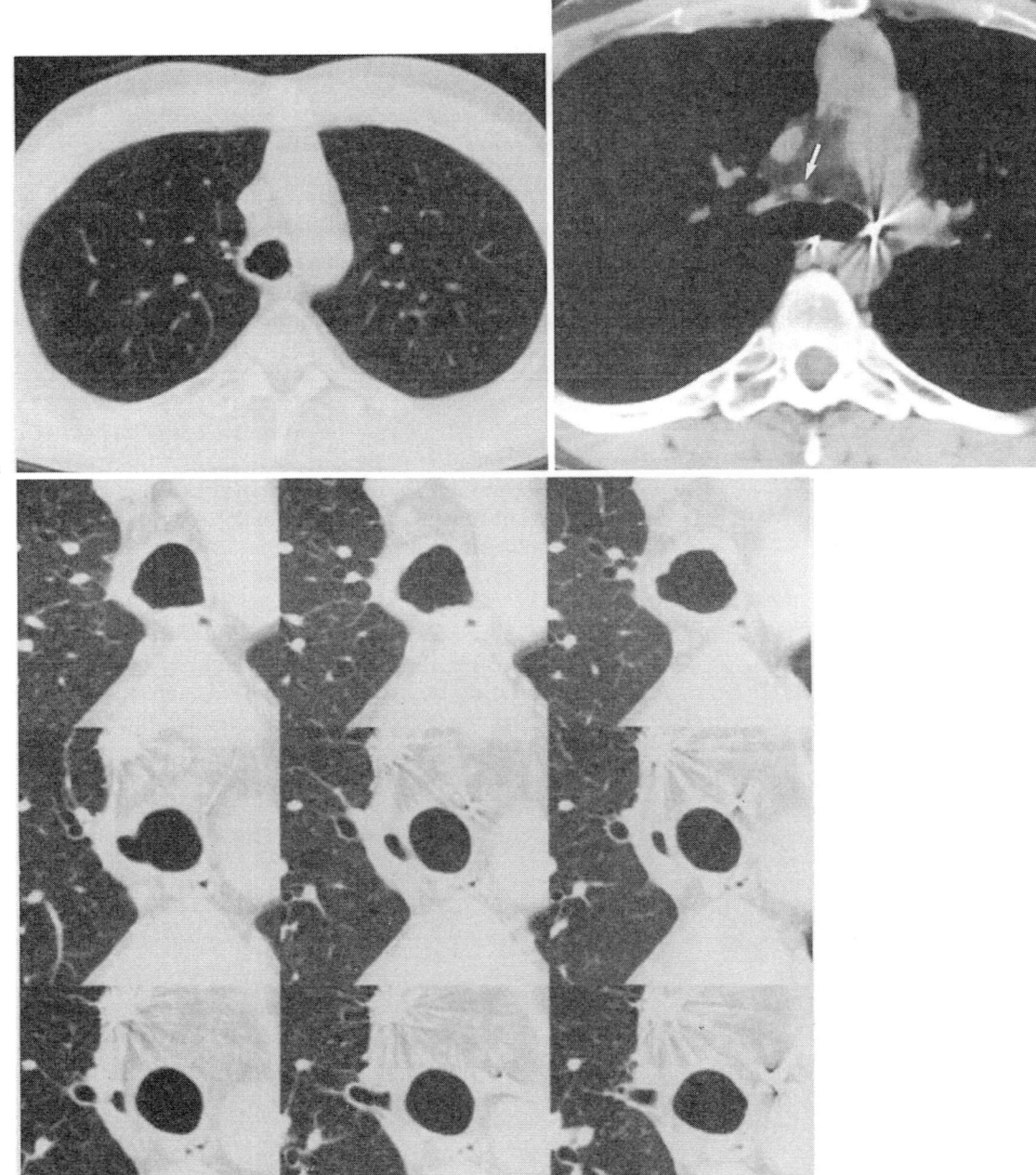

Fig. 5.23. a Eight-millimeter collimated spiral CT section photographed with lung window (L = −700; W = 1500) demonstrating an irregularity about the right lateral wall of the trachea in a patient 10 years following heart-lung transplantation for primary pulmonary hypertension and 7 years following repeat cardiac transplantation for accelerated coronary artery disease. **b** Mediastinal window (L = 40; W = 400) created 3 cm inferiorly demonstrates a rounded mediastinal opacity that might be interpreted as a normal lymph node (*arrow*). **c** Images through the tracheal abnormality obtained with 1-mm collimation, 2.0 pitch, and 1-mm reconstruction interval demonstrate a aberrant tracheal bronchus giving rise to the apical and posterior segmental bronchi of the right upper lobe. **d** Following intravenous contrast administration, the nodular opacity within the mediastinum is enhancing similarly to the pulmonary arteries, this being suggestive of an aberrant right upper lobe pulmonary arterial branch. **e** Curved planar reformation of the proximal tracheal-bronchial tree demonstrates the course of the aberrant right upper lobe bronchus and its position relative to the tracheal carina. **f,g** SSDs of the central pulmonary arteries demonstrate three arterial branches supplying the right upper lobe rather than a single truncus anterior. The identification of this aberrant vasculature may be particularly important if a third mediastinotomy is required in this patient, who undoubtedly has mediastinal adhesions following two prior mediastinotomies

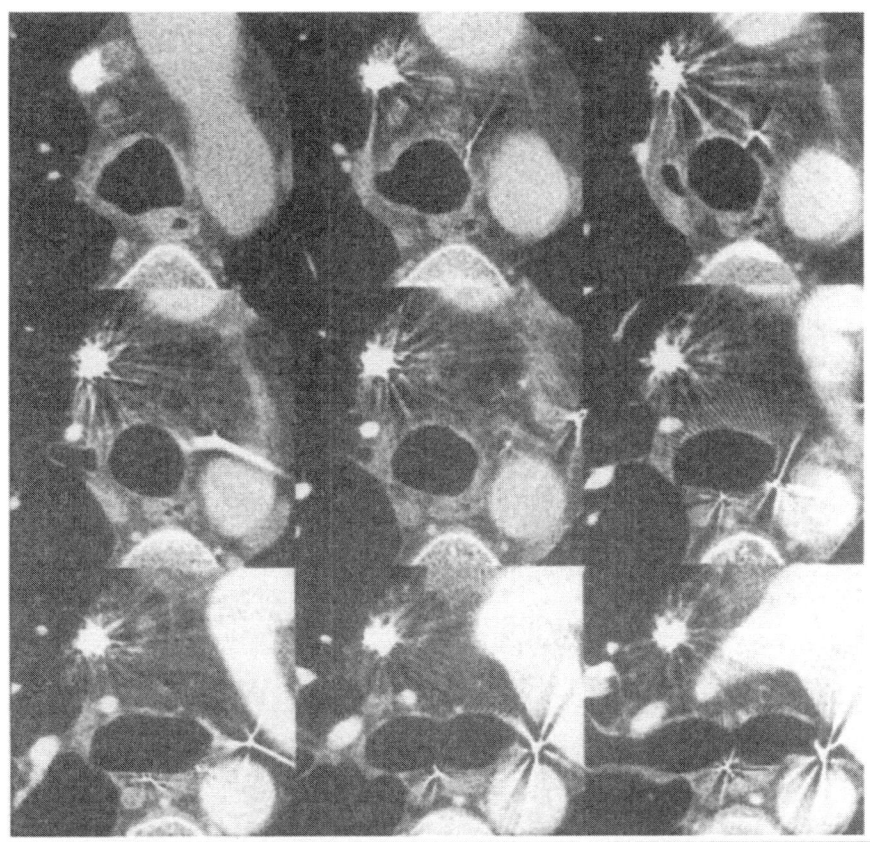

d

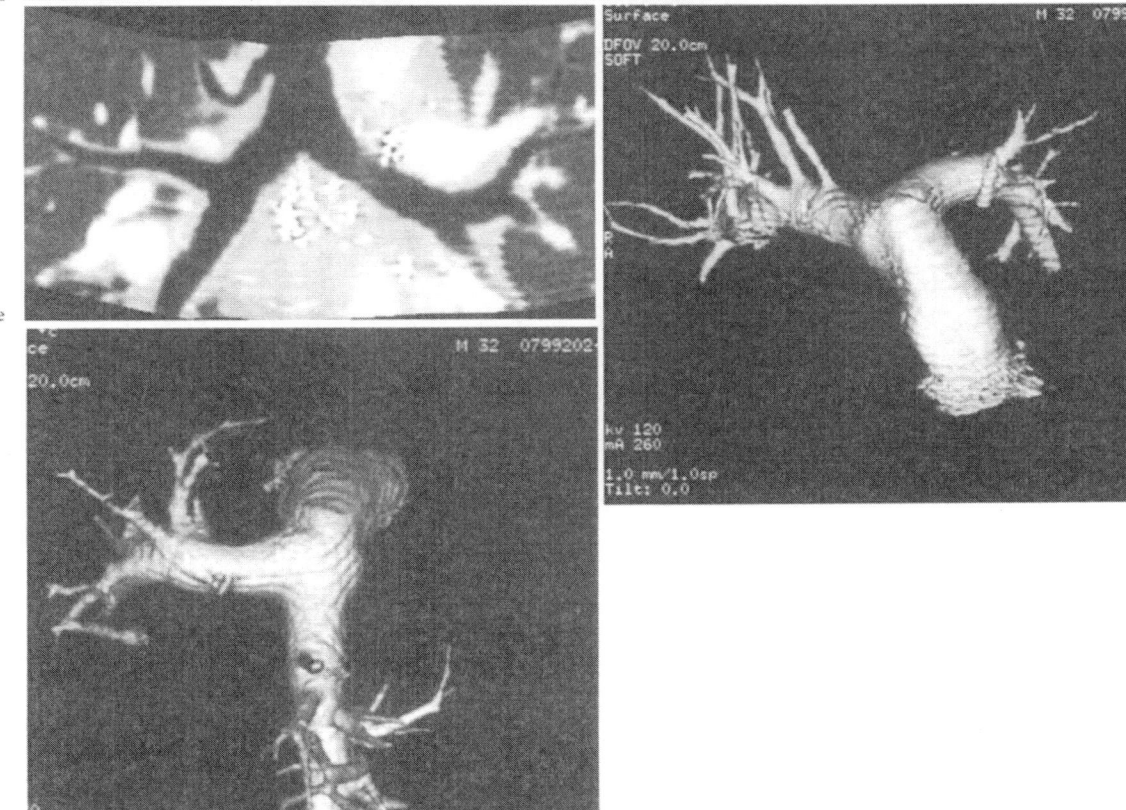

e

f

g

Fig. 5.23d–g

5.6 Limitations of Multiplanar Reformations and Three-Dimensional Renderings

Although the specific limitations of each post-processing technique have been previously described, it is critical to point out that any technique used to view the CT data through any plane other than the transverse plane or projection other than the craniocaudal projection results in an image with anisotropic pixels. The in-plane resolution is defined by the reconstruction kernel and field of view, whereas the through-plane or z-axis resolution is defined by the collimator width, pitch, and interpolation algorithm. Therefore, as the angle of the reformation plane increases relative to the plane of acquisition, spatial resolution decreases. The highest resolution views for evaluating spiral CT scans, regardless of application, are the unedited transverse CT sections. They should always be carefully reviewed at appropriate window and level settings regardless of additional rendering techniques employed.

Additionally, the use of maximum intensity projections and SSDs frequently requires preliminary editing of the CT sections. Whenever editing is employed there is a danger that structures of importance will be inadvertently removed. Renderings generated from edited data should always be reviewed with the source transverse sections.

5.7 Conclusion

Spiral CT data offer considerably greater flexibility for reconstruction than conventional CT. As a result, image quality is highly dependent on the selection of reconstruction parameters as well as the scan parameters. Because spiral CT data are volumetric, multiplanar and 3-D renderings are of higher quality than when created from conventional CT data. As a result these rendering techniques are finding increasing utility as adjuncts to transverse sections for the diagnosis and characterization of thoracic abnormalities. A thorough understanding of the benefits and limitations of these techniques is required prior to relying upon them for diagnosis.

References

Adachi H, Ino T, Mizuhara A, Yamaguchi A, Kobayashi Y, Nagai J (1994) Assessment of aortic disease using three-dimensional CT angiography. J Card Surg 9:673–678

Brink JA, Heiken JP, Balfe DM, Sagel SS, DiCroce J, Vannier MW (1992) Spiral CT: decreased spatial resolution in vivo due to broadening of section-sensitivity profile. Radiology 185:469–474

Brink JA, Heiken JP, Semenkovich J, Teefey SA, McClennan BL, Sagel SS (1994) Abnormalities of the diaphragm and adjacent structures: findings on multiplanar spiral CT scans. AJR 163:307–310

Buckley JA, Scott WW, Siegelman SS et al. (1995) Pulmonary nodules: effect of increased data sampling on detection with spiral CT and confidence in diagnosis. Radiology 196:395–400

Cline HE, Dumoulin CL, Hart HRJ, Lorensen WE, Ludke S (1987) 3D reconstruction of the brain from magnetic resonance images using a connectivity algorithm. Magn Reson Imaging 5:345–352

Cline HE, Lorensen WE, Souza SP et al. (1991) 3D surface rendered MR images of the brain and its vasculature. J Comput Assist Tomogr 15:344–351

Crawford CR, King KF (1990) Computed tomography scanning with simultaneous patient translation. Med Phys 17:967–982

Dillon EH, van Leeuwen MS, Fernandez MA, Mali WPTM (1993) Spiral CT angiography. AJR 160:1273–1278

Drebin RA, Carpenter L, Hanrahan P (1988) Volume rendering. Comput Graphics 22:65–74

Fishman EK, Magid D, Ney DR et al. (1991) Three-dimensional imaging. Radiology 181:321–337

Jurik AG, Albrechtsen J (1994) Spiral CT with three-dimensional and multiplanar reconstruction in the diagnosis of anterior chest wall joint and bone disorders. Acta Radiol 35:468–472

Kalender WA, Seissler W, Klotz E, Vock P (1990) Spiral volumetric CT with single-breath-hold technique, continuous transport, and continuous scanner rotation. Radiology 176:181–190

Kalender WA, Polacin A, Süss C (1994) A comparison of conventional and spiral CT: an experimental study on the detection of spherical lesions. J Comput Assist Tomogr 18:167–176

Keller PJ, Drayer BP, Fram EK, Williams KD, Dumoulin CL, Souza SP (1989) MR angiography with two-dimensional acquisition and three-dimensional display. Radiology 173:527–532

Kobayashi Y (1995) Scanning techniques and three-dimensional reconstruction. In: Adachi H, Nagai J (eds) Three-dimensional CT angiography. Little, Brown and Company, Boston, pp 63–76

Levoy M (1988) Display of surfaces from volume data. IEEE Comput Graph Appl 8:29–37

Magnusson M, Lenz R, Danielsson PE (1991) Evaluation of methods for shaded surface display of CT volumes. Comput Med Imaging Graph 15:247–256

Napel SA (1995) Basic principles of spiral CT. In: Fishman EK, Jeffrey RB (eds) Principles and techniques of 3D spiral CT angiography. Raven Press, new York, pp 167–182

Napel S, Bergin CJ, Paranjpe DV, Rubin GD (1992a) Maximum and minimum intensity projection of spiral CT data for simultaneous 3D imaging of the pulmonary vasculature and airways (abstract). Radiology 185(P):126

Napel S, Marks MP, Rubin GD et al. (1992b) CT angiography with spiral CT and maximum intensity projection. Radiology 185:607–610

Napel S, Rubin GD, Jeffrey RB Jr. (1993) STS-MIP: a new reconstruction technique for CT of the chest. J Comput Assist Tomogr 17:832–838

Ney DR, Fishman EK, Niederhuber JE (1992) Three-dimensional display of hepatic venous anatomy generated from spiral computed tomography data: preliminary experience. J Digit Imaging 5:242–245

Pelc NJ, Colsher JG (1987) Principles of x-ray computed tomography. In: Taveras JM, Ferrucci JT (eds) Radiology. Diagnosis, imaging, and intervention. J.B. Lippincott, Philadelphia Chap. 30, pp 1–11

Polacin A, Kalender WA, Marchal G (1992) Evaluation of section sensitivity profiles and image noise in spiral CT. Radiology 185:29–35

Quint LE, Whyte RI, Kazarooni EA et al. (1995) Stenosis of the central airways: evaluation by using helical CT with multiplanar reconstructions. Radiology 194:871–877

Rémy J, Rémy-Jardin M, Wattinne L, Deffontaines C (1992) Pulmonary arteriovenous malformations: evaluation with CT of the chest before and after treatment. Radiology 182:809–816

Rubin GD (1994) Three-dimensional helical CT angiography. Radiographics 14:905–912

Rubin GD, Costello P (1994) Three-dimensional spiral CT angiography. In: Taveras JM, Ferrucci JT (eds) Radiology: diagnosis, imaging, and intervention. J.B. Lippincott, Philadelphia, pp 1–16

Rubin GD, Jeffrey RB (1994) Spiral CT angiography of the abdomen and thorax. In: Fishman EK, Jeffrey RB (eds) Spiral CT principles, techniques and clinical applications. Raven Press, New York, pp 183–196

Rubin GD, Napel S (1995) Increased scan pitch for vascular and thoracic spiral CT. Radiology 197:316–317

Rubin GD, Silverman SG (1995) Helical CT of the retroperitoneum. Radiol Clin North Am 33:903–932

Rubin GD, Dake MD, Napel S, Jeffrey RBJ (1993a) Three-dimensional CT angiography as an alternative to conventional arteriography in planning and in vivo evaluation of aortic stent grafts. Radiology 189(P):112

Rubin GD, Dake MD, Napel SA, McDonnell CH, Jeffrey RBJ (1993b) Abdominal spiral CT angiography: initial clinical experience. Radiology 186:147–152

Rubin GD, Dake MD, Napel S et al. (1994) Spiral CT of renal artery stenosis: comparison of three-dimensional rendering techniques. Radiology 190:181–189

Rubin GD, Dake MD, Semba CB (1995) Current status of three-dimensional spiral CT scanning for imaging the vasculature. Radiol Clin North Am 33:51–70

Rubin GD, Beaulieu CF, Argiro V et al. (1996) Perspective volume rendering of CT and MR images: applications for endoscopic imaging. Radiology 199:321–330

Rubin GD, Napel S, Leung A (1996) Volumetric analysis of volume data: achieving a paradigm shift. Radiology (in press)

Rusinek H, Mourino MR, Firooznia H, Weinreb JC, Chase NE (1989) Volumetric rendering of MR images. Radiology 171:269–272

Seltzer SE, Judy PF, Adams DF et al. (1995) Spiral CT of the chest: comparison of cine and film-based viewing. Radiology 197:73–78

Silverman PM, Zeiberg AS, Sessions RB, Troost TR, Davros WJ, Zeman RK (1995) Helical CT of the upper airway: normal and abnormal findings on three-dimensional reconstructed images. AJR 165:541–546

Touliopoulos P, Costello P (1995) Helical (spiral) CT of the thorax. Radiol Clin North Am 33:843–861

Vining DJ, Shifrin RY, Haponik EF, Liu K, Choplin RH (1994) Virtual bronchoscopy. Radiology 193(P):261

Vock P, Soucek M, Daepp M, Kalender WA (1990) Lung: spiral volumetric CT with single-breath-hold technique. Radiology 176:864–867

Wang G, Vannier MW (1994a) Longitudinal resolution in volumetric x-ray CT – analytical comparison between conventional and helical CT. Med Phys 21:429–433

Wang G, Vannier MW (1994b) Stair-step artifacts in three-dimensional helical CT: an experimental study. Radiology 191:79–83

Zeman RK, Berman PM, Silverman PM et al. (1995) Diagnosis of aortic dissection: value of helical CT with multiplanar reformation and three-dimensional rendering. AJR 164:1375–1380

6 Volumetric CT in the Evaluation of Focal Pulmonary Disease

D.P. Naidich

CONTENTS

6.1 Introduction

Few technological changes have so rapidly transformed imaging as has the development of continuous volumetric (spiral or helical) CT. Initially described by Kalender et al. (1990) volumetric scanning involves continuous data acquisition while the patient is advanced at a constant rate through the CT gantry. This allows scans then to be reconstructed at arbitrary levels through the selected scan volumes using a variety of interpolation algorithms. The result is an almost limitless set of potential images obtained without interscan delay.

A number of important advantages result from volumetric data acquisition. One is a significant reduction in the time of examination: most commercially available scanners are now capable of imaging the entire thorax in a single breathhold. As important, as documented by Costello et al. (1992), volumetric acquisition consistently reduces contrast media requirements. Furthermore, contrast administration can now be timed more precisely, allowing high-quality images to be consistently obtained at preselected phases of enhancement. Technology also has been developed that provides for initial sampling of select regions of interest as contrast is being administered, allowing image acquisition to be triggered at predetermined levels of tissue enhancement (Silverman et al. 1995). Finally, the ability to retrospectively obtain overlapping reconstructions with-

out the need to rescan patients has led to improved multiplanar imaging as well as the development of a variety of 3D imaging techniques, including the new field of CT angiography and virtual bronchoscopy (Heiken et al. 1993; Ibukuro et al. 1995).

Given these advantages, it is hardly surprising that, to date, volumetric scanning has been successfully applied to imaging nearly all intrathoracic pathology (Naidich 1994). The purpose of this chapter will be to review current indications for the use of volumetric techniques in the evaluation of focal lung disease, with particular emphasis on pulmonary nodules (Table 6.1). Emphasis will be placed first on principles of nodule detection; following this, attention will be directed towards the various uses of volumetric scanning in nodule characterization.

6.2 Nodule Detection

From the outset it has been appreciated that one of the most important uses of volumetric data acquisition would be for detecting pulmonary nodules (Costello et al. 1991; Heywang-Koebrunner et al. 1992; Kalender et al. 1990; Vock and Soucek 1993; Vock et al. 1990). In an early study of 40 patients evaluated with both conventional computed tomography (CCT) and volumetric CT, Heywang-Koebrunner et al. (1992) found that while 245 nodules were identified by both techniques, an additional 22 nodules were only identified with spiral CT whereas only four additional nodules were identified with CCT (Heywang-Koebrunner et al. 1992). Similarly, Remy-Jardin et al. (1993) compared thick-section spiral CT without overlapping reconstructions with conventional CT in 39 patients with suspected pulmonary nodules. Using 10-mm collimation, these authors, too, found that the mean number of nodules identified per patient was significantly higher with spiral CT than with CCT; this was especially true with respect to small peripheral nodules of less than 5 mm. Nonetheless, in only three of 39 patients in whom CCT identified a solitary nodule

D.P. Naidich, MD, Department of Radiology, New York University Medical Center/Bellevue Hospital, 27th Street and 1st Avenue, New York, NY 10016, USA

Table 6.1. Focal lung disease: indications for volumetric CT (modified from NAIDICH and GARAY 1991)

1. Detection
      Pulmonary neoplasia
          Metastatic Dx
          Early lung cancer screening?
2. CT densitometry
      Calcification
          Granulomatous disease (central/diffuse)
          Hamartoma (popcorn)
          Carcinoid tumors (eccentric)
          Bronchogenic carcinoma (eccentric)
      Fat (hamartoma)
      Fluid
          Lung abscess
          Mucoid impaction of the airways
      Contrast enhancement
          Bronchogenic carcinoma
          Carcinoid tumors
          AVMs
3. Morphologic characterization
      Angiocentric disease
          Pulmonary emboli/infarcts
          Pulmonary metastases
          AVMs
      Bronchocentric disease
          Bronchogenic carcinoma
              (+) bronchus sign
          Mucoid impaction/bronchiectasis
              Focal air-trapping
          Bronchopleural fistulae

were additional nodules found. Furthermore, an additional six small nodules not seen by spiral CT were subsequently identified by surgery.

If volumetric CT has been found consistently to identify more lesions than CCT, optimal scan techniques and indications have yet to be established. In particular, it remains unclear what the precise role of overlapping reconstructions should be (BUCKLEY et al. 1995; COLLIE et al. 1994). Theoretically, as established by KALENDER et al. (1994) in a study of phantom spheres of arbitrary diameter and contrast, as compared with CCT, spiral CT should allow greater average contrast and spatial resolution provided that overlapping sections are obtained. This is because while any individual volumetric section will be inferior to corresponding CCT sections due to differences in slice sensitivity profiles, optimal contrast and spatial resolution in CCT studies requires that nodules be precisely centered in the plane of the section. For those nodules that lie between contiguous axial images, contrast and spatial resolution may decline by as much as 50%. In distinction, the contrast and spatial resolution of volumetrically acquired images reconstructed with overlapping reconstruc-

tions may improve small lesion contrast by as much as a factor of 1.8 when compared with CCT (Fig. 6.1).

Despite these calculations, the role of overlapping reconstructions remains controversial. In an early study, COSTELLO et al. (1991), using spiral CT in an

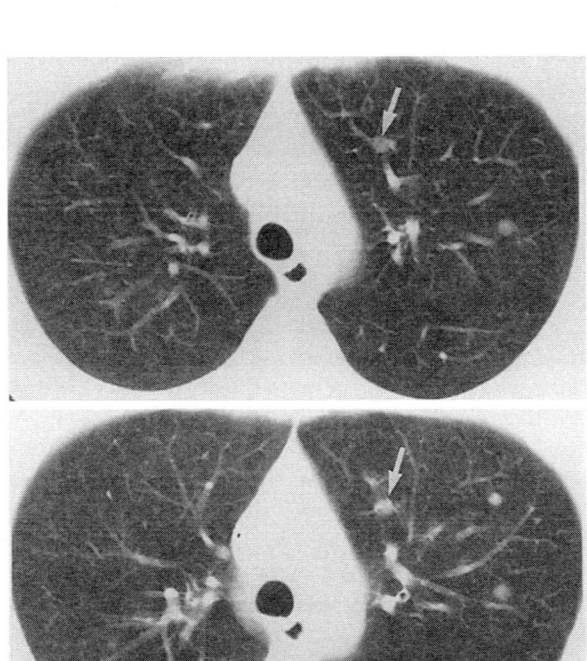

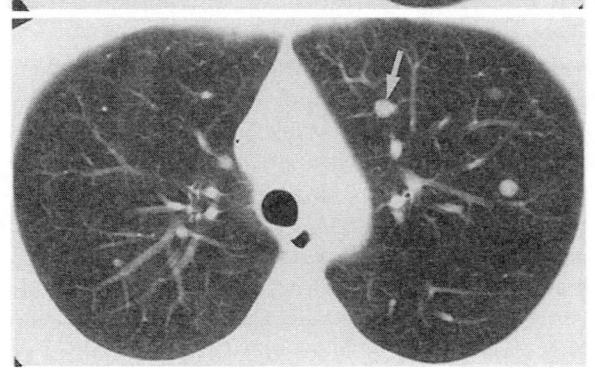

Fig. 6.1a–c. Pulmonary nodule detection: volumetric CT evaluation. **a,b** Contiguous 10-mm sections obtained with a pitch of 1 show multiple pulmonary nodules present in both lungs in a patient with known metastases. Note that while most of these nodules are easily identified, an apparent nodule in the medial portion of the left upper lobe (*arrows*) could be confused with a prominent central vessel. **c** A 10-mm section retrospectively reconstructed from the initial volumetric data centered 5 mm below **a**. A central nodule is now unequivocally present (*arrow*). The ability to retrospectively reconstruct images at any arbitrary level represents one of the most significant advantages of spiral scanning, especially in the detection of pulmonary nodules. (From NAIDICH 1994)

evaluation of 20 patients with suspected pulmonary nodules <1 cm in size, identified four additional lesions when overlapping 8-mm sections were reconstructed every 4 mm. In distinction, COLLIE et al. (1994), in a study evaluating lesion detectability, found that 10-mm sections reconstructed every 5 mm provided no significant advantage compared with scans reconstructed every 10 mm.

More recently, BUCKLEY et al. (1995) retrospectively evaluated 67 spiral CT studies with a total of 116 nodules using four reviewers of varying interpretative skill. Comparing contiguous 8-mm sections with 8-mm sections reconstructed every 4 or 5 mm, these authors showed that significantly more nodules could be identified when overlapping sections were evaluated (583 vs 566, $P < 0.05$): furthermore, they also showed a significant effect on the interpreter's degree of confidence, with more definite nodules and fewer indeterminate nodules identified (482 vs 431 and 101 vs 135, respectively; $P < 0.05$). Although these data appear to suggest that overlapping reconstructions should be consistently used, it should be noted that for experienced readers in this same study the sensitivity for detecting nodules was greater than 90% regardless of whether or not overlapping sections were evaluated! In fact, the most important advantage of the use of overlapping sections appears to lie in a reduction in the number of false-positive nodules, especially for less experienced readers. This problem cannot be overemphasized. In this same study a total of 688 lesions were identified by the four readers: 259 of these proved to be false-positives. Importantly, while 94 (36.3%) were reevaluated as other than nodules when overlapping sections were made available, this still left a sizable percentage of false-positive interpretations. Interestingly, for experienced readers the number of false-positive examinations was greater when overlapping sections were evaluated, suggesting that other factors also were likely influential.

These data cumulatively suggest the following approach to using volumetric CT for detecting nodules: As overlapping reconstructions are time consuming both to generate and to interpret, their routine use is not indicated. Instead, we obtain these retrospectively only in those patients in whom there is an especially high clinical index of suspicion that a nodule(s) is present (for example, patients with known extrapulmonary malignancies with a known predilection for metastasizing to the lungs), and in those in whom detection of additional nodules may lead to a change in clinical management. This includes patients whose initial CT is normal and those

for whom resection of pulmonary metastases is an option.

In addition to these standard techniques, alternative methods of evaluating scans for pulmonary nodules have been proposed. One such approach utilizes cine viewing at a computer workstation in place of film. As shown by SELTZER et al. (1995) in a study of 10-mm collimated spiral images evaluated at 2-mm intervals at frame rates as fast as 10 frames per second, a greater number of simulated nodules was identified with the cine presentation than with film (mean of 0.69 vs 0.58 nodules per case, respectively; $P = 0.006$). The value of this approach awaits further prospective evaluation.

6.3 Nodule Characterization

Although a large number of reports have documented a role for volumetric CT in the identification of pulmonary nodules, relatively few have focused on the role of volumetric data acquisition in characterizing pulmonary nodules. This is somewhat surprising given the large number of studies that have previously been published confirming the value of CCT in assessing focal parenchymal disease, in particular, solitary pulmonary nodules (NAIDICH and GARAY 1991; WEBB 1990). A detailed review of the indications for CT of solitary pulmonary nodules is beyond the scope of the present report: instead, only those aspects of volumetric scanning pertinent to nodule evaluation will be emphasized.

6.3.1 CT Densitometry

From the outset, the potential value of volumetric CT for performing CT densitometry has been identified (KALENDER et al. 1990). Compared with CCT images, volumetric acquisition ensures that contiguous scans will be obtained through the centers of individual nodules. As reproducible sections through the center of lesions are the key to accurate CT densitometry, it is apparent that volumetric acquisition represents an important improvement over conventional high-resolution CT techniques. For anyone who has attempted to obtain contiguous thin sections through small pulmonary nodules in a less than compliant patient, the advantages of volumetric acquisition are clear. By acquiring data in a single breathhold, one can be assured that at least a few representative thin sections will have been attained through the center of a lesion. This is most important for very small lesions where even small differences in respiration between scans may lead to erroneous estimates of the tissue density due to partial volume averaging (Fig. 6.2).

Interestingly, most institutions have abandoned the use of phantom densitometry, despite evidence that comparison of nodules to a standard phantom is still more sensitive than high-resolution CT images alone for detecting calcification (KHAN et al. 1991). In the absence of phantom densitometry, the need for obtaining sections through the center of small lesions is still more critical. Unfortunately, while CT densitometry represents an important component of any evaluation of solitary pulmonary nodules, it is well established that the presence of calcium within nodules as a predictor of benign disease is limited. Approximately 10% of documented lung cancers will have CT evidence of calcification. Although typically these appear as either punctate or eccentric calcifications (and hence are easily identified as likely representing tumoral calcification), in a small percentage of cases lung cancers may be diffusely calcified. Similarly, while the presence of fat within a nodule represents convincing evidence of a hamartoma, this will be present in less than half of cases (SIEGELMAN et al. 1986).

As a consequence, based on an approach first suggested by LITTLETON et al. (1990) using conventional tomography, recent attention has focused on the potential of CT to evaluate patterns of contrast enhancement within nodules (SWENSEN et al. 1992, 1995; YAMASHITA et al. 1995a,b). Based on the assumption that the degree of enhancement within nodules likely represents the vascularity of nodules, which in itself is indicative of malignancy, SWENSEN et al. (1995) evaluated patterns of contrast enhancement in a total of 163 patients with solitary nodules less than 4 cm in size. Following a bolus of 100 cc of intravenous contrast media injected at a constant rate of 2 cc per second, six serial thin-section images were obtained through nodules at 30-s intervals up to 2 min, beginning 30 s after the onset of the injection. In each case a representative CT number was obtained from user-determined regions of interest (ROIs) in order to derive a measurement of peak nodule enhancement. Using this approach, these authors found that malignant neoplasms (median, 40 HU) enhanced to a greater extent than benign lesions (median, 12 HU). Furthermore, using 20 HU as the threshold for identifying a malignant nodule, sensitivity proved to be 100%; specificity,

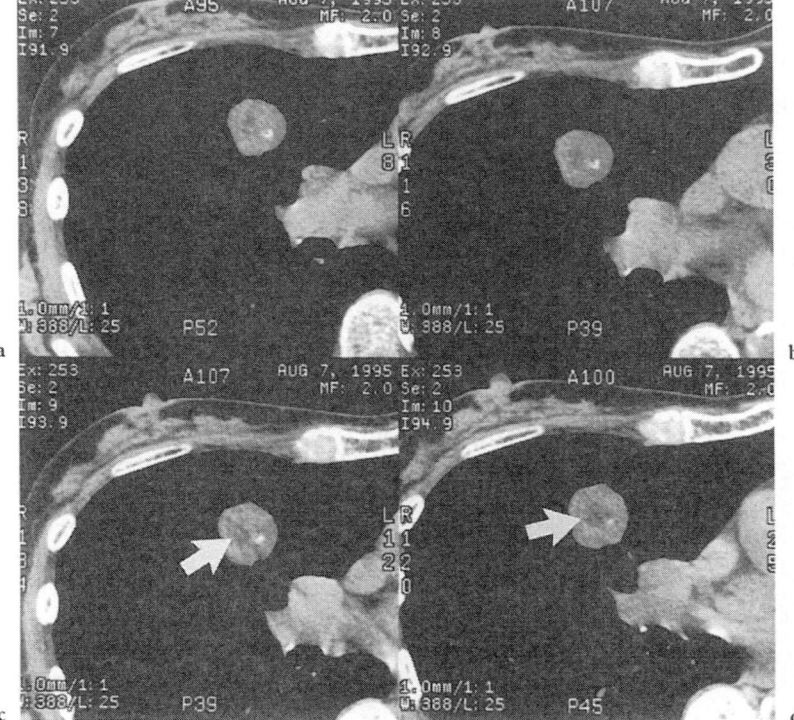

Fig. 6.2a–d. CT densitometry: pulmonary hamartoma. Sequential images obtained through a nodule in the right upper lobe obtained using 1-mm collimation with a pitch of 1. Both fat (*arrows*) and calcium are clearly present within this lesion, findings diagnostic of a pulmonary hamartoma. The ability to obtain 1-mm sections in a single breathhold insures that at least some of the images will be through the center of the lesion, preventing misdiagnoses due to partial volume averaging

76.9%; positive predictive value, 90.2%; negative predictive value, 100%; and accuracy, 92.6% (Figs. 6.3, 6.4).

Similar results have been reported by YAMASHITA et al. (1995a,b). Using 3 cm as a cut-off, these authors evaluated a total of 18 malignant nodules by obtaining axial images at 30 s, 2 min, and 5 mm after the intravenous administration of nonionic contrast media injected at a rate of 2 cc per second (YAMASHITA et al. 1995b). In all cases of malignant nodules there was marked contrast enhancement, always greater than 20 HU. Furthermore, maximum attenuation of these lesions correlated positively with the number of small (0.02–0.10 mm) blood vessels identified histologically.

Surprisingly, despite the apparent success of this technique, these studies all relied on CCT imaging. In fact, the advantages of volumetric data acquisition in this setting should be apparent. In addition to ensuring that scans are obtained through nodules that otherwise may have been missed due to variations in respiration, as importantly, the ability to obtain retrospective overlapping reconstructions ensures that sections through the center of the nodule are obtained, minimizing inaccuracies due to partial volume averaging. Furthermore, the use of retrospective

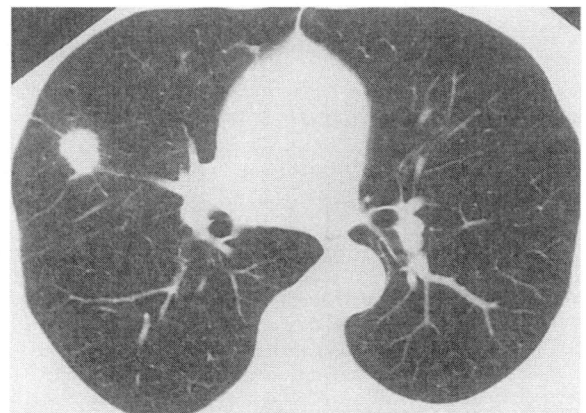

Fig. 6.3a–c. Pulmonary nodule: contrast enhancement – malignant disease. **a** A 5-mm section through the right mid lung shows a spiculated nodule in the right upper lobe with a positive tail sign extending to the pleural surface. **b,c** Select 5-mm sections obtained through this nodule obtained first prior to (**b**) and then 90 s (**c**) following injection of 100 cc of 60% iodinated contrast media at a rate of 2 cc per second. Note that the density measured within the nodule (*lower left corner* of **b** and **c**) changes from a precontrast level of 15 HU to 69.5 HU, indicating considerable vascularity. In initial studies (see text) contrast enhancement greater than 20 HU has been taken as highly suggestive of malignancy. At surgery this proved to be an adenocarcinoma. It should be noted that an optimal method for assessing nodule enhancement has yet to be determined (see text)

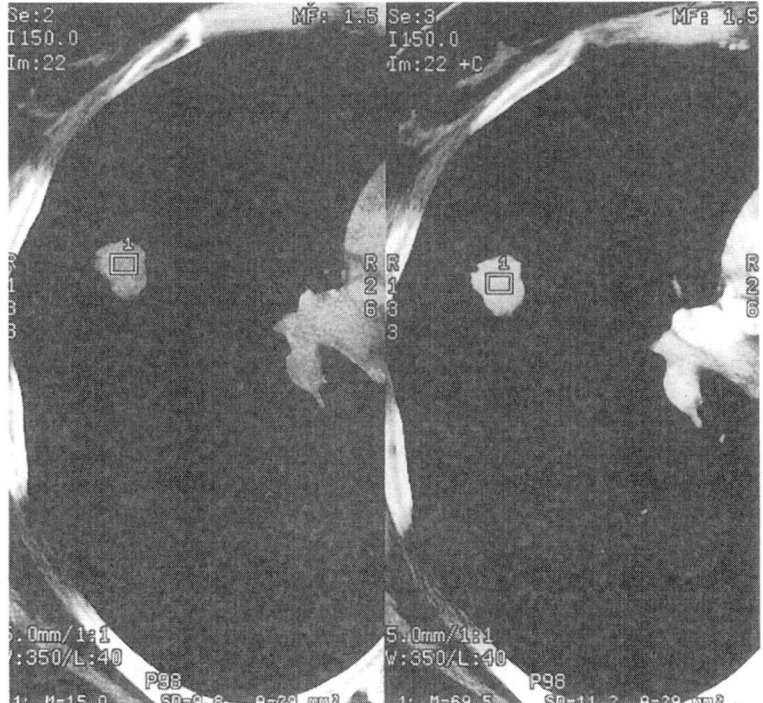

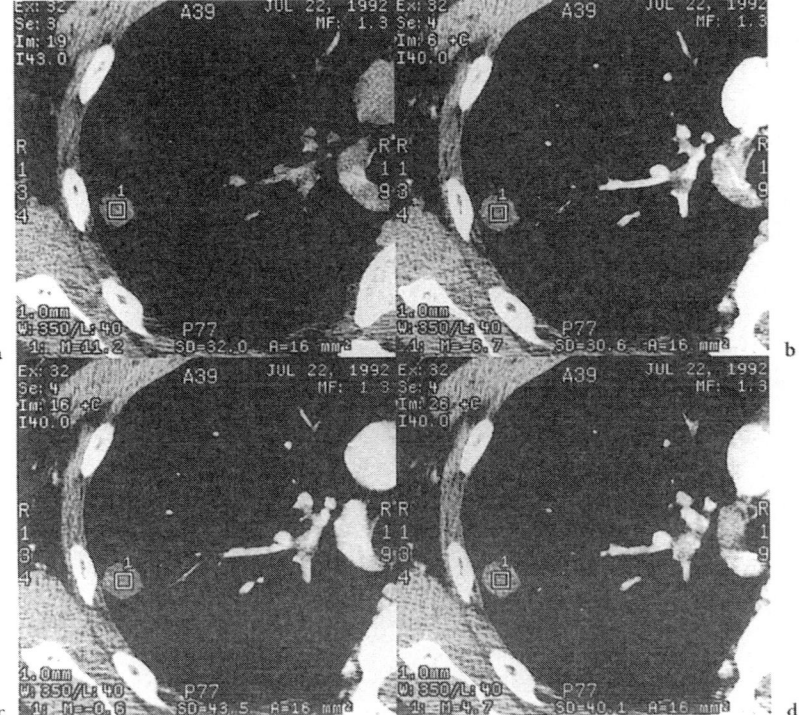

Fig. 6.4a–d. Pulmonary nodule: contrast enhancement – benign disease. Select 1-mm sections obtained at the same level through a small nodule in the right upper lobe first prior to (**a**), then at 30 (**b**), 60 (**c**), and 90 (**d**) s following a bolus of 100 cc of 60% iodinated contrast media injected at a rate of 2 cc per second. Note that the average density within this nodule (lower left corner, **a–d**) never measures more than that mea-sured prior to contrast administration (11.2 HU), confirming absence of vascularity. Cultures from a transthoracic needle aspiration obtained in this AIDS patient confirmed a diagnosis of *Cryptococcus neoformans*. One of the advantages of using volumetric data acquisition to evaluate contrast enhancement is the ability to insure that scans obtained at different times are or are nearly at the exact same level

reconstructions optimizes comparisons between scans taken at different times by allowing more precise identification of sections obtained at the same exact levels.

Despite initial enthusiasm, the role of CT in evaluating patterns of contrast enhancement within nodules remains to be determined. In addition to CT, a number of other modalities are currently under investigation as possible alternative methods for differentiating benign from malignant nodules, including the use both of positron emission tomography with 2-[fluorine-18]fluoro-2-deoxy-D-glucose and magnetic resonance imaging following injection of gadolinium (KONO et al. 1993; PATZ et al. 1993). Given the widespread availability of CT and its well-established role in detecting and characterizing nodules, as against the cost and inaccessibility of positron emission tomography and magnetic resonance imaging scanners, it is likely that a role for helical (or spiral) CT evaluation of contrast enhancement within nodules will become established. In order for this to oc-cur, however, some standardization will be required. In this regard, agreement will have to be reached concerning optimal volume and dose of contrast administration, optimal slice thickness (1 vs 3 mm), algorithms of reconstruction, and the appropriate fields of view. In addition to problems related to scan technique, there is also a need to standardize methods of data evaluation. These include determining the optimal timing of data acquisition, the optimal number of sections to be analyzed, and methods for obtaining representative CT numbers (Figs. 6.3, 6.4).

These caveats aside, there is little doubt that evaluation of patterns of contrast enhancement represents an important new approach to nodule assessment, one in which volumetric data acquisition should play an important role. Currently, as part of an ongoing multi-institutional study, the following approach is recommended: An initial sequence of scans is obtained volumetrically in a single breathhold using 3-mm collimation with a pitch of 1 with overlapping reconstructions obtained every 2 mm, using a standard reconstruction algorithm and a field of view of 15 cm to maximize in-plane spatial resolution (S.J. SWENSEN, personal communication, 1995). Following this, a bolus of between 50 and 175 ml (420 mg I/kg) of intravenous contrast media (300 mg I/ml) is injected at a rate of 2 cc per second; images are then obtained at 60, 120, 180, and 240 s after the start of the injection. For each acquisition the exact same parameters are used as prescribed for the initial nonenhanced sequence of images. From each of these sets of images a minimum of two or three images are selected optimally from the center of the nodule and a representative mean attenuation is then determined using a round or oval ROI, measuring approximately 60% of the diameter of the nodule. While this approach in principle follows the general guidelines set out by initial researchers, it should be emphasized that pending more definitive, multi-institutional trials, numerous methodological modifications may be anticipated. Included among these is a possible role for low-dose CT in minimizing the amount of radiation exposure resulting from repeated scans through the same level, especially in younger patients (ZWIREWICH et al. 1991a).

6.3.2 Morphologic Evaluation

6.3.2.1 Angiocentric Disease

Although volumetric scanning allows more precise morphologic evaluation of lung nodules, largely because of the increased number of contiguous images available for review, in fact little is gained over conventional high-resolution images in assessing most nodule characteristics, including the edge of nodules (smooth versus spiculated), the presence of a halo, and the presence of bubblelike areas of low attenuation. In most series these signs have proved less than definitive in differentiating benign from malignant disease (Gurney et al. 1993; ZWIREWICH et al. 1991a).

In distinction, helical scanning has proved of considerable value in assessing the relationship between focal parenchymal abnormalities and adjacent vessels. In this regard, volumetric CT plays two important and overlapping roles. First, CT defines relationships between focal parenchymal abnormalities and adjacent vessels that cannot be identified on routine chest radiographs. While these findings may be identifiable on routine axial CT images, connec-

tions between nodules and vessels, in particular, may be difficult to establish when 1-mm sections are obtained every 10 mm, as is often the case with high-resolution CT studies. Volumetric high-resolution CT data acquisition through select regions of interest allows confident determination of the hematogenous nature of disease. Included in this category are septic pulmonary emboli and infarcts (including those caused by invasive fungal infections) (Fig. 6.5), hematogenous pulmonary metastases (Fig. 6.6), and the pulmonary vasculitides (GURNEY et al. 1993; NAIDICH and GARAY 1991; PRIMACK et al. 1994).

Additionally, by virtue of its ability to directly visualize blood vessels, CT allows diagnosis of primary vascular pathology including both the pulmonary and systemic circulations. In this category is included pulmonary emboli (both bland and malignant) (Figs. 6.5–6.7), as well as vascular abnormalities seen in association with both acquired and developmental lung disease. This latter group includes arteriovenous malformations (congenital and acquired) and vascular anomalies associated with both intra- and extralobar pulmonary sequestration.

6.3.2.1.1 Pulmonary Emboli/Infarcts. To date, most attention has focused on the role of volumetric CT in

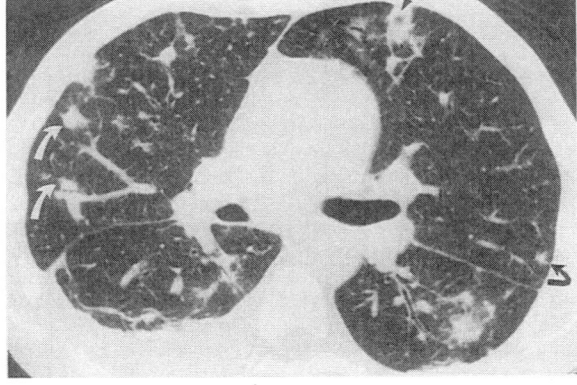

Fig. 6.5. Septic pulmonary emboli. Select 1-mm section obtained through the mid lung shows scattered nodules in both lungs; some are clearly cavitary (*straight arrow*) and many are either associated with peripheral vessels (*curved arrows*) or are subpleural in location associated with a moderate-sized right pleural effusion. This constellation of findings is suggestive of septic pulmonary emboli, in this case confirmed by blood cultures as due to staphylococcal infection. While identification of the relationship between nodules and vessels is frequently easily identified on routine axial images, the use of volumetric acquisition can be of value, especially when small nodules are being assessed

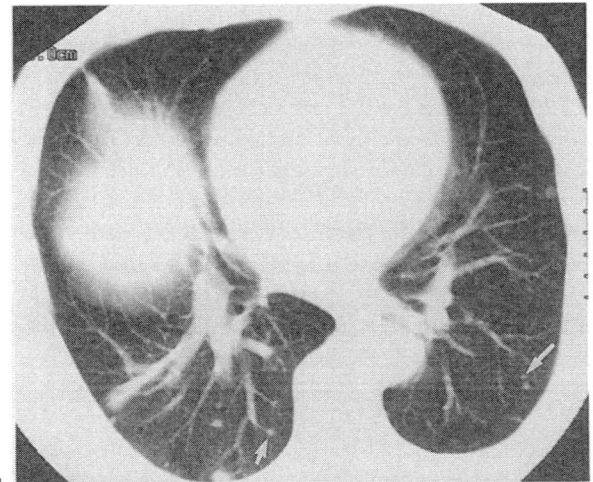

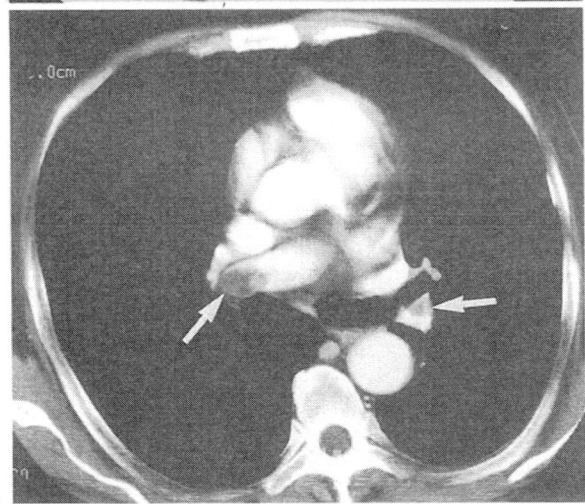

Fig. 6.6a,b. Tumor emboli: adenocarcinoma of the duode-num. **a** A 5-mm section through the lower lobes in a patient with known duodenal carcinoma shows the presence of bilat-eral small, well-defined nodules either adjacent to vessels or subpleural in location (*arrows*). This appearance is strongly suggestive of metastatic disease. **b** Section through the hilum shows discrete filling defects in both the right and the left interlobar pulmonary arteries (*arrows*) consistent with the presence of tumor thrombi. In this case, 10-mm-thick sections were obtained with a pitch of 1 following a bolus of 100 cc of 60% iodinated contrast media following a 20-s delay. Overlap-ping reconstruction every 5 mm were retrospectively obtained only after recognition of intrapulmonary artery filling defects. With the increase in use of volumetric scanners, serendipitous identification of pulmonary thrombi is being increasingly re-ported. One of the advantages of volumetric data acquisition is the ability to retrospectively reconstruct images anywhere within the initial data set without the need to acquire new images or reinject contrast

identifying central pulmonary emboli (RÉMY-JARDIN et al. 1992, 1955a; GOODMAN et al. 1994). As documented by RÉMY-JARDIN et al. (1992) in an early prospective study of 42 patients evaluated with

volumetric CT, there was good correlation between findings at CT and selective pulmonary angiography both in excluding and in identifying central pulmo-nary emboli (Fig. 6.8). Using a combination of signs including direct visualization of intraluminal clot, partial filling defects, "railway tracks," and mural defects, these authors showed that of 23 patients with normal findings on CT, none proved to have angiographic evidence of clot, while a total of 112 central emboli identified by CT (including main, lo-bar, and segmental arteries) corresponded precisely to identical findings on selective angiography. Un-fortunately, in this same study there were a signifi-cant number of false-positive interpretations due to misinterpretation of perivascular areas of decreased attenuation as representing intravascular abnor-malities (RÉMY-JARDIN et al. 1992).

Similar findings have been reported by GOODMAN et al. (1994), who have further emphasized the limita-tions of CT in detecting peripheral thromboem-bolism. In their prospective study of 25 patients with moderate-probability ventilation/perfusion scans, these authors found that while CT had a sensitivity of 91% and a specificity of 86% for segmental and larger pulmonary arteries, sensitivity and specificity de-creased to only 77% and 79%, respectively, when subsegmental emboli were evaluated. It should be emphasized, however, that in this study there were a total of only 14 patients with subsequently verified pulmonary emboli.

Recently, it has been suggested that central emboli may be more accurately evaluated when axial CT images are supplemented by select two-dimensional multiplanar reconstructions, especially for select ar-teries with an oblique course such as the interlobar pulmonary arteries and the middle lobe and lingular arteries (Fig. 6.8) (RÉMY-JARDIN et al. 1995a). Using this approach, these authors showed that among 20 patients with unequivocal pulmonary embolism, 2D reformations improved diagnostic certainty in 13 cases; more importantly, among nine patients with equivocal axial CT studies, 2D reformations allowed confident exclusion of pulmonary embolism in all nine.

Although a potential role for volumetric CT in the assessment of the central pulmonary arteries is likely, precise clinical indications for the use of CT have yet to be defined (GOODMAN et al. 1994). Although CT is of established value in assessing patients with documented central pulmonary emboli as well as patients for whom intravenous contrast administration is contraindicated, and more recently has been shown to be of value in serendipitous

Fig. 6.7a–h. Pulmonary artery sarcoma. **a–d** Enlargements of sequential volumetrically obtained 5-mm sections through the inferior portion of the right hilum show two discrete, otherwise nondescript nodules in the right lower lobe (*arrows* in **b** and **d**). **e–h** Select 5-mm images obtained 20 s following a bolus of 100 cc of 60% nonionic contrast media at a rate of 2 cc per second show the presence of an irregular filling defect within the main (*arrowhead* in **g**) and both the right (*arrows* in **e** and **f**) and left pulmonary arteries. At biopsy this proved to be a primary pulmonary artery sarcoma. Note that at least one of the nodules identified in the right lower lobe has the same density as the tumor noted throughout the right and left main pulmonary arteries (compare *arrow* in **h** with *arrow* in **d**), suggesting that this may actually represent tumor within a focally distended pulmonary artery branch

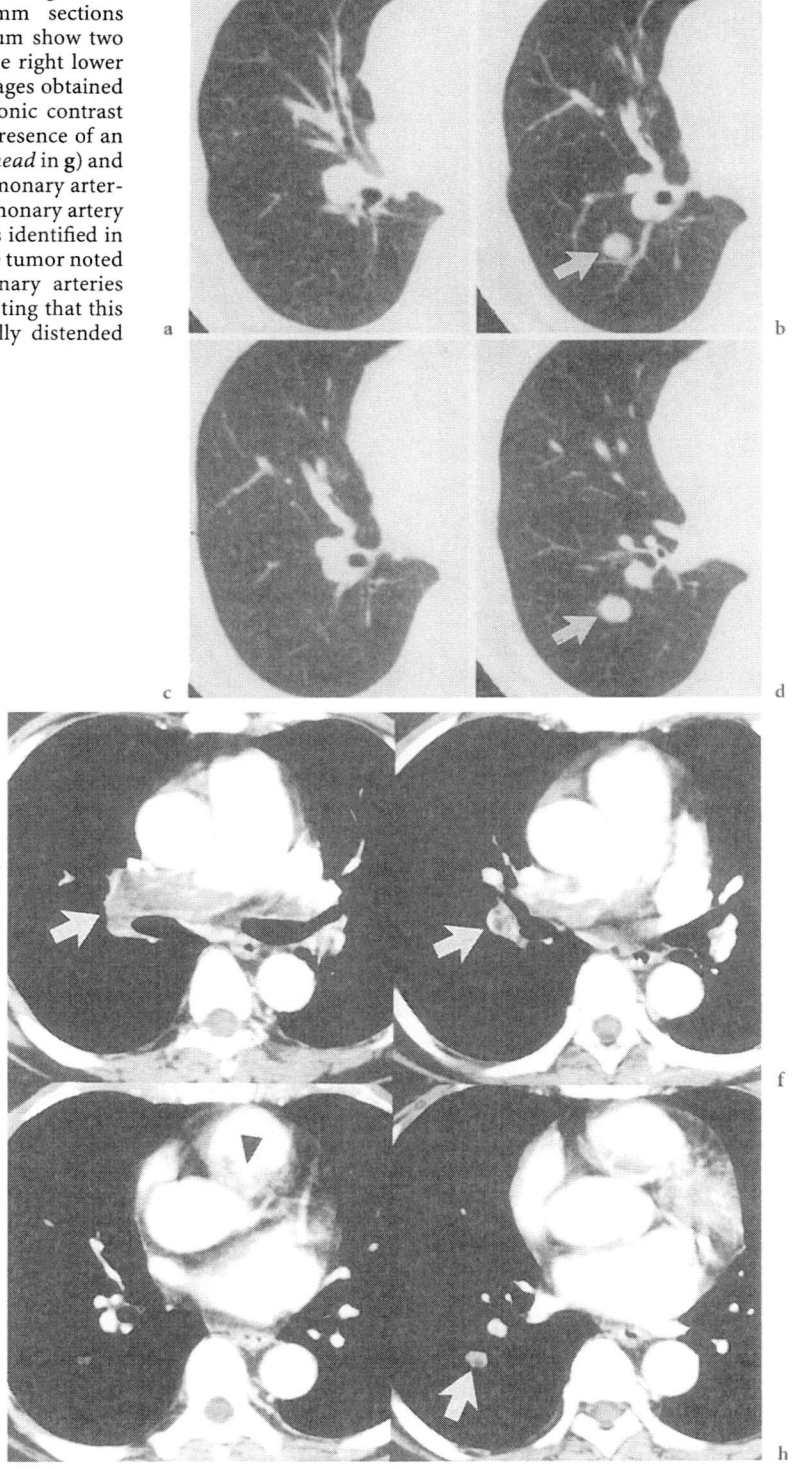

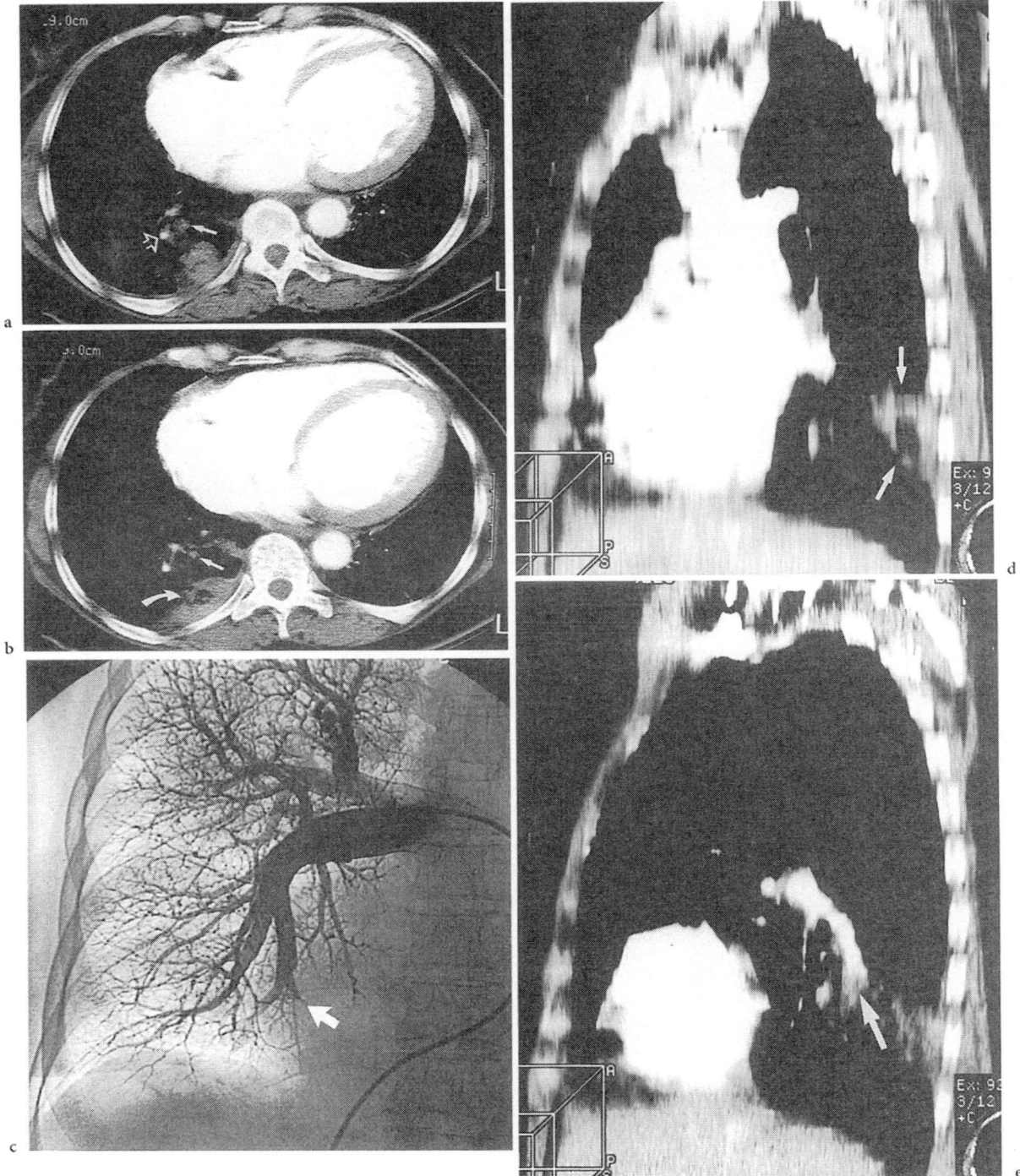

Fig. 6.8a–e. Pulmonary infarction. **a,b** Select 5-mm sections obtained 30 s following a bolus of 100 cc of nonionic contrast media injected at a rate of 3 cc per second with a pitch of 1. A characteristic triangular-shaped subpleural density can be identified in the posterobasilar segment of the right lower lobe (*curved arrow* in **b**). This is associated with a filling defect within the corresponding subsegmental pulmonary artery (*straight arrows* in **a** and **b**). By comparison, note the persistent bright opacification of adjacent subsegmental arteries (*open arrow* in **a**). Note the presence of dilated cardiac chambers in this patient with severe atherosclerotic heart disease.

c Coned-down subtraction view from a selective right main pulmonary angiogram shows that branches of the posterobasilar segmental arteries are cut off (*arrow*), confirming the diagnosis of pulmonary emboli. **d,e** Sagittal reconstructions through the medial portion of the posterobasilar segment of the right lower lobe (**d**) and right hilum (**e**) further confirm the presence of a characteristic subpleural wedge-shaped density consistent with pulmonary infarction (*arrows* in **d**). Note the presence of a filling defect in the distal portion of the right pulmonary artery (*arrow* in **e**)

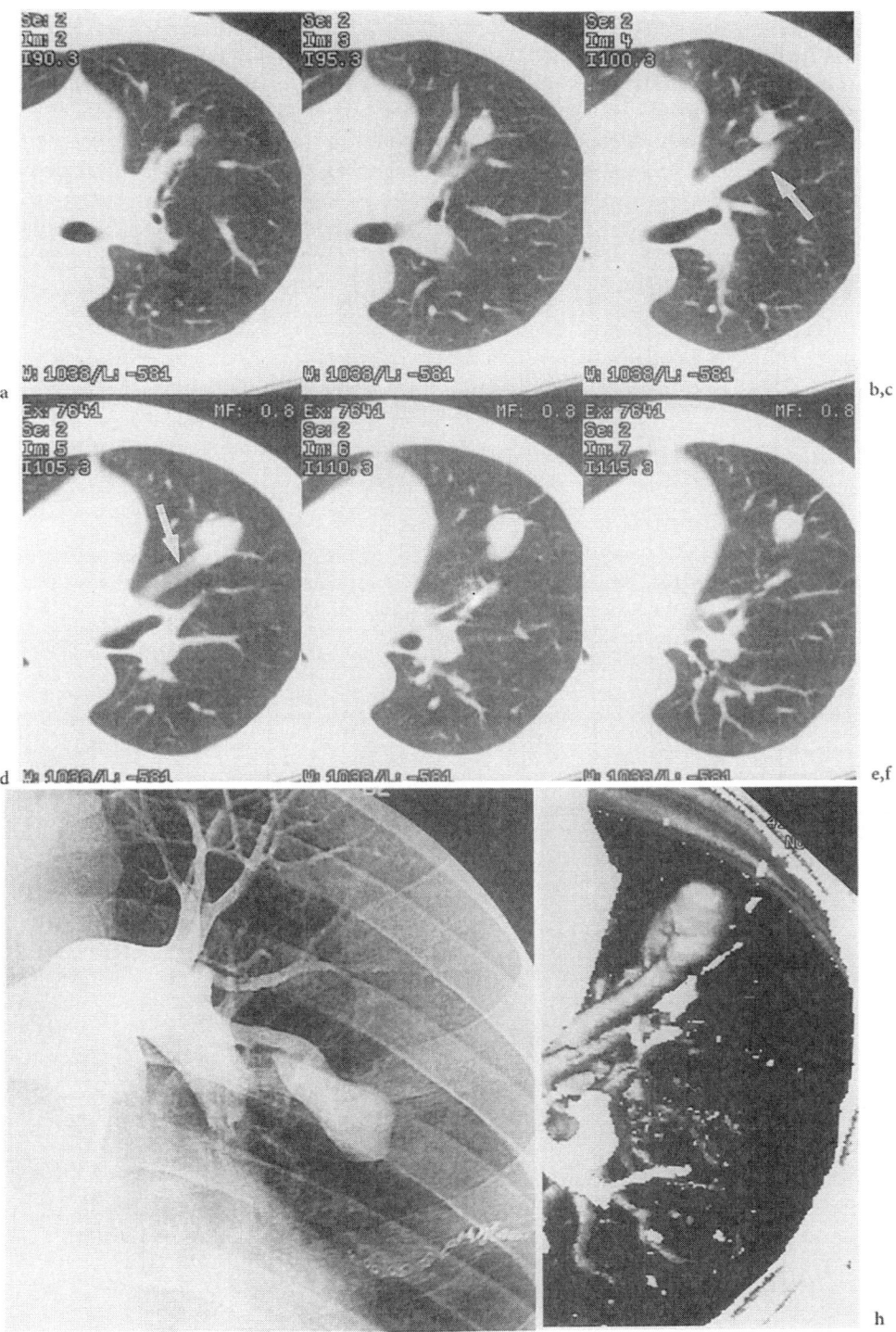

Fig. 6.9a–h. Posttraumatic arteriovenous fistula. a–f Sequential 5-mm helical sections through the left upper lobe show a well-defined nodular density closely related to an enlarged left superior pulmonary vein (*arrows* in **c** and **d**). **g** Coned-down early view from a selective left pulmonary artery injection confirms the presence of an arteriovenous fistula in the left upper lobe with rapid filling of the left upper lobe pulmonary vein. Note the presence of suture material, the result of a previous knife wound several months prior to this admission. **h** 3D surface rendering derived from 5-mm sections reconstructed every 3 mm obtained following a bolus of 100 cc of nonionic intravenous contrast material injected at a rate of 3 cc clearly depicts the enlarged draining pulmonary vein extending to the hilum

diagnosis (WINSTON et al. 1995), as yet no optimal method for performing volumetric CT has been established: this includes choice of scan thickness, rates and quantity of contrast administration, and the need for multiplanar and/or 3D reconstructions. Nor has it been established what role CT will play in any diagnostic algorithm including ventilation/perfusion scintigraphy and pulmonary angiography. Finally, the clinical significance of small peripheral pulmonary emboli detectable

only by pulmonary angiography, especially in the absence of peripheral venous thrombophlebitis, also awaits further prospective evaluation (TELGEN et al. 1995).

6.3.2.1.2 Pulmonary Arteriovenous Malformations.

In addition to identifying intravascular abnormalities, volumetric CT allows detailed assessment of the angioarchitecture of pulmonary arteriovenous malformations (AVMs) (Fig. 6.9). In a study of 109 pa-

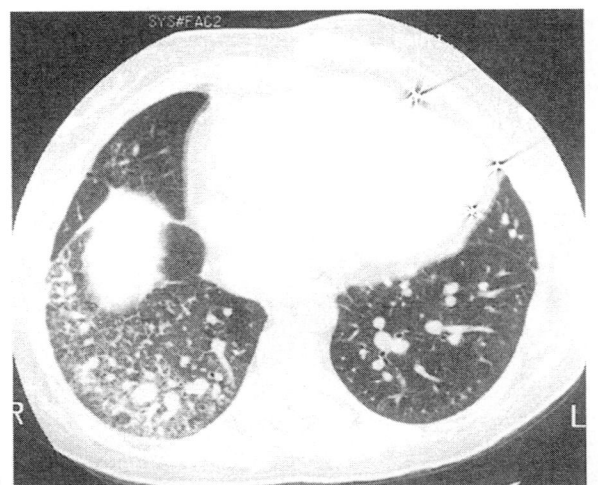

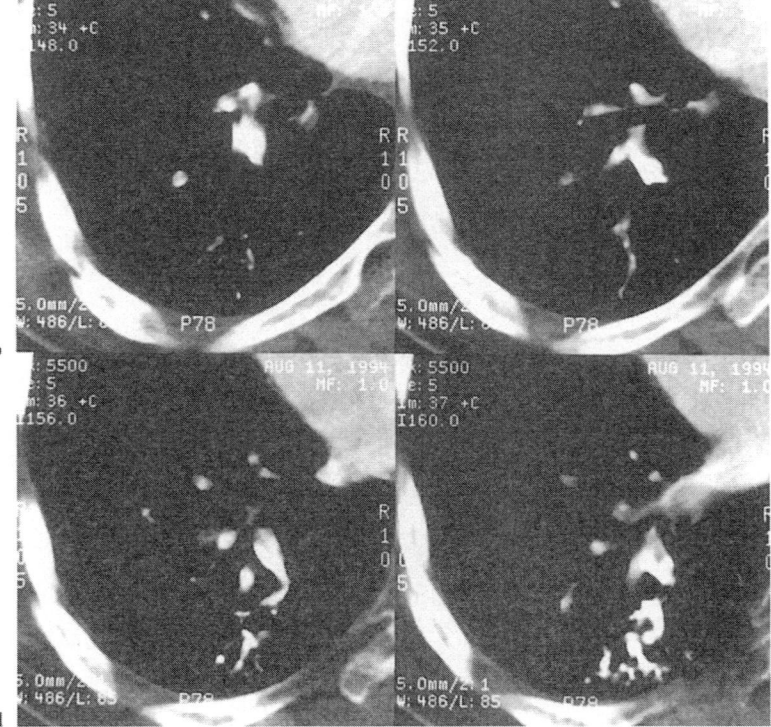

Fig. 6.10a–j. Pulmonary AVMs following a Glenn anastomosis. a 1-mm section through the lower lobes in a 29-year-old female patient with complex congenital heart disease presenting with recurrent hemoptysis following a Glenn (superior vena cava to right pulmonary artery) anastomosis performed 25 years prior to admission for complex congenital heart disease. In these cases, pulmonary AVMs may occur as many as 30 years following surgery. Note the presence of numerous nodular densities in the right lower lobe associated with unilateral ground-glass attenuation. b–i Sequential 5-mm sections obtained through the mid portion of the right lower lobe with a pitch of 2, 20 s following a bolus of 100 cc of nonionic contrast material injected at a rate of 2 cc per second, show diffuse pulmonary AVMs, accounting for this patient's recurrent episodes of hemoptysis. In this case the finding of diffuse ground-glass attenuation throughout the right lower lobe proved to be due to diffuse fibrosis, subsequently confirmed surgically. j 3D surface rendering through the right lower lobe further confirms the presence of AVMs with marked dilatation of the inferior pulmonary vein

Fig. 6.10a–j

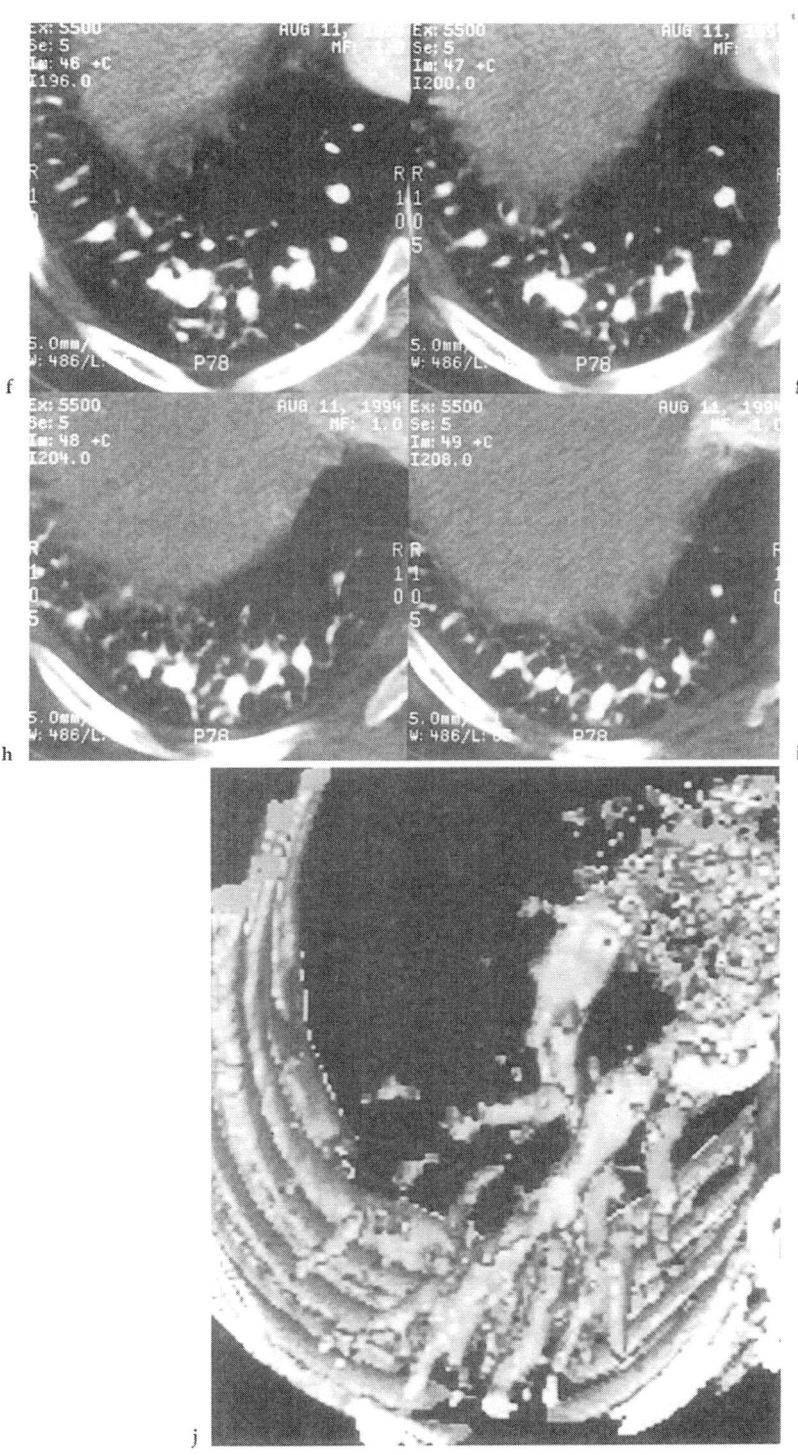

tients with documented AVMs, RÉMY et al. (1992) showed helical CT to be far superior to routine angiography for detecting these lesions [107 (98%) vs 65 (59%), respectively]. In select cases, such as pa- tients with family members with Osler-Weber-Rendu disease, these data suggest that helical CT may replace angiography for the detection of these lesions. Furthermore, helical CT may provide an accurate estimation of the angioarchitecture of AVMs in up to 95% of cases, especially when coupled with 3D reconstructions using shaded-surface displays (REMY et al. 1994). In addition to identifying isolated AVMs, volumetric CT allows evaluation of more extensive arteriovenous shunting, as may occur following vena cava-pulmonary artery (Glenn) shunts (Fig. 6.10).

While most attention has focused on the use of volumetric CT to assess abnormalities of the pulmonary arteries, another important advantage of this

technique is the ability to identify abnormal, anomalous, or hypertrophied systemic vessels, especially the bronchial arteries. These may be hypertrophied and tortuously enlarged in association with a variety of intrapulmonary abnormalties, both congenital and acquired. As documented by KAUCZOR et al. (1994) in a study of 39 patients undergoing pulmonary thromboendarterecomty using spiral CT, dilated bronchial arteries could be identified in 30 (77%) of 39 patients. In our experience, volumetric CT also may be of value in detecting hypertrophied

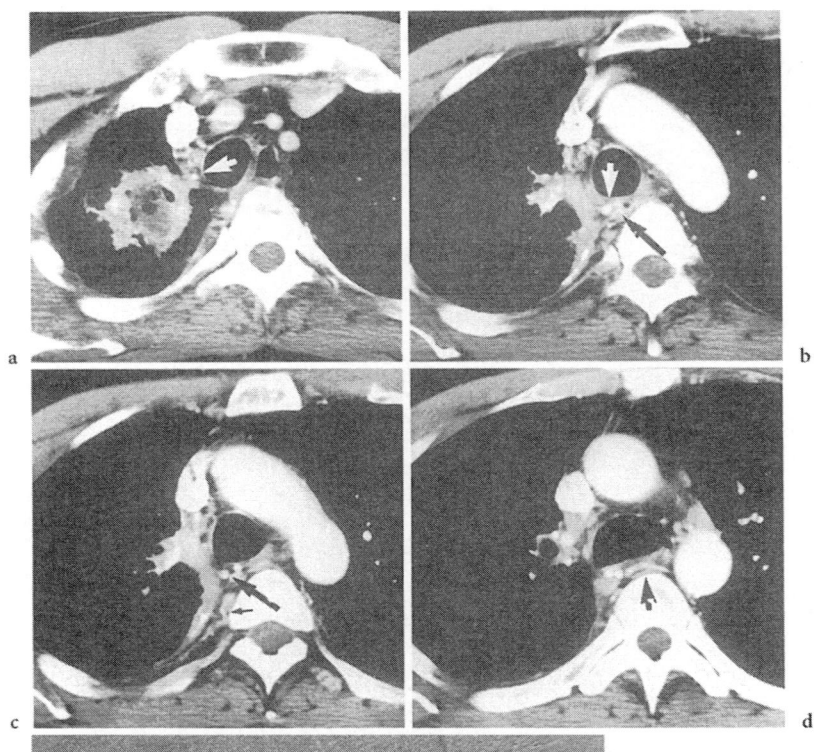

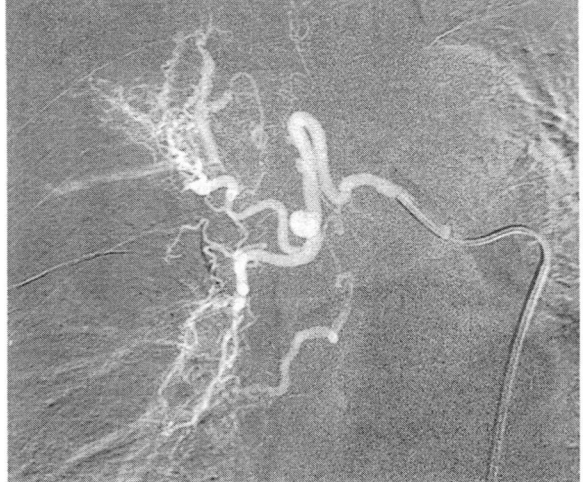

Fig. 6.11a–e. Intracavitary aspergilloma: hypertrophied bronchial arteries. a–d Select 5-mm sections through the upper lobes from above downward in a patient with a right upper lobe cavity presenting with hemoptysis. Following a bolus injection of 100 cc of 60% contrast material injected at a rate of 2 cc per second following a 20-s delay, an enlarged right intercostal-bronchial trunk (*arrow* in **d**) was seen within the posterior mediastinum behind the esophagus, subsequently dividing into a right bronchial (*arrows* in **a–c**) and intercostal arteries (*curved arrows* and *small straight arrow* in **c**). Considerable enhancement of the wall of the abscess cavity is consistent with increased vascularity associated with chronic infection. **e** Coned-down subtraction view from a select right bronchial artery injection confirms the presence of both a hypertrophied right bronchial artery extending into the right upper lobe and a prominent intercostal artery. Biospy and culture confirmed fungal infection due to aspergillus

bronchial arteries in patients with chronic pulmonary fungal infections, especially those presenting with hemoptysis (Fig. 6.11).

6.3.2.2 Bronchocentric Disease

In addition to assessing the relationship between focal lung pathology and vessels, volumetric CT has proved of considerable value in assessing the relationship between focal lung abnormalities and airways. Focal disease for which visualization of airways has proved important include tumors arising from or adjacent to airways, in particular, bronchogenic carcinoma (including bronchoalveolar cell carcinoma), and carcinoid tumors as well as mucoid impaction of the airways.

6.3.2.2.1 Bronchial Neoplasia. Perhaps the most important role of volumetric CT with regard to airway localization has been in the assessment of the likely yield of fiberoptic bronchoscopy (FOB) for diagnosing focal parenchymal abnormalities. The role of FOB in assessing pulmonary nodules is controversial, especially as a means for presurgical staging. In a retrospective evaluation of 33 patients with solitary pulmonary nodules smaller than 4 cm, GOLDBERG et al. (1993) were able to establish a tissue diagnosis in 25 patients, including 23 with lung cancer. However, as none of these patients had bronchoscopic findings precluding surgery, such as contralateral endobronchial metastases, these authors concluded that staging bronchoscopy be abandoned in the evaluation of indeterminate solitary nodules. Similar findings have been reported by TORRINGTON and KERN (1993).

Studies have consistently documented a role for CT in predicting the likely yield of transbronchial biopsy by identifying the presence of a so-called positive bronchus sign (GAETA et al. 1991, 1993; NAIDICH et al. 1988, 1993). In an early retrospective study of 65 nodules evaluated with CT, the yield of transbronchial biopsy was twice that in patients in whom bronchi could be traced to a nodule. It should be emphasized that the role of FOB in the evaluation of solitary nodules is controversial. This is because, depending on the size and location of lesions, the overall diagnostic accuracy of FOB ranges only between 40% and 60% (RADKE et al. 1979; TORRINGTON and KERN 1993).

Volumetric acquisition of 1-mm sections through a single breathhold maximizes visualization of airways even in the periphery of the lung (Figs. 6.12,

6.13). This allows a more confident use of CT both to predict the efficacy of bronchoscopy and to serve as an endoscopic roadmap. Unfortunately, while helical CT has proven of value in predicting the yield of FOB, the impact on diagnostic accuracy may be limited. In one prospective study of 21 focal lesions in 18 patients evaluated first with volumetric CT, the subsequent yield of FOB was not dramatically improved as compared with previous retrospective evaluations (NAIDICH et al. 1993). One exception is those cases in which transbronchial needle aspiration (TBNA) may be preferred (Fig. 6.14). As documented by WANG et al. (1984), in those cases in which the bronchus leading to a nodule or mass is infiltrated with tumor, for lesions larger than 2 cm TBNA may increase the diagnostic yield of FOB by as much as 50%.

In select cases, volumetric data acquisition using thin 1-mm sections also may be of value by demonstrating the relationship between airways and the pleural space or cavities, especially when evaluation is complemented by the use of multiplanar reconstructions (Fig. 6.14). Similarly, volumetric scanning may be of value in assessing the relationship between nodules, masses, and adjacent pleura. KURIYAMA et al. (1994) evaluated 12 patients with documented visceral pleural invasion and five with parietal pleural invasion and found that 2D CT images prospectively identified only two patients in each group, while 3D imaging allowed identification of 11 of 12 patients with visceral pleural invasion and three with parietal pleural invasion. In these authors' experience, the finding of pleural puckering adjacent to peripheral nodules was of particular value (Fig. 6.15). Although these findings are readily apparent with 3D imaging, it should be noted that the true value of 3D images most likely is limited as parietal and, especially, visceral pleural invasion in itself does not preclude surgical resection.

In addition to bronchogenic carcinoma, a relationship between airways and neoplasia has also been noted in patients with carcinoid tumors. Classified as part of the spectrum of neuroendocrine lung neoplasms, carcinoids characteristically arise in close proximity to airways, either growing primarily intraluminally or alternatively extending deeply into adjacent peribronchial tissue. This has led to descriptions of a classic triad of findings of carcinoids as smooth or slightly lobular lesions causing narrowing or obstruction typically of central airways often having eccentric calcifications (NAIDICH and GARAY 1991). Additionally, as carcinoids are highly vascular lesions (often causing hemoptysis both

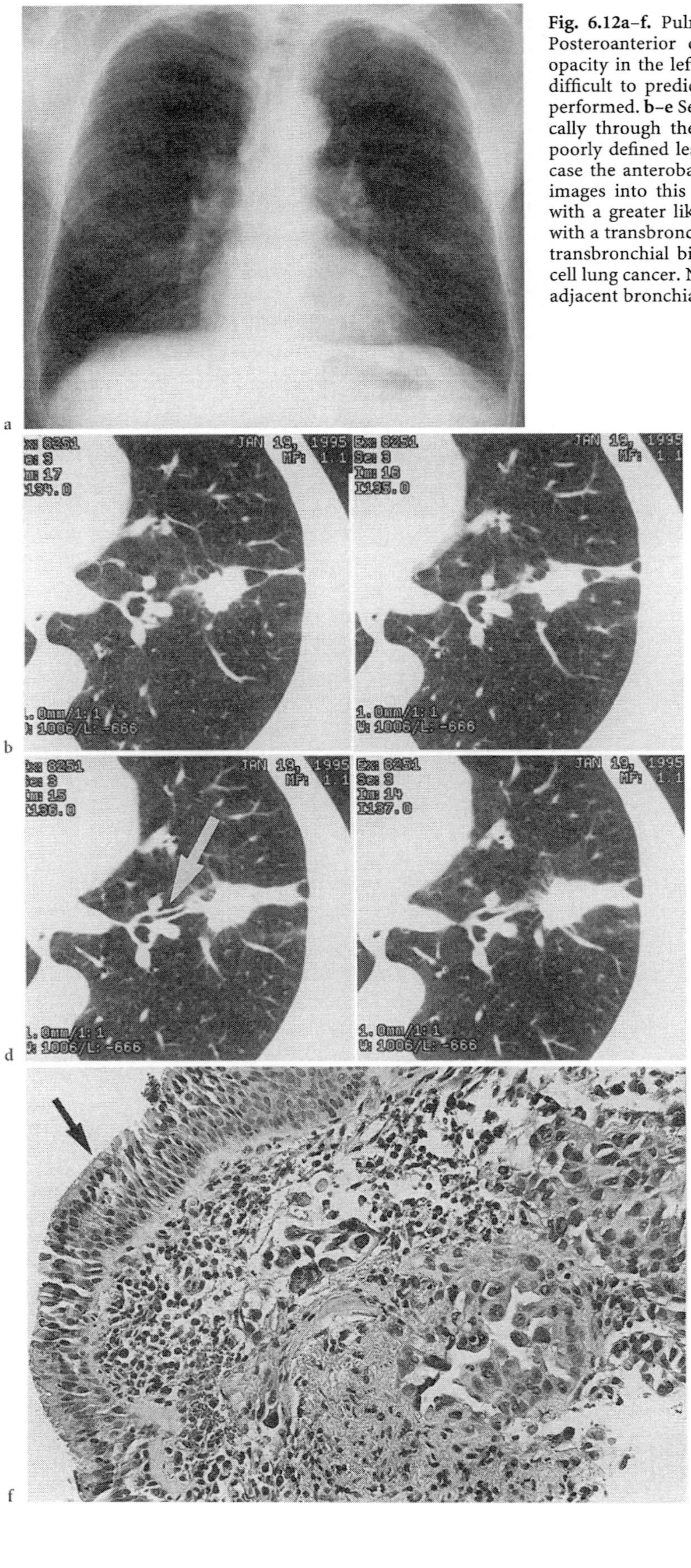

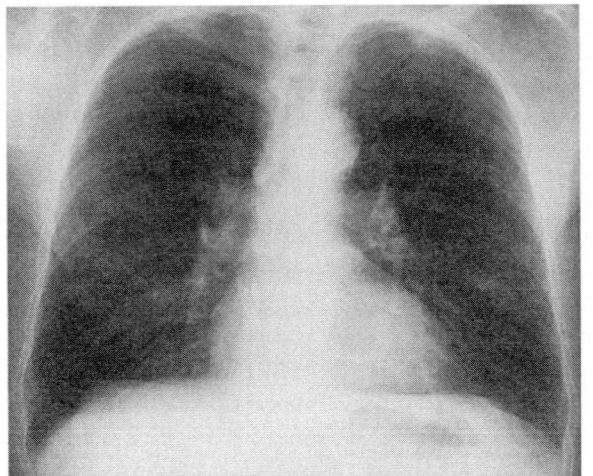

Fig. 6.12a–f. Pulmonary nodule: positive bronchus sign. **a** Posteroanterior chest radiograph shows a poorly defined opacity in the left lower lung field. Based on this image it is difficult to predict whether or not bronchoscopy should be performed. **b–e** Sequential 1-mm sections obtained volumetrically through the left mid lung confirm the presence of a poorly defined lesion in the left lower lobe. Note that in this case the anterobasilar bronchus can be traced on sequential images into this lesion (*arrow*). This appearance correlates with a greater likelihood of obtaining a histologic diagnosis with a transbronchial biopsy. **f** Histologic section obtained by transbronchial biopsy identifying this lesion as a non-small cell lung cancer. Note the close proximity of tumor cells to the adjacent bronchial mucosa (*arrow*)

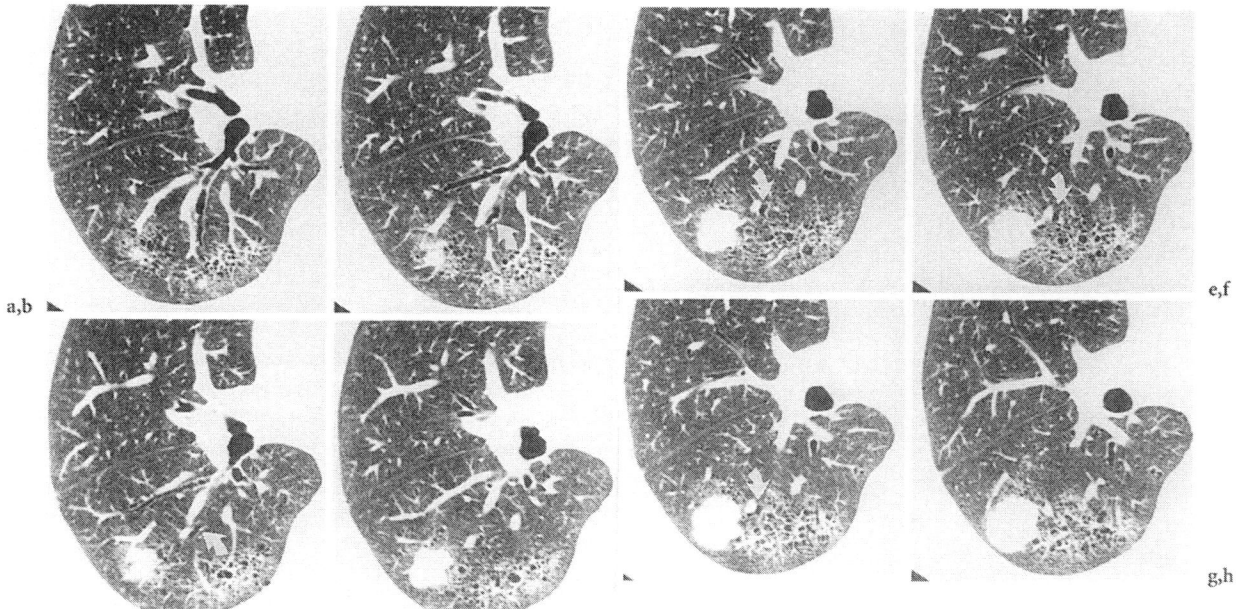

a,b

c,d

e,f

g,h

Fig. 6.13a–h. Pulmonary nodule: negative bronchus sign. **a–h** Sequential 1-mm sections obtained volumetrically through a nodule in the right lower lobe, from below upward. Using spiral CT it is possible to trace central airways even out to the periphery. In this case a branch of the superior segmental bronchus can be identified approximating but never quite reaching he edge of this lesion (*arrows*). Transthoracic needle biopsy confirmed this as a non-small cell lung cancer

Fig. 6.14a–e. Cavitary nodule: evaluation with multiplanar reconstructions. **a–d** Sequential 1-mm sections obtained volumetrically through an ill-defined cavitary infiltrate in the right upper lobe. Note that a peripheral branch of the anterior segmental bronchus of the right upper lobe can be traced to this cavity. **e** Parasagittal reconstruction through the right upper lobe bronchus allows visualization of a much longer portion of the right upper lobe airways, simplifying evaluation. Note again direct communication between the cavity and an adjacent airway (*arrow*)

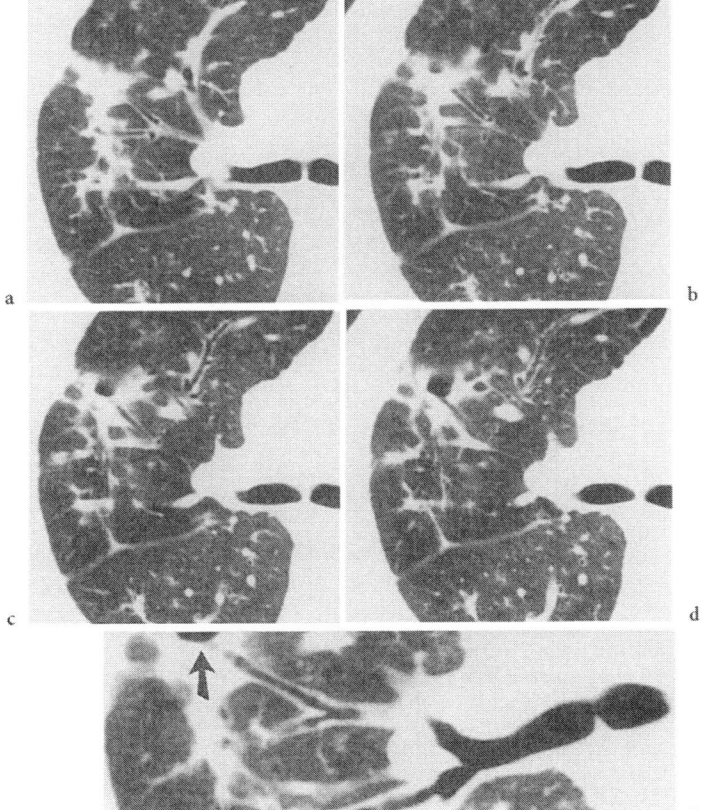

a

b

c

d

e

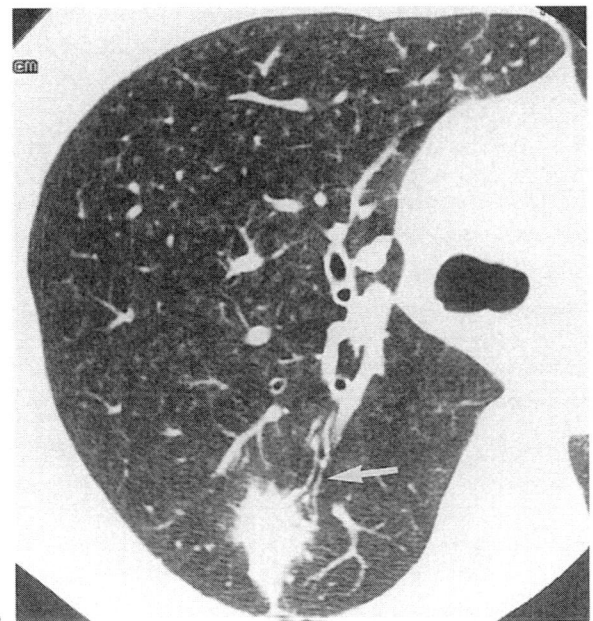

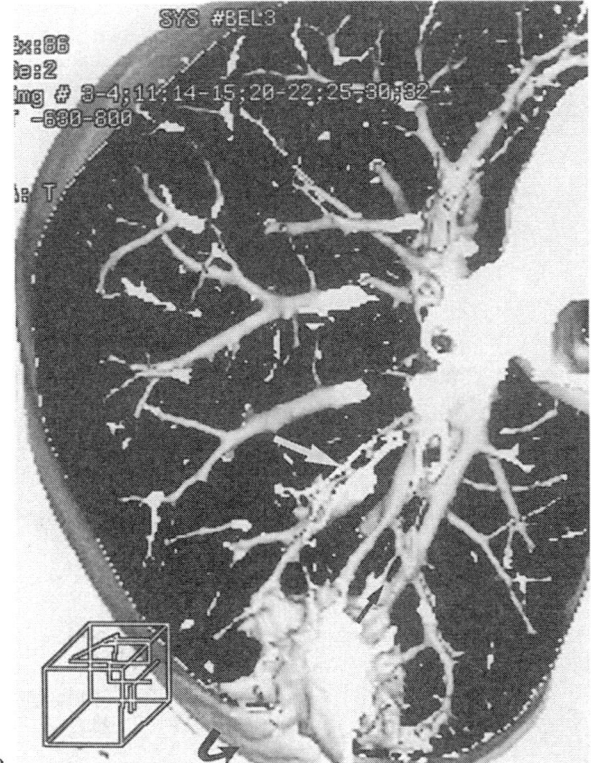

Fig. 6.15a,b. Pulmonary nodule: evaluation with 3D imaging. **a** 1-mm section through the right lung, retrospectively targeted, shows an irregular mass in the posterior segment of the right upper lobe with a positive bronchus sign. Note that posteriorly the mass extends towards the pleural surface. **b** 3D reconstruction shows the mass with an associated vessel and bronchus (*white and black arrows*). In addition. note that the posterior pleural surface is clearly puckered (*curved arrows*). Although in this case parietal pleural involvement was confirmed, the value of this sign has yet to be determined

prior to and, especially, following biopsy), considerable contrast enhancement is usually identifiable following administration of intravenous contrast media. While identification of these features is enhanced by the use of volumetric techniques, it is nonetheless worth emphasizing that many of these findings are frequently absent. In a retrospective study of 31 patients with documented carcinoids (27 typical, 4 atypical) Zweibel et al. (1991) found that 18 (58%) were central while 13 (42%) were peripheral. Furthermore, while calcification was seen in seven (39%) of the central lesions, it was identified in only one (8%) of the peripheral lesions.

It should be noted that in those indeterminate cases for which transthoracic needle biopsy is indicated, volumetric CT is of value by optimizing needle-tip localization in patients undergoing CT-guided percutaneous needle aspiration/biopsy (Silverman et al. 1992).

6.3.2.2.2 Bronchiectasis/Mucoid Impaction. In addition to defining the relationship between pulmonary nodules and airways, volumetric CT may also play an important role in assessing abnormalities of the airways themselves. Although the diagnosis of bronchiectasis typically requires evaluation of the entire lung, focal abnormalities resulting from abnormal dilatation of airways can be evaluated to advantage with volumetric techniques. In patients with mucoid impaction of the airways, for example, differentiation between pulmonary nodules and dilated airways may be problematic (Fig. 6.16). Typically the result of chronic inflammation and decreased clearance of secretions in damaged airways, mucoid impaction may be seen in patients with bronchiectasis from any cause. Less commonly, mucoid impaction may be the result of congenital bronchial abnormalities as occurs in patients with bronchial atresia. Although the appearance of mucus-filled airways generally poses few problems, in select cases accurate identification is usually possible by acquiring images after a bolus of intravenous contrast (Fig. 6.16).

Another potential use of volumetric CT for assessing focal airways and lung is in the identification of both normal and abnormal airway and parenchymal mechanics. To date, a number of reports have emphasized a role for comparison of images obtained both in inspiration and in expiration to allow accurate identification of focal areas of air trapping as well as direct visualization of the central airway mechanics (Hansell et al. 1994; Knudson et al. 1991). In this setting, volumetric CT has two distinct advan-

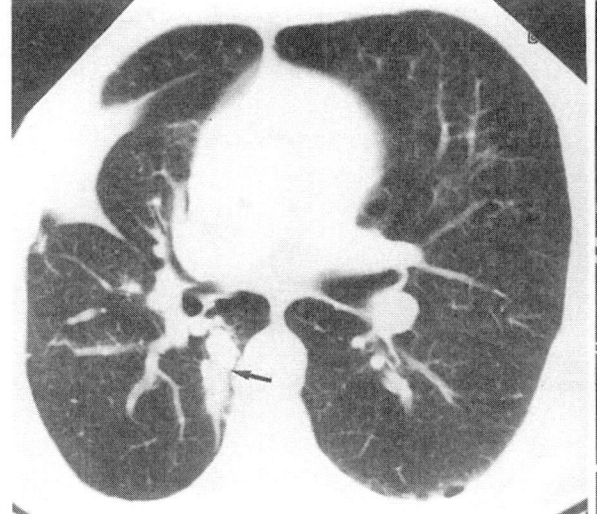
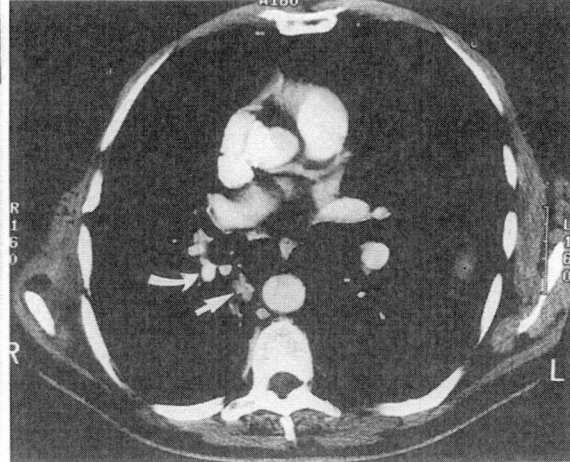
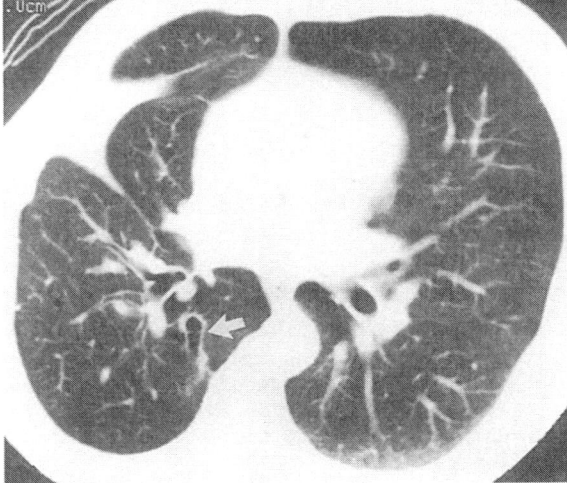

Fig. 6.16a–c. Mucoid impaction: assessment with volumetric CT. **a,b** 5-mm section through the right middle lobe bronchus imaged with both wide and narrow windows in a patient following right upper lobe resection for non-small cell lung carcinoma shows ill-defined nodular densities arrayed linearly in the superior segment of the right lower lobe (*straight arrows*). Although this appearance initially was interpreted as a possible metastasis, note that following a bolus of 100 cc of 60% contrast material injected at a rate of 2 cc per second, there is no evidence of enhancement within these nodules as compared with adjacent hilar vessels (*curved arrow*). This constellation of findings is strongly suggestive of mucoid impaction. **c** Follow-up scan at approximately the same level as shown in **a** and **b** reveals that in place of the previously seen nodules there is a markedly dilated bronchus (*arrow*), confirming the diagnosis of mucoid impaction. Scans obtained slightly more cephalad failed to show evidence of an endobronchial obstructing lesion (not shown)

tages over other methods for acquiring inspiratory/ expiratory images. First, with spiral or helical scanning an entire volume of data is acquired during a single breathhold, potentially providing more accurate identification of focal abnormalities. Second, as images can be retrospectively reconstructed anywhere within the data set, volumetric acquisition assures that sections in the exact same plane can be compared (Fig. 6.17).

6.4 Future Trends

Although emphasis has been placed throughout this review on standard methods of image analysis, it should be noted that other methods for evaluating the parenchyma have been proposed that may have

an impact on the detection and characterization of pulmonary nodules. Recently, NAPEL et al. (1993) have shown that high-resolution CT images of the lung can be obtained using sliding thin-slab maximum intensity projection (STS-MIP) as a technique for enhanced visualization of pulmonary vascular anatomy. Using 1-to 3-mm sections, these authors devised a method for rapidly computing a series of either overlapping maximum (MIP) or minimum (MINIP) intensity projection images through a thin slab of lung retaining a normal superoinferior or axial orientation. This resulted in images of high contrast resolution allowing enhanced visualization either of peripheral blood vessels using MIP reconstructions or bronchi using MINIP reconstructions (Fig. 6.18). Recently, this approach has been validated for detecting micronodules in patients with

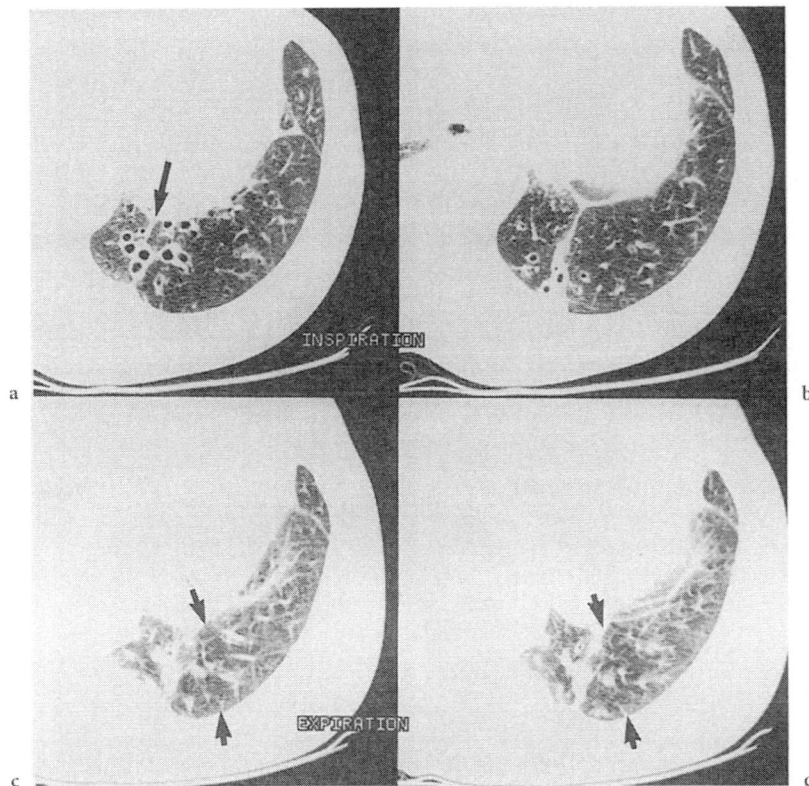

Fig. 6.17a–d. Bronchiectasis: evaluation with inspiratory/expiratory CT. **a,b** Sequential 5-mm sections through the right lower lobe obtained in deep inspiration show dilated, thick-walled bronchi (*arrow* in **a**) associated with a focal area of adjacent decreased lung density, compatible with focal air trapping. **c,d** Sequential 5-mm sections obtained at the same levels as in **a** and **b** obtained at end-expiratory volume show that despite collapse of the previously dilated bronchi there is only limited air trapping, identifiable as an ill-defined area of slightly decreased lung density (*arrows*). A significant advantage of volumetric scanning is the ability to functionally evaluate large areas of the lung during varying phases of respiration, allowing precise comparison of inspiratory/expiratory scans at more than one level

diffuse infiltrative lung disease (REMY-JARDIN et al. 1995b). Still to be considered experimental, this technique offers considerable promise in furthering the boundaries of nodule evaluation with volumetric CT.

Also intriguing is the possibility of using automated segmentation to improve detection of pulmonary nodules. As recently proposed by CROISILLE et al. (1995) using a three-dimensionally seeded region-growing algorithm, it is possible to connect and thus extract vessels from lung images, leaving remaining disconnected nodules more conspicuous. In an analysis of eight patients referred for possible nodules, these authors documented an improved sensitivity of between 58% and 78% for three experienced radiologists using automated vessel subtraction for detection of pulmonary nodules. As important, the proportion of false-positive interpretations decreased from 55% to 12%. While intriguing, the true clinical impact of this technique remains to be assessed.

Another potential application presently under investigation is the use of low-dose volumetric scanning as a means for screening early lung cancer (HENSCHKE et al. 1995). The ability to scan the entire thorax in a single breathhold using mA values as low as 40 makes volumetric scanning a particularly attractive method for early lung cancer detection.

In conclusion, while volumetric scanning has already had a dramatic impact on the use of CT to assess focal lung pathology, the true potential of this modality has yet to be thoroughly explored. Indeed, it is to be anticipated that as further improvements are made in data acquisition as well as computer applications, the number of clinically valuable, cost-effective uses of volumetric CT will continue to expand.

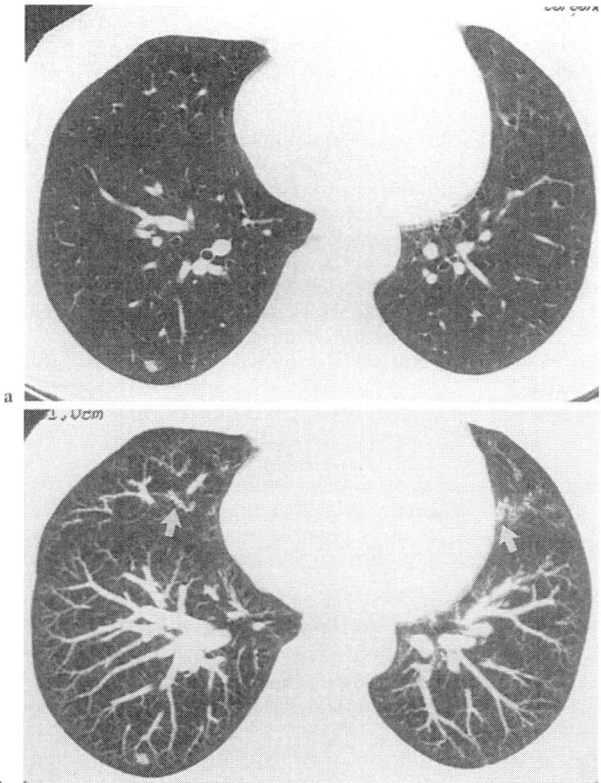

Fig. 6.18a,b. Pulmonary nodules: evaluation with MIP images. **a** 1-mm section through the lung base shows a poorly defined peripheral lung nodule. **b** MIP image generated from a volumetric data set using 1-mm collimation with images reconstructed every 0.5 mm. The advantage of these images is that they enable visualization of most of the vascular tree while maintaining nearly equivalent spatial resolution. In this case the nodule is clearly centrilobular in distribution, consistent with the clinical diagnosis of active tuberculosis. Note that motion artifacts on the transaxial image result in a "beaded vessel" artifact on the MIP image (*arrows*), a potential pitfall in the use of this technique for identifying small, peripheral nodules

References

Buckley JA, Scott WW, Siegelman SS, Kuhlman JE, Urban BA, Bluemake DA, Fishman EK (1995) Pulmonary nodules: effect of increased data sampling on detection with spiral CT and confidence in diagnosis. Radiology 196:395–400

Collie DA, Wright AR, Williams JR, Hashemi-Malayeri BS, Stevenson AJM, Turnbull CM (1994) Comparison of spiral-acquisition computed tomography and conventional computed tomography in the assessment of pulmonary metastatic disease. Br J Radiol 67:436–444

Costello P, Anderson W, Blume D (1991) Pulmonary nodule: evaluation with spiral volumetric CT. Radiology 179:875–876

Costello P, Dupuy DE, Ecker CP, Tello R (1992) Spiral CT of the thorax with reduced volume of contrast material: a comparative study. Radiology 183:663–666

Croisille P, Souto M, Cova M, Wood S, Afework Y, Kuhlman JE, Zerhouni EA (1995) Pulmonary nodules: improved detection with vascular segmentation and extraction with spiral CT. Radiology 197:397–401

Gaeta M, Pandolfo I, Volta S, Russi EG, Baritorom G, Girone G (1991) Bronchus sign on CT in peripheral carcinioma of the lung: value in predicting results of transbronchial biopsy. AJR 157:1181–1185

Gaeta M, Barone M, Russi EG, et al. (1993) Carcinomatous solitary pulmonary nodules: evaluation of the tumor-bronchi relationship with thin-section CT. Radiology 187:535–539

Goldberg SK, Walkenstein MD, Steinbach A, Aranson R (1993) The role of staging bronchoscopy in the preoperative assessment of a solitary pulmonary nodule. Chest 104:94–97

Goodman LR, Curtin JJ, Foley WDM, Mewissen MW, Sagar KB, Lipchik RJ (1994) Helical CT of patients with "unresolved suspicion" of pulmonary embolism: prospective study. Radiology 193(P):262

Grewal RG, Austin JHM (1994) CT demonstration of calcification in cancer of the lung. J Comput Assist Tomogr 18:867–871

Gurney JW, Lyddon DM, McKay JA (1993) Determining the likelihood of malignancy in solitary pulmonary nodules with Bayesian analysis. II. Application. Radiology 186:415–422

Hansell DM, Wells AU, Rubens MB, Cole PJ (1994) Bronchiectasis: functional significance of area of decreased attenuation at expiratory CT. Radiology 193:369–374

Heiken JP, Brink JA, Vannier MW (1993) Spiral (helical) CT. Radiology 189:647–656

Henschke CI, Yankelevitz DF, Libby DM, Smith JP, Pasmantier M, Miiettinen OS (1995) Paradigm for outcomes research: new concepts for lung cancer screening. Radiology 197(P):529

Heywang-Koebrunner S, Lommatzsch B, Fink U, Maayr B (1992) Comparison of spiral and conventional CT in the detection of pulmonary nodules (abstract). Radiology 185(P):131

Ibukuro K, Charnsangavej C, Chasen MH, Cinqualbre AB, Herron DH, Robinson TJ, Wallace S (1995) Helical CT angiography with multiplanar reformation: techniques and clinical applications. Radiographics 15:671–682

Kalender WA, Seissler W, Klotz E, Vock P (1990) Spiral volumetric CT with single-breath-hold technique, continuous transport, and continuous scanner rotation. Radiology 176:181–183

Kalender WA, Polacin A, Suss C (1994) A comparison of conventional and spiral CT: an experimental study on the detection of spherical lesions. J Comput Assist Tomogr 18:167–176

Kauczor H-U, Schwickert HC, Mayer E, Schweden F, Schild HH, Thelen M (1994) Spiral CT of bronchial arteries in chronic thromboembolism. J Comput Assist Tomogr 18:855–861

Khan A, Herman PG, Vorwerk P, Stevens P, Rojas KA, Graver M (1991) Solitary pulmonary nodules: comparison of classification with standard, thin-section, and reference phantom CT. Radiology 179:477–481

Knudson RJ, Standen JR, Kaltenborn WT, Knudson DE, Rehm K, Habib MP, Newell JD (1991) Expiratory computed tomography for assessment of suspected pulmonary emphysema. Chest 99:1357–1366

Kono M, Adachi S, Kusumoto M, Sakai E (1993) Clinical utility of Gd-DTPA-enhanced magnetic resonance imaging in lung cancer. J Thorac Imag 8:18–26

Kuriyama K, Tateichi R, Kumatani T et al. (1994) Pleural invasion by peripheral bronchogenic carcinoma: assessment with three-dimensional helical CT. Radiology 191:365–369

Littleton JT, Durizch ML, Moeller G, Herbert DE (1990) Pulmonary masses: contrast enhancement. Radiology 177: 861–871

Naidich DP (1994) Helical computed tomography of the thorax. Clinical applications. Radiol Clin North Am 32:759–774

Naidich DP, Garay SM (1991) Radiographic evaluation of focal lung disease. Clin Chest Med 12:77–95

Naidich DP, Sussman R, Kutcher WL, Aranda CP, Garay SM, Ettenger NA (1988) Solitary pulmonary nodules: CT-bronchoscopic correlation. Chest 93:595–598

Naidich DP, Harkin TJ, McGuinness G (1993) Helical CT/bronchoscopic correlations (abstract). Presented at the 16th Annual Meeting of the Society of Computed Body Tomography and Magnetic Resonance Imaging, Orlando

Napel S, Rubin GD, Jeffrey RB (1993) Technical note. STS-MIP: a new reconstruction technique for CT of the chest. J Comput Assist Tomogr 17:832–838

Patz EF, Lowe VJ, Hoffman JM (1993) Focal pulmonary abnormalities; evaluation with F-18 fluorodeoxyglucose PET scanning. Radiology 188:487–490

Primack SL, Hartman TE, Lee KS, Müller NL (1994) Pulmonary nodules and the CT halo sign. Radiology 190:513–515

Radke JR, Conway WA, Eyler WR, Kvale PA (1979) Diagnostic accuracy in peripheral lung lesions: factors predicting success with flexible fiberoptic bronchoscopy. Chest 76:176–179

Remy J, Remy-Jardin M, Wattinne L, Deffontaines C (1992) Pulmonary arteriovenous malformations: evaluation with CT of the chest before and after treatment. Radiology 182:808–816

Remy J, Remy-Jardin M, Giraud F, Wattinne L (1994) Angioarchitecture of pulmonary arteriovenous malformations: clinical utility of three-dimensional helical CT. Radiology 191:657–664

Remy-Jardin M, Remy J, Wattinne L, Giraud F (1992) Central pulmonary thromboembolism: diagnosis with spiral volumetric CT with the single-breath-hold technique. Comparison with pulmonary angiography. Radiology 185: 381–387

Remy-Jardin M, Remy J, Giraud F, Marquette CH (1993) Pulmonary nodules: detection with thick-section spiral CT versus conventional CT. Radiology 187:513–520

Remy-Jardin M, Remy J, Cauvain O, Petyt L, Wannebroucq J, Beregi J-P (1995a) Diagnosis of central pulmonary embolism with helical CT: role of two-dimensional multiplanar reformations. AJR 165:1131–1138

Remy-Jardin M, Remy J, Petyt L, Duhamel A (1995b) Sliding thin-slab, maximum-intensity projection in diffuse infiltrative lung disease: clinical value in the detection of a mild micronodular pattern. Radiology 197(P):404

Seltzer SE, Judy PF, Adams DF et al. (1995) Spiral CT of the chest: comparison of cine and film-based viewing. Radiology 197:73–78

Siegelman SS, Khouri NF, Scott WW, Leo FP, Hamper UM, Fishman EK, Zerhouni EA (1986) Pulmonary hamartoma: CT findings. Radiology 160:313–317

Silverman SG, Bloom DA, Seltzer SE, Tempany CMC, Adams D (1992) Needle-tip localization during CT-guided abdominal biopsy: comparison of conventional and spiral CT. AJR 159:1095–1097

Silverman P, Roberts S, Tiffl MC, Brown B, Fox SH (1995) Helical CT of the liver: clinical application of an automated computer technique – SmartPrep – for obtaining images with optimal contrast enhancement. AJR 165:73–78

Swensen SJ, Harms GF, Morin RL, Myers JL (1991) CT evaluation of solitary pulmonary nodules: value of 185-H reference phantom. AJR 156:925–929

Swensen SJ, Morin RL, Schueler BA, Brown LR, Cortese DA, Pairolero PC, Brutinel WM (1992) Solitary pulmonary nodule: CT evaluation of enhancement with iodinated contrast material – a preliminary report. Radiology 182:343–347

Swensen SJ, Brown LR, Colby TV, Weaver AL (1995) Pulmonary nodules: CT evaluation of enhancement with iodinated contrast material. Radiology 194:393–398

Teigen CL, Maus TP, Sheedy PF, Stanson AW, Johnson CM, Breen JF, McKusick MA (1995) Pulmonary embolism: diagnosis with contrast-enhanced electron-beam CT and comparison with pulmonary angiography. Radiology 194: 313–319

Torrington KG, Kern JD (1993) The utility of fiberoptic bronchoscopy in the evaluation of the solitary pulmonary nodule. Chest 104:1021–1024

Vock P, Soucek M (1993) Spiral computed tomography in the assessment of focal and diffuse lung disease. J Thorac Imaging 8:283–290

vock P, Soucek M, Daepp M, Kalender WA (1990) Lung: spiral volumetric CT with single-breath-hold technique. Radiology 176:864–867

Wang KP, Haponik EF, Britt EJ (1984) Transbronchial needle aspiration of peripheral pulmonary nodules. Chest 86:819–823

Webb WR (1990) Radiologic evaluation of the solitary pulmonary nodule. AJR 154:701–708

Winston CB, Wechsler RJ, Slazar AM, Kurtz AB, Spirn PW (1995) Incidental pulmonary emboli detected at helical CT: effect of patient care. Radiology 197(P):303

Yamashita K, Matsunobe S, Takahashi R et al. (1995a) Small peripheral lung carcinoma evaluated with incremental dynamic CT: radiologic-pathologic correlation. Radiology 196:401–408

Yamashita K, Matsunobe S, Tsuda T, Nemoto T, Matsumoto K, Miki H, Konishi J (1995b) Solitary pulmonary nodule: preliminary study of evaluation with incremental dynamic CT. Radiology 194:399–405

Zwiebel BR, Austin JHM, Grines MM (1991) Bronchial carcinoid tumors: assessment with CT of location and intratumoral calcification in 31 patients. Radiology 179: 483–486

Zwirewich CV, Mayo JR, Müller NL (1991a) Low-dose high-resolution CT of lung parenchyma. Radiology 180:413–417

Zwirewich CV, Vedal S, Miller RR, Müller NL (1991b) Solitary pulmonary nodule: high-resolution CT and radiologic-pathologic correlation. Radiology 179:469–476

7 Spiral CT of Parenchymal Lung Disease

M. RÉMY-JARDIN and J. RÉMY

CONTENTS

7.1 Introduction

Over the past decade, thin-section computed tomography (CT) has been widely performed to evaluate patients with respiratory symptoms or pulmonary function abnormalities suggesting restrictive or obstructive syndromes. In the specific area of diffuse infiltrative lung disease (DILD), this CT technique has been shown to provide improved clarity of imaging of parenchymal abnormalities, thus enabling a better and more confident characterization of pathological processes even in severely involved areas (SWIREWICH et al. 1989; MAYO et al. 1987; LEUNG et al. 1991; REMY-JARDIN et al. 1991). By the direct visualization of fine details within the lung, such as septal and polygonal lines, honeycombing, and traction bronchiectasis, thin-section CT enables assessment of parenchymal fibrosis. Moreover, this technique may assist in the evaluation of disease activity by means of accurate depiction of ground glass attenuation (BRAUNER et al. 1992; TERRIFF et al. 1992; LEUNG et al. 1993; REMY-JARDIN et al. 1993a). Owing to the accuracy of thin-section CT, one may

M. RÉMY-JARDIN, MD, PhD, Professor, Department of Radiology, Hospital Calmette, Boulevard Jules Leclerc, 59037 Lille Cédex, France
J. RÉMY, MD, Professor, Department of Radiology, Hospital Calmette, Boulevard Jules Leclerc, 59037 Lille Cédex, France

question the potential diagnostic benefits of spiral CT in evaluating infiltrative and/or destructive lung changes. The reader will easily understand that it is too early to envisage a definitive answer to this question. Nevertheless, a few preliminary results suggest potential clinical applications for spiral CT of the lungs. Therefore, the goal of this chapter is to summarize the current knowledge in respect of two promising developments, i.e., narrow collimation spiral CT and sliding thin slab-maximum (STS-MIP) or -minimum (STS-mIP) intensity projection. Specific applications of the maximum intensity projection in the evaluation of the most peripheral pulmonary vessels are considered in Chap. 11.

7.2 Narrow Collimation Spiral Scanning

In a recent study, ENGELER et al. (1994) evaluated the accuracy of narrow collimation spiral scanning in the diagnosis of interstitial lung disease when four contiguous sections were acquired at three anatomical levels. Furthermore, these authors weighed the potential benefits against the increased radiation dose of multiple scans. For the purpose of their study and considering the results of phantom studies which showed that spatial resolution at 1-mm collimation was similar to that with spiral CT and conventional CT (PARANJPE and BERGIN 1994; RIGAULT et al. 1990), ENGELER et al. introduced the term "volumetric high-resolution CT." They concluded that the use of volumetric high-resolution CT increased the diagnostic accuracy, particularly in respect of bronchiectasis at the lung base, without increasing the peak skin radiation exposure. With the availability of four contiguous scans per anatomical level (i.e., the aortic arch, the carina, and 2 cm above the diaphragm), the subjective confidence in interpretation and the number of motion-free studies also increased. However, the limited experience regarding this specific indication for spiral CT in the thorax does not allow specific recommendations to be made regarding the optimal technique. As pointed out by these authors, more refined protocols can be tailored to individual patients by, for example, increasing the slice thickness to 2 or 3 mm, increasing the number of scans in each set, tilting the gantry to conform to the course of certain parts of the bronchial tree, or using hybrid techniques that incorporate volumetric acquisition and single HRCT scans.

7.3 Sliding Thin Slab-Maximum Intensity Projection

Recent advances in CT have led to the introduction of volumetric scanning, which has the potential to combine the advantages of continuous data acquisition with the use of volume rendering techniques. As previously described (see Chap. 5), the result of maximum intensity projections through slabs of lung parenchyma is to retain the highest attenuated structures within a given slab thickness. Applied to normal lung parenchyma, this technique improves blood vessel conspicuity along greater portions of their lengths. To date, a few potential applications have been investigated, dedicated to the detection of mild forms of micronodular infiltration and bronchiolar abnormalities (REMY-JARDIN et al. 1996a). Through the results of these preliminary investigations, it is possible to underline several advantages and limitations of this technique and to suggest technical guidelines.

7.3.1 Optimal Technique

At the level of a region of interest, a focal spiral CT acquisition can be performed to generate STS-MIP images. From this data set, contiguous transverse CT scans are reconstructed, then stacked to produce slabs of lung parenchyma. On each slab the maximum intensity projection algorithm is applied, enabling projection of the brightest voxels encountered along each ray, thus resulting in an MIP image. According to NAPEL et al.'s (1993) initial description: (a) the first MIP images a slab of a given thickness, referred to as STS-MIP (x); (b) then the computer produces a sequence of overlapping MIP images by advancing the slab along the superoinferior axis of the scanned subvolume.

In the protocol evaluated for detection of lung micronodules (REMY-JARDIN et al. 1996a), the following parameters were selected: 1-mm collimation and a 1 mm/s table feed (i.e., a pitch of 1), 137 kV and 180 mA, and scanning in the superoinferior direction

within a 12-mm scanning volume during a 13-s scanning time. From a preliminary evaluation of five normal volunteers, these authors analyzed the influence of the linear interpolation algorithms (i.e. 180° vs 360°) and the reconstruction kernels (standard, soft, soft detail vs ultra-high) in the structural definition of the normal lung. No major difference in image quality was found between scans reconstructed with the 180° and the 360° linear interpolation algorithms (Fig. 7.1). Similar to conventional CT, reconstruction of STS-MIP images with a high spatial frequency kernel reduces image smoothing and displays more sharply fine parenchymal details in comparison with images reconstructed with standard reconstruction kernels (Fig. 7.2). These results are in agreement with the conclusions drawn by PARANJPE and BERGIN (1994) on the basis of spiral CT scans of the lungs. Despite the lack of major difference in image quality between 180° and 360° linear interpolation algorithms, the former was considered more appropriate for analysis of lung micronodules as it is designed to improve the effects of slice-sensitivity profile broadening. An interesting finding was the observation that reconstruction of STS-MIP images with a 180° linear interpolation algorithm and a high spatial frequency reconstruction kernel reduced the beaded appearance of pulmonary vessels related to partial volume averaging on MIP images (NAPEL 1995). Figure 7.3 illustrates the appearance of normal lung

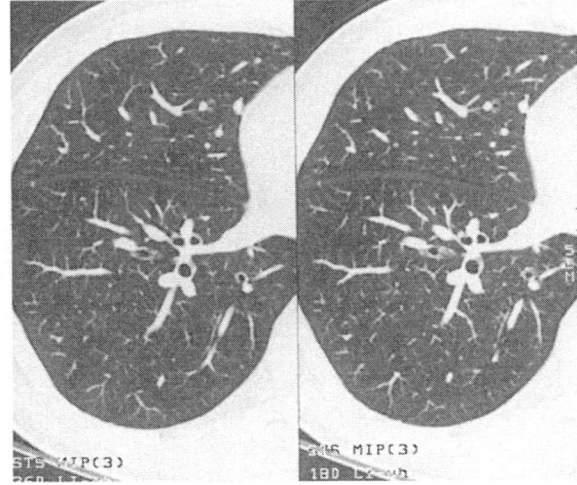

Fig. 7.1. STS-MIP images of lung parenchyma in a 44-year-old adult volunteer (3-mm slab thickness) reconstructed with a 360° (*left*) and a 180° (*right*) linear interpolation algorithm. Both images were photographed with an ultra-high display kernel (*UH*) and similar window settings (window width, 1600 HU; window level, −600 HU). The scans were considered similar

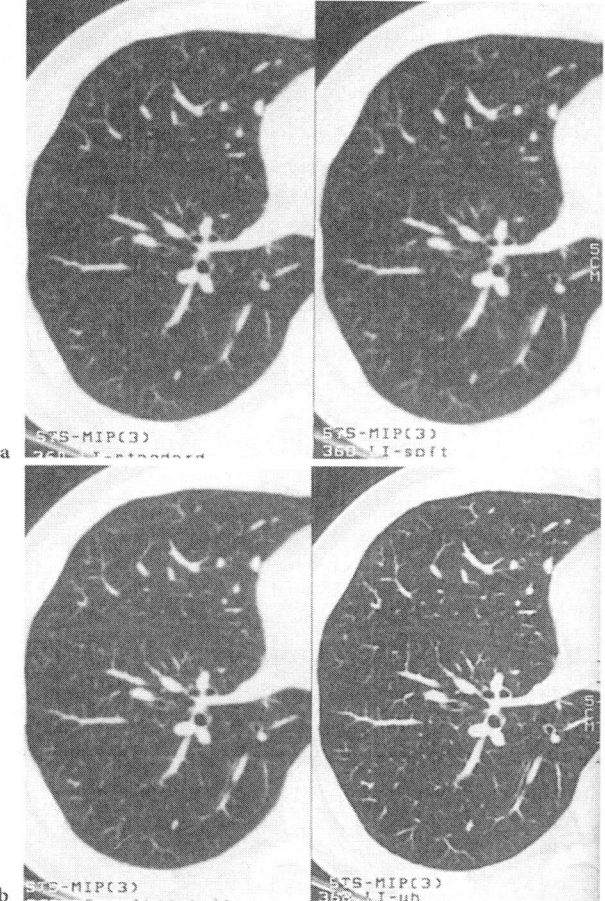

Fig. 7.2a,b. STS-MIP images of lung parenchyma (3-mm slab thickness) reconstructed with a 360° linear interpolation algorithm and four different display kernels: standard (**a**, *left*), soft (**a**, *right*), soft detail (**b**, *left*) and ultra-high (**b**, *right*). Same volunteer as in Fig. 7.1. All the images are photographed at similar window settings (window width, 1600 HU; window level, −600 HU). Structural definition is best on scans photographed with an ultra-high display kernel

parenchyma on STS-MIP images of 3 mm, 5 mm, and 8 mm thickness (Fig. 7.3).

7.3.2 Detection of Micronodules

Although thin-section CT is the most accurate technique for the evaluation of diffuse infiltrative lung disease, a few limitations of this CT technique have been reported with regard to the detection of micronodular infiltration (REMY-JARDIN et al. 1990, 1991). On thin sections, micronodules may be difficult to distinguish from vessels seen on end (when equal in diameter to nearby vessels) and also from points of confluence of abnormal linear areas of at-

tenuation. In this particular setting of lung infiltration, it has been shown that conventional thick sections could take advantage of the superimposition of small nodular lesions. However, an adverse effect of superimposition may be encountered with tiny low attenuated micronodules, which can disappear in a thick collimated scan as they are obscured at that section thickness. This explains why difficulties in confidently assessing micronodular infiltration on conventional CT scans are sometimes encountered in clinical practice.

In order to confirm or rule out radiographic suspicion of micronodular infiltration, REMY-JARDIN et al. (1996a) evaluated 81 consecutive patients suspected of having diffuse infiltrative lung disease. Owing to the complementarity of thin and thick collimated sections in the evaluation of a micronodular pattern

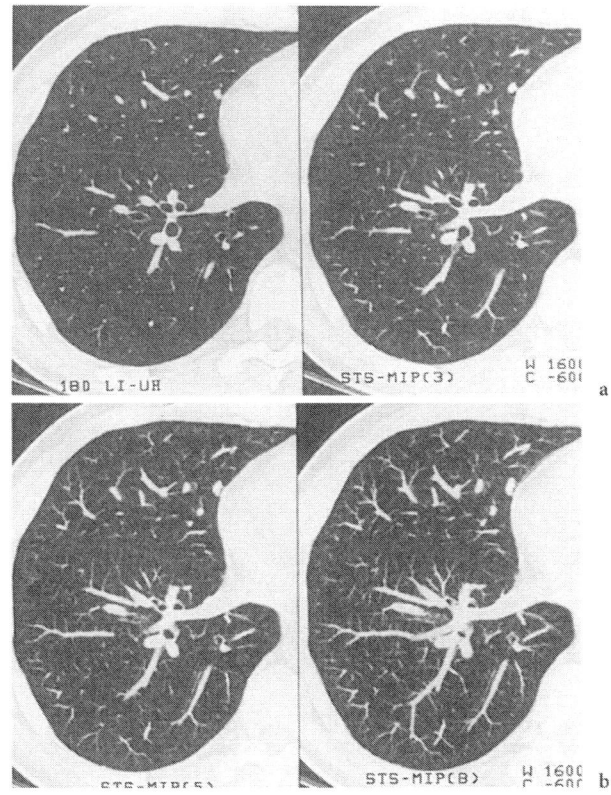

Fig. 7.3a,b. STS-MIP images of lung parenchyma of various thicknesses obtained in the same volunteer as in Fig. 7.1 (180° linear interpolation algorithm; *UH,* ultra-high; window width, 1600 HU; window level, −600 HU). Appearance of normal lung parenchyma on a 1-mm collimation CT scan (**a**, *left*), a 3-mm-thick STS-MIP (**a**, *right*), a 5-mm-thick STS-MIP (**b**, *left*), and an 8-mm-thick STS-MIP (**b**, *right*). Note the progressive increase in vessel trajectories with the slab thickness with a constant high degree of vessel contrast. No beaded appearance of oblique pulmonary vessels

(REMY-JARDIN et al. 1990), each patient underwent both 8-mm and 1-mm conventional CT scans at the level of a region of interest, completed by a focal spiral CT evaluation at the level of this region of interest. Three sets of STS-MIPs were systematically obtained for each patient with a slab thickness of 3 mm, 5 mm, and 8 mm. When conventional CT scans identified micronodules (57% of the study group), their overall conspicuity was increased on STS-MIP images but this visual preference was associated with no diagnostic superiority. Whenever conventional CT scans were interpreted as normal (22% of the study group), STS-MIPs were not shown to depict additional lung abnormalities. However, in the 21% of patients with an inconclusive conventional CT examination, STS-MIPs enabled assessment of micronodular infiltration, taking advantage of the selection of the brightest voxels in a given slab thickness (Fig. 7.4). In this study group, the sensitivity of STS-MIP was found to be significantly higher than that of conventional CT in detecting lung micronodules. However, as STS-MIP images result from a focal spiral CT acquisition, this reconstruction technique is always a second intention diagnostic tool. Therefore, its potential usefulness has to be considered according to the results of conventional CT.

In accordance with the study design, the authors attempted to determine the optimal slab thickness for detection of micronodules. As shown on Fig. 7.4, they observed that a maximum intensity projection over three thin sections was not always sufficient to confidently differentiate tiny micronodules from the background of vascular sections. Moreover, they found that the use of a maximum intensity projection in an 8-mm-thick slab cannot always compensate for the low detectability of tiny micronodules. Therefore, their study suggests that a 5-mm slab thickness could represent the most adequate selection for confident identification of micronodules on STS-MIP images.

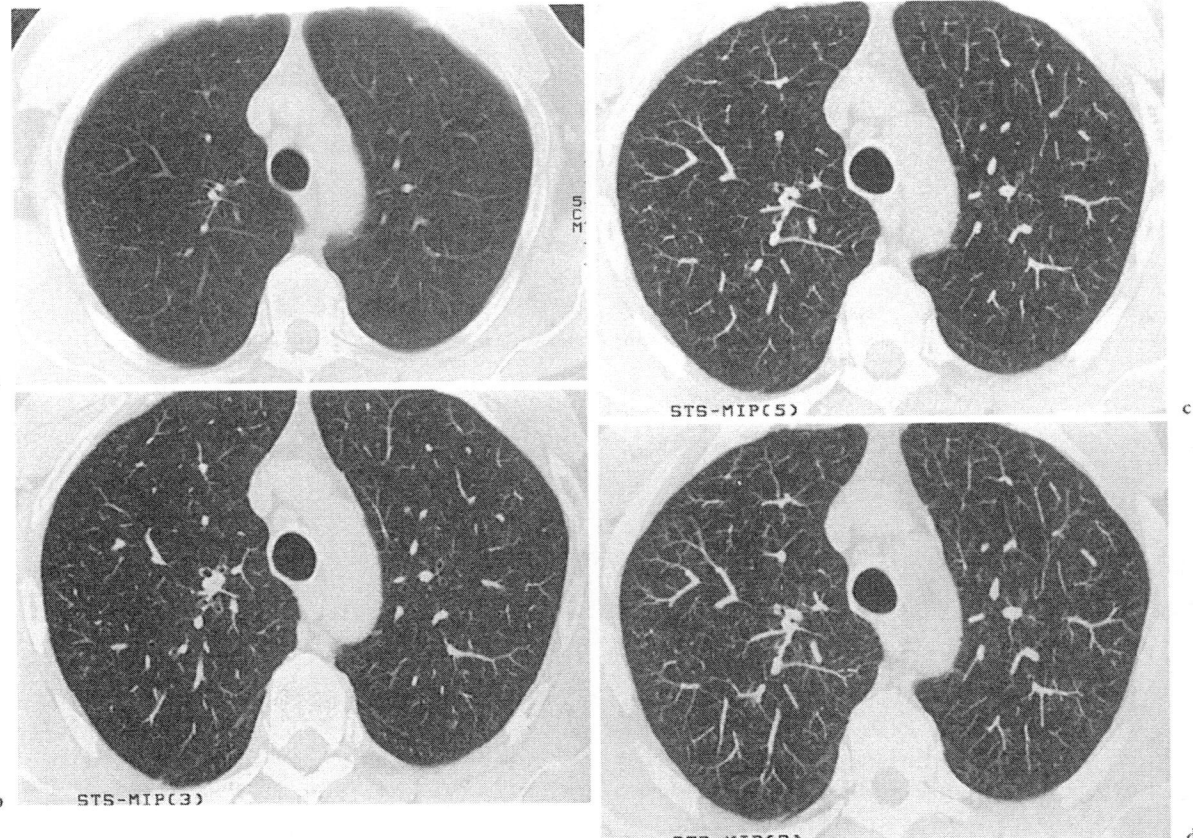

Fig. 7.4a–d. Comparison between an 8-mm collimation CT scan and STS-MIP images obtained at the upper lobe level in a 57-year-old coal worker (180° linear interpolation algorithm; *UH*, ultra-high; window width, 1600 HU; window level, –600 HU). Conventional 8-mm collimation CT scan (**a**) and 3-mm-thick STS-MIP (**b**) are interpreted as inconclusive. Five-mm-thick STS-MIP (**c**) and 8-mm-thick STS-MIP (**d**) demonstrate tiny micronodules with a predominant distribution in the right lung, compatible with simple coal worker's pneumoconiosis

In addition to detection of lung infiltration, an attempt was made to determine whether STS-MIP could help characterize the pattern of lung infiltration. As previously demonstrated by means of pathological-CT correlations, ill-defined centrilobular micronodules are highly suggestive of bronchiolitis (SILVER et al. 1989; MURATA et al. 1986; AKIRA et al. 1992; REMY-JARDIN et al. 1993b) whereas detection of peribronchovascular changes is a useful guide to infiltration of the peripheral compartment of lung interstitium (MUNK et al. 1988; MULLER et al. 1989). As the advantage of STS-MIP over a single thin section is that vessels can be appreciated over a much longer segment of their course, the concurrent improvement in vessel and micronodule conspicuity accounted for the more frequent identification of centrilobular and perivascular changes on STS-MIP images (Fig. 7.5). However, care must be taken to differentiate actual perivascular micronodules from the beaded appearance of MIP artifacts due to partial volume averaging. These artifacts have been described as stair-step vessels and are expected to be found at the level of vessels that pass obliquely through the volume (NAPEL 1995).

These preliminary results suggest that a combination of conventional CT and STS-MIP should be employed to achieve an adequate evaluation of mild forms of micronodular lung infiltration. Since patients cannot be imaged with multiple CT techniques because of the high radiation dosage and time constraints, a focal spiral CT acquisition over a region of interest could complement the conventional CT study performed over the entire thorax.

7.3.3 Detection of Bronchiectasis and Peripheral Mucoid Impactions

Diagnosis of mucoid impaction in peripheral bronchioles on thin-section CT scans is usually based on the identification of short and nontapering tubular areas of attenuation, seen as either single or branching structures (MULLER and MILLER 1995). To date, two studies have evaluated the role of spiral CT in detecting peripheral bronchiectasis and mucoid impaction. REMY-JARDIN et al. (1996a) found that STS-MIP enabled identification of a greater number of bronchiolar changes compared with 1-mm conventional CT scans. These findings are in agreement with those reported by ENGELER et al. (1994) with volumetric scanning. In the latter study, the authors observed that traction bronchiectasis could be accurately differentiated from vessels or small pulmonary

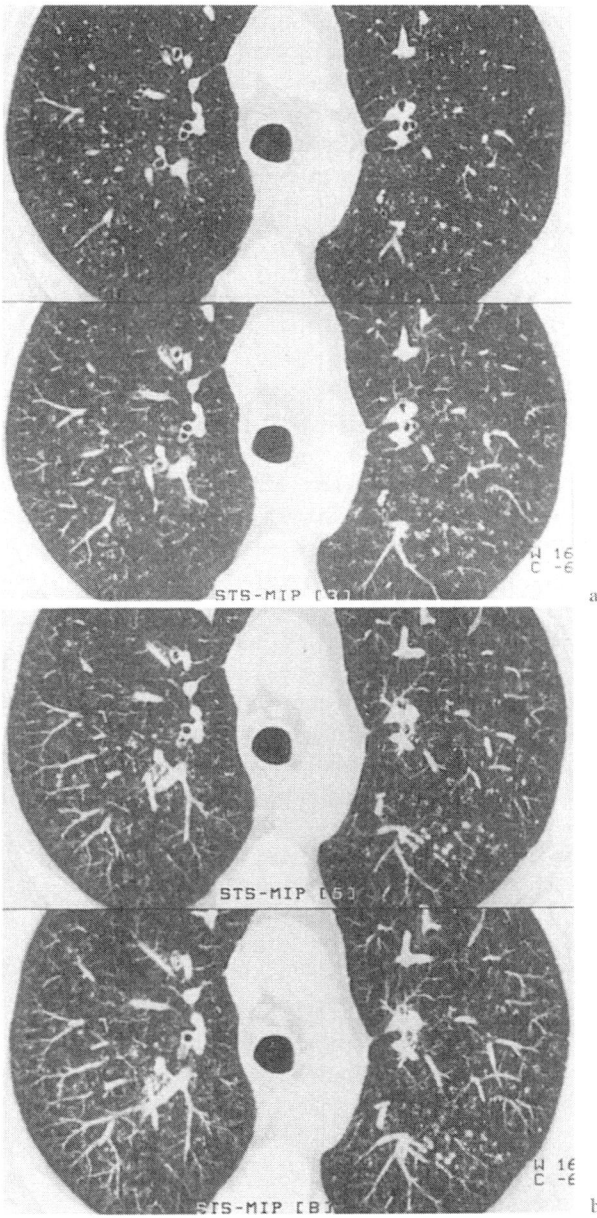

Fig. 7.5a,b. Conventional and STS-MIP images obtained at the right upper lobe level in a 61-year-old coal worker (180° linear interpolation algorithm; *UH*, ultra-high; window width, 1600 HU; window level, −600 HU). Comparison between a conventional 1-mm collimation CT scan (**a**, *top*), a 3-mm-thick STS-MIP (**a**, *bottom*), a 5-mm-thick STS-MIP (**b**, *top*) and an 8-mm-thick STS-MIP (**b**, *bottom*). Parenchymal micronodules are seen to be randomly distributed throughout both lungs on **a**. The centrilobular distribution of micronodules is dramatically demonstrated on **b**. Note the presence of beaded artifacts at the level of oblique vessels in the left lung on **b**

nodules only by examination of four contiguous scans generated from a volumetric CT acquisition. In addition to the specific diagnostic information gained by analyzing an entire set of images of contiguous sections, the authors found that the subjective level of confidence in their interpretations often increased markedly.

7.4 Sliding Thin Slab-Minimum Intensity Projection

The result of the minimum intensity projection (mIP) is to retain low-density structures at the expense of blood vessels. Consequently, this technique results in improved airway visibility along greater portions of their lengths and could help detect mild forms of emphysema. Emphysema is a pathological diagnosis which is diagnosed on the basis of a combination of clinical, functional, and radiographic findings. Whereas radiographic assessment of emphysema requires moderate to severe destruction (THURLBECK and MULLER 1994), it has been shown that CT is effective in the detection and quantification of emphysema (HAYHURST et al. 1984; GODDARD et al. 1982; BERGIN et al. 1986a,b; KREEL 1978; ROSENBLUM et al. 1978; CODDINGTON et al. 1982; FOSTER et al. 1986; MULLER et al. 1988; KLEIN et al. 1992). However, several authors have pointed out that mild emphysema may be missed on CT scans and the severity of emphysema may be underestimated (MILLER et al. 1989; SPOUGE et al. 1993; KUWANO et al. 1990). Therefore, REMY-JARDIN et al. (1996b) designed a study based on pathological-CT correlations to evaluate the ability of STS-mIP to detect emphysema.

7.4.1 Optimal Technique

The spiral CT acquisition consisted of the survey of a limited region of interest located in the lobe to be resected and was obtained at the suspended end-inspiration, without administration of iodinated contrast material. The protocol consisted of a 1-mm collimation and a 1 mm/s table feed (i.e., a pitch of 1), with scanning in the superoinferior direction within a 12-mm volume during a 13-s scanning time. In order to generate STS-mIP images, transverse CT scans were reconstructed from the same data set with a 180° linear interpolation algorithm and a standard reconstruction kernel; these transverse CT scans were then stacked to produce slabs of lung paren-

chyma. The reconstruction process lasted 30 min to generate the three series of STS-mIP images with a slab thickness of 3 mm, 5 mm, and 8 mm. In order to provide comparable material, STS-mIP images were photographed at similar window settings to those used for HRCT scans (500 HU; −850 HU).

The choice of the reconstruction algorithms followed an evaluation of different combinations between 180° and 360° linear interpolation algorithms and standard and high-frequency reconstruction kernels. As shown in Fig. 7.6, the reconstruction of images with a 180° linear interpolation algorithm and a standard kernel was considered the most accurate compromise for depiction of areas of abnormally low attenuation with maximal spatial resolution.

7.4.2 Detection of Emphysema

Evaluating 29 patients without radiographic evidence of emphysema with conventional thin-section CT and STS-mIP immediately before surgery, REMY-JARDIN et al. (1996b) found that volumetric CT could complement the visual inspection of CT images for the recognition of emphysema. When emphysema was identified on thin-section CT scans, as was the case in 45% of the study group, STS-mIPs also demonstrated areas of hypoattenuation which were more conspicuous than on thin-section CT scans (Fig. 7.7). However, this increased conspicuity did not modify the extent scores of emphysema. The subjective superiority of STS-mIP is directly related to the suppression of highly attenuated structures, i.e., vessels and fissures, with a subsequent uniform appearance of the lung parenchyma which was particularly marked on 8-mm-thick slabs. Despite the volumetric approach of STS-mIP, this technique was found to remain compatible with the depiction of morphological features of centrilobular emphysema, such as the clear recognition of small round or confluent areas of low attenuation located near the center of the secondary pulmonary lobule. Among the 16 patients without emphysema on thin-section CT scans (i.e., 65% of the study group), STS-mIP enabled the identification of focal areas of hypoattenuation against the background of the normal lung in four patients with further confirmation of emphysematous changes on histological sections. Comparing the respective sensitivity of STS-mIP (81%) and thin-section CT (62%), the former technique was found to significantly improve emphysema detection. In the remaining 12 patients with normal thin-section CT scans, STS-mIPs correctly excluded emphysema in

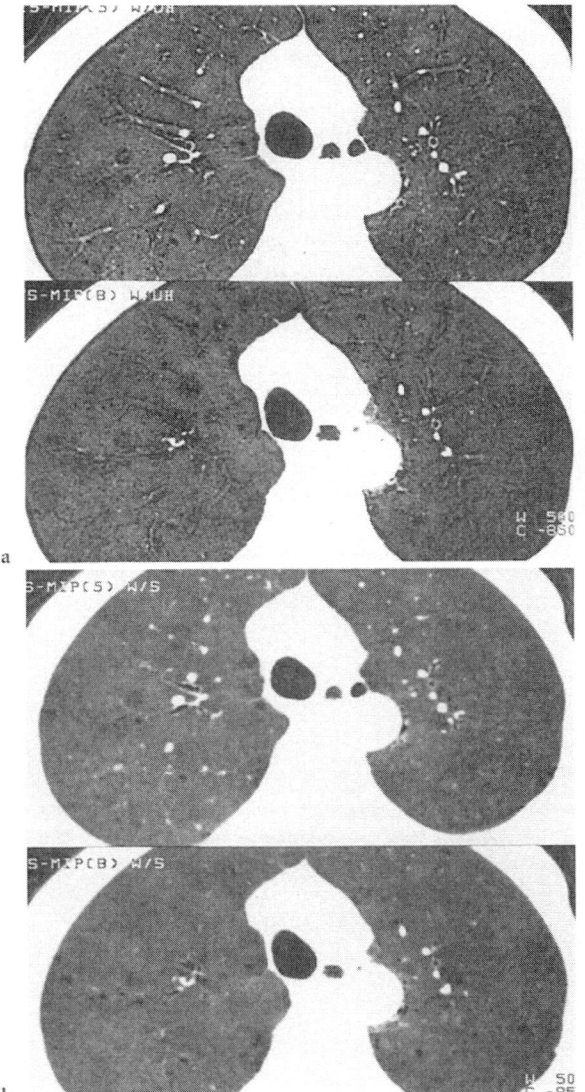

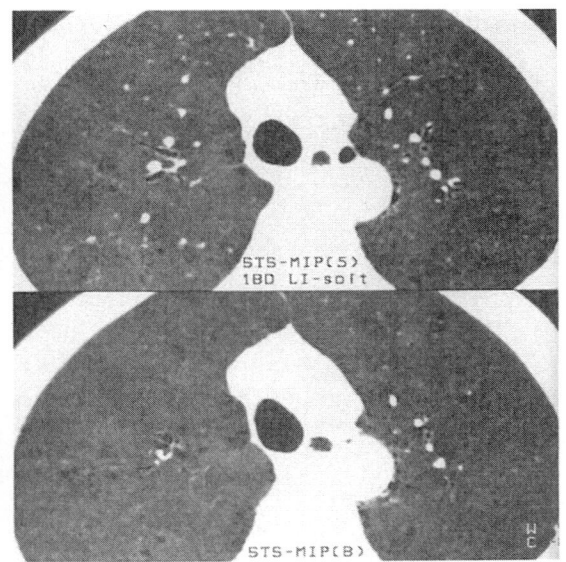

Fig. 7.6a–c. Comparison between different algorithms applied for reconstruction of 5-mm-thick (*top*) and 8-mm-thick (*bottom*) STS-mIPs (window width, 500 HU; window level, −850 HU). **a** STS-mIPs reconstructed with a 360° linear interpolation algorithm (*W*, wide) and a high spatial frequency reconstruction kernel (*UH*, ultra-high). These images show incomplete vascular suppression and multiple hypoattenuated areas around vascular bundles, precluding confident depiction of emphysematous changes. **b** STS-mIPs reconstructed with a 360° linear interpolation algorithm (*W*, wide) and a soft reconstruction kernel (*S*, soft). Compared with **a**, these images show considerable improvement in vascular suppression and depiction of small rounded areas of emphysema, suggesting the superiority of the standard reconstruction kernel. **c** STS-mIPs reconstructed with a 180° linear interpolation algorithm and a soft reconstruction kernel (*S*, soft). Compared with **b**, these images show similar vascular suppression but increased spatial resolution

eight patients but failed to detect minimal emphysematous changes in four. These results suggest that mild forms of emphysema still lie beyond the diagnostic capabilities of this new CT technology. However, it must be pointed out that STS-mIP shares the same limitation as that emphasized with the density mask technique, an alternative diagnostic approach to emphysema with conventional CT based on the quantification of pixels beyond a density threshold (MULLER et al. 1988). When the examination is limited to images taken at full inspiration, it is not possible to distinguish hyperinflation without tissue destruction from emphysema. Care must be taken to avoid misinterpretation of lung morphology in the mIP reconstruction as motion artifacts can mimic

emphysematous changes. Owing to their typical paramediastinal location, cardiac motion artifacts are usually correctly identified. However, breathing artifacts during data acquisition cannot be accurately recognized on STS-mIPs alone; their recognition requires the concurrent analysis of STS-mIP images and individual thin-section CT scans.

In conclusion, these preliminary data suggest that STS-mIP can represent a useful complement to conventional thin-section CT in the detection of mild forms of emphysema. However, this technique requires further comparison with other promising alternatives such as the density mask technique at full expiration (KNUDSEN et al. 1991) to define their respective clinical applications.

158   M. Rémy-Jardin and J. Rémy

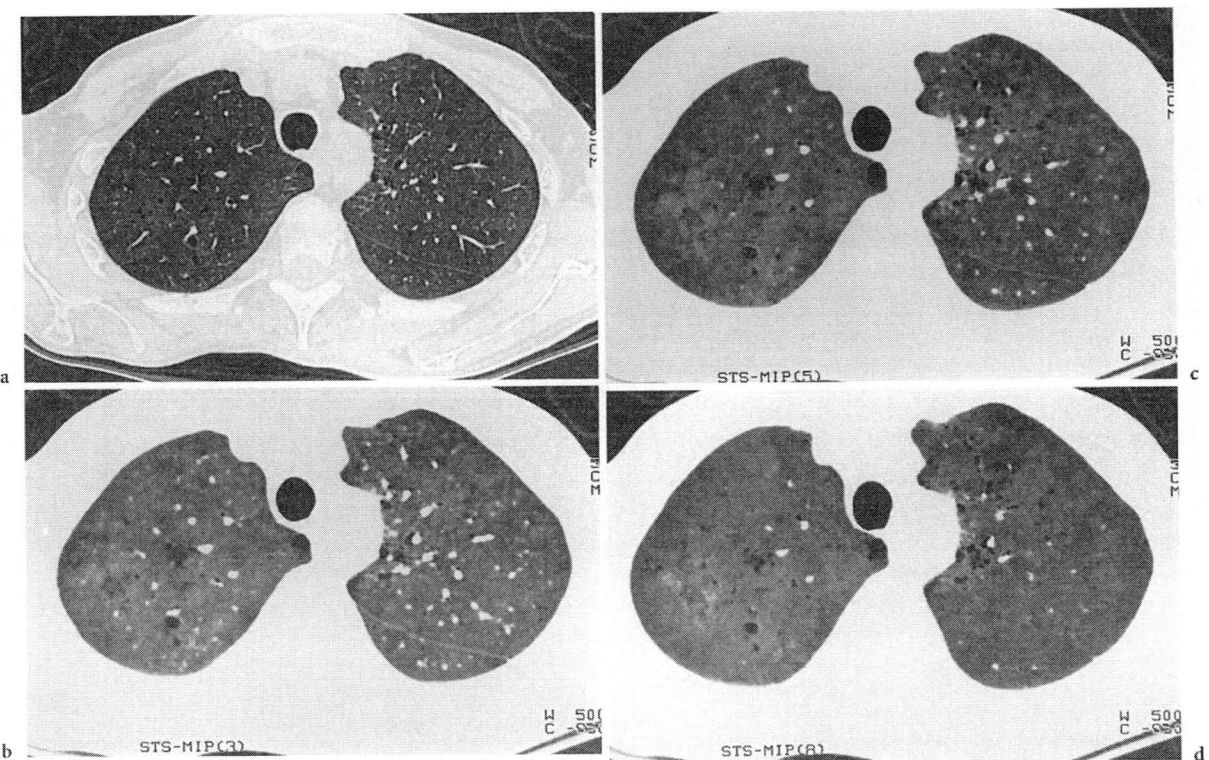

Fig. 7.7a–d. Detection of emphysema in a 37-year-old smoker (180° linear interpolation algorithm; soft reconstruction kernel). The conventional 1-mm collimation CT scan (**a**) shows tiny hypoattenuated areas suggestive of emphysema and mild cylindral bronchiectases on both lungs (window width, 1600 HU; window level, –600 HU). Note the increased conspicuity of parenchymal and bronchial abnormalities on STS-mIPs of 3-mm thickness (**b**), 5-mm thickness (**c**), and 8-mm thickness (**d**). Mild ground glass attenuation is easier to detect on STS-mIPs (window width, 500 HU; window level, –850 HU)

References

Akira M, Kita N, Higashihara T, Sakatani M, Kozuka T (1992) Summer-type hypersensitivity pneumonitis: comparison of high-resolution CT and plain radiographic findings. AJR 158:1223–1228

Bergin CL, Muller N, Nichols DM et al. (1986a) The diagnosis of emphysema: a computed tomographic-pathologic correlation. Am Rev Respir Dis 133:541–546

Bergin CL, Muller NL, Miller RR (1986b) CT in the quantitative assessment of emphysema. J Thorac Imaging 1:94–103

Brauner MW, Lenoir S, Grenier PH, Cluzel P, Battesti JP, Valeyre D (1992) Pulmonary sarcoidosis: CT assessment of lesion reversibility. Radiology 182:349–354

Cardoso WV, Sekhon HS, Hyde DM, Thurlbeck WM (1993) Collagen and elastin in human pulmonary emphysema. Am Rev Respir Dis 147:975–981

Coddington R, Mera SL, Goddard PR, Bradfield JWB (1982) Pathological evaluation of computed tomography images of the lungs. J Clin Pathol 35:536–540

Engeler CE, Tashjian JH, Engeler CM, Geise RA, Holm JC, Ritenour ER (1994) Volumetric high-resolution CT in the diagnosis of interstitial lung disease and bronchiectasis: diagnostic accuracy and radiation dose. AJR 163:31–35

Foster WL, Pratt PC, Roggli VL, Godwin JD, Halvorsen RA, Putman CE (1986) Centrilobular emphysema: CT-pathologic correlation. Radiology 159:27–32

Goddard PR, Nicholson EU, Laszlo G, Watt I (1982) Computed tomography in pulmonary emphysema. Clin Radiol 33:379–387

Hayhurst MD, Flenley DC, McLean A (1984) Diagnosis of pulmonary emphysema by computerised tomography. Lancet II:320–322

Kim WD, Eidelman DH, Izquierdo JL, Ghezzo H, Saetta MP, Cosio MG (1991) Centrilobular and panlobular emphysema in smokers. Two distinct morphologic and functional entities. Am Rev Respir Dis 144:1385–1390

Klein JS, Gamsu G, Webb WR et al. (1992) High-resolution CT diagnosis of emphysema in symptomatic patients with normal chest radiographs and isolated low diffusing capacity. Radiology 182:817–821

Knudsen RJ, Standen JR, Kaltenborn WT et al. (1991) Expiratory computed tomography for assessment of suspected pulmonary emphysema. Chest 99:1357–1366

Kreel L (1978) Computed tomography of the thorax. Radiol Clin North Am 16:575–584

Kuwano K, Matsuba K, Ikeda T et al. (1990) The diagnosis of mild emphysema. Correlation of computed tomography and pathology scores. Am Rev Respir Dis 141:169–178

Leopold JG, Gough J (1957) The centrilobular form of hyper-trophic emphysema and its relation to chronic bronchitis. Thorax 12:219–235

Leung AN, Staples CA, Muller NL (1991) Chronic diffuse infil-trative lung disease: comparison of diagnostic accuracy of high-resolution CT and conventional CT. AJR 157:693–696

Leung AN, Miller RR, Muller NL (1993) Parenchymal opacification in chronic infiltrative lung diseases: CT-pathologic correlation. Radiology 188:209–214

Mayo JR, Webb WR, Gould R et al. (1987) High resolution CT of the lungs: an optimal approach. Radiology 163:507–510

Miller RR, Muller NL, Vedal S, Morrison NJ, Staples CA (1989) Limitations of computed tomography in the assessment of emphysema. Am Rev Respir Dis 139:980–983

Muller NL, Miller RR (1995) Diseases of the bronchioles: CT and histopathologic findings. Radiology 196:3–12

Muller NL, Staples CA, Miller RR, Abbound RT (1988) "Den-sity mask": an objective method to quantitate emphysema using computed tomography. Chest 94:782–787

Muller NL, Kullnig P, Miller RR (1989) The CT findings of pulmonary sarcoidosis: analysis of 25 patients. AJR 152:1179–1182

Munk PL, Muller NL, Miller RR, Ostrow DN (1988) Pulmonary lymphangitic carcinomatosis: CT and pathologic findings. Radiology 166:705–709

Murata K, Otoh H, Todo G et al. (1986) Centrilobular lesions of the lungs: demonstration by high-resolution CT and pathologic correlation. Radiology 161:641–645

Napel SA (1995) Principles and techniques of 3D spiral CT angiography. In: Jeffrey RB, Fishman EK (eds) Spiral CT. Raven Press, New York, pp 167–196

Napel S, Rubin GD, Jeffrey RB (1993) STS-MIP: a new recon-struction technique for CT of the chest. J Comput Assist Tomogr 17:832–838

Paranjpe DV, Bergin CJ (1994) Spiral CT of the lungs: optimal technique and resolution compared with conventional CT. AJR 162:561–567

Pratt PC (1987) Role of conventional chest radiography in diagnosis and exclusion of emphysema. Am J Med 82:998–1006

Rémy-Jardin M, Degreef JM, Beuscart R, Voisin C, Remy J (1990) Coal worker's pneumoconiosis: CT assessment in exposed workers and correlation with radiographic find-ings. Radiology 177:363–371

Rémy-Jardin M, Rémy J, Deffontaines C, Duhamel A (1991) Assessment of diffuse infiltrative lung disease: comparison of conventional CT and high-resolution CT. Radiology 181:157–162

Rémy-Jardin M, Giraud F, Rémy J, Copin MC, Gosselin B, Duhamel A (1993a) Importance of ground glass attenua-tion in chronic diffuse infiltrative lung disease: pathologic-CT correlation. Radiology 189:693–698

Rémy-Jardin M, Rémy J, Gosselin B, Becette V, Edme JL (1993b) Lung parenchymal changes secondary to cigarette smoking: pathologic-CT correlations. Radiology 186:643–651

Rémy-Jardin M, Rémy J, Artaud D, Deschildre F, Duhamel A (1996a) Diffuse infiltrative lung disease: clinical value of sliding-thin-slab maximum intensity projection CT scans in the detection of mild micronodular patterns. Radiology 200:333–339

Rémy-Jardin M, Rémy J, Gosselin B, Copin MC, Wurtz A, Duhamel A (1996b) Sliding-thin-slab, minimum intensity projection technique in the diagnosis of emphysema: histopathologic-CT correlation. Radiology 200:665–671

Rigault H, Marchal G, Baert AL, Hupke R (1990) Spiral scan-ning: phantom studies and patient material. In: Fuchs WA (ed) Advances in CT. Springer, New York Berlin Heidel-berg, pp 65–76

Rosenblum LJ, Mauceri RA, Wellestein DE, Bassano DA, Cohen WN, Heitzman ER (1978) Computed tomography of the lung. Radiology 129:521–524

Silver SF, Muller NL, Miller RR, Lefcoe MS (1989) Hypersensi-tivity pneumonitis: evaluation with CT. Radiology 173:441–445

Snider GL (1994) Pathogenesis and terminology of emphy-sema (letter to the editor). Am J Respir Crit Care Med 149:1382–1383

Snider GL, Kleinerman J, Thurlbeck WM, Bengali ZH (1985) The definition of emphysema: report of a National Heart, Lung and Blood Institute, Division of Lung Diseases work-shop. Am Rev Respir Dis 132:182–185

Spouge D, Mayo JR, Cardoso W, Muller NL (1993) Panacinar emphysema: CT and pathologic findings. J Comput Assist Tomogr 17:710–713

Swirewich CV, Terriff B, Muller NL (1989) High spatial fre-quency (bone) algorithm improves quality of standard CT of the thorax. AJR 153:1169–1173

Terriff BA, Kwan SY, Chan-Yeung MM, Muller NL (1992) Fibrosing alveolitis: chest radiography and CT predictors of clinical and functional impairment at follow-up in 26 patients. Radiology 184:445–449

Thurlbeck WM, Muller NL (1994) Emphysema: definition, imaging and quantification. AJR 163:1017–1025

8 Spiral CT of the Trachea and Main Bronchi

C.M. Schaefer-Prokop and M. Prokop

CONTENTS

8.1 Introduction

Bronchoscopy serves as one of the first-line methods for evaluation of tracheobronchial pathology and is often considered the "gold standard." Any other imaging technique such as spiral CT will have to be compared with this endoscopic technique.

Bronchoscopy provides direct visualization of the mucosa and includes the option to acquire a specimen for histopathologic evaluation. There are, however, important constraints. Bronchoscopy does not provide information about the extraluminal extent of disease, the relationship to adjacent mediastinal structures, and the presence of mediastinal lymph nodes. Bronchoscopy provides unlimited visualization of the tracheal wall and the main bronchi, with

C.M. Schaefer-Prokop, MD, Department of Radiology I, Hannover Medical School, 30623 Hannover, Germany
M. Prokop, MD, Department of Radiology I, Hannover Medical School, 30623 Hannover, Germany

the exception of the proximal subglottic trachea (0.5–1 cm), in which bronchoscopic evaluation is difficult. Submucosal disease without intraluminal extension may be missed and increased secretion of mucus can obscure pathology. High-grade stenoses (<5 mm) cannot be passed by standard bronchoscopes. In these cases, no information about the length of the stenosis and about the poststenotic bronchi can be obtained. Anatomic orientation may be difficult in patients with congenital variants, or with tumor-induced or postoperative alterations of the anatomy.

Magnetic resonance imaging (MRI) still has a very limited role in the assessment of the trachea and bronchi. It may be useful in tumor staging and in performing longitudinal sections of the trachea.

At present, CT is the cross-sectional technique of choice for imaging of the tracheobronchial system. It is superior to bronchoscopy in detecting the presence and extent of extraluminal disease. The air column within trachea and bronchi serves as an excellent negative contrast medium for visualization of the surface of the tracheobronchial lumen. However, breathing effects and stair-step artifacts on longitudinal reformats limit the evaluation of small, focal intraluminal pathology with standard CT. Spiral CT, with its capability for continuous volume acquisition during a single breathhold, provides a superb tool to visualize even minor intra- and extraluminal pathology in the trachea and main bronchi. Spiral CT can visualize the tracheobronchial system distal to an airway obstruction. Findings, however, are often nonspecific and require biopsy. Spiral CT and bronchoscopy are therefore complementary methods for the diagnostic workup of tracheobronchial disease.

8.2 Spiral CT Data Acquisition and Evaluation

In standard CT, image quality is dependent on image noise and spatial resolution within the transaxial scan plane (xy resolution). Through-plane resolution (z-axis resolution) usually is of importance only if small structures such as endobronchial lesions have to be evaluated in areas where the course of the bronchi is oblique to the scan plane. Stair-step artifacts will occur whenever 3D reconstructions or 2D reformats are performed. For most indications, however, diagnosis can be readily made on the transaxial sections.

In spiral CT, xy resolution is identical to that in standard CT given identical scanning parameters (KALENDER and POLACIN 1991). Image noise will in addition depend on the raw data interpolation employed and will increase with narrower slice collimation. The z-axis resolution is directly related to the effective slice thickness. The smaller the effective

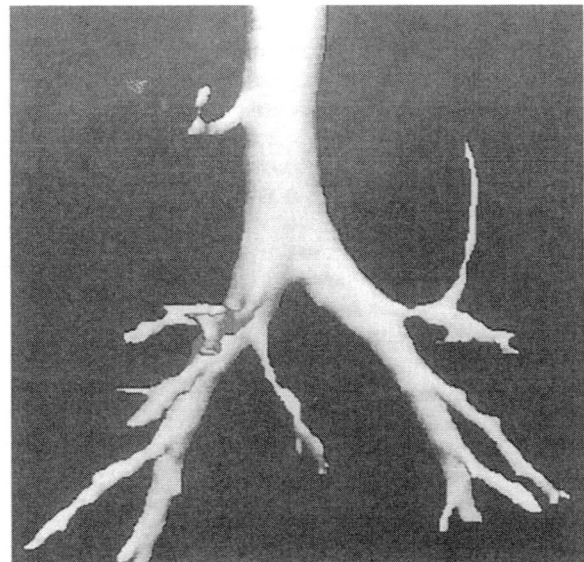
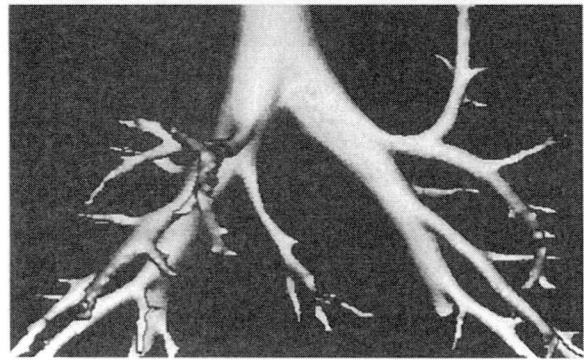

Fig. 8.1. SSD of the tracheobronchial tree of a pig: comparison of scan protocol A (**a**) and protocol B (**b**) with the scan parameters SC/TS/RI = 5/8/2 (**a**) and 1/2/1 (**b**). Note the superior visualization of the bronchi with smaller effective slice thickness. Improvement is especially obvious for the segmental and subsegmental bronchi and bronchi with a horizontal course

slice thickness, the more precise are 2D reformats or 3D reconstructions (Fig. 8.1). Measurements of the craniocaudal extent of a lesion or the craniocaudal diameter of a bronchus depend heavily on a high z-axis resolution if lesions or bronchi are smaller than 1 cm in size.

8.2.1 Scanner Technology and z-Axis Resolution

The available z-axis resolution will depend (a) on the required scan range and (b) on the scanner technology (Table 8.1). For a given scanner type and a limited scan time (usually 24–30 s), scan range and z-axis resolution are inversely proportional. The z-axis resolution can be improved by employing 180° raw data interpolation and using a high pitch factor. However, both 180° interpolation and pitch factors close to 2 will increase the likelihood of periodic wall irregularities ("serrations") due to pulsation effects. These effects increase from the trachea to the lower lobe bronchi. Recent advances in scanner technology could further improve z-axis resolution by increasing the speed of tube rotation or by employing more than one detector array (split detector systems).

8.2.2 Scan Protocols

Imaging of the trachea and central airways will rarely be confined to these regions but will frequently include an examination of the whole chest (Table 8.2, protocol A). Optimum evaluation of the region of interest, however, will often require a targeted scan with minimum effective slice thickness for the highest possible z-axis resolution and a field of view (FOV) of 15–25 cm for high xy resolution (Table 8.2, protocol B). At present, only split detector systems are able to acquire data from the whole chest (protocol A) at a resolution that is sufficient to omit a second scan (protocol B). Depending on the pathology, a scan of only a limited part of the trachea or bronchi will suffice for protocol B, although more often trachea and carina or carina and central bronchi will have to be imaged together. Transaxial images will have to be reconstructed with at least a 50% overlap for either protocol in order to fully utilize the advantages of spiral CT. Suggestions for scan parameters are given in Table 8.2.

Due to their fixed positions within the mediastinum, the trachea and carina are only slightly affected by flat respiration. Scans in suspended respiration are therefore not mandatory. Scans during a specific

Table 8.1. Influence of scanner technology on z-axis resolution using the minimal effective slice thickness for a required scan length of some 12 cm (central airways) at a maximum scan time of 32 s and a pitch of 2. The effective slice thickness was calculated according to POLACIN et al. (1992)

RS	Detector	TI	SP	SC	TS	Pitch	ST
1 s	Single	24 s	360° LI	5 mm	10 mm/s	1	8.3 mm
1 s	Single	24 s	180° LI	3 mm	5 mm/s	2	4.5 mm
1 s	Single	32 s	180° LI	2 mm	4 mm/s	2	3.4 mm
0.75 s	Single	32 s	180° LI	1.5 mm	3 mm/s	2	2.5 mm
1 s	Split	32 s	180° LI	1 mm	4 mm/s	2	1.7 mm

RS, Rotation speed of scanner tube; TI, total scan time; SP, slice profile; SC, slice collimation; TS, table speed; ST, effective slice thickness (full width at tenth area)

Table 8.2. Scan protocols for scanners with 1-s tube rotation and single detector array

Protocol	Anatomic region	TI	L	SC	TS	RI	Pitch
A	Whole chest	30	24	4–5	8	4	1.6–2
B	Trachea/bronchi	30	6–12	1–2	2–4	1–2	1.5–2

TI, Scan time (s); L, scan range (cm); SC, slice collimation (mm); TS, table speed (mm/s); RI, reconstruction interval (mm)

respiratory maneuver can assist in the diagnosis of abnormal tracheal wall compliance. If the whole chest is examined or the bronchi are included in the scan range, scans are obtained at full inspiration in order to avoid motion-related artifacts. Axial sections from spiral CT are less vulnerable to breathing effects than axial sections from standard CT. However, even slight respiratory motions may markedly impair the evaluation of 2D reformats or 3D reconstructions from a spiral CT data set.

In clinical practice, most patients can handle a period of 30 s in suspended inspiration, given a sufficiently careful instruction and a short period of hyperventilation prior to the scan. Endonasal inflation of oxygen may also be helpful. It is advantageous to start the spiral scan at the lower level and to scan towards the apex of the lungs: if the patient starts to breathe close to the end of the scan, artifacts are less pronounced since apical lung structures and the trachea are less affected by diaphragmatic motions.

The patient is scanned in the supine position. When the region of primary concern is the extrathoracic trachea, the patient's arms are positioned at the side, with the shoulders pulled down as far as possible. For the mediastinal portion of the trachea or the central bronchi, the patient's arms are positioned above the head to eliminate streak artifacts from the arms and shoulder.

8.2.3 Contrast Administration

Intravenous injection of contrast medium has not been shown to directly assist in the diagnosis of tracheal or bronchial masses. However, the differentiation between a vessel and a mass will often depend on contrast administration. This is especially important if deep transmural biopsy is to be performed in masses that impinge on trachea or bronchi. Spiral CT yields constantly high and homogeneous intravascular contrast given an optimized bolus technique (see Chap. 4).

8.2.4 Image Evaluation

The primary volume data set from a spiral CT scan consists of overlapping transaxial images. Multiplanar 2D reformats also take advantage of these data without any reduction of information. 3D rendering techniques such as surface or volume rendering have to reduce the data in order to transform them into a two-dimensional image. 3D techniques provide a comprehensive display of the anatomic situation and are well suited for image presentation to the referring physicians, but cannot serve as a basis for diagnosis. Acceptable results require a high z-axis resolution (protocol B).

8.2.4.1 Primary Cross-sectional Data Set

Overlapping transaxial images provide the highest morphologic detail and are indispensable for diagnosis. Detection of subtle tracheobronchial findings is best when axial images are viewed interactively in a cine display.

Multiplanar reformatting is required to display a lesion in a second plane in order to define its craniocaudal extent. Optimal results are achieved when cut planes are interactively adjusted to the anatomic situation. A (semi-)coronal reformat of the trachea and main bronchi appears to provide the best information. Additional planes adapted to the pathology may be useful for evaluation of lesions and the origins of branching lobar bronchi. Irregularly curve-shaped planes may be necessary to display trachea and main bronchi along their axis.

8.2.4.2 Minimum Intensity Projections

Minimum intensity projection (mIP) imaging is a simple 3D volume rendering technique that is able to project the tracheobronchial air column into a viewing plane (see Chap. 5). For each ray that passes a predefined volume of interest (VOI), the minimum CT number encountered on its path is displayed. The technique is very vulnerable to varying width of VOI and to partial volume effects. Both severely limit the clinical usefulness of mIP.

Even minor partial volume averaging (>10% soft tissue within an endoluminal voxel) leads to an increase in CT numbers towards the level of surrounding lung and, thus, to underestimation of the airway caliber. This effect grows with increasing effective slice thickness, decreasing bronchial diameter, and horizontal course of a bronchus (Fig. 8.2). Therefore, peripheral bronchi can hardly be visualized. For the mediastinal portion of the central airways, the vulnerability to partial volume effects can be markedly reduced if a narrow VOI is employed that excludes overlying lung tissue. Under this condition, mIP images provide a good overview of the anatomy and gross pathology of trachea and central bronchi.

There are, however, a large number of pitfalls. Depending on the VOI, the trachea can be obscured on an anteroposterior view by an air-filled esophagus. Under unfavorable conditions, high-grade stenoses are imaged as pseudo-occlusions (Fig. 8.3). The intraluminal growth of eccentric tumors is generally underestimated and may even be completely

missed (Figs. 8.4, 8.5). Intraluminal structures of higher density (e.g., stents) are not displayed. Wall irregularities are only seen in a mIP if imaged in profile.

Many of these problems can be overcome by creating "sliding thin slab mIP" (STS-mIP) images. These are an overlapping sequence of mIP images that are based on only a few transaxial sections each. Small structures are displayed with higher detail and obscuring partial volume effects are reduced. The clinical value of this technique, however, is not yet clear.

8.2.4.3 Shaded Surface Display

Shaded surface displays are based on a surface rendering technique that requires the definition of a binary object in three-dimensional space. This is usually done by selecting a certain threshold range of

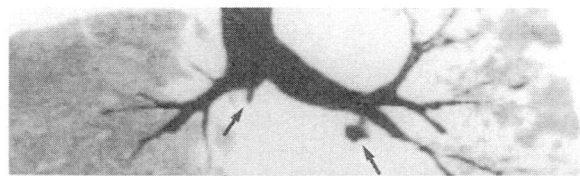

Fig. 8.2. Anteroposterior mIP image in a patient with bilateral small anastomotic dehiscences (*arrows*) after lung transplantation and a left-sided pulmonary infiltration. Note the improved display of the bronchi down to the subsegmental level on the left side due to the increased density of the surrounding parenchyma. Also note that the visualization of bronchi deteriorates if they run horizontally and not perpendicularly to the scan plane (protocol B: SC/TS/RI = 2/2/1)

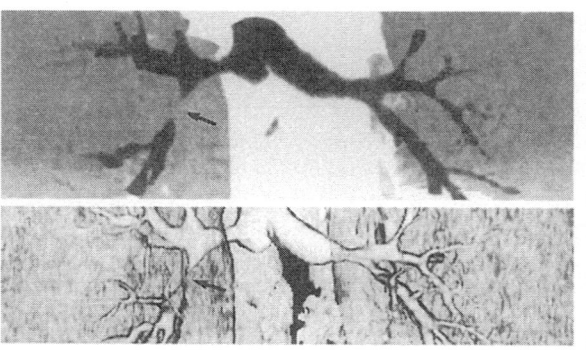

Fig. 8.3. Comparison of mIP (**a**) and an advanced volume rendering technique (**b**) in a patient with bilateral strictures of the main bronchi and a high-grade stenosis of the intermediate bronchus that is imaged as a "pseudo-occlusion" (*arrow*) due to partial volume effects (protocol B: 2/2/1)

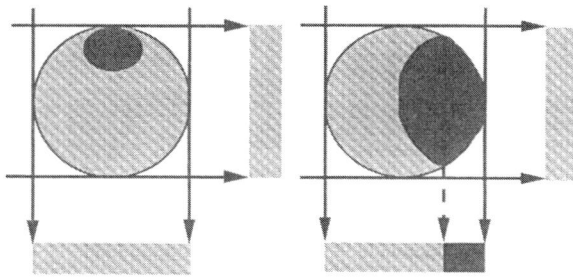

Fig. 8.4. The visualization of an intraluminal tumor is highly dependent on tumor size and projection effects. A mIP will show a tumor only if there is no superimposed intrabronchial air

CT numbers to be included in this object. A realistic "3D look" is obtained by casting rays onto the object surface and assigning gray levels to each surface point according to the locally reflected or scattered light (voxel gradient shading). SSD leads to a further reduction of information from the primary data set, since no attenuation values are preserved and CT values outside the threshold range are not displayed. Depending on the threshold range, a positive or negative cast of the air column or an endoscopic view of the inner surface of the tracheobronchial system is produced (Fig. 8.6).

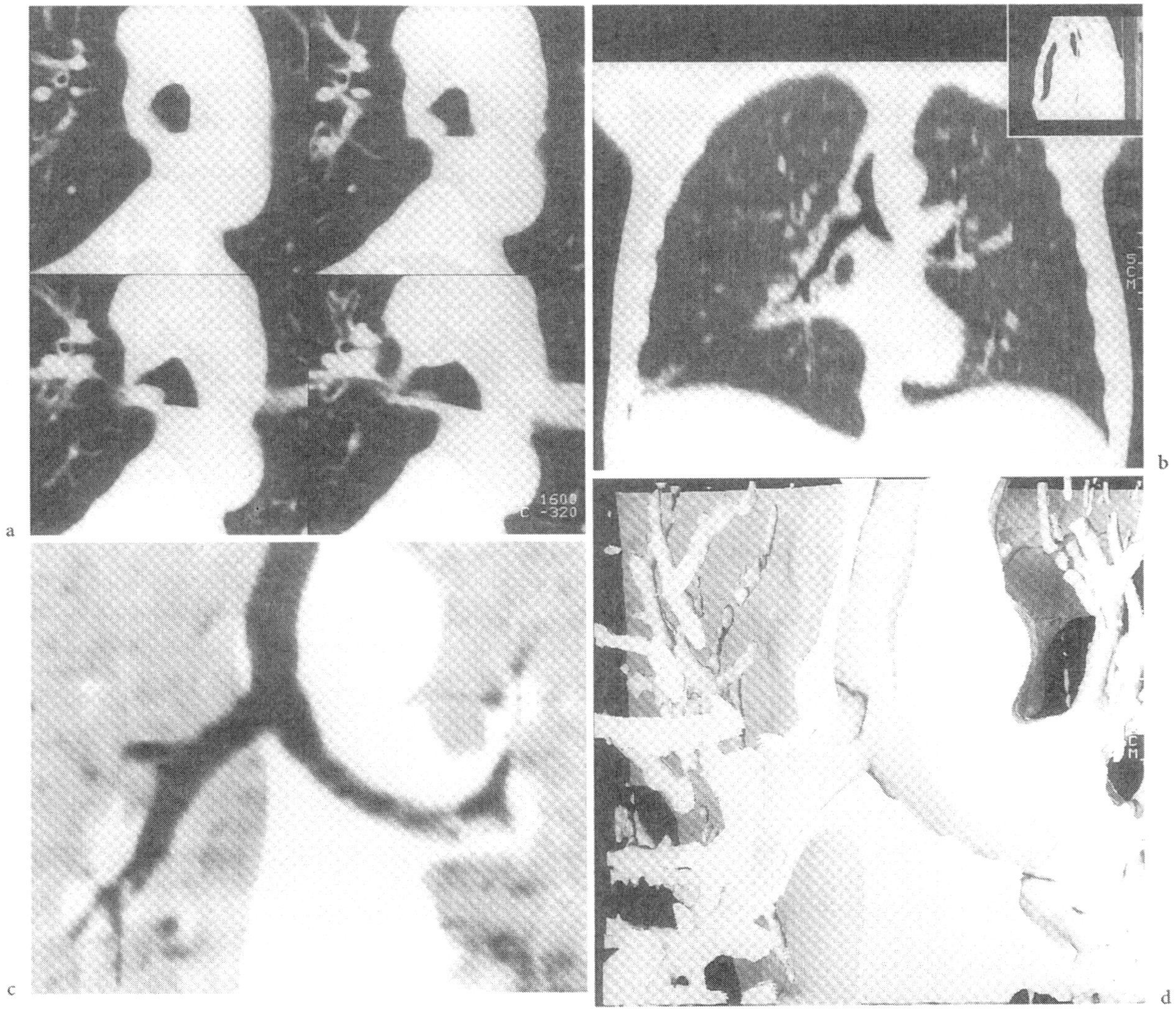

Fig. 8.5. Axial sections (**a**), coronal reformats (**b**), mIP (**c**) and SSD (**d**) in a patient with a carcinoid tumor of pericarinal location. Note that SSD is superior to mIP for demonstration of intraluminal tumors (protocol A: 5/8/4)

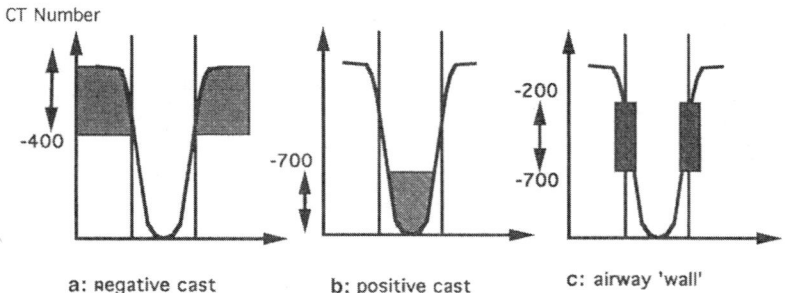

CT Number

-400

-200

-700

a: negative cast   b: positive cast   c: airway 'wall'

Fig. 8.6. Depending on the threshold range, a negative (**a**) or positive cast (**b**) of the air column or a view of the "wall" of the tracheobronchial system (**c**) is produced

8.2.4.3.1 Mediastinal Soft Tissue "Block" (Negative Cast).

Inclusion of all pixel values above a single pre-defined *lower* threshold below that of fatty tissue (e.g., −400 HU) produces an image of the mediastinal soft tissue block. The air-filled tracheobronchial tree is hidden within this block and is made visible by cut functions (Fig. 8.7a). The cuts have to be tailored to the individual course of the bronchi. The diameter of the airway is heavily dependent on the selected threshold.

8.2.4.3.2 Tracheobronchial "Cast" (Positive Cast).

Inclusion of all pixel values below a preselected *upper* threshold (e.g., −700 HU) produces a three-dimensional positive "*cast*" of the air column. The surface of this cast reflects the inner surface of the airways (Fig. 8.7b). The tracheobronchial wall itself is not imaged. The diameter of a "bronchus" is determined by the selected threshold level. A flexible adjustment of the threshold is necessary depending on bronchus size and surrounding tissue in order to produce a realistic 3D reconstruction: In airways surrounded by soft tissue, the density of airway borders increases with decreasing diameter, and in airways surrounded by ventilated lung parenchyma, the density of the bronchial wall decreases with decreasing diameter.

The segmentation of airways from lung parenchyma has still to be done interactively and is error-prone and time-consuming. There are attempts to replace the interactive editing by computer algorithms that automatically detect borders and extract the VOI.

8.2.4.3.3 Tracheobronchial "Wall."

Inclusion of all pixel values within a preselected *threshold* range of, for example, −200 to −700 HU produces an image of the air/soft tissue interface. This results in an image that resembles the tracheobronchial wall (Fig. 8.7c). The *outer* diameter of this structure correlates best with the true bronchial diameter. However, one must always keep in mind that this "wall" is a simple visu-

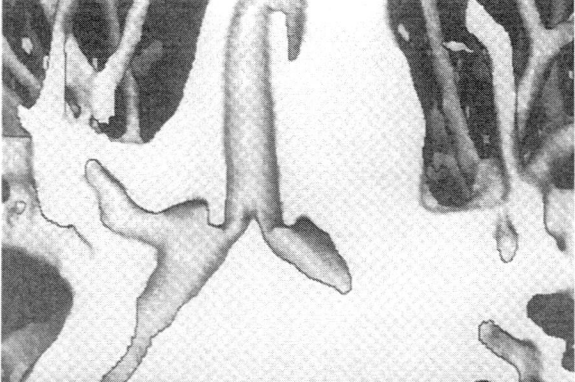

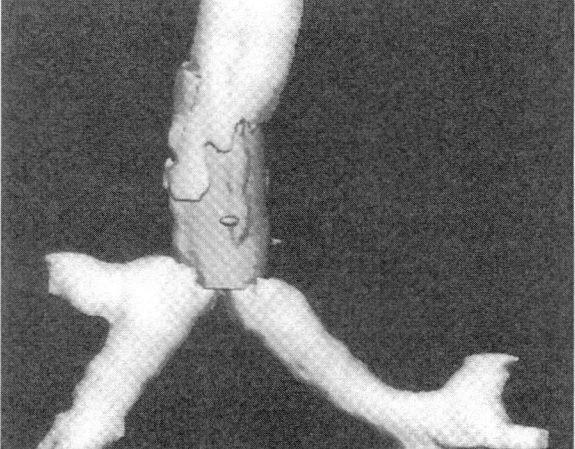

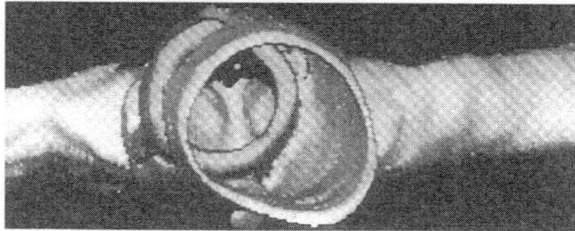

Fig. 8.7. Patient who received a tracheal stent for tracheomalacia after heart-lung transplantation with tracheal anastomosis: negative cast (**a**), positive cast (**b**), and view of the "airway wall" looking into the trachea (**c**). Note that the stent is displaced caudally and is riding on the carina, resulting in a partial obstruction of the air flow into the main bronchi. The stent is also slightly tilted and causes a protrusion of the tracheal wall (protocol A: 5/8/4)

alization trick that does not correspond to the real wall structures.

8.2.4.3.4 "Bronchoscopic" View. Bronchoscopic images can be obtained with method A ("mediastinal block") if the viewing distance for the SSD is not infinity (parallel projection) but the view point is placed inside the trachea or bronchi (central projection). By moving the view point along a path through the tracheobronchial system, "CT bronchoscopy" or "virtual bronchoscopy" can be performed. The strong threshold dependence of the luminal diameter can be reduced if advanced volume rendering techniques are used that do not require a fixed threshold value but instead employ a density-dependent lookup function to assign opacity to the tracheobronchial wall. The observer may then interactively move through the airways. Visualization of up to fifth order bronchi is possible with appropriate scan parameters (effective slice thickness ≤3 mm). Semitransparent display of the airway wall allows for simultaneous visualization of adjacent vascular structures. It is an excellent planning tool for transbronchial procedures.

8.3 Clinical Applications

Diseases affecting the trachea and main bronchi can be divided into those that cause focal disease and those that result in diffuse disease. While most focal diseases tend to produce decreased airway diameter, diffuse diseases result in both enlargement and narrowing of the airway. CT has become the radiologic examination of choice for investigating tracheobronchial disorders. In the following, advantages and limitations of spiral CT technology with respect to particular disease groups will be described and further outlined by typical image examples.

8.3.1 Normal Anatomy of the Trachea and Main Bronchi

The trachea is a fibromuscular and cartilaginous tube of 10–12 cm length. It extends from the lower border of the cricoid cartilage to the bifurcation at the tracheal carina. The trachea is a midline structure except for its few inferior centimeters, which incline slightly to the right. The shape of the intrathoracic portion of the trachea, which is about 6–9 cm in length, varies between persons and at different levels in the same person, and may assume a horseshoe, elliptical, or circular configuration. In 50%, the normal posterior tracheal membrane protrudes slightly into the tracheal air column.

Computed tomography is the method of choice to assess diameters and cross-sectional areas of the airways. Table 8.3 lists the dimensions of the normal adult trachea. The dimensions and shape of the trachea change with various respiratory maneuvers: At normal end-expiration the trachea narrows only slightly, while during a forced expiratory maneuver or coughing the posterior tracheal membrane invaginates to greatly reduce the cross-sectional area of the trachea, whereas the lateral and anterior walls are minimally altered. During a Valsalva maneuver, the diameter of the extrathoracic trachea increases by 2–4 mm while the intrathoracic trachea remains unchanged in size.

The tracheal wall is visible on CT scans as a distinct thin line against the background of mediastinal fat. It is obscured when lung parenchyma or vessels contact the trachea. Distinct calcifications of the cartilage rings of the trachea are a common finding after the age of 40 years. The trachea divides into the two mainstem bronchi at the carina. In children the angles are symmetric, but in adults the right main bronchus has a more vertical course than the left main bronchus. The right upper lobe bronchus

Table 8.3. Normal anatomic dimensions of trachea and main bronchi

	Trachea			Main bronchi	
	Total	Extrathoracic	Intrathoracic	Right	Left
Length	10–12 cm	2–4 cm	6–9 cm	2.2–2.5 cm	5 cm
	Area	Coronal	Sagittal	Right	Left
Cross-section Male Female	272 ± 33 mm² 194 ± 35 mm²	19 ± 2 mm 16 ± 2 mm	20 ± 2 mm 17 ± 2 mm	15 mm	13 mm

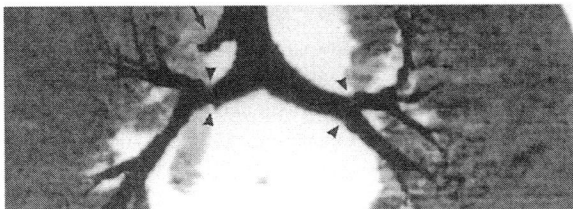

Fig. 8.8. Anteroposterior mIP in a patient with a tracheal bronchus (*arrow*) that was ligated during bilateral lung transplantation. Note the wall irregularities at the site of anastomosis (*arrowheads*) in both main bronchi (protocol B: 2/3/2)

arises more proximally than the left upper lobe bronchus.

The right main bronchus and its divisions into the right upper lobe bronchus and intermediate bronchus are outlined posteriorly by lung parenchyma so that the posterior walls are seen as a thin stripe. On an mIP in the anteroposterior viewing direction, this area always shows an air–lung contrast. The region is a sensitive area in which to look for masses, such as lymphadenopathy. On the left side, the lower lobe pulmonary artery intervenes between the lung and the bronchial tree, and only a small tongue of lung can invaginate between the left lower lobe artery and the descending aorta to contact the posterior wall of the left mainstem bronchus.

8.3.2 Anatomic Variants and Anomalies

In general, the tracheobronchial branching pattern is remarkably uniform. Most variations have no clinical relevance, although they may be confusing to the bronchoscopist searching for landmarks. Ectopic or accessory bronchi may arise from the right lower trachea (tracheal bronchus, Fig. 8.8) or from the medial wall of the intermediate bronchus (cardiac bronchus). A tracheal bronchus can represent an aberrant origin of the apical segment of the right upper lobe bronchus or be a truly supernumerary bronchus. Patients are asymptomatic or show recurrent pulmonary infections or other abnormalities of the tracheobronchial tree. Unilateral absence of a lung or lobe is a rare congenital abnormality sometimes associated with tracheo-esophageal fistula or esophageal atresia.

Vascular rings may cause slight obstruction of the upper trachea. This usually results in respiratory problems only during exercise. The most common forms are an aberrant right subclavian artery, a right aortic arch with aberrant left subclavian artery or a

double aortic arch. A "pulmonary sling" is caused by an anomalous left pulmonary artery. This rare anatomic variant is frequently associated with respiratory problems. The left pulmonary artery courses around the right main bronchus and between the lower trachea and the esophagus to reach the left lung (Fig. 8.9). In more than 50% of cases, respiratory problems, however, are not due to the external compression by vascular structures but rather to an associated tracheal anomaly. The tracheal cartilage may form a completely closed ring ("napkin ring") instead of being connected posteriorly by a membranous band.

Spiral CT. Most anomalies can already be detected with the screening protocol A. They are often incidental findings. In conditions that require operative treatment, targeted scans (protocol B, if necessary with i.v. contrast) are indicated. The napkin ring anomaly in the pulmonary sling syndrome may be diagnosed with separate spiral scans in full inspiration and expiration.

Multiplanar reformats and SSD images are warranted only in complex cases. Simultaneous display of tracheal lumen and vascular structures are possible with SSD images that combine CTA and tracheobronchial "casts" (Fig. 8.9).

8.3.3 Tracheal Enlargement

Most of the disorders that enlarge the trachea have in common the loss of normal cartilaginous support in the wall of the trachea due to trauma (long-term intubation), defective cartilage formation (Ehlers-Danlos syndrome), or a number of chronic inflammatory conditions, including cystic fibrosis, immune deficiency states, and recurrent childhood infections (Table 8.4). Tracheomegaly has also been described as a complication of diffuse pulmonary fibrosis in

Table 8.4. Causes of tracheal enlargement

Trauma: long-term intubation
Defective cartilage formation: Ehlers-Danlos syndrome
Chronic inflammatory conditions:
   Recurrent childhood infections
   Immune deficiency states
   Cystic fibrosis (mild enlargement only of sagittal
     diameter)
Traction: upper zone or diffuse pulmonary fibrosis
   (e.g., sarcoidosis, fibrosing alveolitis, histoplasmosis)
Congenital tracheobronchomegaly:
   Mounier-Kuhn syndrome

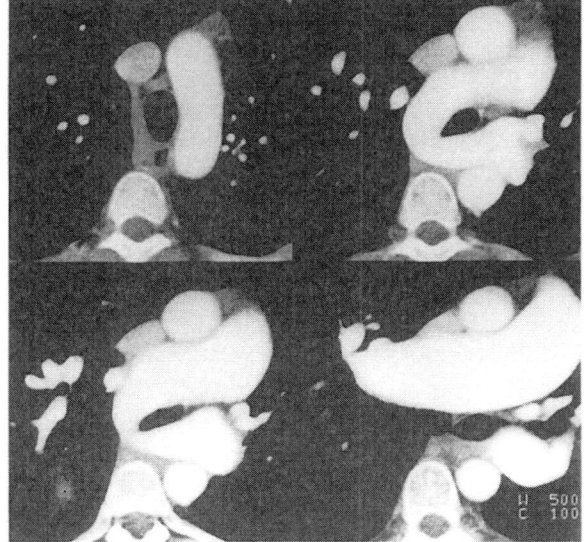

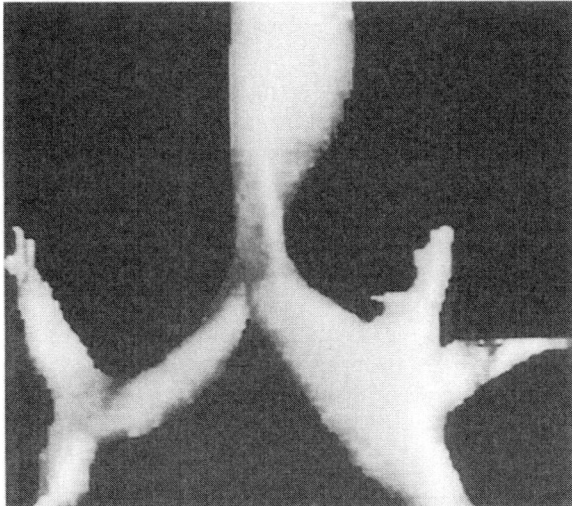

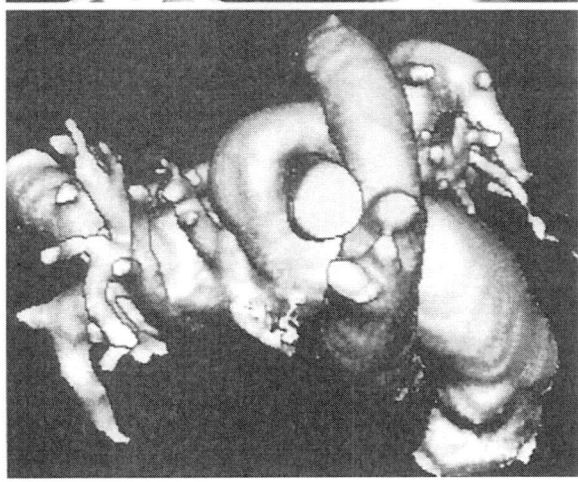

Fig. 8.9. Patient with idiopathic pulmonary hypertension and pulmonary sling syndrome: axial sections (**a**), SSD of mediastinal vessels and main airways seen from above (**b**) and SSD of the trachea and main bronchi rotated 45° RPO (**c**). **a** and **b** demonstrate the normal course of the right and the atypical course of the left pulmonary artery; **c** shows the subsequent external compression of the lower trachea and left main bronchus (protocol A: 5/8/4)

patients with at least moderate restrictive lung disease and prolonged illness.

Mounier-Kuhn syndrome is a rare congenital condition with tracheobronchomegaly. Dilatation may affect just the trachea (>3 cm in diameter) or extend into the main stem bronchi (>2.4 cm in diameter) and lobar and segmental bronchi. Protrusion of redundant musculomembranous tissue between the cartilaginous rings results in an irregularly corrugated and scalloped appearance of the air column and is described as "tracheal/bronchial diverticulosis."

Spiral CT. Most cases of tracheomegaly are probably underdiagnosed. While the diagnosis of enlarged tracheobronchial diameter can be securely made by standard CT, spiral CT (protocol B) in expiration and inspiration is advantageous for quantitative measurement of tracheobronchial diameters and the assessment of abnormal wall compliance. Measurements on axial CT sections may overestimate the tracheal diameter if the head position is elevated during the scan or if the trachea is elongated in older individuals. Diameters should therefore be measured in 2D reformats that are chosen perpendicular to the trachea or main bronchi.

The typical appearance of tracheobronchial diverticulosis is more easily appreciated in orthogonal reformats than in axial images alone. The most common location for diverticuli is on the posterior tracheal wall.

Usually, SSD and mIP images do not add information. They may even be irritating because the diameter of the airways in these images is dependent on the size of the VOI and the selected threshold.

8.3.4 Nonneoplastic Tracheal Narrowing

Tracheal narrowing may affect a long or short segment, and can be caused by extrinsic or intrinsic processes (Tables 8.5, 8.6). It may be part of a generalized pulmonary or systemic disorder or may be confined to the trachea. Several of the diseases that destroy the cartilage temporarily result in an enlarged trachea but finally cause a narrowed trachea once fibrosis and healing occur.

Nonneoplastic tracheal narrowing due to extrinsic processes is most commonly due to vascular rings (see Fig. 8.9) or to external compression by an enlarged thyroid gland (Fig. 8.10). Depending on whether the thyroid is enlarged uni- or bilaterally, the trachea is pushed anteriorly, laterally, or posteriorly.

The following intrinsic processes are characterized by a smooth, sharply defined narrowing of the airway without wall thickening. Due to a typical CT morphology, they usually pose no diagnostic problem.

A *saber sheath* trachea is characterized by the sudden marked reduction of the coronal tracheal diameter (less than two-thirds of the sagittal diameter) at the beginning of the intrathoracic portion of the trachea. It is commonly associated with chronic obstructive lung disease and occurs almost exclusively in male patients. The narrowing usually affects most of the intrathoracic segment of the trachea. Tracheal ring calcification is common, and the anterior arch of the trachea is abnormally narrow. Additional wall flaccidity indicates upper airway dysfunction.

The *ischemic damage* of the tracheal wall from a *cuffed endotracheal or tracheostomy tube* can result in a circumscribed, mostly smooth fibrotic narrowing (Fig. 8.11). Strictures occur at the location of the cuff or at the tracheostomy site.

After *lung transplantation*, strictures occur due to *postischemic fibrosis*. Patients may develop one or multiple strictures. Locations of predilection are the anastomotic sites in trachea or main bronchi, the intermediate bronchus, or the upper lobe bronchi (Figs. 8.12, 8.13). Strictures are usually concentric with smooth wall contours and may be severe. Frequently they are preceded by a wall dehiscence at the site of anastomosis. Endoluminal fibrin layers pose a differential diagnostic problem and may be diagnosed only from air bubbles that get caught under them.

Tracheal narrowing that is accompanied by an irregular, sometimes nodular wall thickening can be caused by a number of rather uncommon disorders (Table 8.6). The narrowing can have various appearances ranging from eccentric to concentric and may be smooth, irregular, nodular, or even masslike. The

Table 8.5. Nonneoplastic tracheal narrowing without wall thickening

a) *Intrinsic*	
Saber sheath trachea	Sudden reduction of coronal tracheal diameter (<2/3 of the sagittal diameter)
	Trachea is abnormally narrow anteriorly
	Involves whole intrathoracic trachea
	Wall flaccidity leading to upper airway dysfunction
	Mostly male patients
	± Chronic obstructive lung disease
	± Tracheal ring calcification
Ischemic damage from a cuffed endotracheal or tracheostomy tube	Circumscribed, mostly smooth fibrotic narrowing
	Location of the cuff or at the tracheostomy site
Postischemic fibrosis after lung transplantation	One or multiple strictures
	Sites of predilection: bronchial anastomoses, intermediate bronchus, upper lobe bronchi
	Smooth, concentric tracheal narrowing
b) *Extrinsic*	
Vascular structures	Aortic ectasia; aneurysm
	Aberrant right subclavian artery
	Right aortic arch with aberrant left subclavian artery
	Double aortic arch
	Pulmonary sling
Thyroid	Upper third of the trachea
	Uni- or bilateral compression
	Smooth tracheal contour
	Frequently tracheal displacement

Table 8.6. Nonneoplastic tracheal narrowing with irregular/nodular wall thickening

Tracheo(broncho)pathia Osteo(chondro)plastica	Inferior trachea ± main stem bronchi Long segment Extensive polynodular thickening: anterior and lateral tracheal wall; posterior wall spared; ± calcifications
Relapsing polychondritis	Destruction of the cartilaginous rings by recurrent episodes of inflammation leading to: 1) Cicatricial fibrosis and stenosis 2) Rarely, flaccid walls and malacia
Scleroderma	Proximal trachea Smooth tracheal narrowing
Wegener's granulomatosis	1) Subglottic region: smooth or irregular tracheal narrowing, 3–4 cm long, + irregular thickening of tracheal rings/laryngeal cartilages 2) Distal airways (main stem or lobar bronchi): stenotic lesions (rare)
Ulcerative colitis	Irregular thickening of tracheobronchial walls Mostly concentric narrowing ± calcifications in destroyed cartilage
Amyloidosis	1) Multiple concentric and eccentric strictures Mural nodular masses ± calcifications/ossifications 2) Single submucosal mass mimics neoplasm (less common)
Sarcoid	Tracheal involvement is rare and always associated with laryngeal involvement: 1) Intrinsic granulomatous disease of trachea and main bronchi 2) Extrinsic compression (rare) by mediastinal lymphadenopathy or extensive mediastinal fibrosis
Infections	Tuberculosis Scleroma (*Klebsiella rhinoscleromatis*) Fungal infection: histoplasmosis, coccidioidomycosis, mucormycosis, candidiasis, necrotizing aspergillosis
Granulomatous repair	Inflammation or radiation therapy Longer tracheal segment, wall irregularities leading to biopsy for differentiation from neoplasm

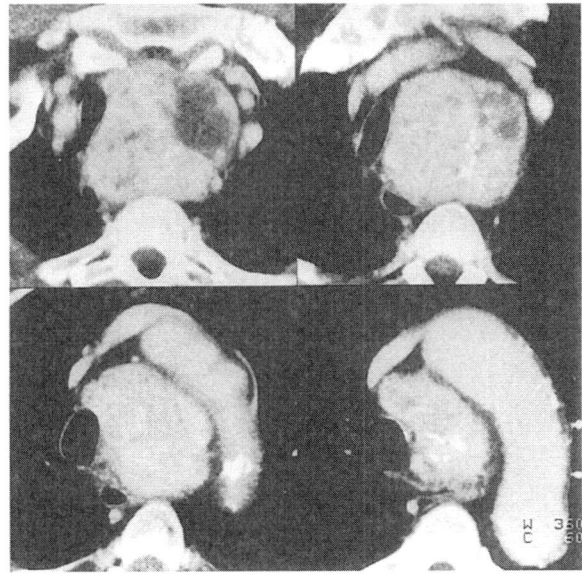

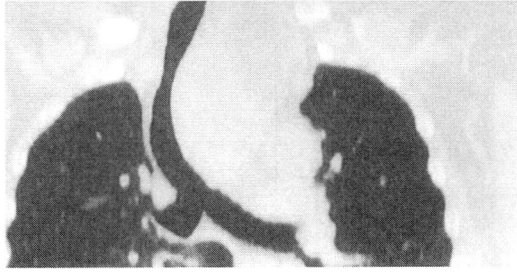

Fig. 8.10. Axial scans (**a**) and coronal reformat (**b**) in a patient with a large left-sided goiter and displacement and compression of the trachea. Note the superior demonstration of the tracheal deformation in the coronal reformat (protocol A: 5/8/4)

only distinguishing feature is the location of the narrowed segment. CT morphology is otherwise nonspecific, and diagnosis requires clinical information and histologic examination (KWONG et al. 1992).

Depending on the etiology, exact knowledge of the length of the narrowing, of involvement of lobar bronchi, and of segments with abnormal wall compliance is essential to determine the appropriate

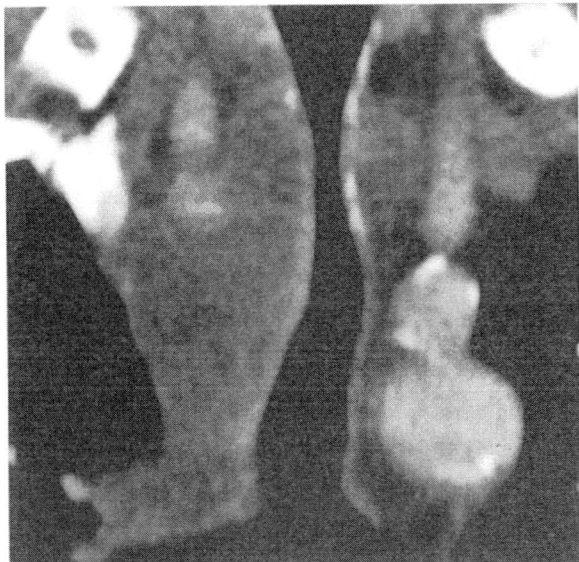

Fig. 8.11. Coronal reformat of a smooth infraglottic tracheal stenosis after tracheotomy. Note some distinct wall calcifications (protocol A: 5/8/4)

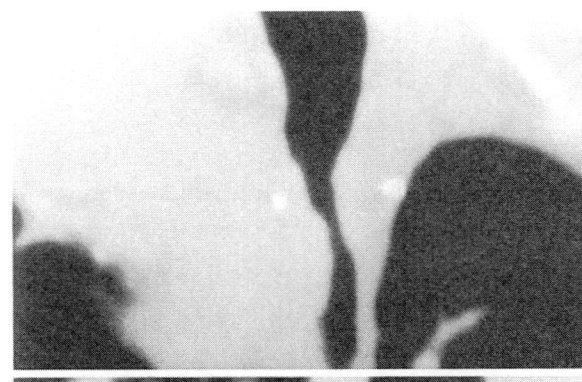
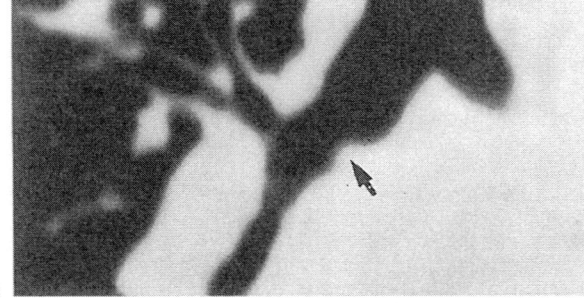

Fig. 8.12. Patient after lung transplantation with a longstanding asymmetric stenosis of the intermediate bronchus: reformats along the long axis of the right main bronchus and intermediate bronchus in a sagittal (**a**) and coronal (**b**) plane. The stenosis is more pronounced in the sagittal plane (**a**). Note the slight indentation of the main bronchus at the site of the anastomosis (*arrow* in **b**) (protocol B: 2/2/1)

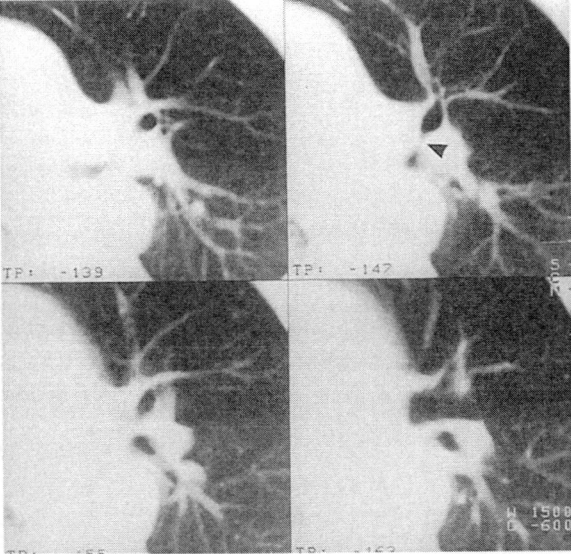
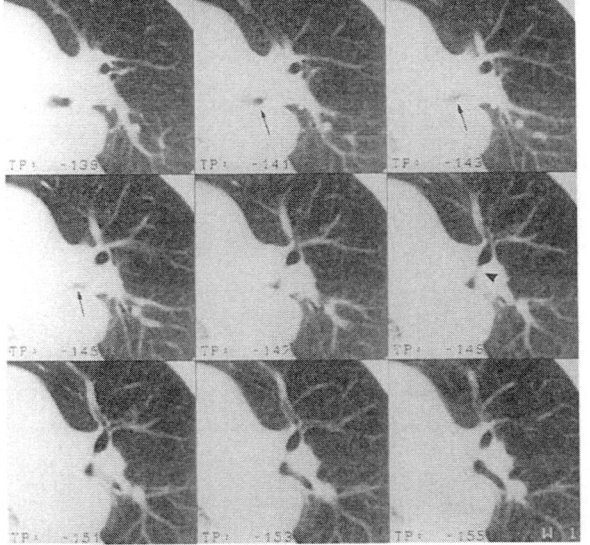

Fig. 8.13. Axial sections from a standard CT (contiguous 8-mm slice collimation) (**a**) and a spiral CT (protocol A: 5/8/4) (**b**) in a lung-transplanted patient. While the high-grade upper lobe stricture is easily seen with both techniques (*arrowheads*), the additional moderate stricture of the left main bronchus can only be appreciated on the spiral scan (*arrows* in **b**)

therapeutic concept. Therapeutic options include bronchoscopic dilatation, stent implantation, and surgery.

Spiral CT. Tracheal narrowing usually requires no special CT technique for making the diagnosis. Spiral scans, however, will be able to demonstrate the craniocaudal extent to better advantage. Chest scans according to protocol A will provide the necessary information and will allow for reformats or SSD images of sufficient quality (Figs. 8.9–8.11). Only rarely will mIP be useful for image presentation. Cases with marked anterior narrowing due to saber sheath trachea may be missed on mIP images.

Coned-down spiral scans according to protocol B will better demonstrate irregular thickening of the tracheal wall. They are essential to fully assess eccentric or very short, membrane-like narrowings that are difficult to assess with standard CT. Protocol B is always recommended if involvement of the central bronchi is suspected (Fig. 8.12). In order to demonstrate wall instability, an additional scan in full expiration should be performed. Longitudinal 2D reformats are the superior display mode for defining the length of tracheal/bronchial stenosis (Figs. 8.11, 8.12). The minimum diameter is most accurately assessed on reformats perpendicular to the tracheal or bronchial longitudinal axis. A recently published paper described an accuracy of 94% for spiral CT including multiplanar reformats as compared to 91% for standard CT for the detection of stenosis of the central airways (Figs. 8.12, 8.13) (QUINT et al. 1995). Three-dimensional SSD serves as a comprehensive display, and mIP may be useful only for concentric stenoses. With both mIP and SSD, high-grade stenoses are frequently overestimated and displayed as pseudo-occlusions (Fig. 8.3).

Spiral CT obtained with thin sections provides high morphologic detail to characterize the morphology of a stenosis (eccentric versus concentric, smooth versus irregular) and to exclude an extraluminal soft tissue component that raises the suspicion of malignancy. Involvement of the mucosa remains an imaging task for bronchoscopy.

8.3.5 Neoplastic Narrowing

8.3.5.1 Benign Lesions

Benign neoplasms of the trachea and central bronchi include a number of rare etiologies (Table 8.7). Most of these tumors have no distinctive radiographic characteristics, and definite diagnosis has to be based on histopathologic findings. The major task of CT is to exclude extratracheal or extrabronchial extension. The presence of any extraluminal extension virtually excludes a benign histology as benign neoplasms do not invade the tracheal wall. Nonspecific signs of benign tumors are their sharply defined contours, a polypoid, broad-based, and occasionally pedunculated morphology, and a size of under 2 cm (Fig. 8.14).

Intraluminal collections of *mucus* in the trachea or major bronchi may simulate an intraluminal tumor. This finding can be made more frequently in old and sick patients with a diminished cough reflex. It can be expected that more mucus globs will be seen with spiral CT. Curvilinear and small dot-like densi-

Table 8.7. Benign neoplasms of the trachea and main bronchi

Chondroma, Chondroblastoma	Areas of calcification
Hamartoma	Areas of calcification (popcorn) and/or fatty tissue Cystic collections of fluid Rarely centrally located (8%)
Lipoma	Fat density (characteristic)
Fibroma Paraganglioma Myoblastoma Hemangioendothelioma Neurofibroma Leiomyoma	Noncharacteristic
Hemangioma	Strong contrast enhancement Often associated with cutaneous hemangiomas Mostly located in the subglottic region Second most common tracheal tumor in childhood
Intratracheal goiter	Early contrast enhancement
Squamous cell papilloma	Noncharacteristic, usually part of JLP (see below)
Juvenile laryngeal papillomatosis (JLP)	Multiple endobronchial/parenchymal masses Most lesions arise in the larynx Distal spread in 5%

Common sign: no Extraluminal extension of disease

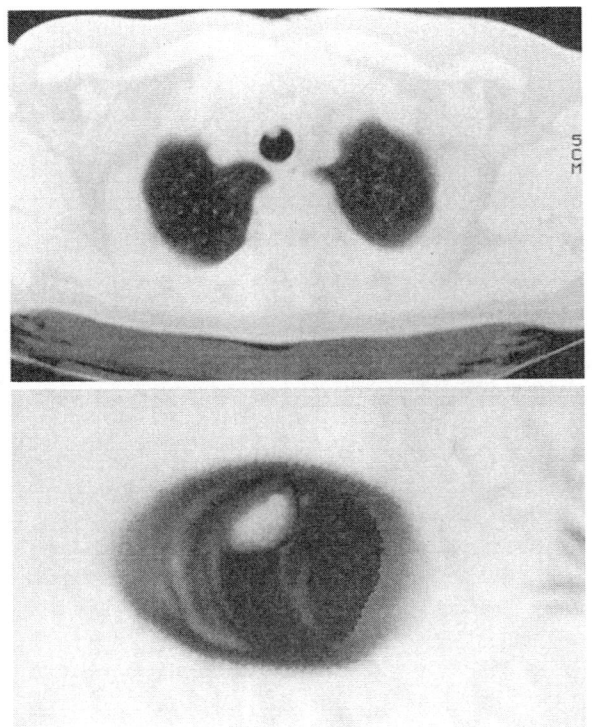

Fig. 8.14. Axial section (a) and "endoscopic" SSD (b) of a small tracheal papilloma (protocol B: 3/5/3)

ties hanging into the intraluminal air are characteristic features. Mucus usually has a lower than soft tissue density dependent on partial volume effects. The majority of mucoid pseudotumors are found in the area of the tracheal bifurcation. In doubtful cases, a repeat scan after vigorous coughing can prove the mucoid origin of a lesion.

8.3.5.2 Primary Malignant Neoplasms

8.3.5.2.1 Tracheal Tumors. Primary tracheal tumors are very rare (Table 8.8). Malignant tumors of laryngeal and bronchial origin are, respectively, at least 75 and 180 times more common than those arising in the trachea (WEBER and GRILLO 1978). They are insidious in onset, and symptoms often manifest only in late stages of the disease unless there is hemoptysis. The tracheal lumen is frequently more than 75% occluded before symptoms appear. Thus, most malignant tumors are advanced at the time of diagnosis. Only rarely does one encounter a small lesion in CT.

The three most frequent tumor types (squamous cell carcinoma, adenoid cystic carcinoma, and mucoepidermoid tumors) grow exophytically and infiltratively, usually over a length of 2–4 cm, although up to 10 cm of submucosal spread is occasionally seen and usually underestimated with CT. Approximately 10% of malignant tracheal neoplasms are circumferential, a finding that is not seen with benign tumors. CT morphology of the intraluminal soft tissue mass is nonspecific. Thus, bronchoscopic biopsy is always required. Invasion into adjacent lymph nodes and mediastinal structures is common (>40%). CT is the method of choice to assess the extratracheal component, invasion of vascular structures, and the presence of lymphadenopathy. For surgical planning, it is essential to determine whether tumors of the upper trachea involve the adjacent infraglottic portion of the larynx and whether tumors of the lower trachea extend into the main bronchi. Early tumor involvement can only be visualized on CT scans if thickening of airway walls adjacent to the tumor is present.

8.3.5.2.2 Tracheal/Bronchial Adenomas. Adenomas constitute only about 0.6%–1.2% of neoplasms of the tracheobronchial system. Cylindromas (= adenoid cystic carcinomas) make up only 6%–12% of bronchial adenomas, but account for 95% of tracheal adenomas. The majority (85%) of bronchial adenomas are carcinoid tumors (Tables 8.8, 8.9). Carcinoid tumors are low-grade carcinomas and are locally invasive. They may present as defined endobronchial lesions or extend extraluminally in the surrounding lung parenchyma. They can also metastasize to regional lymph nodes and to distant sites (liver, skeleton). They arise most often at bifur-

Table 8.8. Malignant neoplasms of the trachea

Primary	Secondary
Squamous cell carcinoma (>50%)	Bronchial carcinoma
Mucoepidermoid carcinoma	
Adenoma (= 95% adenoid cystic carcinoma)	Thyroid Esophagus
Very rare: sarcomas, adenocarcinomas, chondrosarcomas, plasmocytoma, histiocytoma, small cell carcinoma	Lymphoma Kaposi sarcoma Metastases (melanoma, breast carcinoma, renal cell carcinoma, colorectal carcinoma)

Table 8.9. Malignant neoplasms of the main bronchi

Primary	Secondary
Bronchial carcinoma Adenoma (= 85% carcinoid)	Metastases (melanoma, breast carcinoma, renal cell carcinoma, colorectal carcinoma) Esophagus Lymphoma Kaposi sarcoma

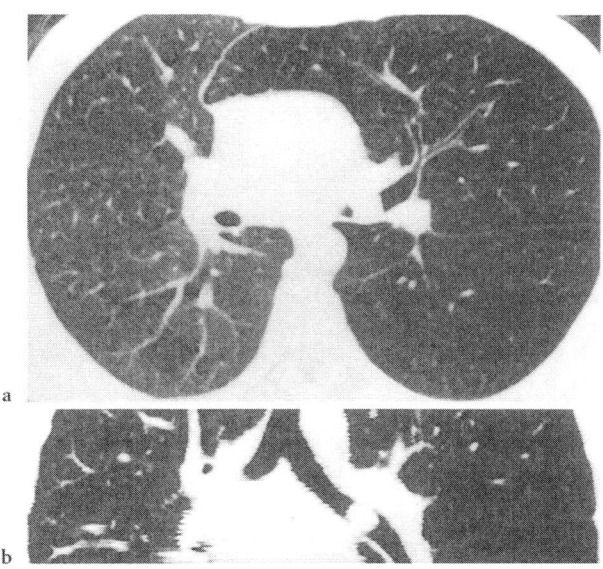

Fig. 8.15. Axial section (a) and coronal reformat (b) in a patient with a carcinoid occluding the main bronchus and leading to air trapping in the left lung (protocol B: 2/2/1)

cations of the central bronchi and present with bronchial obstruction (Fig. 8.15).

8.3.5.3 Bronchial Carcinoma

The most common malignant tumor to be encountered in the region of the trachea and main bronchi is a bronchial carcinoma from a lobar bronchus that invades adjacent tracheobronchial structures (Fig. 8.16, Table 8.9). The therapeutic approach depends on the involvement of hilar and mediastinal lymph nodes and on the local tumor extent. Invasion of the main bronchus usually classifies the tumor as T2. The uncommon superficially growing tumor with an invasive component limited to the bronchial wall and a superficial proximal extension to the main bronchus is still classified as T1. Tumor growth in the main bronchus within 2 cm of the carina represents

stage T3a, which is still amenable to tracheobronchial sleeve resection (Fig. 8.17). Tracheal involvement represents stage T3b or T4 and precludes surgical treatment.

The decision on whether a lobectomy or a pneumonectomy is required for complete tumor resection is particularly important in patients with diminished pulmonary function who cannot tolerate a pneumonectomy. Transfissural tumor growth, cen-

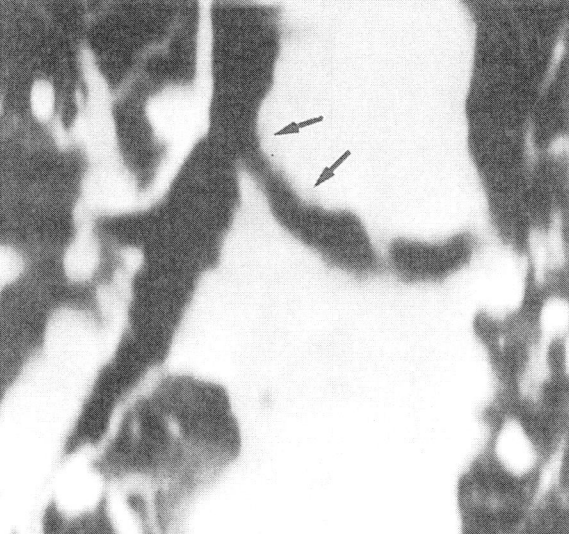

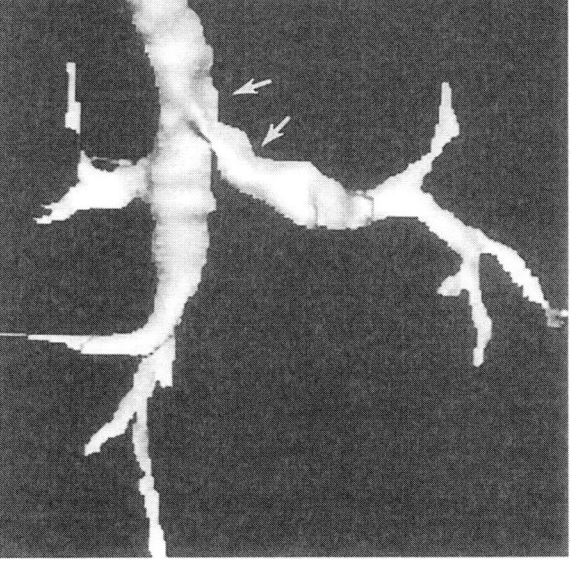

Fig. 8.16a,b. Patient after resection of the left upper lobe: a recurrent bronchial carcinoma infiltrates the lower trachea and left main bronchus. Both coronal reformat (a) and SSD (b) demonstrate the irregular narrowing of the pericarinal airways (protocol A: 5/8/4). Note the lower detail visibility in the reformat and SSD due to the relatively large slice thickness in protocol A

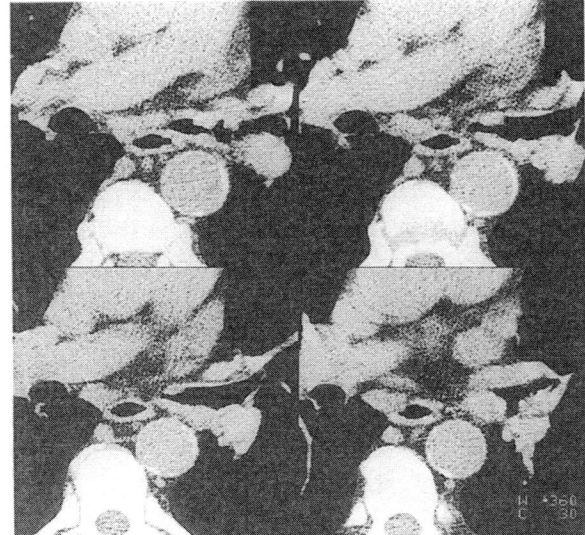

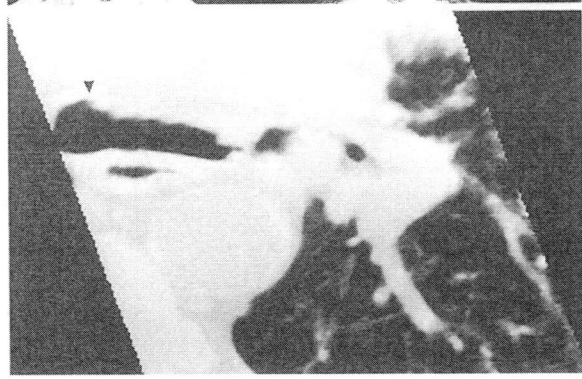

Fig. 8.17. Bronchial carcinoma with longstanding infiltration of the bronchial wall: axial sections (**a**) and reformat along the long axis of the left main bronchus (**b**). The reformat demonstrates the extent of endoluminal tumor growth and the presence of tumor infiltration along the anterior wall, almost reaching the carina (*arrowhead*) (protocol B: 2/2/1)

tral pulmonary artery involvement, and invasion of a main bronchus or of both the upper and lower bronchi preclude bronchoplasty and require pneumonectomy.

Computed tomographic signs suggestive of bronchial involvement are the presence of abnormal soft tissue within the bronchus, a reduced caliber of the airway associated with irregular wall thickening (Figs. 8.16, 8.17). Due to the relatively low accuracy of CT for delineation of invasion of the main bronchi and of pulmonary artery involvement, surgeons frequently rely on bronchoscopy or on the findings during thoracotomy (QUINT et al. 1987).

On axial sections of obliquely oriented bronchi (left main bronchus), the assessment of craniocaudal airway caliber and wall thickness is difficult due to

partial volume effects. Thin sections improve the sensitivity of standard CT (KWONG et al. 1992). Yet, submucosal extension from an adjacent bronchial lesion with tumor invasion into, but not through the bronchial wall may lead to false-negative findings at both CT and bronchoscopy (NAIDICH et al. 1987). To date MRI has not demonstrated advantages over CT in this respect (WEBB et al. 1991). Intraluminal ultrasonography provides excellently detailed visualization of intramural tumor growth; however, more experience is needed to assess its value.

8.3.5.4 Secondary Malignant Neoplasms

Neoplasms may secondarily involve the trachea and main bronchi by invasion from adjacent organs or by metastasizing from distant sites. Extrinsic lesions can displace, compress, or encase the trachea or bronchi, compromising the airway diameter to the extent that symptoms of airway obstruction occur. Soft tissue density within the tracheal or bronchial lumen is a secure sign of direct tumor invasion (Figs. 8.18–8.20). CT can determine the degree of compromise of the airway and show advanced disease with mediastinal involvement. Blurring of the interface between the tracheal or bronchial wall and adjacent organs, e.g., esophagus or thyroid, has been demonstrated to be an unreliable sign of tumor infiltration.

8.3.5.4.1 Laryngeal Tumors. CT was found to be superior to bronchoscopy for evaluation of the subglottic laryngeal region within the cricoid cartilage (GAMSU et al. 1981). Subglottic extension of laryngeal carcinoma into the trachea or extension of a tracheal tumor to the undersurface of the true vocal cords indicates the need for both laryngectomy and resection of the proximal trachea.

8.3.5.4.2 Thyroid Tumors. Blurring of the interface between the outer layers of the tracheal wall and the thyroid was found to be an unreliable CT sign for the determination of tumor invasion (GAMSU and WEBB 1982).

8.3.5.4.3 Esophageal Tumors. Esophagotracheal or esophagobronchial fistuli frequently occur in patients with advanced esophageal tumors and tracheobronchial involvement (Fig. 8.18). The task of CT is to demonstrate the presence, location, and extent of pathologic air collections, to delineate the fistula itself, and to assess potential complications such as abscess formation.

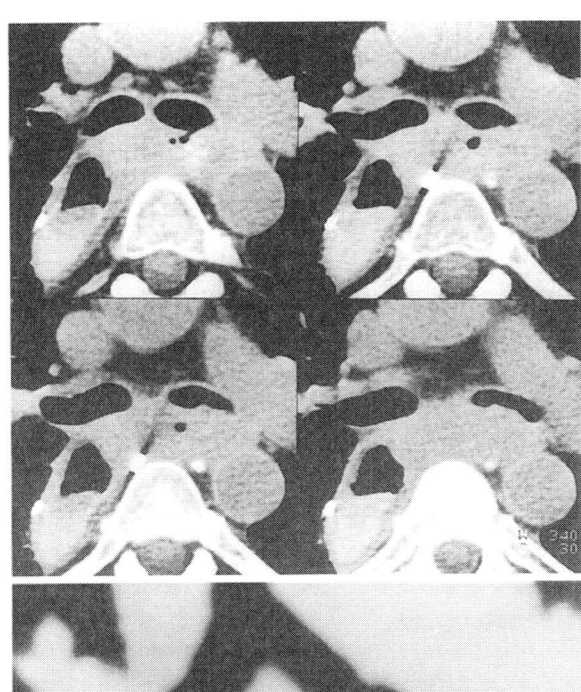

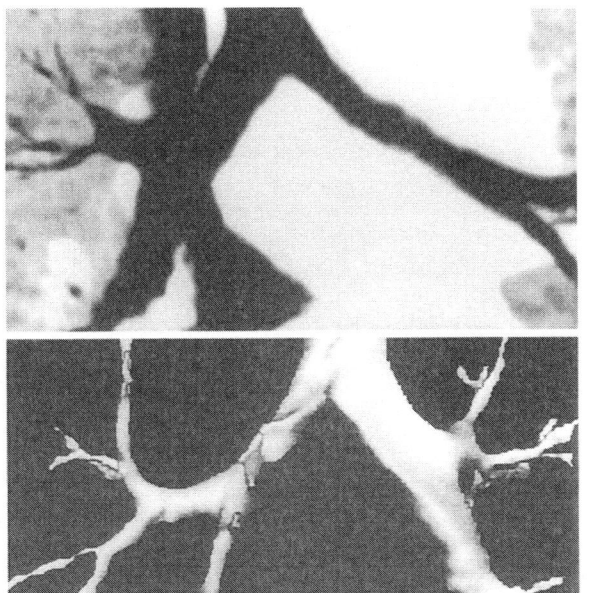

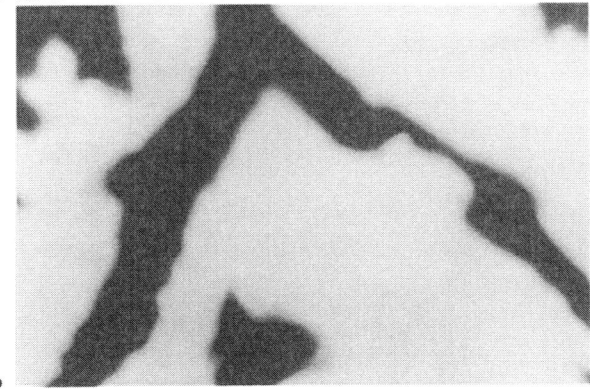

Fig. 8.18. Axial sections (**a**), reformat (**b**), mIP (**c**), and SSD in the posteroanterior orientation (**d**) in a patient with a recurrent esophageal tumor that infiltrates the left main bronchus (fistula) and encases the right main bronchus. The images demonstrate that SSD is the superior modality for comprehensive display. While intraluminal infiltration is seen well on the reformat and the SSD, it is underestimated on the mIP. Due to projection effects, the compression of the right bronchus is not seen in the reformat and the mIP (protocol B: 2/2/1)

8.3.5.4.4 Metastases. In patients with endotracheal metastases from distant tumors, CT is helpful to define the tumor extent and to decide on the therapeutic consequences, i.e., surgery, radiation therapy, laser resection, or stenting (Fig. 8.20). The most common extrathoracic tumors associated with endobronchial metastases are carcinomas of the breast, kidney, colon, rectum and melanomas. Differentiation of etiology is not possible based on CT morphology. Bronchoscopic biopsy is needed for histologic proof.

8.3.5.4.5 Lymphoma. Hodgkin's disease (HD) may manifest as a solitary endobronchial mass associated with regional lymphadenopathy. The possibility of an endobronchial manifestation should be considered in patients with atelectasis and known lymphoma. Non-Hodgkin's lymphoma (NHL) affects the central airways more rarely than HD. In advanced stages,

8.3.5.4.6 Extrinsic Compression. Mediastinal tumors or extensive lymphadenopathy may lead to airway compression. In 55% of children with newly diagnosed HD, tracheobronchial compression occurs. CT is important to identify patients at risk for symptomatic and occasionally life-threatening airway compression.

8.3.5.5 Spiral CT

The detection of large tumors rarely poses a problem with standard CT techniques. An optimum assessment of small tumors, intrabronchial lesions, or tumor infiltration into critical adjacent structures will always require spiral scans with maximum spatial resolution (protocol B) and intravenous contrast injection.

Compared with bronchoscopy, the sensitivity of

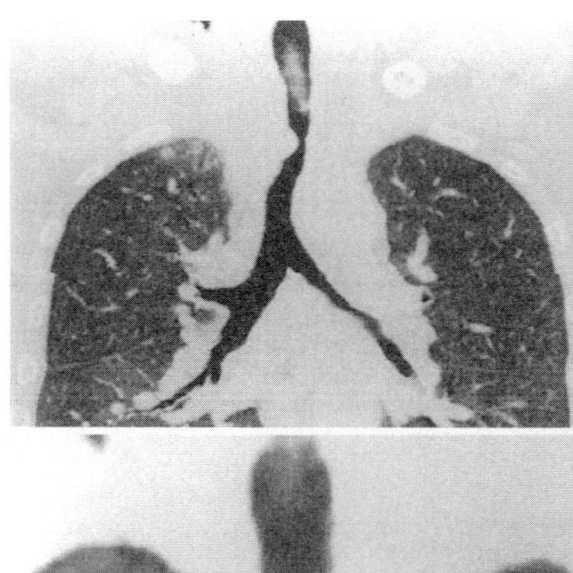

a

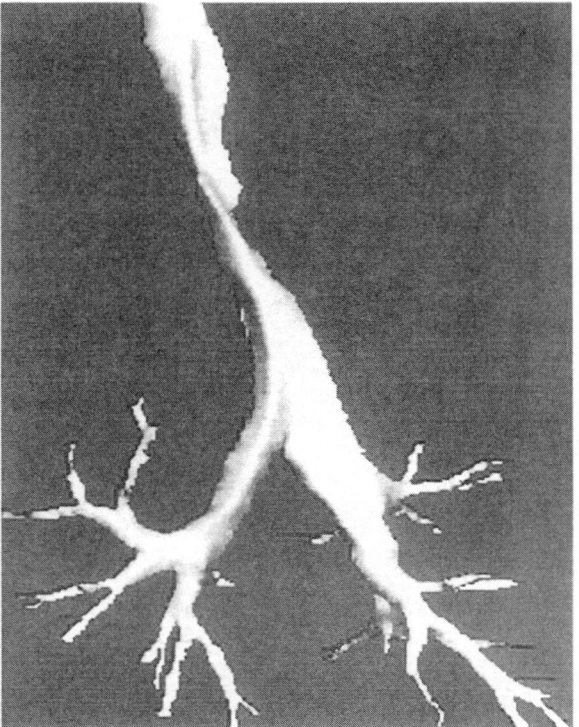

c

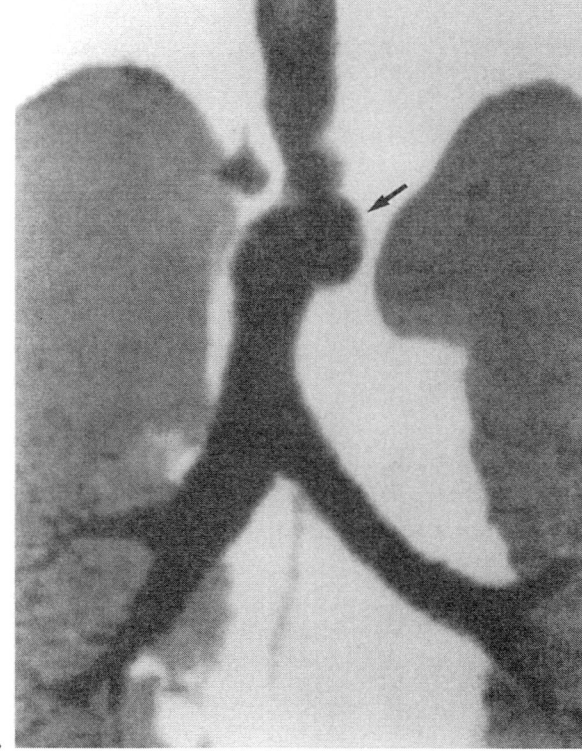

b

Fig. 8.19. Coronal reformat (a), mIP (b), and posteroanterior SSD (c) in a patient with an esophageal tumor that is infiltrating the trachea and compressing the left main bronchus. The contours of the trachea are obscured in the anteroposterior mIP by the air-filled dilated esophagus (*arrow*). The intraluminal tumorous filling defect is well demonstrated on the coronal reformat and the SSD (protocol B: 1/2/1)

nosis of tumors in the trachea and main bronchi has been reported to be 94% (KWONG et al. 1993). Few lesions were missed and all of them were small and located in the main bronchi. The diagnostic performance of standard CT can be further improved using thin-slice collimation (2–5 mm). Thus, the advantage of spiral CT will be not so much the detection of lesions but an improved description of tumor location, extent, and relationship to adjacent structures. Contrast injection does not provide additional information about the character of a tracheobronchial lesion but facilitates visualization of the adjacent vessels. To what extent the assessment of tumor infiltration into critical structures will be improved using

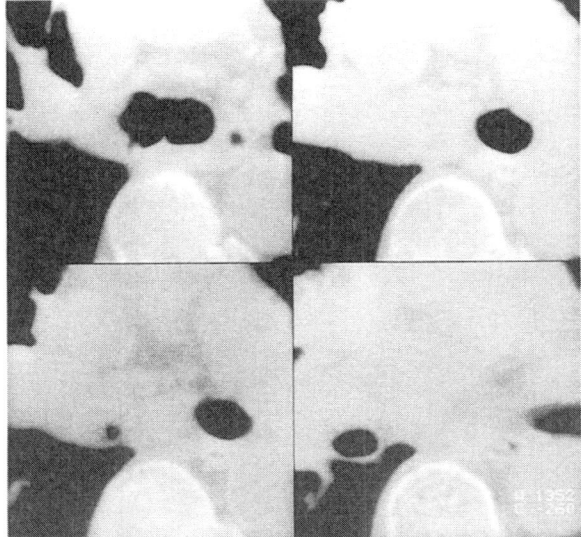

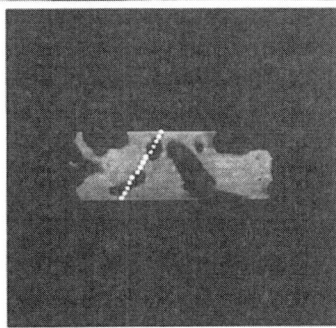

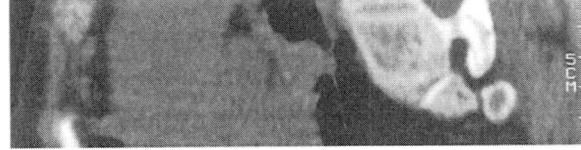

Fig. 8.20. Axial sections (a) and reformat (b) in a patient with an occluding metastasis of a hypernephroma in the right main bronchus that was successfully treated by laser therapy. The reformat is superior to the axial sections for delineating the craniocaudal extent of the tumorous occlusion (protocol A: 5/5/3)

high-resolution spiral CT with intravenous contrast is not yet clear. CT is not able to differentiate between (smooth) thickening of the airway wall caused by edema, inflammation, or submucosal tumor. Only the presence of a slight wall irregularity, an intraluminal filling defect, or extraluminal tumor extension are indicators of endobronchial tumor spread (Figs. 8.17–8.19). The detection of these subtle findings is improved by spiral CT. Despite general limitations of morphologic criteria, spiral CT is expected to increase the accuracy for staging tracheobronchial tumors.

Diagnosis is made on the basis of overlapping axial scans and, if necessary, reformats that are tailored to the location of the lesion and the anatomic course of the bronchi (Figs. 8.5, 8.17) (SCHAEFER et al. 1991). Axial scans provide the most detailed visualization with simultaneous demonstration of intra- and extraluminal tumor portions, airways, and soft tissue structures.

Three-dimensional surface displays (SSDs) are valuable for providing a comprehensive display of a focal lesion relative to the branching bronchi (Figs. 8.5, 8.16, 8.18) (SCHAEFER et al. 1991; COSTELLO 1994; NEWMARK et al. 1994). This is especially helpful when assessing a tumor that leads to only subtotal occlusion of the airways and can be visualized in a 3D SSD as a filling defect (Fig. 8.5). Complete occlusion of main or lobar bronchi leads to a cut-off of one or several bronchi in SSDs without direct visualization of the tumor itself. The feasibility of laser therapy can be assessed by display of the course of the bronchi distal to the lesion (straight path of laser beam) (Fig. 8.20). SSD "casts" are very sensitive to tumor-related deformation of the walls of the trachea and main bronchi (Figs. 8.16, 8.18, 8.19), a sign that appears to correlate with wall infiltration. Bronchoscopic views will be most interesting prior to deep biopsy or laser therapy to determine the relationship of the site of intervention to vessels and lung parenchyma (VINING et al. 1994).

Minimum intensity projections are only suited for display of circular tumor stenoses (Fig. 8.3), not for focal intraluminal tumors (Fig. 8.5) (RÉMY-JARDIN et al. 1994).

8.3.6 Wall Defects

Tracheobronchial wall defects may be congenital (tracheo-esophageal fistulas with or without esophageal atresia), be caused by trauma (penetration injury) or neoplastic infiltration (esophageal tumor), be iatrogenic (intubation) or occur as a complication after lung transplantation (Table 8.10). Bronchoscopy and CT provide complementary diagnostic information: CT is superior to bronchoscopy for its ability to outline pathologic mediastinal air collections, to determine connections to the pleural, esophageal, or pulmonary space, and to diagnose complications such as absess formation (SEMENKOVICH et al. 1995). Bronchoscopy with the option of direct visualization of the airway wall shows mucosal necrosis and is superior to CT in the diagnosis of impending wall rupture when the ad-

Table 8.10. Tracheal wall defects

Congenital:	Tracheo-esophageal fistulas with or without esophageal atresia
Trauma:	Penetration injury
Iatrogenic:	Intubation
Neoplastic infiltration	Esophageal tumor
Postsurgical:	Anastomotic dehiscence after lung transplantation

wall irregularities, small air collections, and fine fistulas.

Diagnosis is based on overlapping axial images and multiplanar reformats (SCHAEFER et al. 1993). Coronal reformats and anteroposterior mIP images improve the visualization of the cranial and caudal wall of the main bronchi, where wall discontinuities can easily be missed due to partial volume effects (Fig. 8.21). Thin-slab mIP images are an excellent

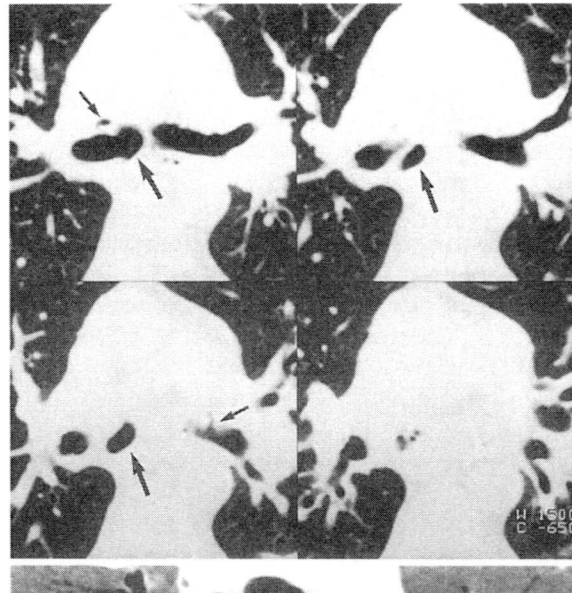

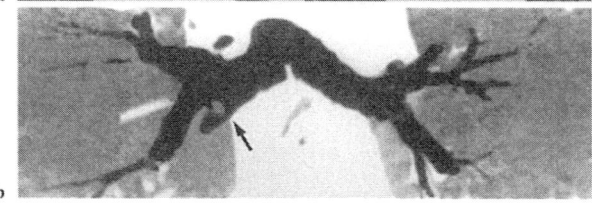

Fig. 8.21. Axial sections (**a**) and mIP (**b**) in a patient with bilateral dehiscences: while the small pseudodiverticuli (*small arrows*) usually heal without sequelae, we found that the large outpouching typically seen at the caudal wall of the right main bronchus (*large arrows*) predisposes to the development of strictures. Due to projection effects, the left-sided dehiscence is not seen on the anteroposterior mIP (protocol B: 2/3/2)

ventitial sleeve is still intact and an air leak is not yet present. Radiographic signs of a tracheobronchial fracture include a large pneumothorax, a pneumomediastinum, and disturbed ventilation of the lung distal to the fracture. All these signs, however, are nonspecific and often overshadowed by other injuries.

Spiral CT. Large dehiscences will be seen independent of CT technique. Spiral CT (protocol B) is superior to standard CT for detection of subtle

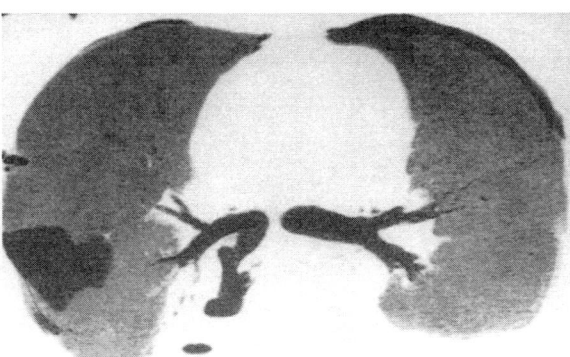

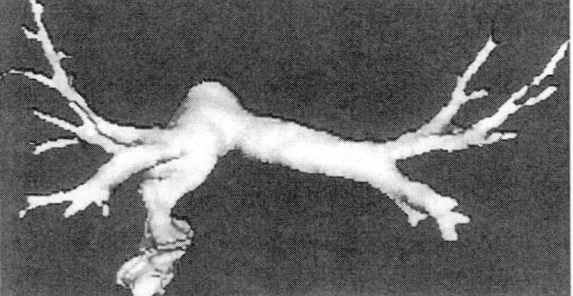

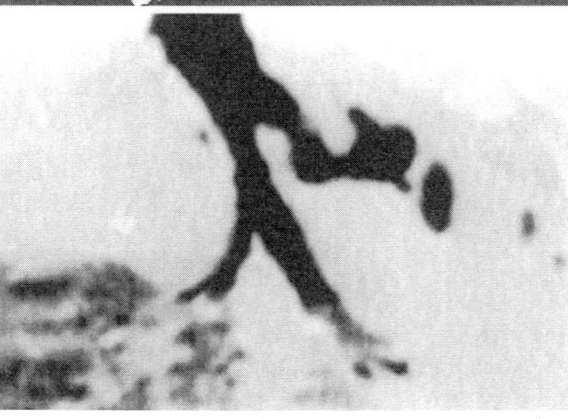

Fig. 8.22. Sagittal reformat (**a**), mIP (**b**), and SSD (**c**) in a lung transplanted patient that developed a large dehiscence with a bronchopleural fistula. All three techniques demonstrate the broad wall defect and the extent of the extrabronchial air collection. The dorsocaudal extension of the air collection is best seen on the reformat, while the relationship to branching bronchi is best demonstrated on the mIP and SSD (protocol B: 2/2/1)

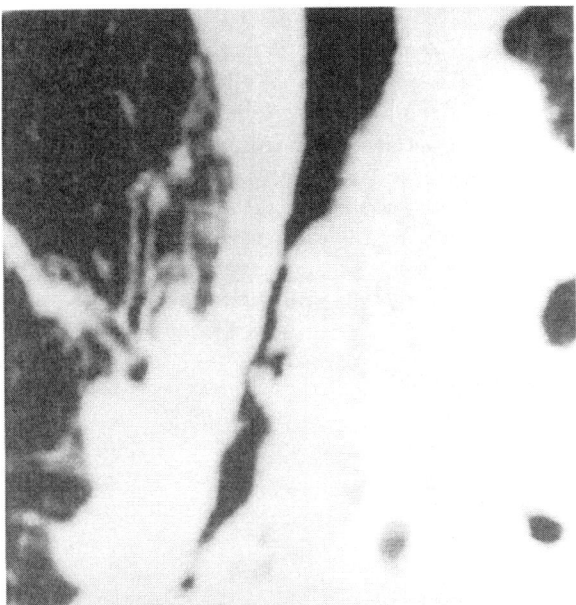

Fig. 8.23. Sagittal reformat along the long axis of the lower trachea, right main bronchus, and intermediate bronchus in a patient with an extensive infiltrating esophageal tumor. Note the superb delineation of subtotal occlusion by endoluminal tumor growth (protocol B: 1/2/1)

mode for display of small extraluminal air collections ventral or dorsal to the wall of the main bronchi (Fig. 8.22). SSDs are mainly suited for a comprehensive display of large extraluminal air collections. SSDs still lack sufficiently detailed visualization to be used for diagnosis or to show fine pathology.

8.3.7 Evaluation Before/After Interventional Procedures

Laser photoresection is a palliative treatment for various obstructive tracheobronchial diseases. A straight passage from the lesion to the bronchus distal to the obstructed area is important in order not to penetrate the tracheobronchial wall during laser therapy (Fig. 8.23). Knowledge of vascular structures adjoining the tracheobronchial lesions is of importance to the endoscopist to reduce the risk of accidental damage to adjacent major vessels and subsequent exsanguination (PEARLBERG et al. 1985). Because laser photoresection is only able to remove endoluminal obstruction, presence of predominantly extraluminal tumor compression on CT correlates with a poor response to laser therapy (ZWIREWICH et al. 1988).

Patients with tracheobronchial dyskinesias, obstructing nonresectable tumors, acquired esophagorespiratory fistulas, or circumscribed fibrotic strictures are candidates for bronchoscopic insertion of an endotracheal or endobronchial stent. Complications from stent placement include primary misplacement, stent migration (Fig. 8.7), airway obstruction, wall penetration, and recurrent stenosis. Y-shaped tracheal stents are less prone to dislocation (Fig. 8.24).

Spiral CT. The highest possible z-axis resolution (scan protocol B) is mandatory for the workup before laser resection or stent placement because realistic measurements are required. Spiral CT is markedly superior over conventional CT for this imaging task.

Prior to laser therapy, spiral CT is the method of choice to assess the relative contribution of intraluminal and extraluminal tumor to the obstruction, and to determine vascular structures adjacent to the planned area of photoresection. Multiplanar reformats along the axis of the obstructed airway best demonstrate the direction in which the photoresection has to be performed. Endoscopic views with semitransparent walls may be of value for planning laser therapy because of their "realistic" display of the anatomic relationship between airways, lesion, and vascular structures.

Both quantitative measurements (made on axial scans and multiplanar reformats) and three-dimensional reconstructions for anatomic visualization represent an excellent data base for planning

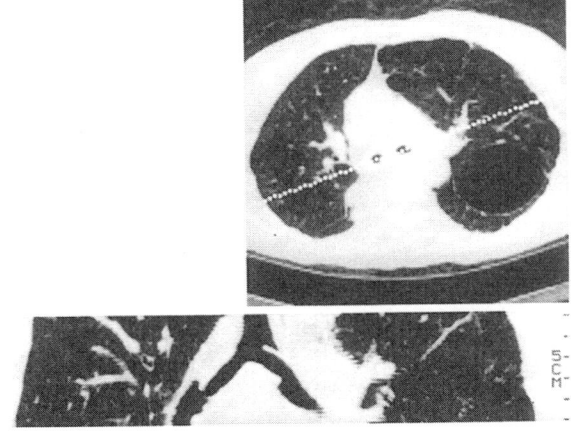

Fig. 8.24. Coronal reformat in a patient after lung transplantation and placement of a bifurcate stent: note the protrusion of the upper end of the stent into the tracheal lumen (protocol B: 2/2/1)

and manufacturing individual stents tailored to the specific anatomic situation (ALBES et al. 1994). This may be necessary in patients with multiple stenoses in the main or lobar bronchi (e.g., due to large or multifocal tumors or due to postischemic strictures after lung transplantation). In patients with esophagorespiratory fistulas, the configuration and diameter of the involved airway can be accurately assessed. The location and dimension of the fistula can be demonstrated if there is air within the fistula or if oral iodinated contrast is applied that enters the fistula. Based on the measurement of the distance between the fistula and the carina, bifurcate tracheal stents with appropriately mounted foam cuffs can be selected (Fig. 8.25).

Spiral CT is well suited for diagnosis of immediate complications of stenting such as a suboptimal stent placement or wall perforation, and for noninvasive control of late complications such as stent migration or luminal obstruction due to tumor recurrence or granulation tissue. Control examinations after laser therapy or stent implantation verify the reestablishment of a satisfactory airway diameter or successful occlusion of a fistula.

Multiplanar reformats perpendicular to the long axis of the stent provide the most accurate assess-

ment of stent position and luminal compromise due to tumor recurrence or granulation tissue. Reformats along the long axis of the stent and perpendicular to the origins of the branching lobar bronchi are best suited to outline the stent position in its relationship to the orifices of the branching lobar bronchi. Stent migration and dislocation with obstruction of a bronchus can be clearly diagnosed (Figs. 8.7, 8.24).

Endoscopic views of the inner surface of the airways demonstrate the in situ situation of the airways after stent implantation or laser therapy (Fig. 8.7c).

8.3.8 Evaluation After Tracheobronchoplastic Surgery

With constantly improving surgical techniques, there is an increasing number of patients who undergo bronchoplastic surgery. Underlying etiologies include neoplastic diseases, strictures after transplantation, and circumscribed narrowings of other etiology. The derangement of the bronchial branching pattern can be very complex and difficult to assess on axial images.

Spiral CT. Spiral CT with SSDs or even bronchoscopic views will aid in determining the exact postoperative anatomy and may improve orientation for the surgeon and bronchoscopist.

8.4 Summary

Spiral CT with its multiprojectional approach provides an excellent tool for imaging of focal lesions in their relationship to branching bronchi and adjacent mediastinal structures. Diagnosis is mainly based on overlapping axial sections and 2D reformats that are adjusted to the anatomic situation. 3D surface display serves as a comprehensive means of presentation of pathologic findings to bronchoscopists and surgeons. Endoscopic views may be helpful for planning interventional procedures such as laser therapy or transbronchial biopsies. They are also an excellent teaching tool. CT will continue to have limited accuracy for the detection of submucosal tumor spread or mucosal alterations. CT morphology of the various tracheal and bronchial tumors and diffuse diseases also lacks specificity in spiral CT. The sensitivity for the detection of small lesions in the main bronchi and the characterization of lesions with respect to location and morphology are considerably improved with the spiral CT technique.

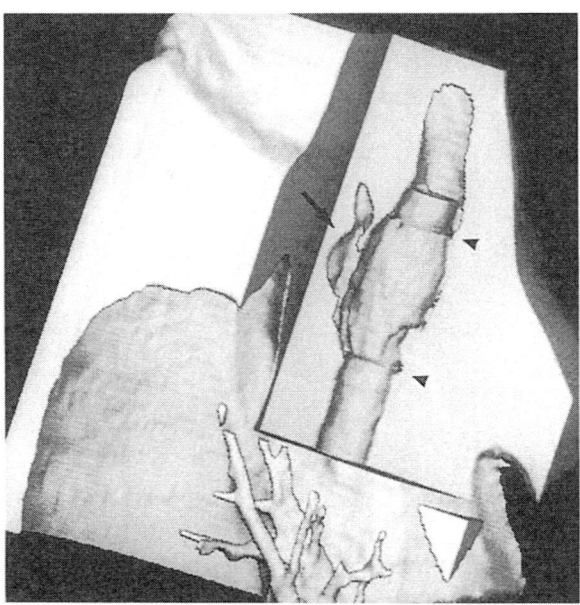

Fig. 8.25. SSD in a patient that received a tracheal stent for treatment of an infiltrating esophageal tumor with tracheoesophageal fistula. *Arrowheads* mark the upper and lower end of the foam cuff that is in an optimum position to occlude the fistula (*long arrow*). The sagittal cut plane demonstrates the air-filled trachea as a negative cast within the mediastinal soft tissue "block" (protocol B: 3/5/2)

References

Albes JM, Prokop M, Gebel M, Donow C, Schäfers HJ (1994) Bifurcate tracheal stent with foam cuff for tracheo-esophageal fistula: utilization of reconstruction modes of spiral computed tomography. Thorac Cardiovasc Surg 42:367–369

Costello PH (1994) Spiral CT of the thorax. Semin Ultrasound CT MR 15:90–106

Gamsu G, Webb R (1982) Computed tomography of the trachea: normal and abnormal. AJR 139:321–326

Gamsu G, Webb R, Shallit JB, Moss AA (1981) CT in carcinoma of the larynx and piriform sinus: value of phonation scans. AJR 136:577

Kalender WA, Polacin A (1991) Physical performance characteristics of spiral CT scanning. Med Phys 18:910–915

Kwong JS, Müller NL, Miller RR (1992) Diseases of the trachea and main stem bronchi: correlation of CT with pathologic findings. Radiographics 12:645–657

Kwong JS, Adler BD, Padley SPG, Müller NL (1993) Diagnosis of diseases of the trachea and main bronchi: chest radiography vs CT. AJR 161:519–522

Naidich DP, Lee JJ, Garay SM, McCauley DI, Aranda CP, Boyd AD (1987) Comparison of CT and fiberoptic bronchoscopy in the evaluation of bronchial disease. AJR 148:1–7

Newmark GM, Conces DJ, Kopecky (1994) Spiral CT evaluation of the trachea and bronchi. J Comput Assist Tomogr 18:552–554

Polacin A, Kalender WA, Marchal G (1992) Evaluation of section sensitivity profiles and image noise in spiral CT. Radiology 185:29–35

Pearlberg JL, Sandler MA, Kvale P, Beute GH, Madrazo BL (1985) Computed-tomographic and conventional linear-tomographic evaluation of tracheobronchial lesions for laser photoresection. Radiology 154:759–762

Quint LE, Glazer GM, Orringer MB (1987) Central lung masses: prediction with CT of need for pneumonectomy versus lobectomy. Radiology 165:735–738

Quint LE, Whyte RI, Kazerooni EA et al. (1995) Stenosis of the central airways: evaluation by using helical CT with multiplanar reconstructions. Radiology 194:871–877

Rémy-Jardin M, Rémy J, Petyt L, Wannebroucq (1994) Spiral CT tracheobronchography with multiplanar and 3D reformations (abstract). Radiology 193(P):261

Schaefer CM, Prokop M, Döhring W, Schäfers HJ, Galanski M (1991) Spiral CT of the tracheobronchial system: optimized technique and clinical applications (abstract). Radiology 181(P):274

Schaefer CM, Prokop M, Zink C, Galanski M (1993) Spiral CT of anastomotic complications after lung transplantation (abstract). Radiology 189(P):263

Semenkovich JW, Glazer HS, Anderson DC, Arcidi JM, Cooper JD, Patterson GA (1995) Bronchial dehiscence in lung transplantation: CT evaluation. Radiology 194:205–208

Vining DJ, Shifrin RY, Haponik EF, Liu K, Choplin RH (1994) Virtual bronchoscopy (abstract). Radiology 193(P):261

Webb WR, Gatsonis C, Zerhouni EA, Heelan RT, Glazer GM, Francis IR, McNeil BJ (1991) CT and MR imaging in staging non-small cell bronchogenic carcinoma: report of the radiologic diagnostic oncology group. Radiology 176:705–713

Weber AL, Grillo HC (1978) Tracheal tumors: a radiological, clinical, and pathological evaluation of 84 cases. Radiol Clin North Am 16:227–246

Zwirewich CV, Müller NL, Lam SCT (1988) Photodynamic laser therapy to alleviate complete bronchial obstruction: comparison of CT and bronchoscopy to predict outcome. AJR 151:897–901

9 Spiral CT of the Bronchial Tree

P. Grenier and C. Beigelman

9.1 Introduction

High-resolution computed tomography (HRCT) has gained wide acceptance as the imaging modality of choice in the evaluation of most airway lesions. On the other hand, spiral CT provides considerable improvement over conventional CT due to its ability to utilize thin collimation to detect subtle airway pathology, while eliminating the recording gaps that result from slight variations in breath-holding. Currently, both spiral volumetric and HRCT techniques can be used in combination for good assessment of focal or diffuse, proximal or distal airway disease.

9.2 Technique of Examination

Adequate assessment of airway morphology necessitates that the section thickness approximate the size of the airways under evaluation.

P. Grenier, MD, Department of Radiology, Hôpital de la Salpétrière, 47, boulevard de l'Hôpital, 75641 Paris Cédex 13, France
C. Beigelman, MD, Department of Radiology, Hôpital de la Salpétrière, 47, boulevard de l'Hôpital, 75641 Paris Cédex 13, France

9.2.1 Lobar and Segmental Bronchi

Using spiral CT, all lobar and segmental airways can be routinely identified during a 20-s breath-hold using 3-mm collimation. Once acquired, axial planes can be reconstructed as necessary every 1 or 2 mm. The potential of applying this technique for multiplanar and three-dimensional (3D) reconstructions can be readily appreciated, since it provides benefit by both simplifying and reinforcing interpretation of otherwise complex anatomy (NAIDICH et al. 1993). Several reconstruction techniques can be used:

1. 3D surface-rendering techniques using double-thresholding segmentation enable separation of air from other tissues. By this means, the bronchial tree, emphysema, and other air-containing structures are reformated. The voxels are assigned a gray value according to the shaded-surface display. However, with this technique, voxels containing a volume-averaging effect are not correctly classified and structures included in their volume can be falsely eliminated.

2. 3D volume-rendering techniques enable the bronchial tree to be displayed by selecting only voxels of a minimum density (minimum intensity projection) along a virtual ray tracing.

3. Multiplanar reformation (MPR) can be obtained rapidly in coronal, sagittal, oblique, or curved viewing angles, from cross-sectional images or from the 3D shaded-surface display. This technique has the advantage over 3D images of slicing the volume of interest. By contrast to the 3D display, it is able to visualize all the densities included in the acquired volumes: air, calcium, contrast medium, soft tissues, and fat. It provides a better visualization and therefore better comprehension of the intraluminal morphology of the airways than 3D images.

One pitfall of CT with the MPR technique is the necessity for patients to cooperate fully in regard to lack of motion, including the ability to hold their breath. Examinations performed during free breathing are usually of limited diagnostic use.

The 3D and MPR displays enable a better analysis of vertical and oblique bronchi by synthetically showing the overall shape and junction between normal and diseased areas. They can help in the planning of the surgical or endoscopic appproach because the lesion is shown in a viewing angle that can simulate the surgical approach (ADACHI et al. 1993; MERGO et al. 1994; RÉMY-JARDIN et al. 1994). Virtual reality imaging of the airways has been used for viewing spiral CT thin sections of the chest from the perspective of a bronchoscopist. Virtual bronchoscopy would allow physicians a "fantastic voyage," flying through, around, and into the central airways, including lobar and segmental bronchi, for inspection of abnormalities. This technique is currently under clinical evaluation but preliminary results indicate that virtual bronchoscopy enables accurate prediction of bronchial involvement by mediastimal tumors, evaluation of areas of bronchial stenosis and bronchiectasis, and discovery of unsuspected anatomic variants (VINING et al. 1994).

9.2.2 Subsegmental and Distal Bronchi

Since most of the subsegmental bronchi as well as their homologous pulmonary arteries run obliquely to the scanning plane, the attenuation of the pulmonary artery creates a partial volume effect on the adjacent bronchus, blurring it margins. Reducing slice thickness (to 1–3 mm) decreases this partial volume effect and provides better delineation of the bronchial wall and lumen.

Because of constraints of time and radiation dose, spiral acquisition using thin collimation (1–3 mm) cannot be performed over the whole chest from the apex of the lungs to the diaphragm. Localization of volumetric scanning with 1- to 3-mm collimation must be selected and limited to the region of interest. The pitch may be as close as possible to 1 and axial images are reconstructed every 1 mm. Visualization of the overlapped thin axial images in a cine-loop allows the bronchial divisions to be followed from the segmental origin to the distal bronchial lumens down to the smallest bronchi which can be identified on thin-section images (2 mm in diameter). This viewing technique helps indicate the segmental and subsegmental distribution of any airway lesion and may serve as a road map for the endoscopist (NAIDICH 1994).

Multiplanar reformation and 3D imaging of subsegmental bronchi can be performed with spiral acquisition but the results are very inconsistent. Slid-

ing thin-slab-minimum intensity projection (STS-mIP) is another technique that can be recommended for imaging small bronchi (NAPEL et al. 1993). This technique is a specific implementation of maximal intensity projection which consists of: (a) restriction of the volume in the projection direction to a thin slab that is only several voxels in depth; (b) the perspective is identical for each mIP image in the sequence; and (c) the slabs overlap by a relatively large fraction of the slab thickness.

In the caudocranial direction, STS-mIP is particularly simple to compute because mathematical rotations and interpolations are not required and, consequently, blurring caused by interpolation cannot occur. However, this technique may be extended to other perspectives (anteroposterior, lateral, or oblique) if desired. The advantage of STS-mIP for assessing airways is that the overall bronchial size can be better demonstrated compared with viewing the individual sections. This ability to completely visualize the size of the bronchus is best appreciated in the assessment of bronchiectasis. However, the exact physical relationship of mucus plug or bronchial tumors in the bronchus may be lost. Indeed, some endobronchial lesions may potentially be suppressed by the projection process. For instance, when restricted to the caudocranial direction, STS-mIP may not show a filling defect when the lesion is located on the superior or inferior surface of the airway (NAPEL et al. 1993). The use of composite images from both the minimum and the maximum intensity projection is currently under evaluation.

9.3 Bronchial Stenosis

Spiral CT can improve detection, evaluation of extent, and characterization of bronchial stenoses. It may orientate the endoscopist and serve as a guide for the taking of a biopsy specimen.

9.3.1 Detection

Computerized tomography has been considered a reliable method to demonstrate tumoral lesions of the bronchi (NAIDICH et al. 1987). MAYR et al. (1989) evaluated the performance of conventional CT with 8-mm collimation in detecting endobronchial tumors. In 121 of the 142 patients included in their study, the presence of an endobronchial mass was confirmed at bronchoscopy with biopsy or at surgery. Using two independent observers, the sensitivity and specificity of CT for diagnosing normal or narrowed bronchial lumens were 91%–94% and 99%, respectively. Owing to lower scan thickness (3 mm), spiral CT can reduce volume averaging and, in this way, can detect subtle bronchial tumors localized on lobar, segmental, or subsegmental bronchi which would have been missed using only conventional CT (Fig. 9.1).

Although CT is effective in the detection of endobronchial disease and bronchiectasis, its role in the investigation of hemoptysis has been controversial. Although HAPONIK et al. (1987) found that CT did not have a sufficient impact on case management to warrant its routine use, NAIDICH et al. (1990) advocated its use as a screening technique. However, three recent prospective studies emphasized the complementary roles of CT and bronchoscopy in maximizing the diagnostic yield for malignant disease and bronchiectasis in patients with hemoptysis. MILLAR et al. (1992) showed that CT contributed to a diagnosis in 20 of 40 (50%) patients with hemoptysis in whom both chest radiograph and fiberoptic bronchoscopy results had been normal. Concerning their series of 91 patients with hemoptysis, SET et al. (1993) reported that CT detected all bronchial tumors seen at bronchoscopy and seven others, five of which were beyond bronchoscopic range. CT was unable to demonstrate early mucosal abnormalities, bronchitis, squamous metaplasia, and a benign papilloma, all found at bronchoscopy.

In the study by McGUINNESS et al. (1994), which included 57 patients, all seven cases of bronchial tumors were diagnosed by both CT and fiberoptic bronchoscopy. CT proved particularly valuable in diagnosing bronchiectasis and aspergilloma, while fiberoptic bronchoscopy was better able to detect bronchitis and mucosal lesions. These authors concluded that the high sensitivity of CT in identifying both the intraluminal and the extraluminal extent of central lung cancers in conjunction with its contribution to diagnosing bronchiectasis suggests that CT scans should be obtained prior to bronchoscopy in all patients with hemoptysis. Using spiral CT, the recommended protocol could be based on the combination of: (a) 1.5-mm collimation HRCT scans with 10-mm interspacing over the upper and lower parts of the lung, and (b) spiral volumetric acquisition with 3- to 5-mm collimation, and a pitch of 1–1.6 from the carina to the inferior pulmonary vein during breath-holding.

9.3.2 Evaluation of Extent

Multiplanar reformation and 3D images of lobar and segmental airways may prove valuable in patients with bronchial stenosis from central tumors as well as from inflammatory diseases or fibrosis after surgery or interventional endoscopic treatment (Fig. 9.2). Main clinical applications include localization

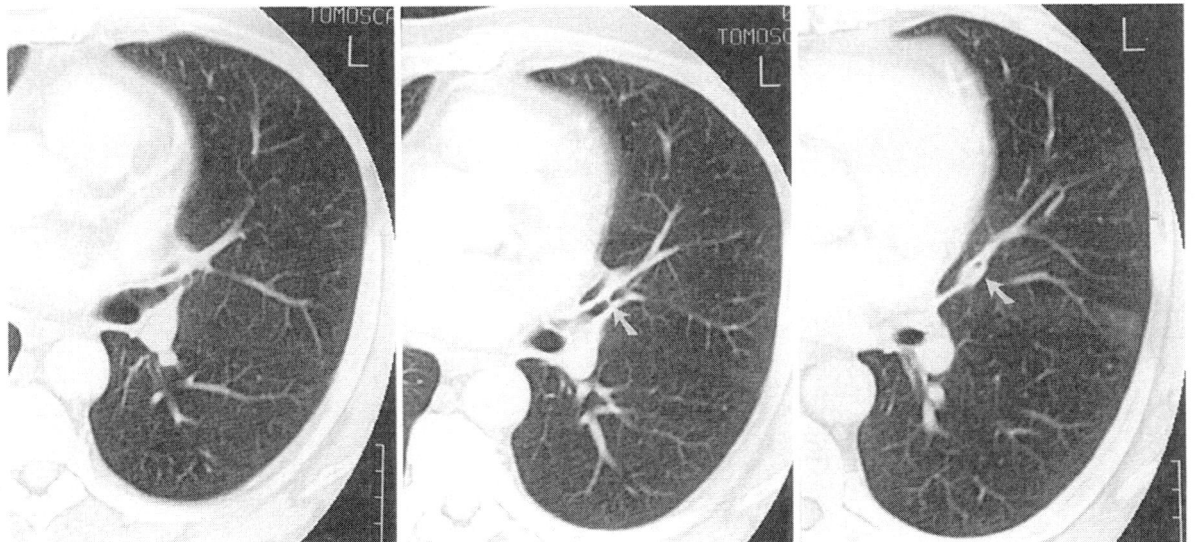

Fig. 9.1a–c. Detection of a bronchial tumor of the lingular bronchus with spiral volumetric acquisition using 5-mm collimation reconstructed every 3 mm. **a** Axial scan at the level of the lower part of the left upper lobe bronchus: the origin of the lingular bronchus appears normal. **b** Axial scan 3 mm below **a**: a web stenosis is present in the lumen of the lingular bronchus (*arrow*). **c** Scan 6 mm below **b**: incomplete filling of the dilated lumen of the bronchus distal to the stenosis (*arrow*)

and measurement of bronchical stenosis, control of laser therapy, and stent localization. Because of the orientation of the images along the long axis of the bronchus, the lengths of stenotic segments are depicted more clearly with MPR. A thin horizontal web seen on CT images with MPR can be invisible on the axial images. CT with MPR and 3D provides information that allows more precise, directed bronchoscopy, including demonstration of the length of a stricture and depiction of additional areas

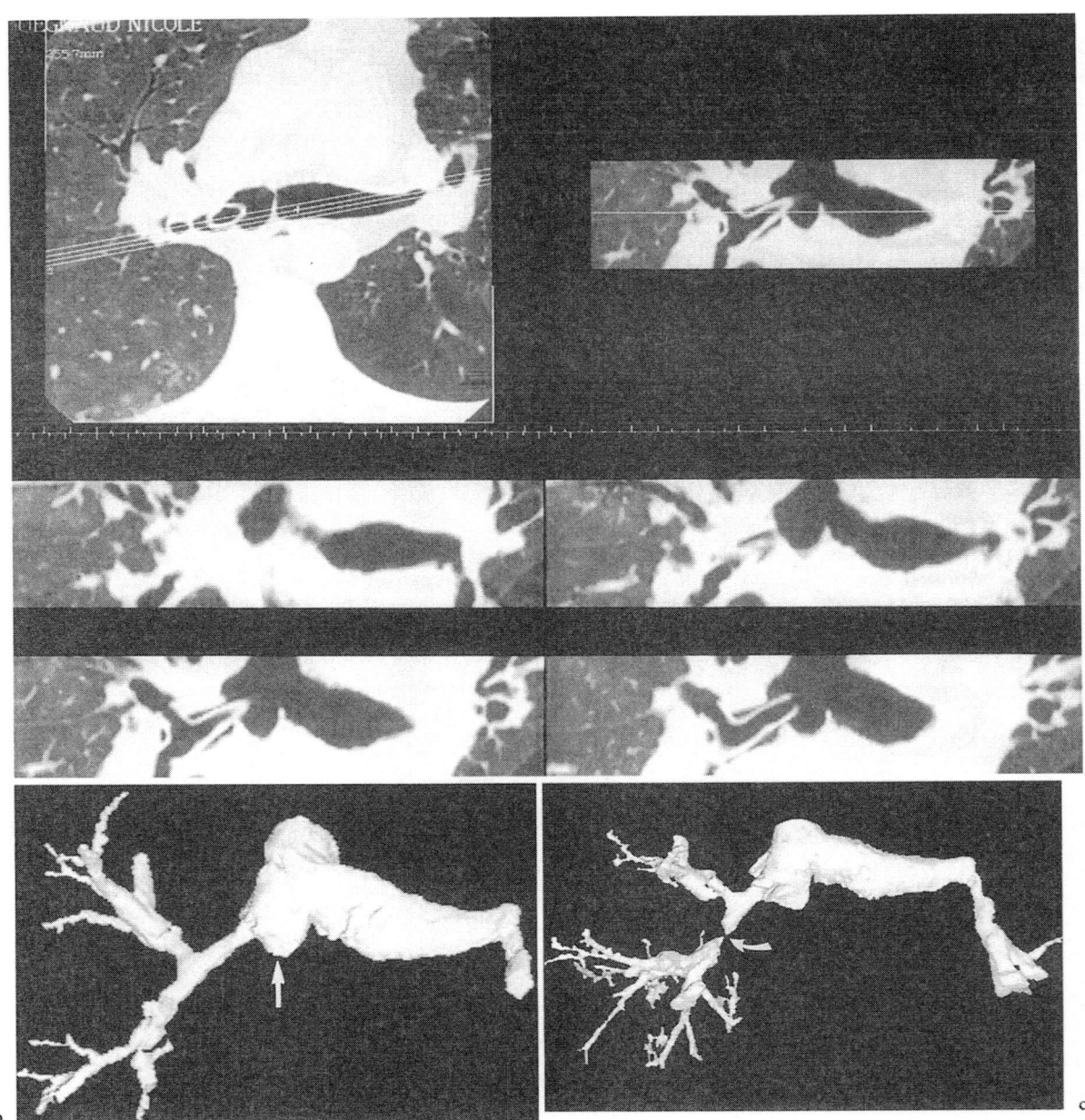

Fig. 9.2a–c. Bronchial stenosis occurring after bilateral lung transplantation and treated with stenting. **a** MPR in a coronal oblique plane selected on an axial scan. The position and morphology of the stent and its relationship with the bronchial stenosis are perfectly assessed. **b** 3D shaded-surface display of the bronchial tree. This image represents the air content of the bronchial tree and the lumen of the bronchial stent. Note the ectasia of the native main bronchus proximal to the bronchial anastomosis (*arrow*). **c** Control of the 3D shaded-surface display 3 months later: appearance of a stenosis of the intermediate bronchus distal to the lower part of the stent (*arrow*). (Courtesy of Dr. Arrivé)

of stricture beyond an area of narrowing that is not traversable by the bronchoscope (QUINT et al. 1995). This capacity is particularly important in patients who are prone to multiple strictures, such as those with Wegener's granulomatosis or relapsing polychondritis. It may also be easier to measure the degree of stenosis at CT with MPR compared with the view obtained at bronchoscopy. In addition, whereas the extraluminal extent of an abnormality is not visible at bronchoscopy, it can generally be demonstrated at CT.

RÉMY-JARDIN et al. (1994) demonstrated that MPR selected on 3D shaded-surface display images can depict airway changes either not seen or incompletely evaluated with fiberoptic bronchoscopy. For these authors, MPRs selected on shaded-surface display were superior to minimum intensity projection images in the evaluation of airway changes. By using minimum intensity projection, even when the results have been improved by projecting together only a small number of sections, eccentric stenoses and small tumors can disappear from the projection. Because of their high susceptibility to a partial volume effect, minimum intensity projections provide only relative information about bronchus diameter and shape. Absolute measurements are not possible, particularly for stenosis. Indeed, a high-grade stricture can appear as a pseudo-occlusion depending on the size of the underlying volume of interest (SCHAFFER-PROKOP et al. 1994).

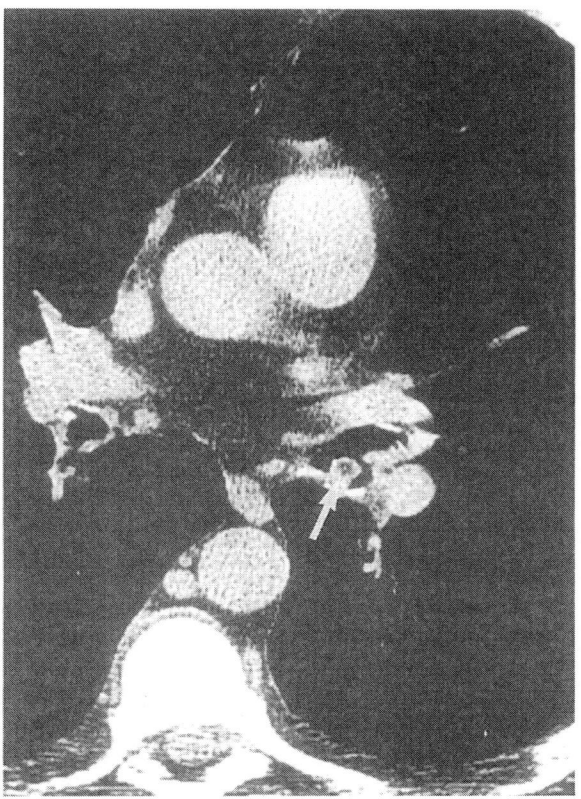

Fig. 9.3. Endobronchial hamartoma detected with spiral volumetric acquisition using 5-mm collimation and a pitch of 1, reconstructed every 3 mm. A 4-mm endobronchial tumor is growing from the posterior wall of the origin of the left lower lobe bronchus. A fat collection is visualized within the center of the tumor (*arrow*). (Courtesy of Dr. Brauner)

9.3.3 Characterization

Analysis of the shape, content, density, and anatomic relationships of the lesion on the successive contiguous thin sections obtained by spiral CT can contribute to determining the precise etiology of a bronchial stenosis. For instance, demonstration of fat within an endoluminal mass is characteristic of a hamartoma (AHN et al. 1994) (Fig. 9.3). When central or popcorn calcifications are associated with fat, the diagnosis of hamartoma becomes highly probable. Fat density is also a major CT finding seen in the very uncommon endobronchial lipoma (MENDELSOHN et al. 1983).

Broncholithiasis, a condition in which peribronchial calcified nodal disease erodes into or distorts an adjacent bronchus, is most reliably diagnosed with spiral CT (CONCES et al. 1991). Actually, CT can demonstrate: (a) a calcified endobronchial or peribronchial lymph node, which is the key radiological finding; (b) bronchopulmonary complications due to obstruction (including atelectasis,

pneumonia, bronchiectasis, and air trapping); and (c) the absence of an associated soft tissue mass. Difficulty in determining the relationship between lymph node and bronchus due to volume averaging is easily circumvented by spiral thin-collimation CT with reconstruction of axial images every 1–2 mm and MPR. Bronchial stenosis, which can result from fibrosing hilitis, is generally considered a late complication of granulomatous infection, especially histoplasmosis or tuberculosis. The abundant fibrosis may compress and invade any hilar structure, notably the bronchial tree. By depicting calcification within the hilar mass in conjunction with bronchial narrowing, CT can strongly suggest the diagnosis (GRENIER et al. 1993) (Fig. 9.4). Focal or diffuse bronchial stenosis can be observed in several inflammatory diseases, such as sarcoidosis, Wegener's granulomatosis, amyloidosis, and relapsing polychondritis (IM et al. 1988; DAVIS et al. 1989). CT can demonstrate regular or irregular narrowing

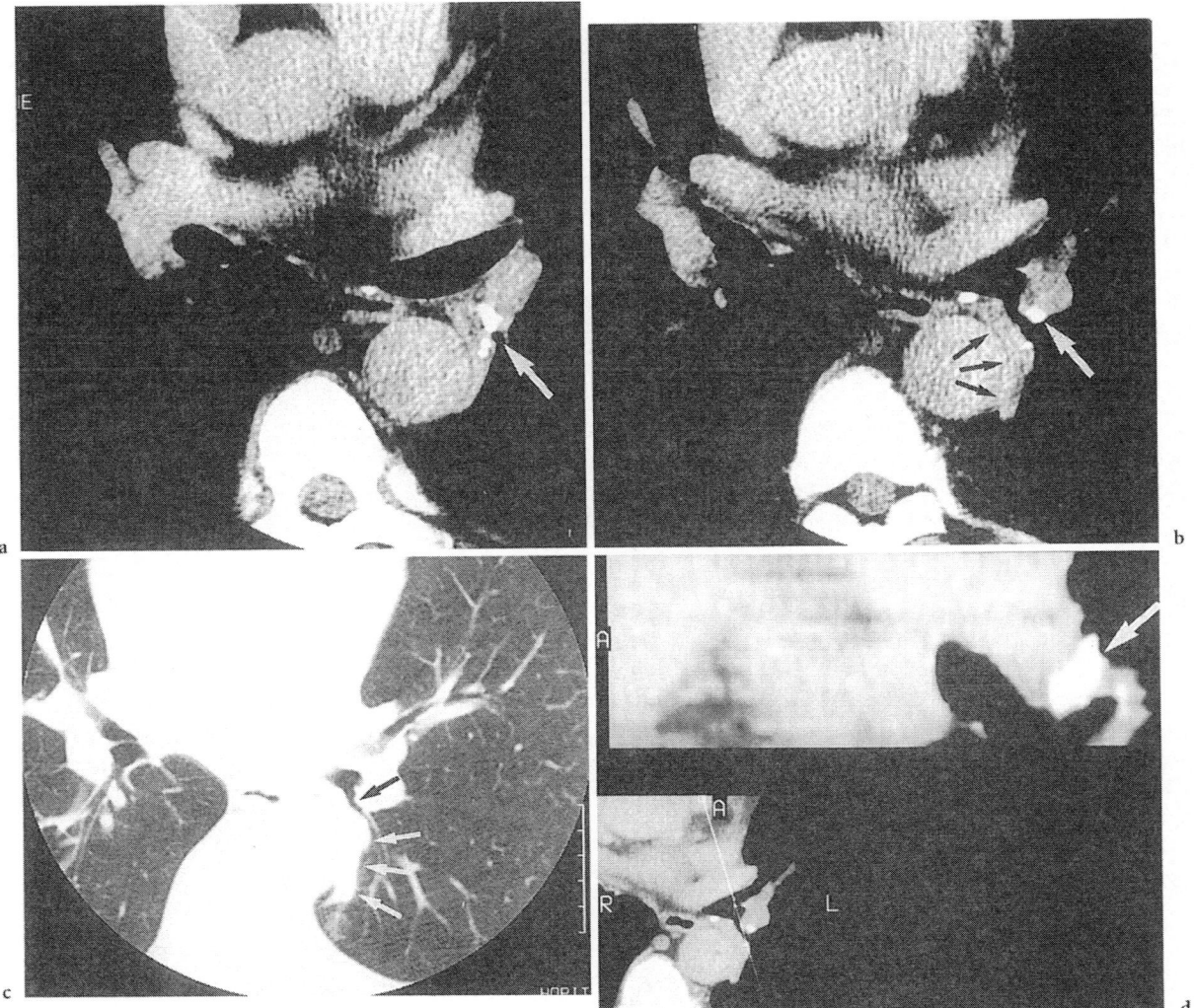

Fig. 9.4a–d. Calcified fibrosing hilitis of the left lung detected with spiral volumetric acquisition using 3-mm collimation and a pitch of 1, reconstructed every 2 mm. There is stenosis of the superior segmental bronchus of the left lower lobe bronchus (*black arrow* in c), and complete obstruction of the medial subsegment with distal atelectasis (*white arrows* in c; *black arrows* in **b**). Peribronchial calcifications are seen on axial (a, b, c) and coronal oblique (d) reformations at the superior and lateral part of the bronchus (*white arrows* in a, b, and d). a,b Axial slices; mediastinal windows. c Axial slice; lung windows. d Coronal oblique reformation; mediastinal windows

of the airways, thickening of the bronchial wall, sometimes with dense calcium deposits, or extrinsic airway compression by enlarged nodes.

9.3.4 Guiding Transbronchial Biopsy

Computerized tomography can be useful to the bronchoscopist when bronchial tumors are not visible, to guide the taking of transbronchial biopsy specimens (NAIDICH et al. 1988; ZACHAROPOULOS et al. 1990; GAETA et al. 1991). In a series of 27 patients with solitary pulmonary nodules associated with a positive CT bronchus sign, GAETA et al. (1993) showed that the diagnostic contribution of transbronchial biopsy depends upon the type of tumor–bronchus relationship and the biopsy technique performed. Thus, the ability to make a definitive diagnosis after bronchial forceps biopsy and bronchial brushing was much better for lesions characterized by a bronchus cut-off or bronchus contained within the tumor. Transbronchial needle aspiration was best able to provide a diagnosis in patients with a bronchus compressed by the tumor or with a thickening and narrowing of the bronchus leading to the tumor. Spiral CT using thin collimation (1–2 mm) could be particularly contributive to demonstrating the relationship between the bronchial tree and peripheral carcinomatous lung lesions, and in this way to help plan the transbronchial approach.

9.4 Bronchial Fistula

A bronchopleural fistula is an abnormal communication between a bronchus and the pleural space that may lead to large persistent air leaks and/or pleural infection. It is most commonly caused by necrotizing pneumonia, but traumatic origins are also frequent. Contiguous HRCT, as provided by spiral thin-collimation CT, is the most accurate technique to identify peripheral bronchopleural fistulas (WESTCOTT and VOLPE 1995).

The presence of gas in cavitated hilar adenopathy adjacent to the airways is highly suggestive of a nodobronchial fistula which is generally a consequence of infection (GRENIER et al. 1993). *Mycobacterium tuberculosis* is the organism most frequently involved, with the fistula resulting from erosion of caseous peribronchial lymph nodes into the tracheobronchial tree and occasionally into the esophagus as well. Direct visualization of the sinus tract, between the bronchial lumen and the hypertrophied cavitated lymph node and/or esophagus, can be helpful in planning therapy, but often remains difficult, particularly in cases of peripheral fistulas. Even the use of contiguous sections (spiral thin-collimation CT) only rarely permits direct visualization of the sinus tract. Congenital bronchoeso-phageal fistula can also be seen in adults (IM et al. 1991).

9.5 Congenital Abnormalities of the Airways

Congenital anomalies of the bronchial branching pattern involve: (a) the usual number of bronchi in ectopic locations; (b) the accessory cardiac bronchus, which is a true supernumerary anomalous bronchus; (c) bronchial atresia; and (d) lobar hypoplasia. These kinds of anomalies may be detected radiologically as an asymptomatic incidental finding. Ectopic bronchi, particularly the tracheal bronchus or accessory cardiac bronchus, can be revealed by hemoptysis or recurrent infection, as secretions can be retained with resultant inflammation and hypervascularity. Invasive tracheobronchography

can no longer be considered the optimal procedure for detecting developmental anomalies of the airways. All these abnormalities can be analyzed by CT (MORRISSON 1988; McGUINNESS et al. 1993). From a single data acquisition using spiral volumetric scanning, the developmental abnormalities can be diagnosed and the airways reconstructed by using MPR and 3D imaging techniques (Fig. 9.5).

A focal mucoid impaction projecting into a hyperinflated and oligemic segment or lobe, discovered in an asymptomatic adult, is highly suggestive of the diagnosis of bronchial atresia. The segmental or lobar hyperinflation distal to the atretic bronchus, which develops early in life as a result of collateral ventilation, is easily identified on CT scans (RÉMY-JARDIN et al. 1989). Spiral CT using thin collimation is particularly useful in making the diagnosis, since the bronchoscopy is usually interpreted as being normal. MPR enables the visualization of the linear opacities connecting the bronchocele and the bronchial tree, corresponding to the atretic bronchial segment (Fig. 9.6).

9.6 Bronchiectasis

The widely accepted technique for assessing the presence, type, and distribution of bronchiectasis is HRCT, whose accuracy is comparable to that of bronchography. GRENIER et al. (1986) obtained a sensitivity of 96% and a specificity of 93% in the detection of bronchiectasis, whereas several other studies demonstrated that use of conventional 10-mm collimation CT scans results in a sensitivity of 60%–80% and a specificity of 95%–100% (MULLER et al. 1984; PHILLIPS et al. 1986; SILVERMAN and GODWIN 1987). The HRCT protocol recommended for patients suspected of having bronchiectasis is based on 1.5-mm collimation scans with 10-mm interspacing over the chest from the apex of the lung to the diaphragm. Slice interspacing can be reduced to 5 mm over the most suspicious pulmonary areas (GRENIER et al. 1990). In addition, the gantry can be inclined 20° cranially, as it improves CT analysis of segmental or subsegmental bronchi (RÉMY-JARDIN and RÉMY 1988).

This protocol is not able to definitively eliminate potential pitfalls, which include: (a) artifacts that result from both respiratory and cardiac motion, which degrade bronchial imaging, particularly in paracardiac areas; (b) the possibility of overlooking areas of focal bronchiectasis, located exclusively in skipped areas; and (c) the difficulty of

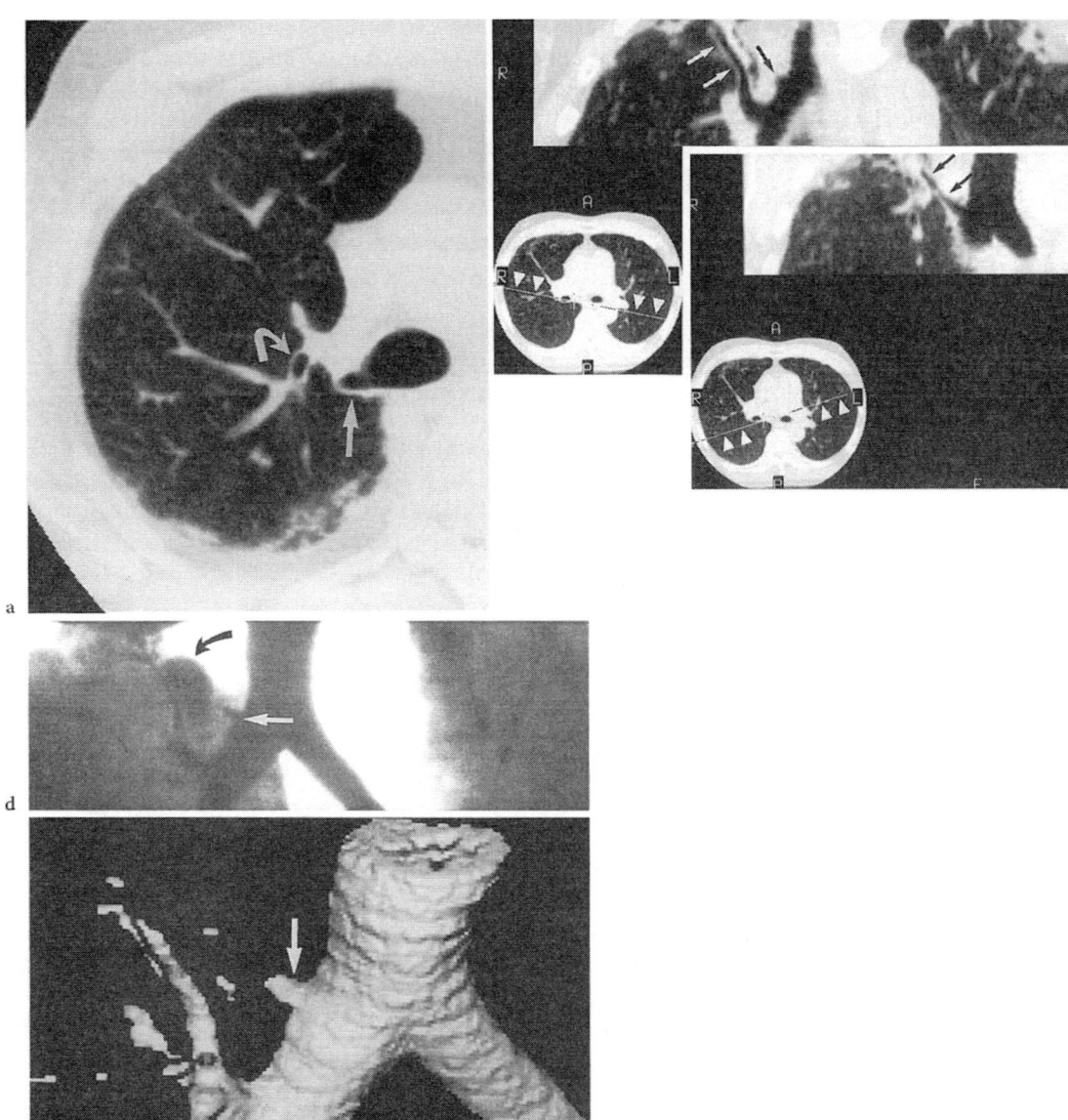

Fig. 9.5a–e. Recurrent infection in the apex of the right lung due to a tracheal bronchus visualized by means of spiral volumetric acquisition using 5-mm collimation and a pitch of 1, reconstructed every 3 mm. **a** Axial CT scan targeted on the right lung at the level of the distal part of the trachea: the origin of the ectopic right tracheal bronchus is clearly seen (*arrow*). In this image, the origin of the bronchus lying adjacent to the ectopic bronchus is impossible to assess (*curved arrow*). Note the paraseptal emphysema along the mediastinal pleura. **b,c** Coronal oblique reformated images selected from an axial scan (*arrowheads, bottom left*). In **b,** the origin of the ectopic bronchus (*black arrow*) can be seen. The bronchus section seen in **a** (*curved arrow*) corresponds to the normal superior segmental bronchus of the right upper lobe (*white arrows, top*). By changing the obliquity of the coronal reformation (**c,** *bottom left*), the ectopic bronchus can be visualized along its entire length (*black arrows, top*). This ectopic bronchus ventilates part of the superior segment of the right upper lobe, which is consolidated. **d** Coronal mIP display of the airways: the origin of the tracheal bronchus (*white arrow*) and normal bronchi are visualized. The abnormal lucency (*curved black arrow*) adjacent to the origin of the tracheal bronchus corresponds to the projection of the paraseptal emphysematous changes noted in **a. e** 3D shaded-surface display of the tracheobronchial tree. The left oblique anterior view optimizes the visualization of the origin of the tracheal bronchus (*arrow*) from the posterolateral aspect of the carina

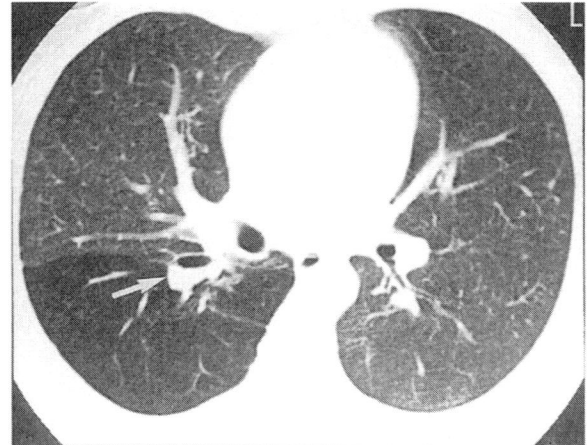

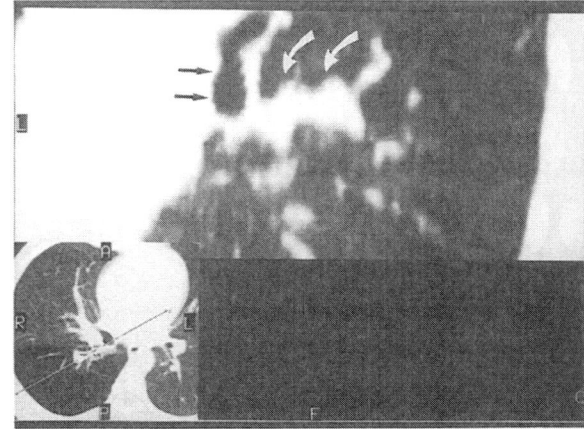

Fig. 9.6a,b. Atresia of the superior segmental bronchus of the right lower lobe detected with spiral volumetric acquisition using 3-mm collimation and a pitch of 1, reconstructed every 2 mm. **a** Axial CT scan: note the dilated bronchus (*arrow*) containing an air-fluid level associated with a hyperinflated and hypoattenuated superior segment of the right lower lobe. The origin of the segmental bronchus is not seen. **b** Longitudinal oblique reformation (*bottom left*) displays the mucoid impaction (*curved arrows*) proximal to the atretic segment of the bronchus. The *black arrows* point to the lumen of the intermediate bronchus

perceiving the slight dilatation of mild cylindrical bronchiectasis.

Spiral CT could contribute to reducing some of these pitfalls. Motion degradation of bronchial images can be reduced by using interpolation algorithms to reconstruct axial images after spiral scanning. In addition, volumetric acquisition during breath-holding eliminates the potential risk of missing small subtle bronchiectasis in areas skipped by interspacing between HRCT scans (Fig. 9.7).

The CT criteria for diagnosing cylindrical bronchiectasis include a bronchial diameter greater

than that of the accompanying pulmonary artery, lack of tapering of the bronchial lumen, and visualization of bronchi in the periphery of the lungs. However, the true value of seeing a bronchus with a diameter greater than that of the adjacent pulmonary artery for diagnosing cylindrical bronchiectais was recently called into doubt by LYNCH et al. (1993), who demonstrated that 16 (59%) of 27 healthy volunteers had at least one dilated bronchus at CT. In addition, theoretically, the small diameter of pulmonary arteries within an oligemic parenchymal zone may lead to a false-positive diagnosis of bronchiectasis, while large pulmonary arteries in a zone with vasodilation due to pulmonary blood flow redistribution or pulmonary hypertension may lead to a false-negative result. LYNCH et al. (1993) advanced that bronchiectasis should be diagnosed only when there is evidence of lack of tapering of the bronchus. Lack of bronchial tapering was the most sensitive finding indicating bronchiectasis in the study by KANG et al. (1995); it was present in 37 (79%) of the 47 pathologically proven bronchiectatic lobes. Usually, the lack of bronchial tapering in bronchiectasis is difficult to perceive on successive spaced HRCT scans. The assessment of this finding should be improved by using spiral CT with thin collimation and viewing the contiguous scans in a cine-mode (VAN DER BRUGGEN-BOGAARTS et al. 1994).

Another weakness of HRCT in diagnosing bronchiectasis is mucoid impaction filling bronchiectatic bronchi that can simulate pulmonary nodules or masses. Typically, the diagnosis of dilated bronchi filled with pus, secretions, or mycetoma is based on the recognition on a few successive slices of the segmental distribution of the corresponding densities, and the observation of the homologous pulmonary arteries, whose diameters are smaller than those of the dilated filled bronchi (GRENIER et al. 1993). Sometimes the segmental distribution of the densities cannot be correctly perceived on successive HRCT scans and pulmonary arteries are not recognized because of intense vasoconstriction in hypoventilated areas. Using spiral CT with thin collimation over the suspicious areas provides a multiplanar display of the radiopaque tubular structures converging toward the hilum in a segmental or subsegmental distribution, corresponding to bronchiectasis (Fig. 9.8).

Bronchiolitis is common in patients with bronchiectasis, including inflammatory and obliterative bronchiolitis. CT findings of bronchiolitis include centrilobular nodular or linear branching opacities, patchy areas of decreased lung attenuation due to

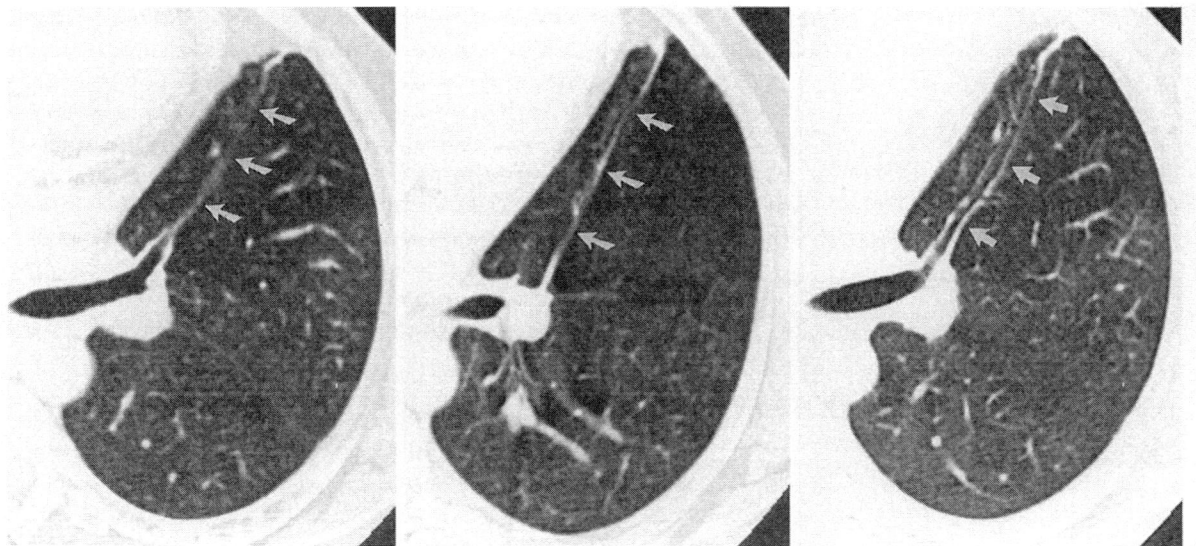

Fig. 9.7a–c. Mild cylindrical bronchiectasis in the lingula. **a,b** Axial oblique HRCT scans with 1.5-mm collimation and 5-mm interspacing. A linear density is seen from the origin of the lingular bronchus to the pleura (*arrows*). The lumen of the bronchus is not seen. Note the hypoattenuated area within the anterior part of the left upper lobe. **c** Spiral volumetric acquisition using 3-mm collimation and a pitch of 1, reconstructed every 2 mm. The lack of distal tapering of the bronchial lumen provides the diagnosis of bronchiectasis (*arrows*)

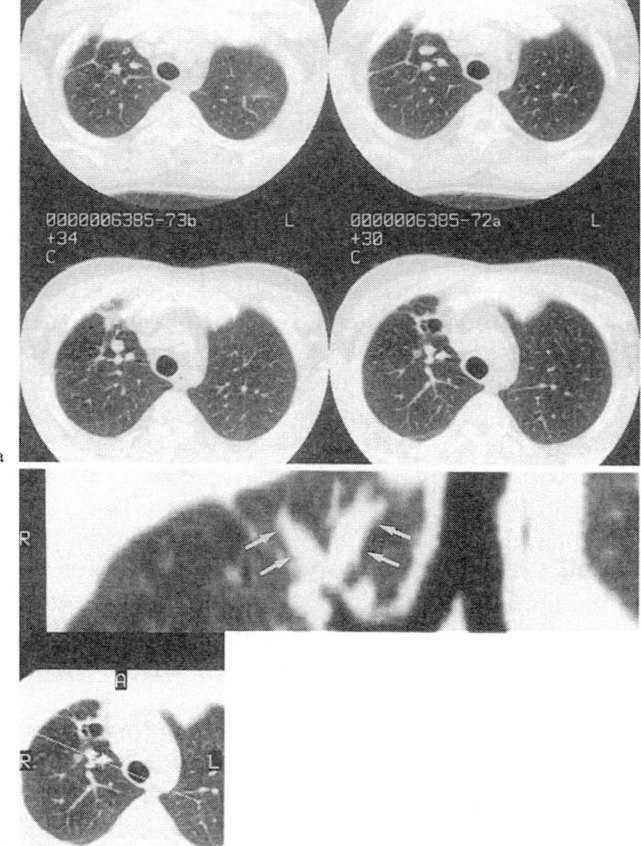

Fig. 9.8a,b. Mucoid impaction of the superior subsegmental bronchi of the right upper lobe detected with spiral volumetric acquisition using 5-mm collimation and a pitch of 1, reconstructed every 3 mm. **a** Contiguous axial CT scans. The nature of the nodules of the anterior part of the superior segment of the right upper lobe cannot be evaluated. Note linear opacities and paracicatricial emphysema due to sequelae of tuberculosis. **b** Longitudinal oblique reformation (*bottom left*): the tubular shapes of the opacities (*arrows*) converging towards the lumen of the superior segmental bronchus of the right upper lobe provide the diagnosis of mucoid impaction in dilated subsegmental bronchi, and suggest the presence of inflammatory bronchial stenosis

focal air trapping and decreased perfusion, and bronchiolectasis (WEBB 1994). Volumetric scanning with thin collimation can be helpful in the diagnosis of peripheral bronchiole plugging, which could be accurately distinguished from vessels or small pulmonary nodules by examination of contiguous scans (ENGELER et al. 1994).

Because of constraints of time and radiation dose, spiral CT cannot be used over the entire chest and volume scanning may be selected over the most suspicious areas. ENGELER et al. (1994) used thin-collimation spiral scanning to obtain four contiguous HRCT images at three different levels of the lungs (arch, carina, basis). The accuracy in diagnosing bronchiectasis was improved with a 2.8-fold increase in integral radiation exposure compared to that obtained with the standard technique without any modification of the exposure peak.

Surgery is still performed on some patients when bronchiectasis is localized. In such cases, accurate assessment is required on a segmental basis. Indeed, the surgeon must identify with certainty which segments are diseased, since modern surgical techniques frequently permit preservation of one or more normal pulmonary segments from a lobe in which bronchiectasis is present. Therefore, it may be

helpful to use HRCT and spiral CT in combination. We recommend performing HRCT scans with 1.5-mm collimation and 10-mm interspacing over the upper and lower parts of the lungs, where segmental and subsegmental bronchi run mainly perpendicular to the scan plane. Spiral CT scanning with 3-mm collimation is selected from 15 mm above the carina, in a caudal direction, during a 20-s breath-hold over the lung areas where segmental and subsegmental bronchi run mostly parallel to the scan plane (Fig. 9.9). Images are reconstructed every 2 mm. A pitch of 1.6 provides an increase in the lung volume examined during the scan time and reduces the radiation without any remarkable degradation of image quality. By angling the gantry 20° cranially, the segmental and subsegmental bronchi of the superior and anterobasal segments of lower lobes, anterior and posterior segments of the right upper lobe and culmen, and segments of the right middle lobe and lingula can be included within the lung volume imaged by spiral scanning (Fig. 9.10).

As compared to HRCT, spiral thin-collimation CT reduces interobserver variability and improves the diagnostic accuracy of segmental and subsegmental distribution of bronchiectasis (COCHE et al. 1995).

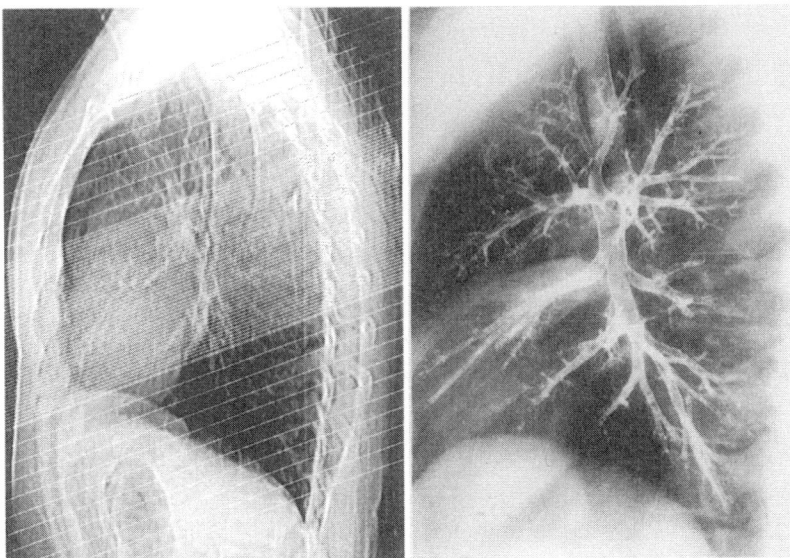

a   b

Fig. 9.9a,b. Proposed CT protocol for patients suspected of having bronchiectasis. a The lateral scout view of the chest represents the positions of both 1.5-mm collimation slices with 10-mm interspacing over the upper and lower parts of the lungs, and the spiral volumetric acquisition with 3-mm collimation reconstructed every 2 mm over the middle part of the lungs. The 20° cranial angulation of the gantry is also repre-sented. b Lateral view of a right bronchogram of a different patient shows that the subsegmental bronchi of the anterior and posterior segmental bronchi of the right upper lobe, the segmental bronchi of the middle lobe, and the superior and anterobasal segmental bronchi of the right lower lobe are included in the lung volume scanned by the spiral acquisition illustrated in a

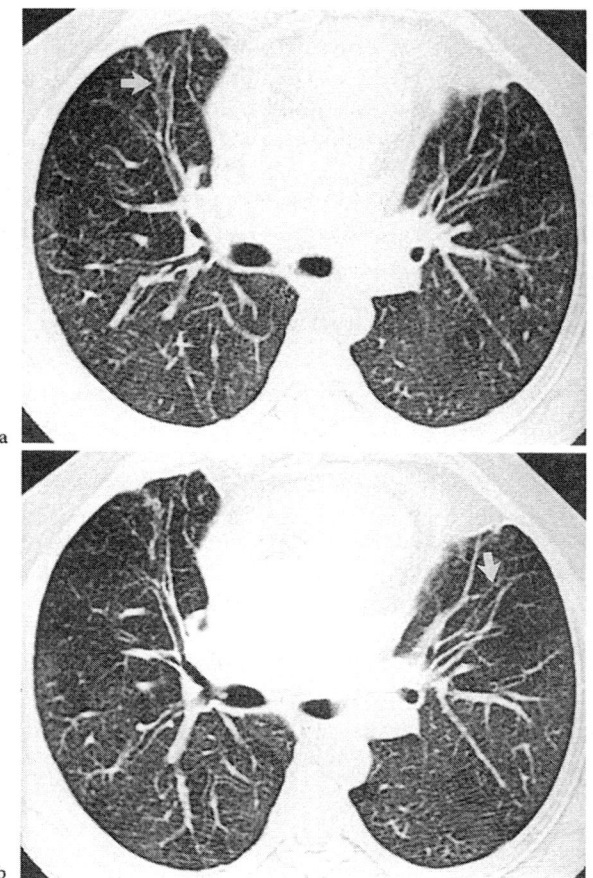

a

b

Fig. 9.10a,b. Bronchiectasis viewed in two successive scans (3-mm collimation) obtained with spiral volumetric CT, reconstructed every 2 mm, at the level of the right upper lobe bronchus. In **a**, varicose subsegmental bronchiectasis is seen within the anterior segment of the right upper lobe (*arrow*). In **b**, varicose subsegmental bronchiectasis is observed within the anterior segment of the upper division of the left upper lobe (culmen) (*arrow*)

9.7 Small Airway Diseases

The diagnosis of small airway disease is challenging for the clinician, as there are no pathognomonic clinical, functional, or radiographic features. At a functional level, the small airways contribute very little to normal airway resistance. As a result, widespread obliteration of these small airways is needed before there is any obvious functional impairment and clinical manifestations. Recently, conventional HRCT scans performed at suspended full expiration have been used to demonstrate air trapping in patients with emphysema, asthma, bronchiectasis, and bronchiolitis (EBER et al. 1993; HANSELL et al. 1994; STERN and FRANK 1994). Expiratory scans may show

evidence of air trapping even in the absence of morphologic abnormalities recognizable on inspiratory scans.

Normally at expiration, the lung density increases while lung cross-section areas decrease. When air trapping is present, lung density fails to increase while lung cross-section areas fail to decrease as normally expected (WEBB et al. 1993). The decreased attenuation in affected areas is, in part, due to underperfusion as a consequence of hypoventilation (hypoxic vasoconstriction). In cases in which there is global involvement of the small airways, a lack of regional homogeneity of the lung density may be lost and there is a uniform decrease in attenuation of the lung parenchyma. Furthermore, sections taken at end expiration may appear unremarkable in patients with particularly severe and widespread involvement of the small airways. In these patients, the most striking features are a paucity of pulmonary vessels and a lack of change of the cross-sectional areas of the lungs at comparable levels on inspiratory and expiratory scans. Although air trapping can be seen in subjects with normal pulmonary function tests, the extent and intensity of air trapping assessed on expiratory scans have been shown to correlate with the degree of airway obstruction (HANSELL et al. 1994; STERN et al. 1994).

A suggested protocol for HRCT scanning in cases of suspected small airway disease is 1.5-mm collimation every 10-mm section in full inspiration followed by 1.5-mm/30-mm sections obtained at end expiration. Spiral HRCT may also be used to search for air trapping during active expiration. Only small motion-related degradation of images acquired during dynamic expiration is visible because the interpolation algorithm used to reconstruct images reduces the movement-related artifacts (Fig. 9.11). The spiral HRCT technique may consist of a 15-mm-thick lung volume selected in the region of interest with 1.5-mm collimation and a pitch of 1 for the caudocranial increment of the table. Ten slices are obtained during the 10-s period as the patient performs a forced expiratory maneuver. The series of ten images can be viewed in a cine view in which the ten individual images can be rapidly displayed in a sequential fashion. In an unpublished series of 49 patients with suspicion of small airway disease, we compared dynamic expiration using spiral CT vs suspended end-expiration CT for assessing air trapping. In 35 patients, air trapping was noted on expiratory HRCT scans. Air trapping scores, established subjectively based on the extent and intensity of air trapping on dynamic expiratory CT scans, were superior in 16

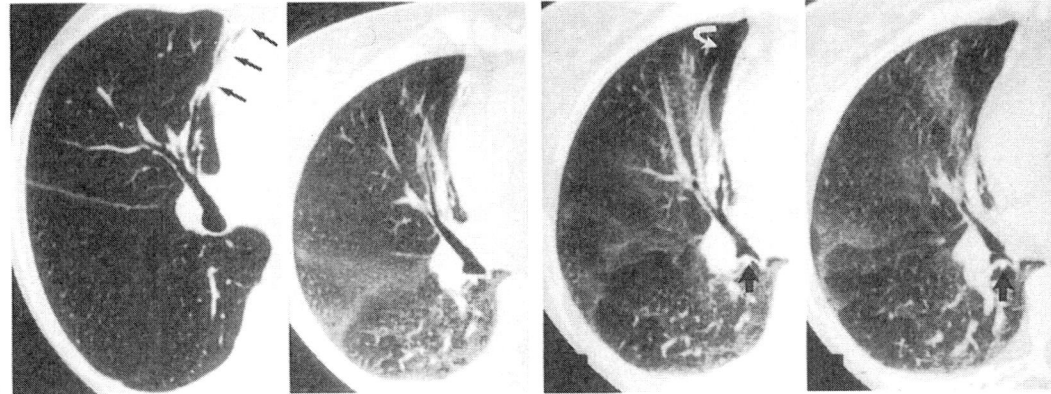

Fig. 9.11a,b. Air trapping at expiration-HRCT scan targeted on the right lung at the level of the right middle lobe bronchus. **a** *Left*: HRCT scan at suspended inspiration; *right*: HRCT scan at suspended end-expiration. Presence of subsegmental atelectasis is observed in the anteromedial segment of the middle lobe (*arrows*). Air trapping is seen within another subsegment close to the atelectatic lung. **b,c** Spiral volumetric acquisition with 1.5-mm collimation during a forced expiratory maneuver. Hyperlucency due to air trapping (*curved white arrow*) is more clearly illustrated than in **a**. Note the deformation with an anterior convexity of the posterior wall of the intermediate bronchus during active expiration (*black arrows*)

patients (46%) (Fig. 9.12), equal in 11 (31%), and inferior in eight (23%) as compared to those obtained on static expiration scans. Motion-related artifacts spoiled dynamic expiration scan interpretation in only three cases.

Although the reasons for the improvement provided by dynamic expiratory CT examinations remains partly unclear, one explanation could be "pendelluft." This phenomenon could result in a paradoxical decrease in attenuation within a partially obstructed lung, which may empty more slowly during rapid expiration, accentuating the attenuation differences (STERN and WEBB 1993). In addition, the lack of change in cross-sectional areas of the lungs during exhalation is easier to perceive on the cine view of CT scans obtained during active expiration than on suspended end-expiratory scans. Therefore, a complementary dynamic expiration study using the spiral technique could improve evaluation of air trapping at CT.

9.8 Dynamic Changes of Airways

Dynamic alterations in the appearance and caliber of the airways can also be evaluated when images of the central airways are obtained in both deep inspiration and expiration. This technique enables detailed evaluation of both regional and global bronchial physiologic mechanisms. The assessment of bronchial calibers and section areas has been proven use-ful experimentally in evaluating noninvasively and in vivo the airway resistance and response (bronchoconstriction and bronchodilatation) to the effects of different types of stimuli, including histamine, inhaled anesthesia, and hypoxia (BROWN et al. 1991, 1993; HEROLD et al. 1991; ZERHOUNI et al. 1993). Recent studies performed in asthmatic subjects and normal controls showed that HRCT can demonstrate changes in airway lumen diameter and airway wall thickness induced by bronchoprovocation (ABERLE et al. 1994; KEE et al. 1994). Use of spirometry and respiratory-gated spiral CT is required to be sure that volumetric scanning is performed at the controlled lung volume (RÉMY-JARDIN et al. 1992). Overlapped reconstructions of thin sections after a volumetric acquisition enable comparison of CT scans before and after stimulation at the same anatomic level.

One limitation for measuring airway cross-sections on HRCT scans is the change of orientation of bronchi with respect to the axial plane from one scanning to another. This limitation could be circumvented by 3D reconstruction of the bronchial tree which permits the location of a central axis of each bronchus to be calculated. This central axis can then be used to measure the true cross-sectional area by reconstructing a section perpendicular to the central axis. In this way, the technique enables the measurement of airway cross-sections, regardless of their orientations, and provides a more accurate area measurement (WOOD et al. 1994).

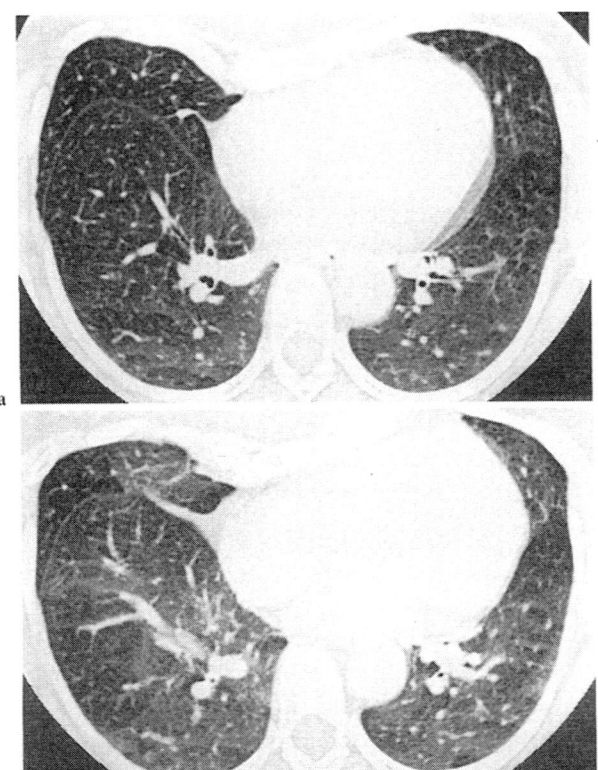

Fig. 9.12a,b. Small airway disease. **a** HRCT scan performed at suspended end-expiration at the level of the inferior pulmonary veins. **b** Spiral HRCT scan obtained approximately at the same anatomic level as **a** during a forced expiratory maneuver. The mosaic pattern due to the lack of homogeneity of lung density is better perceived in **b** than in **a**. Hypoattenuated areas in the lungs correspond to oligemia due to air trapping. In addition, in **b**, note that the calibers of the segmental bronchi in the lower lobes are smaller than on the scan obtained at suspended end-expiration (**a**)

References

Aberle DR, Goldin J, McNitt-Gray MF, Greaves SM, Kleerup E, Tashkin DP (1994) CT of airway reactivity in patients with asthma after bronchoprovocation testing. Radiology 193(P):368

Adachi S, Kono M, Takemura T, Itouji E, Kusumoto M, Sakai E (1993) Evaluation of 3D spiral CT bronchoscopy in patients with lung cancer. Radiology 189(P):264

Ahn JM, Im JG, Seo JW, Han HS, Yoon HK, Kim WS (1994) Endobronchial hamartoma: CT findings in three patients. AJR 163:49–50

Brown RH, Herold CJ, Hirshman CA, Zerhouni EA, Mitzner W (1991) In vivo measurements of airway reactivity using HRCT. Am Rev Respir Dis 144:208–212

Brown RH, Mitzner W, Zerhouni E, Hirshman CA (1993) Direct in vivo visualization of bronchodilation induced by inhalational anesthesia using high-resolution computed tomography. Anesthesiology 78:295–300

Coche E, Lucidarme O, Lenoir S, Beigelman C, Grenier P (1995) Bronchiectasis: assessment by spiral CT with thin collimation compared with high-resolution CT. Radiology 195(P):250

Conces DJ, Tarver RD, Vix VA (1991) Broncholithiasis: CT features in 15 patients. AJR 157:249–254

Davis SD, Berkmen YM, King T (1989) Peripheral bronchial involvement in relapsing polychondritis: demonstration by thin-section CT. AJR 153:953–954

Eber CD, Stark P, Bertozzi P (1993) Bronchiolitis obliterans on high-resolution CT: a pattern of mosaic oligemia. J Comput Assist Tomogr 17:853–856

Engeler CE, Tashjian JH, Engeler CM, Geise RA, Holm JC, Ritenour ER (1994) Volumetric high-resolution CT in the diagnosis of interstitial lung disease and bronchiectasis: diagnostic accuracy and radiation dose. AJR 163:31–35

Gaeta M, Pandolfo I, Volta S et al. (1991) Bronchus sign on CT in peripheral carcinoma of the lung: value in predicting results of transbronchial biopsy. AJR 157:1181–1185

Gaeta M, Barone M, Russi EG et al. (1993) Carcinomatous solitary pulmonary nodules: evaluation of the tumor-bronchi relationship with thin-section CT. Radiology 187:535–539

Grenier P, Maurice F, Musset D, Menu Y, Nahum H (1986) Bronchiectasis: assessment by thin-section CT. Radiology 161:95–99

Grenier P, Lenoir S, Brauner M (1990) Computed tomographic assessment of bronchiectasis. Semin US CT MR 11:430–441

Grenier P, Cordeau MP, Beigelman C (1993) High-resolution computed tomography of the airways. J Thorac Imaging 8:213–229

Hansell DM, Wells AU, Rubens MB, Cole PJ (1994) Bronchiectasis: functional significance of areas of decreased attenuation at expiratory CT. Radiology 193:369–374

Haponik EF, Britt EJ, Smith PL, Bleecker ER (1987) Computed chest tomography in the evaluation of hemoptysis: impact on diagnosis and treatment. Chest 91:80–85

Herold CJ, Brown RH, Mitzner W, Links JM, Hirshman CA, Zerhouni EA (1991) Assessment of pulmonary airway reactivity with high resolution CT. Radiology 181:369–374

Im JG, Chung JW, Han SK, Han MC, Kim CW (1988) CT manifestations of tracheobronchial involvement in relapsing polychondritis. J Comput Assist Tomogr 12:792–793

Im JG, Lee WJ, Han MC, Chi JG, Han JK, Kim CW (1991) Congenital broncho-oesophageal fistula in the adult. Clin Radiol 43:380–384

Kang EY, Miller RR, Müller NL (1995) Bronchiectasis: comparison of preoperative thin-section CT and pathologic findings in resected specimens. Radiology 195:649–654

Kee ST, Fahy JV, Derong C, Webb WR, Gamsu G (1994) Use of CT to measure changes in airway lumen diameter and airway wall thickness after induced bronchoconstriction and bronchodilatation in asthmatic subjects. Radiology 193(P):367

Lynch DA, Newell JD, Tschomper BA, Cink TM, Newman LS, Bethel R (1993) Uncomplicated asthma in adults: comparison of CT appearance of the lungs in asthmatic and healthy subjects. Radiology 188:829–833

Mayr B, Ingrisch H, Häussinger K, Huber RM, Sunder-Plassmann L (1989) Tumors of the bronchi: role of evaluation with CT. Radiology 172:647–652

McGuinness G, Naidich DP, Garay SM, Davis AL, Boyd AD, Mizrachi HH (1993) Accessory cardiac bronchus: CT features and clinical significance. Radiology 189:563–566

McGuinness G, Beacher JR, Harkin TJ, Garay SM, Rom WN, Naidich DP (1994) Hemoptysis: prospective high-resolution CT/bronchoscopic correlation. Chest 105:1155–1162

Mendelsohn SL, Fogelman D, Zwanger-Mendelsohn S (1983) Endobronchial lipoma demonstrated by CT. Radiology 148:790

Mergo PJ, Fenton J, Ross PR, Staab EV (1994) Three-dimensional CT of the tracheobronchial tree: correlative study with bronchoscopy in 30 cases. Radiology 193(P):261

Millar AB, Boothroyd AE, Edwards D, Hetzel MR (1992) The role of computed tomography (CT) in the investigation of unexplained haemoptysis. Respir Med 86:39–44

Morrison SC (1988) Demonstration of a tracheal bronchus by computed tomography. Clin Radiol 39:208–209

Müller NL, Bergin CJ, Ostrow DN, Nichols DM (1984) Role of computed tomography in the recognition of bronchiectasis. AJR 143:971–976

Naidich DP (1994) Helical computed tomography of the thorax. Clinical applications. Radiol Clin North Am 32:759–773

Naidich DP, Lee JJ, Garay SM, McCauley DI, Aranda CP, Boyd AD (1987) Comparison of CT and fiberoptic bronchoscopy in the evaluation of bronchial disease. AJR 148:1–7

Naidich DP, Sussman R, Kutcher WL, Aranda CP, Garay SM, Ettenger NA (1988) Solitary pulmonary nodules: CT-bronchoscopic correlation. Chest 93:595–598

Naidich DP, Funt S, Ettenger NA, Arranda C (1990) Hemoptysis: CT-bronchoscopic correlations in 58 cases. Radiology 177:357–362

Naidich DP, Webb WR, Müller NL (1993) Thoracic computed tomography: current concepts. In: Potchen EJ, Grainger RG, Greene R (eds) Pulmonary radiology. Saunders, Philadelphia, pp 386–404

Napel S, Rubin GD, Jeffrey RB Jr (1993) STS-MIP: a new reconstruction technique for CT of the chest. J Comput Assist Tomogr 17:832–838

Phillips MS, Williams MP, Flower CDR (1986) How useful is computed tomography in the diagnosis and assessment of bronchiectasis? Clin Radiol 37:321–325

Quint LE, Whyte RI, Kazerooni EA et al. (1995) Stenosis of the central airways: evaluation by using helical CT with multiplanar reconstructions. Radiology 194:871–877

Rémy-Jardin M, Rémy J (1988) Comparison of vertical and oblique CT in evaluation of bronchial tree. J Comput Assist Tomogr 12:956–962

Rémy-Jardin M, Rémy J, Ribet M, Gosselin B (1989) Bronchial atresia: diagnostic criteria and embryologic considerations. Diagn Intervent Radiol 1:45–51

Rémy-Jardin M, Rémy J, Marquette CH, Wattinne L, Giraud F, Tonnel AB (1992) Central airways in asthmatics and control subjects: evaluation with spirometric-gated spiral CT. Radiology 185(P):131

Rémy-Jardin M, Rémy J, Petyt L, Wannebroucq J (1994) Spiral CT tracheobronchography with multiplanar and 3D reformations. Radiology 193(P):261

Schaffer-Prokop C, Prokop M, Galanski M (1994) Minimum and maximum intensity projections for evaluation of spiral CT data of the chest. In: Polieser H, Lechner G (eds) Advances in CT. III. 3rd European Scientific User Conference, Somaton Plus CT, Vienna, April 1994, Springer, Berlin Heidelberg New York, pp 269–275

Set PAK, Flower CDR, Smith IE, Cahn AP, Twentyman OP, Shneerson JM (1993) Hemoptysis: comparative study of the role of CT and fiberoptic bronchoscopy. Radiology 189:677–680

Silverman PM, Godwin JD (1987) CT-bronchographic correlations in bronchiectasis. J Comput Assist Tomogr 11:52–56

Stern EJ, Frank MS (1994) Small-airway diseases of the lungs: findings at expiratory CT. AJR 163:37–41

Stern EJ, Webb WR (1993) Dynamic imaging of lung morphology with ultrafast high-resolution computed tomography. J Thorac Imaging 8:273–282

Stern EJ, Webb WR, Gamsu G (1994) Dynamic quantitative computed tomography. A predictor of pulmonary function in obstructive lung diseases. Invest Radiol 29:564–569

Van der Bruggen-Bogaarts BA, Van der Bruggen HM, Van Waes PF, Lammers JJ (1994) Assessment of bronchiectasis with 40-second breath-hold spiral CT: a feasible alternative to high-resolution CT? Radiology 193(P):261

Vining DJ, Shifrin RY, Haponik EF, Liu K, Choplin RH (1994) Virtual bronchoscopy. Radiology 193(P):261

Webb WR (1994) High-resolution computed tomography of obstructive lung disease. Radiol Clin North Am 32:745–757

Webb WR, Stern EJ, Kanth N, Gamsu G (1993) Dynamic pulmonary CT: findings in healthy adult men. Radiology 186:117–124

Westcott JL, Volpe JP (1995) Peripheral bronchopleural fistula: CT evaluation in 20 patients with pneumonia, empyema, or postoperative air leak. Radiology 196:175–181

Wood SA, Mitzner W, Zerhouni EA (1994) Quantifying the changes in cross-sectional area during inspiration and expiration with use of 3D airway tree segmentation. Radiology 193(P):368

Zacharopoulos G, Adam A, Ind PW (1990) The positive bronchus sign in patients with known lung cancer. Eur J Radiol 10:130–133

Zerhouni EA, Herold CJ, Brown RH et al. (1993) High-resolution computed tomography – physiologic correlation. J Thorac Imaging 8:265–272

10 Spiral CT of Pulmonary Embolism

M. Rémy-Jardin and J. Rémy

CONTENTS

10.1 Introduction

With variable symptoms and a nonspecific radiographic appearance, pulmonary embolism is a frequent and often undiagnosed cause of mortality and morbidity for which the availability of an accurate, noninvasive screening examination is highly desirable. Until recently, various noninvasive imaging procedures have been used to detect pulmonary embolism, including ventilation-perfusion scanning (PIOPED Investigators 1990) (HULL et al. 1985; SPIES et al. 1986; HANSON and COLEMAN 1989; STEIN et al. 1993; SOSTMAN et al. 1994), magnetic resonance (MR) imaging (WHITE et al. 1987; OVENFORS and BATRA 1988; SHAH et al. 1989; SCHIEBLER et al. 1993; LOUBEYRE et al. 1994; SOSTMAN et al. 1993b), and conventional computed tomography (CT) (SINNER 1978; GODWIN et al. 1980; OVENFORS et al. 1981; SINNER 1982; DI CARLO et al. 1982; BREATNACH and STANLEY 1984; CHINTAPELLI et al. 1988; KALEBO and WALLIN 1989; VERSCHAKELEN et al. 1993). The Lack of specificity of ventilation-perfusion imaging and the limitations of conventional CT and MR imaging provide an explanation why pulmonary angiography remains the usual standard in the detection of pulmonary embolism. However, this procedure carries a significant incidence of morbidity and mortality (PIOPED Investigators 1990), which justifies the current search for an accurate and noninvasive diagnostic modality.

Recent improvements in scanner technology have led to the introduction of spiral CT and ultrafast CT, and several studies have already evaluated the role of these newly developed CT technologies in the recognition of central pulmonary emboli (REMY-JARDIN et al. 1992; TEIGEN et al. 1993; BLUM et al. 1994; REMY-JARDIN et al. 1995c; TEIGEN et al. 1995; GOODMAN et al. 1995; SENAC et al. 1995). Whatever the new CT technique used, accurate detection of central pulmonary embolism requires optimal vascular opacification in order to demonstrate the presence of vascular signs of pulmonary thromboembolism. The purpose of this chapter is to review the use of spiral CT to demonstrate pulmonary embolism, with special emphasis on the protocol parameters and the scan interpretation.

M. RÉMY-JARDIN, MD, PhD, Professor, Department of Radiology, Hospital Calmette, Boulevard Jules Leclerc, 59037 Lille Cedex, France
J. RÉMY, MD, Professor Department of Radiology, Hospital Calmette, Boulevard Jules Leclerc, 59037 Lille Cedex, France

10.2 Data Acquisition

As the diagnostic information is directly dependent on the quality of spiral CT images, great emphasis must be placed on meticulous data acquisition. As reported for the evaluation of many other vessels, spiral CT angiography of the pulmonary arteries results from a focal spiral CT examination which is usually preceded by conventional non-contrast CT scans over the entire thorax. The interest of this preliminary sequential CT examination is threefold. First, it enables analysis of the pleura and lung parenchyma for depiction of any associated abnormalities such as pleural effusion and/or parenchymal infarction. Second, noncontrast scans are helpful for identifying calcified hilar lymph nodes, which can hamper analysis of enhanced CT scans, and also calcified thrombi, which might be missed on enhanced images. Third, it enables accurate localization of the anatomical volume of interest prior to spiral CT scanning. This conventional CT examination can be performed with thin collimated scans at 15-mm intervals. The advantage of selecting a narrow collimation for noncontrast scans is mainly related to the possibility of detecting additional changes, such as areas of ground glass attenuation, which could be missed on thick collimated scans in cases of unsuspected chronic pulmonary embolism.

With regard to the spiral CT protocol, the radiologist has to choose a first group of parameters including the height of the region of interest, the optimal collimation, and the speed of the table feed. These parameters cannot be selected without taking into consideration the patient's clinical status. Therefore, their selection always results from a compromise between the technical imperatives for an optimal spatial resolution and the patient's breath-hold tolerance. From a practical point of view, there are two major protocols for data acquisition: (a) one enabling an optimal CT examination of pulmonary arteries but requiring a 20-s breath hold; (b) a second protocol enabling evaluation of dyspneic patients in only 10 s but at the expense of spatial resolution, as further reviewed below.

10.2.1 Selection of the Volume of Interest

Scanning of 10 cm from the aortic arch to the level of the inferior pulmonary veins enables imaging of the main, lobar, and segmental arteries of the upper, mid, and lower lobes during the spiral CT sequence in every patient. In order to include the target vasculature within the scan volume, care must be taken to obtain the same degree of ventilation during the spiral CT sequence as is obtained during the preliminary localizing scans. Otherwise, variations in diaphragmatic excursion may displace structures of interest out of the spiral scan volume. In our experience, scanning in the craniocaudal direction seems well suited for coverage of the desired volume of interest even if the patient does not strictly reproduce the inspiratory level of the noncontrast scans. This is due to the fact that there is a lower excursion of the lung in the apices compared with the bases. Consequently, in the event of a mild to moderate difference in the inspiratory levels between the sequential and spiral acquisitions, there will be a lower risk of misregistration than when starting scanning at the level of the lower lobes in the caudocranial direction.

10.2.2 Collimation and Table Feed

The radiologist must select the collimation and the speed of the table feed with two imperatives in mind. The first is to find a compromise between the patient's respiratory status and the duration of the breath hold necessary for the evaluation of the pulmonary vasculature in a single CT examination. The second is to scan the patient with the narrowest collimation in order to reduce, as far as possible, partial volume effects. The latter point is of great concern for accurate evaluation of the peripheral pulmonary arteries.

Since 1992, a collimation varying from 3 mm to 5 mm has been reported in the literature (RÉMY-JARDIN et al. 1992; KAUCZOR et al. 1994; SCHWICKERT et al. 1994; BLUM et al. 1994; GOODMAN et al. 1995). In our initial report (RÉMY-JARDIN et al. 1992), a 5-mm collimation and a 5 mm/s table feed, i.e., a pitch ratio of 1:1, were selected. Of the 42 patients included in this study, 83% were able to hold their breath for the entire scanning duration. GOOMAN et al. (1995) selected a similar protocol in a study of 20 patients and reported good quality of spiral CT scans. However, 5-mm collimation has the drawback of partial volume effects at the level of small vessels which may limit detection of segmental filling defects. In order to overcome this technical limitation, a 3-mm collimation and a 5 mm/s table feed, i.e., a pitch ratio of 1.7:1 may be used; this was found to improve spatial resolution at the level of segmental arteries, as suggested by a lower number of peripheral arterial branches coded as nonanalyzable (RÉMY-JARDIN et al. 1995c). It is worthy of note that this selection does not modify the patient's breath-hold duration or the anatomical coverage.

In dyspneic patients otherwise capable of maintaining apnea, one must try to acquire data in a shorter period of time. This can be achieved by selecting a thicker collimation and/or increasing the speed of the table feed. A 10-mm collimation and a 10 mm/s table feed could help cover the region of interest in a reduced interval of time compared to the usual protocol. However, according to previous considerations, this would severely limit the spatial resolution. This is why we favor increasing the speed of the table feed to 10 mm/s while selecting a 5-mm collimation, i.e., a pitch ratio of 2:1. Another scanning protocol has recently been proposed by GOODMAN et al. (1995); this consists in two 12-s breath holds with a 6-s pause for breathing with a pitch ratio of 1:1 (5-mm collimation; 5 mm/s table feed). This protocol probably requires highly cooperative patients in order to avoid misregistration artifacts after the breathing interval. Moreover, a good quality of arterial enhancement in the second subvolume requires a constant injection of contrast material throughout the entire study, thus including the breathing interval, with a subsequent increase in the total iodine load.

A particular clinical situation is represented by sedated and intubated patients referred from intensive care units. This clinical situation does not hamper accurate evaluation of pulmonary arteries as it is possible to scan these patients with the "optimal" protocol, i.e., a 3-mm collimation and a 5 mm/s table feed. Such a technique is possible by means of simple cooperation between the radiologist and the referring clinician, the latter maintaining mechanically the patient in inspiratory apnea during data acquisition. Therefore, the spiral CT examination can be adequately performed at deep inspiration during 20 s without motion artifacts.

10.2.3 Duration of Breath Hold

The duration of breath hold is deduced from the three parameters previously selected. According to the patient's clinical status, a 10- to 20-s breath hold is required to scan the pulmonary vasculature. Hyperventilation before the start of the examination, usually consisting in a few deep respiration excursions prior to scanning, is usually recommended as it facilitates prolonged breath holding. In our clinical practice, the patients are instructed by the CT technologist on the breath-holding technique immediately before the beginning of the spiral acquisition.

Should breathing commence toward the end of the study, mild degradation of lung images related to motion artifacts is usually observed, but the central pulmonary arterial vasculature remains interpretable on mediastinal window settings. However, one may encounter pseudo-arterial filling defects at the level of segmental arteries due to motion along the z-axis during data acquisition, as further described below. It is therefore mandatory for the radiologist to interpret spiral CT scans with a precise knowledge of the conditions under which the examination has been undertaken.

When searching for pulmonary embolism in sedated patients under artificial ventilation, we recommend that the referring physician be asked to manually hold the patient's breath for 15–20 s in deep inspiration. In our experience, this technique provides excellent results with regard to the quality of mediastinal images and enables an accurate analysis of the central pulmonary vasculature in patients referred from intensive care units.

10.2.4 Inspiratory Apnea

Whenever possible, the patients should be scanned with breath holding after a maximum inspiration owing to the direct relationship between the degree of arterial opacification and the level of pulmonary arterial resistance. From physiological studies, it has been demonstrated that pulmonary resistance increases at high states of lung inflation as lung inflation causes the small alveolar vessels to be compressed (GREEN 1977). The end result is an increase in the resistance to flow in all vessels exposed to alveolar pressure, which facilitates high-quality arterial opacification.

Difficulty in being able to obtain a deep inspiration is not an exceptional situation in patients with suspected pulmonary embolism. The most common cause is the chest pain induced by pleural effusion (REMY-JARDIN et al. 1995c). In such situations, several physiological considerations suggest that we should ask the patient to stop breathing near end-expiration. As demonstrated by HOWELL et al. (1961) and HUGHES et al. (1968), pulmonary vascular resistance increases not only at high states of lung inflation but also at low levels of inflation. There is, thus, a U-shaped curve of pulmonary vascular resistance versus lung inflation. The high vascular resistance at low states of inflation is assumed to be caused by narrowing of extra-alveolar vessels, those arteries and veins which are not directly exposed to alveolar pressure and which run through the lung parenchyma (GREEN 1977). Consequently, scanning the patient at expiration during the spiral sequence helps maintain high levels of pulmonary resistance and thus a good quality of arterial opacification.

10.3 Contrast Material Administration

The aim of the spiral protocol is to start scanning while the target vascular structures are opacified and to ensure a constant degree of pulmonary arterial opacification during the entire sequence. An adequate examination of the pulmonary arteries requires selection of the most appropriate contrast agent and timing of injection but also careful monitoring of the venous access.

10.3.1 Concentration and Rate of Injection

The combination of an automated injection of contrast medium with the use of spiral CT yields excellent arterial opacification while using a smaller amount of iodine than is usually recommended with sequential CT (REMY-JARDIN et al. 1991; COSTELLO et al. 1992; KAUCZOR et al. 1994; SCHWICKERT et al. 1994). To date, several approaches have been reported for the diagnosis of pulmonary embolism with spiral CT, selecting either a low-concentration and high-flow protocol or a high-concentration and low-flow protocol. In every case, the radiologist aims at finding a compromise between the quality of arterial enhancement and the total amount of iodine injected to the patient (Fig. 10.1).

Injection of a highly concentrated contrast agent (i.e., 350–400 mg/ml) usually results in streak artifacts as the level of the subclavian and brachiocephalic veins and also at the level of the superior vena cava (Fig. 10.2). In this latter location, radiating artifacts can significantly degrade quality in the adjacent right main pulmonary artery, which may hamper detection of intraluminal changes. A means of reducing the superior vena cava artifacts might be to scan from caudal to cranial with cessation of inflow of contrast when scanning the superior mediastinum. However, this is contrary to the usual recommendation for spiral CT angiography in that the bolus duration must be as long as the scan time to obtain consistent arterial opacification throughout the en-

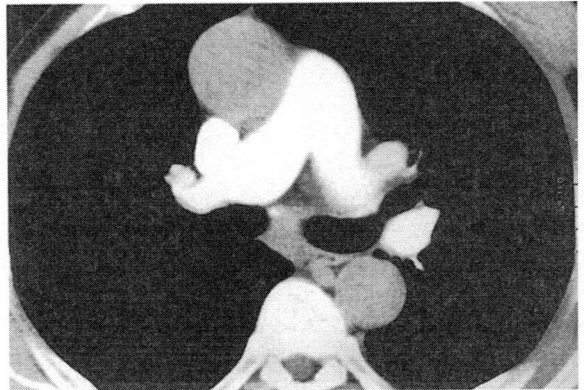

Fig. 10.1. Spiral CT scan (5-mm collimation; 5 mm/s table feed) obtained in a 60-year-old man at the level of the tracheal bifurcation. There is a high degree of contrast enhancement of the right and left pulmonary arteries without artifacts at the level of the superior vena cava (inspiratory apnea; 120 cc of 20% ionic contrast material; 5 cc/s)

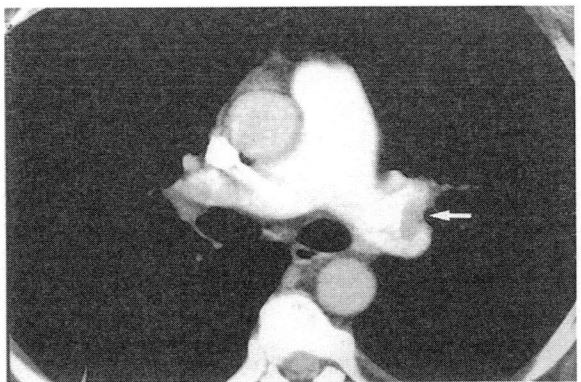

Fig. 10.2. Spiral CT scan (3-mm collimation; 6 mm/s table feed) obtained in a 55-year-old man at the level of the tracheal bifurcation (inspiratory apnea; 90 cc of 38% ionic contrast agent; 3 cc/s). Streak artifacts around the superior vena cava inherent to the injection of a highly concentrated contrast agent hamper analysis of the right main pulmonary artery. Pulmonary arterial opacification is sufficient for the depiction of the large thrombus in the left main pulmonary artery (*arrow*) without the high degree of contrast enhancement shown on Fig. 10.1

tire scan (NAPEL 1995; RUBIN and JEFFREY 1995). Cessation of injection before the end of data acquisition results in a suboptimal enhancement of the pulmonary arteries on the last levels imaged with a risk of false-positive or false-negative diagnosis of pulmonary embolism. Another solution to reduce the streak artifacts may be to administer the contrast material at a low rate (i.e., 2–3 ml/s), which is a common recommendation when using a highly concentrated material. Whereas the overall quality of vascular opacification obtained with this protocol is usually sufficient for depiction of large emboli (Fig. 10.2), a low rate of injection is not always compatible with identification of emboli at the level of segmental arteries.

These limitations have led us to favor low-concentration and high-flow protocols. The lowest concentration reported for the evaluation of pulmonary arteries has been 120 mg/ml, injected at a rate of 7 cc/s (RÉMY-JARDIN et al. 1992). This protocol resulted in a high degree of vascular opacification in the majority of cases (74%), thus enabling confident depiction of all central pulmonary emboli. However, 24% of mediastinal images showed a quality of arterial enhancement sufficient for the analysis of pulmonary arteries but without the high degree of contrast enhancement previously quoted. Whereas this protocol remained compatible with the detection of emboli in main and lobar arteries, there was a potential risk of missing thrombi in segmental branches. This preliminary experience over a 2-year period led us to increase the iodine concentration in subsequent routine examinations (RÉMY-JARDIN et al. 1995c). Our current protocol consists in the administration of 120–140 cc of 24%–30% contrast agent [ionic (80%); nonionic (20%)] at a rate of 4–5 cc/s. However, the ideal concentration of contrast material for low-concentration and high-flow protocols has not yet been definitely determined. With the aim of optimizing the total iodine burden administered to every patient, several authors have used 15% iodinated contrast agents administered at 4–5 cc/s in both clinical (SCHNYDER et al. 1995; SENAC et al. 1995) and experimental (WOODARD et al. 1995) studies, and have reported good results.

Although use of dilute contrast material has been advocated by several authors, it does entail certain risks. The first drawback is the septic risk inherent to any dilution maneuver. The second flaw is the instability of the solution obtained after mixing contrast medium with a saline solution, as pointed out by contrast medium manufacturers. The choice between ionic and nonionic contrast agents is dependent on economic constraints. In our clinical practice, the main indications for use of nonionic material are a previous history of allergic reaction, cardiac and/or renal insufficiency, and pulmonary hypertension, whereas ionic material is largely used in the remaining patients. It is worthy of note that low-concentration ionic contrast media usage is particularly well tolerated by patients: over the past 5 years, we have encountered no severe drug reactions among the recipients of such agents.

10.3.2 Scan Delay

The scan delay is the interval of time between administration of contrast material and commencement of scanning. In patients with normal right ventricular outflow, an 8- to 10-s scan delay usually provides sufficient latitude that the pulmonary arteries are almost always well opacified. For patients with right-sided heart failure and patients with pulmonary hypertension, a longer start delay is required, varying between 10 and 15 s. As recently pointed out by SOSTMAN et al. (1993b) it is important to be aware that the presence of pulmonary hypertension per se does not have a direct correlation with pulmonary blood flow until right-sided heart failure supervenes. However, a rather inhomogeneous distribution of velocities across the arterial lumen with reverse flow in mid systole to late systole has been shown on cine phase contrast MR images of pulmonary arteries in the presence of pulmonary hypertension (SOSTMAN et al. 1993a,b).

In these cases, owing to the impossibility of predicting the scan delay, a time-density curve may be obtained to determine the transit time from the venous site to the pulmonary arteries. This technique consists in obtaining serial scans at the level of the main pulmonary arteries every 4 s after injection of a limited amount of contrast material (e.g., 20 cc), which enables one to obtain plots of enhancement in the target arteries as a function of time. It is then possible to calculate the time needed to reach the peak of the curve, which represents the higher attenuation value in the pulmonary artery. The time of maximal opacification of the pulmonary artery provides a guide for more precise timing of the final bolus. However, proper application of this test requires selection of the same rate of injection as is intended for use in the actual study. This technique has proven to be reliable but it results in a slight increase in the radiation dose and the total amount of iodine injected to the patient and adds several minutes to the examination. In our clinical practice, test injections are not systematically performed unless the patient's clinical status raises the likelihood of delayed peak opacification of the pulmonary arteries. An alternative is to visually monitor contrast enhancement during the early stages of contrast injection, as recently evaluated by SILVERMAN et al. (1995) for liver examinations. This method provides a mechanism by which the time of scan initiation can be individualized based on the actual enhancement of anatomical structures. When a desired level of enhancement is reached for a particular structure, a transition is made to routine diagnostic spiral imaging series.

Choosing an improper scan delay may lead to artifacts that are easily depicted as they typically affect the top or the bottom of the subvolume scanned. If the scan delay is too short, there is insufficient time to allow adequate opacification of the pulmonary arteries on the first images, which results in pseudo-filling defects (RÉMY-JARDIN et al. 1992; TEIGEN et al. 1993) (Fig. 10.3). On the other hand, if one selects too long a scan delay, there is not enough contrast material left at the bottom of the selected subvolume and one cannot determine whether hypoattenuation areas at the level of pulmonary arterial branches correspond to technical limitations or actual filling defects (Fig. 10.4). When suboptimal arterial opacification inherent to an inadequate scan delay is observed in a limited portion of the volume of interest, it is usually recommended that the initial examination be supplemented by a second and short acquisition

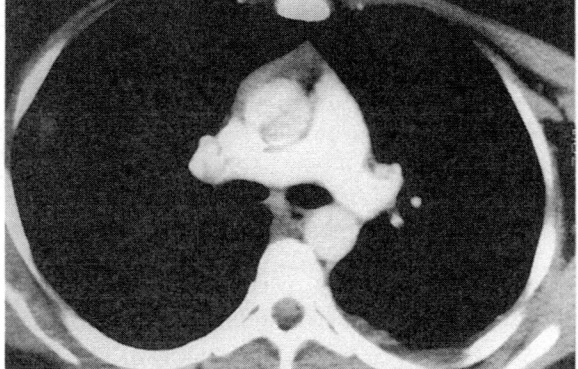

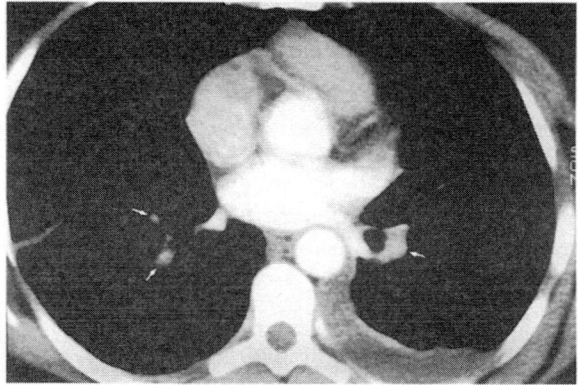

Fig. 10.4. Spiral CT scans at the level of the tracheal bifurcation (a) and pulmonary inferior veins (b) in a 30-year-old woman with left-sided chest pain and mild hemoptysis (5-mm collimation; 5 mm/s table feed; inspiratory apnea; 100 cc of a 12% ionic contrast agent; 7 cc/s). Selection of a long start delay (12 s) without increasing the total amount of contrast material injected has no adverse consequences on the quality of pulmonary arterial opacification on the first levels imaged (a; excellent quality of arterial enhancement) but is incompatible with adequate opacification at the bottom of the selected subvolume (b). Note the hypoattenuated areas at the level of the right and left pulmonary arterial sections (*arrows*): Filling defects? Technical limitation?

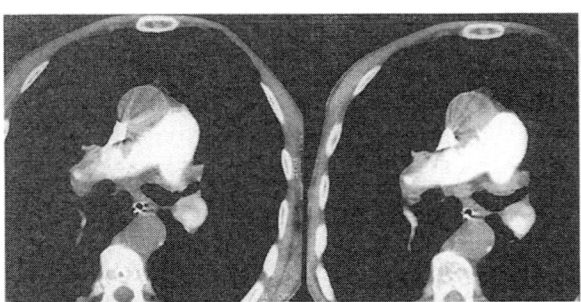

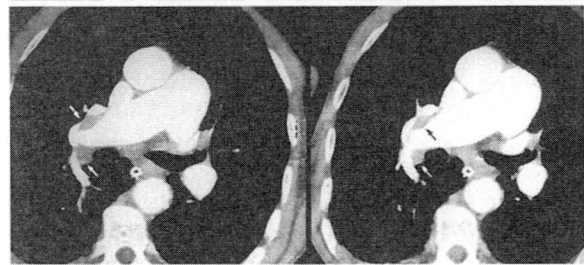

Fig. 10.3a,b. Spiral CT scans obtained in a 73-year-old man first seen with acute onset of shortness of breath. **a** Contiguous spiral CT scans (3-mm collimation; 6 mm/s table feed) at the level of the right bronchus intermedius (inspiratory apnea; 120 cc of a 24% nonionic contrast agent; 5 cc/s). Pseudo-filling defects at the level of the proximal part of the right pulmonary artery and left interlobar pulmonary artery are due to the choice of too short a start delay (7 s) in this patient with pulmonary hypertension. **b** Spiral CT scans obtained at the same level as **a**, with a start delay of 13 s. The homogeneous opacification of the right and left pulmonary arteries enables exclusion of any partial filling defects. Note the presence of a mural thrombus at the level of the right interlobar pulmonary artery (*black and white arrows*), suggesting chronic pulmonary thromboembolic disease

throughout this subvolume after proper modification of the start delay. At the expense of an additional but limited scanning time and a limited amount of contrast material, this may help avoid any further diagnostic procedure.

10.3.3 Venous Access

A power injection is mandatory to obtain a homogeneous and constant level of arterial enhancement through the entire spiral sequence. However, by nature of the rapid administration of contrast material, care must be taken to carefully adapt the rate of injection to the site of administration, especially when selecting high-flow protocols. In the majority of spiral CT examinations, a 18- or 20-gauge catheter is inserted into a medially located antecubital vein through which the contrast bolus is safely injected at a rate varying between 2 and 5 cc/s. From a practical point of view, it is worthy of note that the contrast material can be administered with the patient's arm positioned along the thorax without artifacts on the target anatomy. This ensures a safer injection as it enables control of venous access during the injection with a subsequent possibility of immediately stopping the injection in the event of extravasation. In addition, it improves progression of the injected material through the systemic veins as venous compression at the thoracobrachial junction is avoided.

When an antecubital vein is not accessible, a more peripheral venous access can be used. While such access remains compatible with spiral CT angiography of the pulmonary arteries, care must be taken to avoid extravasation from a small and fragile peripheral vein. This requires two precautions: (a) reduction of the rate of injection to avoid any venous damage, and (b) an increase in the start delay by 4–6 s to allow sufficient time for the contrast material to opacify the pulmonary arteries on the first levels imaged.

When the patient is referred from an intensive care unit, central venous access is often available and may be used for the administration of the contrast material. It is then mandatory to verify the maximal rate of injection acceptable for a given catheter (often 4–5 cc/s). Because of the central location of the tip of the catheter, usually at the level of the superior vena cava, a shorter scan delay can be selected, resulting in a shorter injection period.

10.4 Image Reconstruction

As recommended by POLACIN et al. (1992), data must be reconstructed with a 180° linear interpolation algorithm whether using a pitch of 1 or a pitch of greater than 1. The effects of data processing on detection of filling defects are illustrated in Fig. 10.5. Overlapped transverse CT scans are then reconstructed. A greater number of images may be needed for depiction of small emboli. As recently demonstrated for detection of spherical lesions (KALENDER et al. 1994), the contrast exhibited by a small lesion strongly depends on its location within the slice. If only one image is calculated per slice width, the inherent advantage of spiral CT is not exploited sufficiently. According to KALENDER et al., two to four

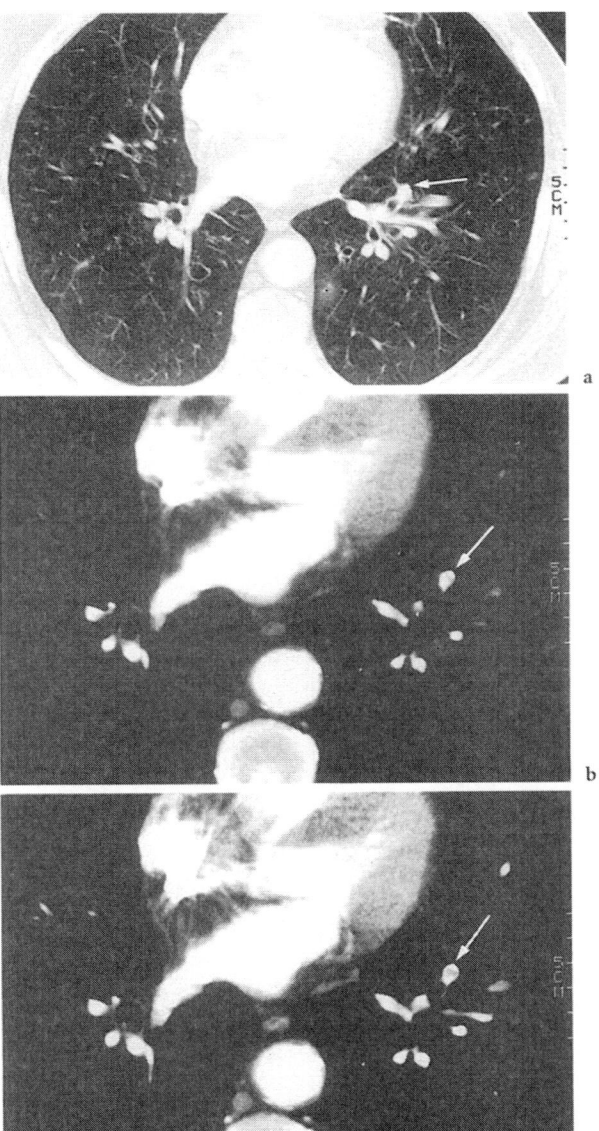

Fig. 10.5a–c. Spiral CT scans (5-mm collimation; 5 mm/s table feed) obtained in a 60-year-old patient with chronic obstructive pulmonary disease and acute worsening of dyspnea (inspiratory apnea; 140 cc of 24% ionic contrast agent; 5 cc/s). **a** Transverse CT scan viewed at lung window settings (1600 HU; −600 HU) at the level of the lower lobes shows bilateral bronchiectasis. The *arrow* indicates the anterior segmental artery of the left lower lobe. **b,c** Transverse CT sections viewed at mediastinal window settings (350 HU; 50 HU) at the same level as that of **a**, reconstructed with a 180° linear interpolation algorithm (**b**) and a 360° linear interpolation algorithm (**c**). Note the improved delineation of the partial filling defect located at the level of the left lower lobe segmental artery (*arrow*) on **b**

images per nominal slice width should be calculated to generate images with high contrast which could help identify partial filling defects within segmental arteries. The overlapping sections are easily reviewed on a page display.

10.5 Interpretation

In order to be able to confidently interpret vascular signs of pulmonary embolism at the level of main, lobar, and segmental arteries, familiarity with central and peripheral bronchovascular anatomy is required (OSBORNE et al. 1984; JARDIN and RÉMY 1986). In order to help distinguish arterial from venous sections, we have found it useful to photograph on separate sets the CT scans taken at lung and mediastinal window settings, both reconstructed with similar increments. As previously emphasized, one should follow KALENDER et al.'s recommendations regarding reconstruction of several images per slice to achieve the theoretical optimum of spatial resolution.

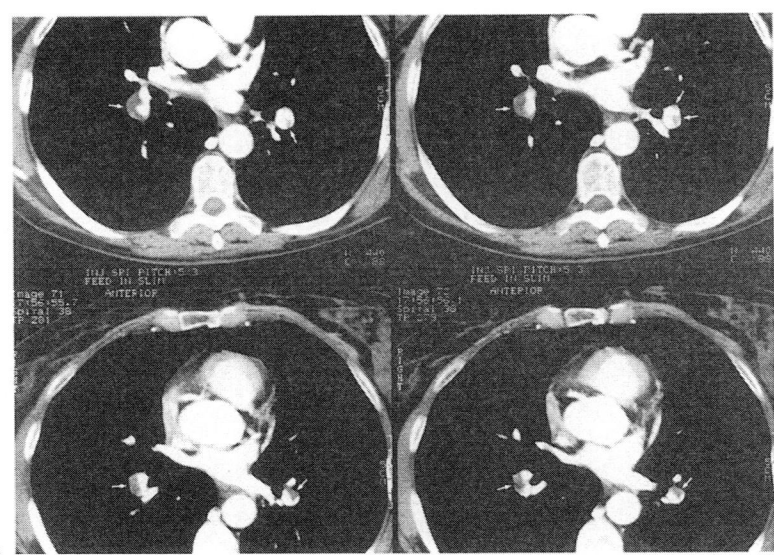

a

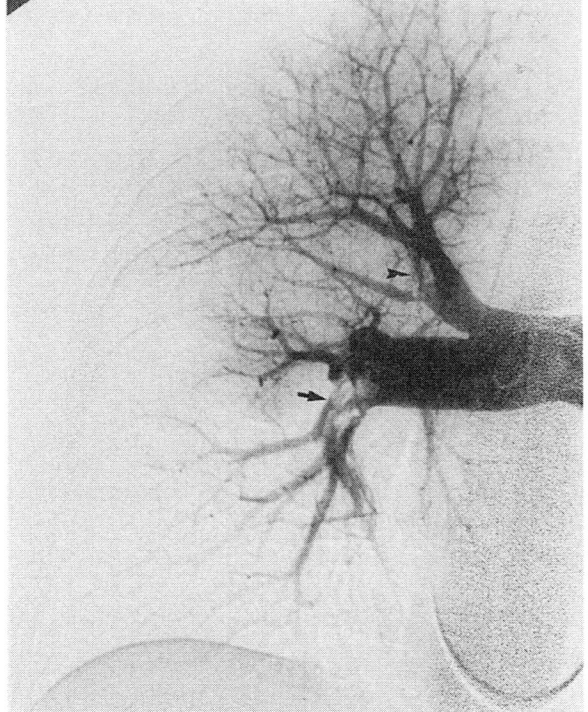

b

Fig. 10.6a, b. Massive pulmonary embolism in 54-year-old woman first seen with acute shortness of breath. **a** Contiguous spiral CT scans (3-mm collimation; 5 mm/s table feed; inspiratory apnea; 120 cc of 24% nonionic contrast agent; 5 cc/s). Presence of multiple partial filling defects (*arrows*) at the level of the right and left pulmonary arteries. **b** Frontal digital pulmonary angiogram obtained 6 s after injection shows intraluminal filling defects in the right upper (*arrowhead*) middle, and lower lobe (*arrow*) pulmonary arteries. (From CAUVAIN et al., 1996)

10.5.1 CT Signs of Acute Pulmonary Embolism

It is possible to demonstrate the presence of pleural effusion and/or peripheral lung consolidation when scanning patients with acute pulmonary embolism but these CT findings are of limited diagnostic value. The most reliable CT feature allowing definitive diagnosis of pulmonary embolism is the demonstration of intravascular clot(s).

The presence of vascular signs of pulmonary embolism is usually evaluated on the basis of the slightly modified Sinner's description (SINNER 1982): (a) a partial filling defect is defined as central or marginal intraluminal areas of low attenuation surrounded by variable amounts of contrast medium with regular or irregular borders; (b) a complete filling defect is defined as an intraluminal area of low attenuation that is not surrounded by contrast medium and that occupies the entire arterial section; (c) the "railway track sign" is the finding of thromboembolic masses seen floating freely in the lumen, allowing the flow of blood between the wall of the vessel and the thrombus and/or embolus; (d) mural defects are defined by peripheral areas of low attenuation within arterial sections (Figs. 10.6, 10.7).

10.5.2 CT Signs of Chronic Pulmonary Embolism

Direct visualization and delineation of a thrombotic clot, sometimes calcified, is the most specific vascular finding on CT scans in this disease (Fig. 10.8). With this direct criterion alone, SCHWICKERT et al. (1994) found that the diagnosis of chronic thromboembolism was possible with CT in 53 of 75 patients. Although nonspecific, indirect signs contribute to the correct diagnosis of chronic pulmonary embolism and are expected to increase the diagnosis of chronic thromboembolic pulmonary hypertension. Indirect signs of chronic pulmonary embolism can be derived from angiographic findings and include: (a) an irregular or nodular arterial wall in central and peripheral branches; (b) abrupt narrowing of the vessel diameter (Fig. 10.9); and (c) abrupt cutoff of distal lobar or segmental artery branches (SCHWICKERT et al. 1994). TEIGEN et al. (1993) considered emboli as chronic if they were eccentric and contiguous with the vessel wall or if they demonstrated evidence of recanalization. Additional diagnostic findings have previously been described with conventional CT and also can be depicted on spiral CT scans (SHAH et al. 1989). They include dilatation of the main pulmonary arteries, decrease in the caliber of small branches, and narrowing of the periph-

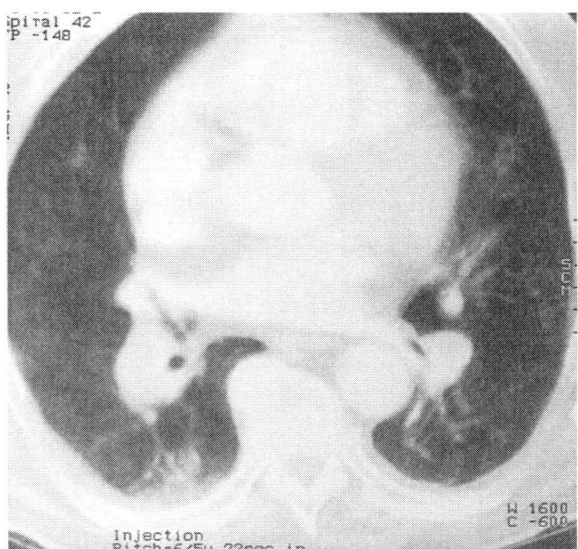

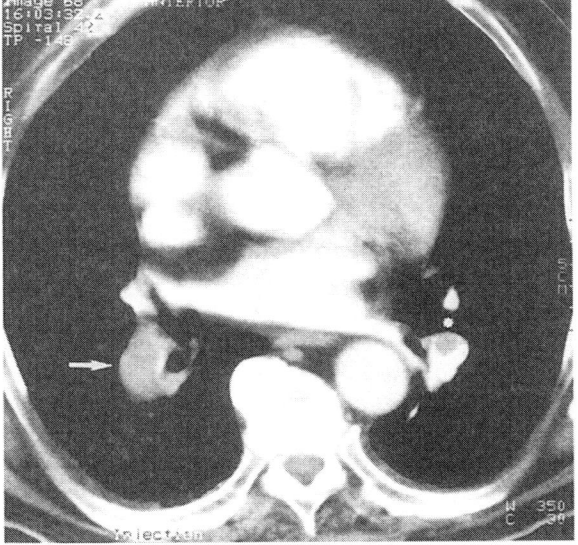

Fig. 10.7a,b. Spiral CT scan (3-mm collimation; 5 mm/s table feed) in a 60-year-old man with acute onset of shortness of breath and a previous history of chronic obstructive pulmonary disease (120 cc of 24% nonionic contrast agent; 5 cc/s). a Transverse CT section at the level of the bronchus intermedius (window width, 1600 HU; window center, −600 HU). The presence of motion artifacts within the lung parenchyma is due to scanning while the patient was breathing quietly. **b** Same anatomical level to that shown on **a** (window width, 350 HU; window center, 50 HU). Massive pulmonary embolism [complete filling defect at the level of the right lower lobe pulmonary artery (*arrow*); partial filling defect at the level of the left lower lobe pulmonary artery (*star*)] can be confidently depicted despite the absence of apnea during data acquisition. There is absence of major motion artifact on this CT section. (From CAUVAIN et al., 1996)

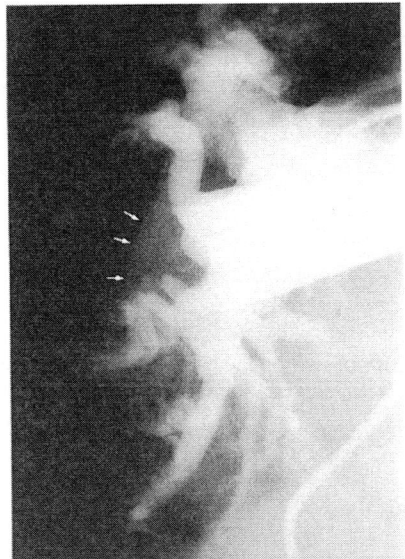

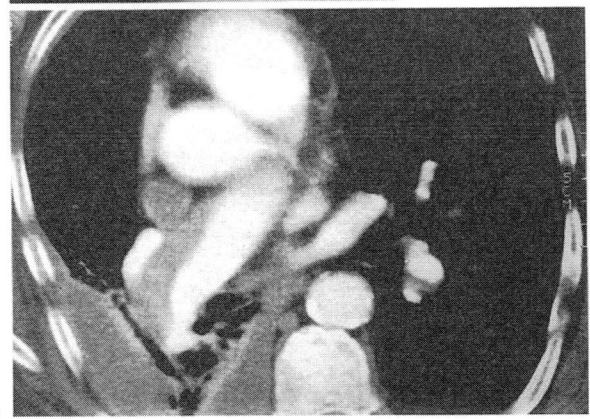

low. CT can also depict changes at the level of the systemic arterial circulation, the collateral supply of the occluded pulmonary arterial bed. The most common findings on CT scans consist of dilated bronchial arteries which can be detected as tortuous and/or dotted vascular section in their mediastinal and/or hilar pathways (see also Chap. 11). Enlargement of the internal mammary arteries is also easily detectable on CT scans, especially in cases of asymmetric or unilateral systemic supply.

Vascular changes in chronic pulmonary embolism may be accompanied by attenuation changes in the lung parenchyma. SCHWICKERT et al. (1994) reported pleura-based areas of high attenuation, most often located distal to thrombotically altered vessels, which did not enhance after administration of contrast agent. These areas can be interpreted as residual infarctions following pulmonary embolism that have

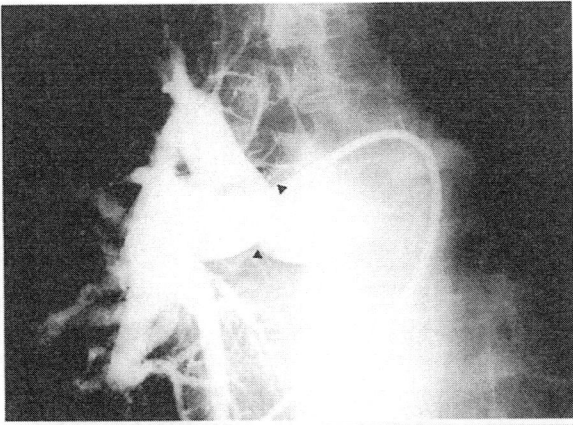

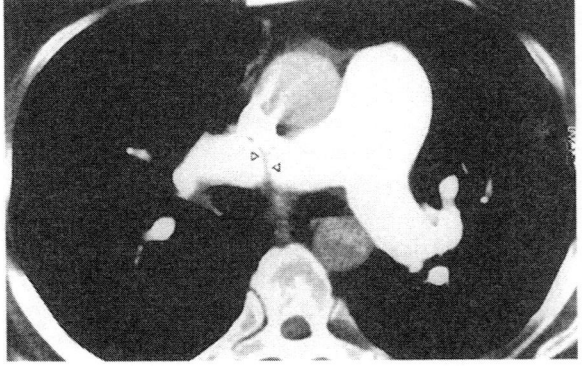

Fig. 10.8a,b. Images obtained in a 56-year-old man with chronic thromboembolic pulmonary hypertension. **a** Right posterior oblique pulmonary angiogram obtained 5 s after injection of contrast material shows a substantial distance between the outer border of the vessel (*arrows*) and the edge of the column of contrast material, suggesting a thrombus. Note dilated and tortuous vessels and right lower lobe atelectasis. **b** Spiral CT scan (inspiratory apnea; 90 cc of 30% nonionic contrast agent; 3 cc/s) obtained at the level of the right interlobar pulmonary artery confirms a large mural thrombus in the right pulmonary artery. Note the finding, similar to that in **a**, at the level of the left lower lobe pulmonary artery. (From RÉMY-JARDIN et al. 1992)

eral pulmonary vessels. On transverse CT scans, correct assessment of changes in vascular diameter requires consideration of the orientation of the vessels relative to the CT plane, thereby avoiding misinterpretation of partial volume effects as vascular changes. In this particular clinical setting, transverse CT scans can be efficiently completed with multiplanar reformations, as further described be-

Fig. 10.9a,b. Images obtained in a 54-year-old woman with pulmonary hypertension and suspected chronic pulmonary thromboembolism. Narrowing of the dilated right main pulmonary artery is depicted as a band of decreased attenuation on (**a**) the right oblique pulmonary angiograms (*arrowheads*) and (**b**) the spiral volumetric CT scan (*arrowheads*) (spiral volumetric CT scan obtained with 90 ml of 30% contrast material; excellent quality of arterial opacification). (From RÉMY-JARDIN et al. 1992)

already been replaced by fibrotic scar. Another parenchymal finding in chronic pulmonary embolism is regional, sharply demarcated areas of hyperattenuation (TARDIVON et al. 1993; SCHWICKERT et al. 1994). By means of correlations with lung scintiscans and single-photon emission computed tomography scans, it is possible to confirm that these areas of hyperattenuation are related to redistribution of blood flow at the level of nonoccluded pulmonary arterial bed (KING et al. 1994). In addition, the presence of regional hyperdensities has recently been shown to correlate closely with dilated feeding segmental arteries, confirming that hyperattenuated lung parenchyma represents hyperperfused lung in chronic pulmonary embolism (SCHWICKERT et al. 1995).

10.5.3 Accuracy of Spiral CT for the Detection of Acute Pulmonary Embolism

The first blinded, prospective study of 42 patients compared spiral CT with pulmonary angiography for the detection of acute pulmonary embolism (REMY-JARDIN et al. 1992). The total number of main, lobar, and segmental emboli detected with spiral CT was determined for each lung and compared with a unilateral pulmonary angiogram. In this study, branches obscured by partial volume averaging were excluded. Of the 42 patients, 23 had a CT scan negative for pulmonary embolism. All of these patients had a normal pulmonary angiogram. In the remaining 19 patients, spiral CT identified 112 pulmonary emboli (8 main, 28 lobar and 76 segmental). In 18 of these 19 (95%) patients, pulmonary emboli were identified at angiography. The overall sensitivity and specificity of spiral CT for detecting central pulmonary embolism were 100% and 96%, respectively. In a larger series of 72 patients, we have recently reported a sensitivity of 91% and a specificity of 86% (REMY-

JARDIN et al. 1995c). In this protocol, we did not exclude arterial branches with partial volume averaging and this accounts for the lower sensitivity and specificity compared with our initial study.

Similar results have been reported in the literature whether using spiral CT (GOODMAN et al. 1995; SENAC et al. 1995; VAN ROSSUM et al. 1995) or electron-beam CT (TEIGEN et al. 1993, 1995) for the diagnosis of acute central pulmonary embolism (Table 10.1). It is important to emphasize that both imaging modalities reasonably extend the range of depiction of pulmonary embolism down to the segmental level but not beyond it. Experimentally induced pulmonary emboli in second- to fourth-division pulmonary arteries have also been reliably detected by electron beam CT (GERAGHTY et al. 1992; STANFORD et al. 1994; WOODARD et al. 1995). GOODMAN et al. (1995) found a 75% interobserver agreement as to the presence or absence of central pulmonary emboli on the CT scan of a given lung. In the analysis of their results, these authors pointed out that in the PIOPED study, reviewers of angiography agreed on the presence of thrombi in 98% of lobar vessels and 90% of segmental vessels. Whereas they did not comment on the low interobserver agreement observed in their study, they concluded that consensus interpretation of two experienced reviewers, if feasible, appeared to be helpful. We agree with them that, on the grounds of basic anatomical knowledge and appropriate protocol selection, depiction of emboli is improved by the experience of the reviewer. However, this is not specific to spiral CT as a consensus reading of angiograms and/or scintigrams is also known to improve detection of central emboli.

Several specific advantages of spiral CT over pulmonary angiography have been reported recently. The only diagnostic angiographic signs of acute pulmonary embolism are the identification of an intravascular filling defect surrounded by contrast

Table 10.1. Accuracy of fast scanning techniques in the diagnosis of acute central pulmonary embolism

Study	Sensitivity (%)	Specificity (%)	Prevalence
RÉMY-JARDIN et al. (1992)	100	96	43
TEIGEN et al. (1993)	95	80	85
TEIGEN et al. (1995)	75	98	38
RÉMY-JARDIN et al. (1995c)	91	86	54
GOODMAN et al. (1995)	86	92	35
VAN ROSSUM et al. (1995)	97	98	24
SENAC et al. (1995)	86	100	64

material or the delineation of the trailing edge of a thrombus obstructing a vessel (STEIN et al. 1967). Complete obstruction of a pulmonary artery without visualization of the trailing edge of the thrombus is not diagnostic of acute pulmonary embolism as it can also be observed in various clinical situations such as chronic pulmonary embolism or hilar tumoral or inflammatory infiltration. Other manifestations which can also occur in a variety of pulmonary parenchymal diseases include decreased local perfusion, crowded vessels, delayed venous return from the affected area, and shunting away from the involved lung (BOOKSTEIN and SILVER 1974). By means of transverse imaging, spiral CT is able to provide direct visualization of the thrombus when the latter cannot be detected on pulmonary angiograms. When comparing the results at the level of 112 thromboemboli depicted with both techniques, we observed that spiral CT and pulmonary angiography similarly identified the intraluminal filling defect in 48% of cases while the pulmonary angiogram showed only indirect signs of pulmonary embolism in 52% of cases (RÉMY-JARDIN et al. 1992). Moreover, CT allows concurrent evaluation of other chest abnormalities that may mimic symptoms of pulmonary embolism. In two of the 60 patients evaluated by TEIGEN et al. (1995), the pulmonary angiogram was prospectively read as positive for pulmonary embolism whereas the electron-beam CT scans were read as negative for this diagnosis. In one of these two patients, the CT scan demonstrated a large mass that encased the truncus anterior with no enhancement of the right upper lobe vessels, therefore suggesting that the vascular occlusion seen on the angiogram was due to a malignant process rather than pulmonary embolism (further confirmed by

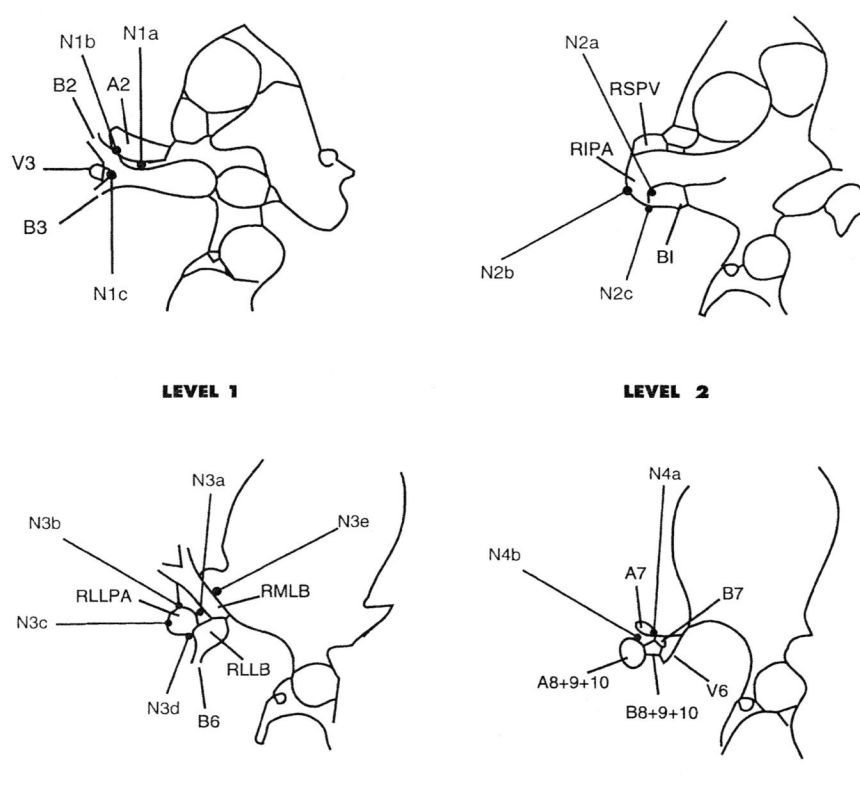

Fig. 10.10. a Schematic diagram of pulmonary lymph nodes of the right hilum at four levels. *Level 1:* lymph nodes at the level of the right upper lobe bronchus (upper lobe group: *N1a–N1c*). *Level 2:* lymph nodes at the level of the right bronchus intermedius (interlobar group: *N2a–N2c*). *Level 3:* lymph nodes at the level of the right middle lobe bronchus (middle lobe group: *N3a–N3e*). *Level 4:* lymph nodes at the level of the proximal ramification of the right common basal bronchus (lower lobe group: *N4a, N4b*). *RSPV,* right superior pulmonary vein; *RIPA,* right interlobar pulmonary artery; *BI,* bronchus intermedius; *RMLB,* right middle lobe bronchus; *RLLB,* right lower lobe bronchus; *RLLPA,* right lower lobe pulmonary artery. **b** Frequency of identification of pulmonary lymph nodes of the right hilum. *Levels* and *abbreviations* are as for **a.** (From RÉMY-JARDIN et al. 1995a)

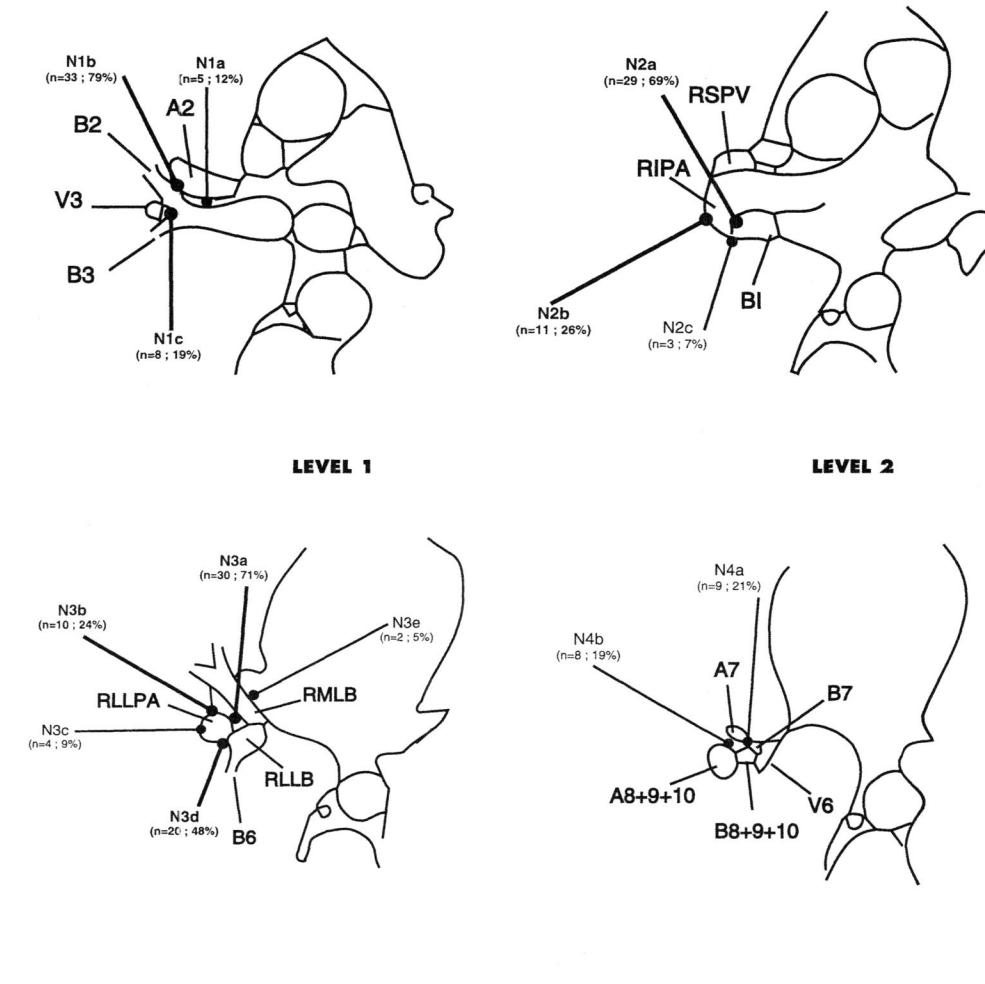

Fig. 10.10b

LEVEL 1

LEVEL 2

LEVEL 3

LEVEL 4

biopsy). In the second patient, vascular changes in the right upper lobe were attributed to chronic pulmonary embolism on angiograms whereas the findings at CT were diagnosed as postirradiation vascular changes.

The introduction of fast scanning techniques has also led to the observation of false-negative angiograms. TEIGEN et al. (1995) reported that one patient with a positive electron-beam CT scan and a negative pulmonary angiogram had a small segmental embolus at CT. The region of this embolus was poorly depicted with pulmonary angiography and, although unproven, this was retrospectively considered to represent a false-negative angiographic finding.

10.6 Interpretative Pitfalls

A number of interpretative pitfalls exist in assessing enhanced spiral CT images and certain caveats have to be heeded. However, it is important to keep in mind that their recognition becomes less and less problematic as the radiologist gains experience with spiral CT of the pulmonary vasculature (TEIGEN et al. 1993).

10.6.1 Bronchovascular Segmental Anatomy

As previously pointed out, precise knowledge of the bronchovascular segmental anatomy is mandatory in order to avoid misinterpretation between arteries and veins on spiral CT scans. An accurate identification of segmental arteries requires a meticulous analysis of both mediastinal and lung window settings to name the arteries according to their relationship to the bronchi: the segmental arteries are always seen near the accompanying branches of the bronchial tree. From a practical point of view, we recommend to follow the path of the pulmonary arteries on contiguous sections so that a poorly enhanced pulmonary vein cannot be mistaken for an occluded pulmonary artery. Moreover, differences between blood and contrast medium flows at the time of early venous enhancement may be responsible for pseudo-

filling defects. At the level of venous sections, one may observe a dense peripheral rim of contrast medium surrounding a central hypoattenuated area, the latter corresponding to the venous return not yet opacified.

10.6.2 Hilar Lymph Nodes

Knowledge of the size and location of hilar lymph nodes is of great importance when analyzing enhanced images as they may mimic the appearance of pulmonary emboli (Rémy-Jardin et al. 1992; Teigen et al. 1993). However, it is now possible to

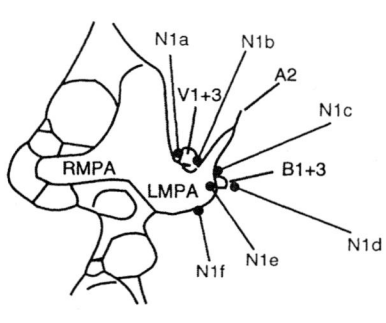

LEVEL 1

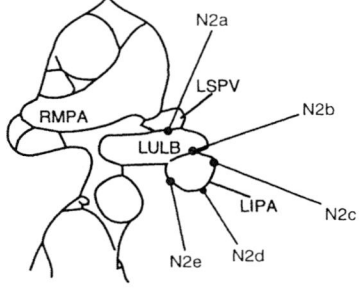

LEVEL 2

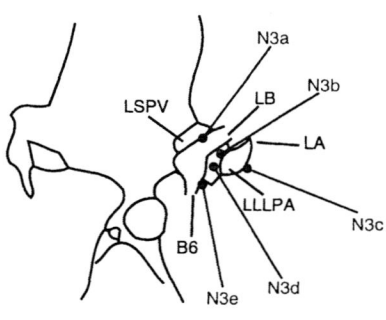

a   **LEVEL 3**

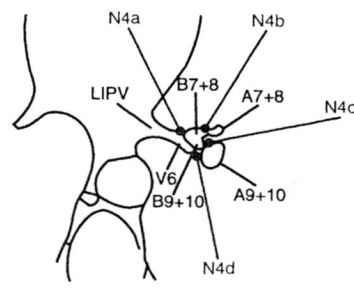

LEVEL 4

Fig. 10.11. a Schematic diagram of pulmonary lymph nodes of the left hilum at four levels. *Level 1*: lymph nodes at the level of the left pulmonary arterial arch (culminal group: *N1a–N1f*). *Level 2*: lymph nodes at the level of the left upper lobe bronchus (interlobar group: *N2a–N2e*). *Level 3*: lymph nodes at the level of the lingular bronchus (lingular group: *N3a–N3e*). *Level 4*: lymph nodes at the level of the proximal ramifications of the left common basal bronchus (lower lobe group: *N4a–N4d*).

RMPA, right main pulmonary artery; *LMPA*, left main pulmonary artery; *LULB*, left upper lobe bronchus; *LSPV*, left superior pulmonary vein; *LIPA*, left interlobar pulmonary artery; *LB*, lingular bronchus; *LA*, lingular artery; *LLLPA*, left lower lobe pulmonary artery; *LIPV*, left inferior pulmonary vein. **b** Frequency of identification of pulmonary lymph nodes of the left hilum. *Levels* and *abbreviations* are as for **a**. (From Rémy-Jardin et al. 1995a)

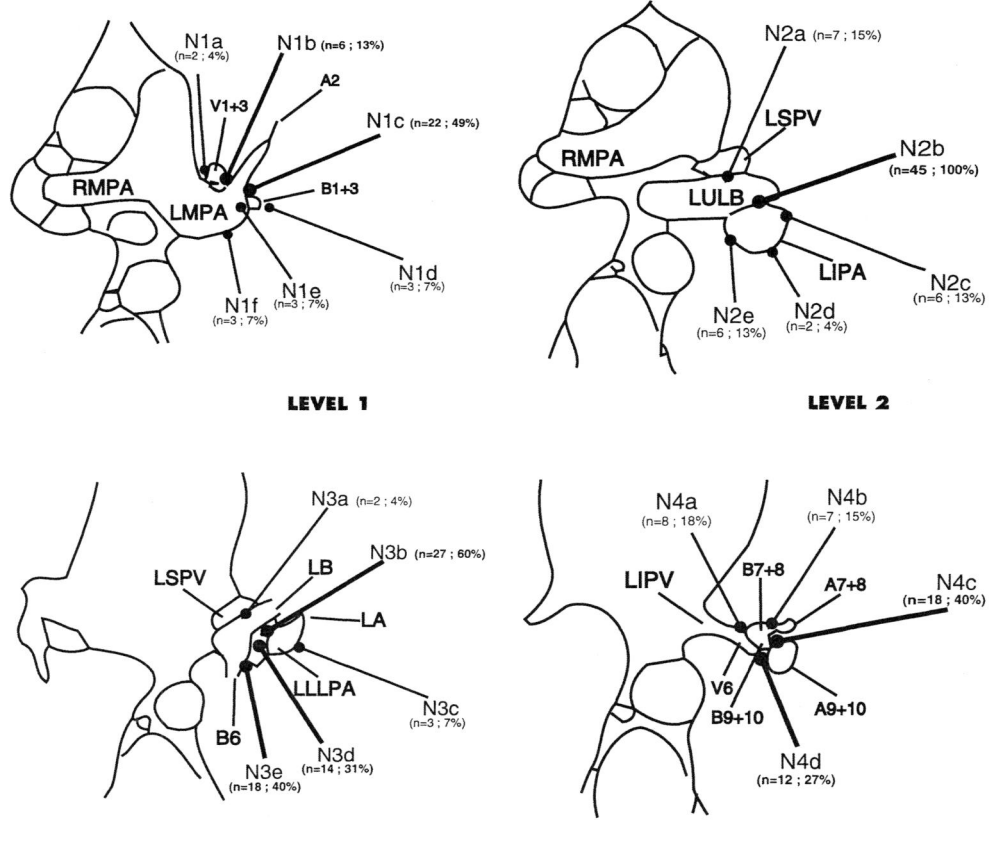

Fig. 10.11b

recognize on CT scans specific relationships between hilar lymph nodes and proximal bronchovascular structures, especially with pulmonary arterial branches.

Using a slightly modified version of the classification of SONE et al. (1983), hilar lymph nodes can be conveniently divided into four groups in the right lung (i.e., the upper lobe, interlobar, middle lobe, and lower lobe groups) and into four groups in the left lung (i.e., the culminal, interlobar, lingular, and lower lobe groups) (RÉMY-JARDIN et al. 1995a) (Figs. 10.10, 10.11). By means of surgical sampling, it was possible to confirm that these areas actually correspond to lymphatic structures. They were shown to be composed of conglomerates of small lymph nodes either histologically normal or presenting with slight sinusal hyperplasia. Although not sampled during thoracotomy, peribronchovascular connective tissue and/or hilar bronchial vessels are most likely to be part of the hypoattenuated areas imaged on CT scans.

At the level of the right and left upper lobe groups, most hilar hypoattenuated areas are identified adjacent to the lateral borders of the pulmonary arteries, as previously emphasized in anatomical descriptions (ROUVIERE 1929; SARRAZIN et al. 1974; NAGAISHI 1972; YAMASHITA 1978; CHANG and ZINN 1976; RIQUET 1992, 1993). The most common right upper lobe site (79%) can be seen as a linear area of hypoattenuation, lateral to the truncus anterior and usually located in the region between the upper lobe bronchus and the anterior segmental artery (Fig. 10.12a). At the level of the culminal group, a triangular area of hypoattenuation can be detected lateral to the anterior segmental artery of the left upper lobe in 49% of the cases but also lateral to the left pulmonary arterial arch in 7% of cases (Fig. 10.12b).

At more caudal levels, most hypoattenuated areas display a different arrangement on CT scans as they are mainly located lateral to bronchi and medial to pulmonary arterial branches. At the level of the right interlobar group, a triangular area of hypoattenuation is observed in 69% of cases between the bronchus intermedius and the medial aspect of the interlobar artery. However, in 26% of cases, a linear area of hypoattenuation can also be seen lateral to the right interlobar artery, which corresponds to the most caudal prolongation of lymph nodes situated superior to the interlobar pulmonary artery. The latter group, described as part of the right upper lobe group by SONE et al. (1983) or as the inferior part of Borrie's lymphatic sump (NOHL 1972; BORRIE 1952), has previously been described on CT scans as low-density soft tissue collections, sometimes mimicking hilar adenopathy or thrombus of the right pulmonary artery (ASHIDA et al. 1987). In 7% of the cases, it is possible to observe a triangular area of hypoattenuation posterior to the right interlobar artery and immediately adjacent to the superior aspect of the apical segmental artery of the right lower lobe. At the level of the left interlobar group, a rim of hypoattenuation is a constant finding along the anteromedial border of the left interlobar pulmonary artery. In 13% of cases a focal area of hypoattenuation can also be depicted lateral to the left interlobar pulmonary artery, while additional hypoattenuated zones can be found posterior (4%) or medial (13%) to the left interlobar arterial wall. These CT findings are in agreement with anatomical descriptions which have previously emphasized that the left interlobar artery is encircled by lymph nodes (NAGAISHI 1972; SONE et al. 1983).

At the level of the right middle lobe and lingular groups, the most striking feature is the high prevalence of hypoattenuated areas in intimate relation to the medial perimeter of pulmonary arterial branches. On both sides, the most frequent sites of hypoattenuation are found interposed between the lateral walls of proximal bronchi (the right middle lobe bronchus and the proximal part of the right lower lobe bronchus, and the lingular bronchus and the proximal part of the left lower lobe bronchus) and the medial walls of their corresponding pulmonary arteries, confirming the importance of the "lymphatic sump" on both sides (NOHL 1972; BORRIE

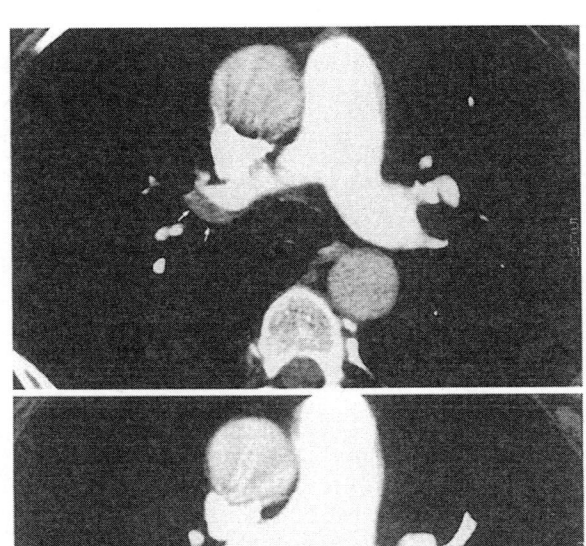

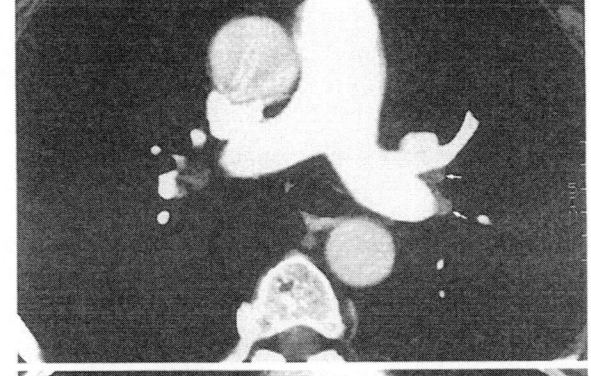

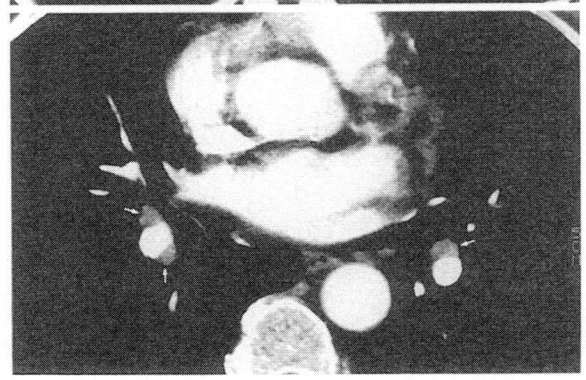

Fig. 10.12. Spiral CT scans obtained in a 66-year-old coal miner (inspiratory apnea; 130 cc of a 30% ionic contrast agent; 5 cc/s) at the level of the right upper lobe bronchus (**a**), the left main pulmonary artery (**b**), and the right middle lobe bronchus (**c**). Hypoattenuated areas (*arrows*) in close contact with pulmonary arterial branches should not be misinterpreted as segmental filling defects. Normal findings on the pulmonary angiogram confirmed that these areas corresponded to hilar lymph nodes

1952) (Fig. 10.12c). At the level of the right and left lower lobe groups, most lymph nodes are interposed between segmental bronchi and their corresponding arteries, or are identified in the angle of bifurcation of segmental arteries.

Such a compartmentalization is necessarily arbitrary and we may sometimes encounter difficulties in clearly defining distinct boundaries between hilar nodal stations. Moreover, we must keep in mind the fact that the anatomical landmarks used for this classification of hilar lymph nodes may vary among patients, thus explaining why a strict application of this classification may sometimes be difficult. In our investigation, we measured the maximum short axes of hilar hypoattenuated areas on enhanced CT scans. Such measurements provide only an approximation of lymph node size as these areas are not exclusively related to lymphatic tissue. Moreover, short-axis measurements may be distorted because of variable nodal orientation. Despite these limitations, we observed that a uniform short-axis threshold of 3 mm, except around the left lower lobe pulmonary artery, could be used to distinguish normal patients from those with enlarged hilar lymph nodes. This threshold should be considered only as an interim standard until similar data are collected in a larger population.

10.6.3 Hemodynamics of Pulmonary Circulation

Physiological data must also be integrated in the spiral volumetric CT evaluation of vascular enhancement as arterial opacification on spiral CT scans is highly dependent on the physiological conditions under which the studies are performed. Several cases of unilateral increased pulmonary vascular resistance due to extensive airspace consolidation have led to false-positive diagnosis of pulmonary embolism. We observed such a case with a 21-year-old woman presenting with left-sided chest trauma and suspicion of right pulmonary embolism (RÉMY-JARDIN et al. 1992). The asymmetry in arterial perfusion was explained by a slow flow through the left basilar arteries owing to ipsilateral pleural effusion and posterior lung consolidation whereas normally circulating right pulmonary arteries appeared abnormally hypoattenuated (Fig. 10.13). For similar reasons, two false-positive diagnoses of emboli in segmental lower lobe arteries were made in patients with atelectasis or consolidation and pleural effusions (GOODMAN et al. 1995). This also caused unilateral slow flow through lower lobe pulmonary arteries and the impression of emboli contralateral to pleuro-parenchymal disease. In both studies, angiographic examinations demonstrated slow but unobstructed flow through these vessels. Similarly, we must keep in mind that any cause of unilaterally increased vascular resistance may lead to asymmetry in pulmonary arterial opacification.

Table 10.2 summarizes the various causes of unilateral nonopacification or faint opacification of a pulmonary artery which have been previously described on angiograms and lung scans (SAGEL and GREENSPAN 1970; WORSLEY et al. 1993). The best way to demonstrate on CT scans the patency of a unilateral faintly opacified pulmonary artery is to perform a second spiral CT acquisition with a longer scan delay to suppress flow phenomena at the level of this vessel. It is worthy of note that patients with congestive heart failure may have a circumferential collar of low-attenuation material around a proximal segmental artery secondary to perivascular edema. As previously pointed out by TEIGEN et al. (1993), this finding should not be mistaken for chronic pulmonary embolism.

10.6.4 Obliquely Oriented Arteries

The pulmonary artery branches which are oblique to the transverse CT images may be poorly demonstrated and sometimes represent relatively "blind areas" with CT. The percentage of inadequately visualized arteries has been reported to vary between 4% and 7% of the vascular zones, with the right middle lobe and lingular arteries being primarily affected (RÉMY-JARDIN 1992; TEIGEN et al. 1993). Several other obliquely oriented vessels, such as the anterior segmental arteries of the upper lobes and the apical segmental arteries of the lower lobes, also may be problematic owing to their incomplete depiction in the plane of the scan (RÉMY-JARDIN et al. 1995b,c). The interpretative difficulties encountered at the level of these vessels on transverse CT scans can be

Table 10.2. Causes of unilateral nonopacification or faint opacification of a pulmonary artery (modified from SAGEL and GREENSPAN 1970; WORSLEY et al. 1993)

1. "Occult" pulmonary artery
2. Unilateral pulmonary artery obstruction of extrinsic, mural or endoluminal origin
3. Unilateral increase in pulmonary vascular resistance, secondary to:
   - Proximal or distal bronchial obstruction
   - Bronchiolar obstruction
   - Parenchymal destruction
   - Extensive airspace consolidation
   - Pleural restrictive or expansive process
   - Conditions with elevated venous pressure
4. Hemithoracic shunting of blood from the systemic to the pulmonary circulation following surgical anastomoses of Blalock, Waterston, Potts and Glenn

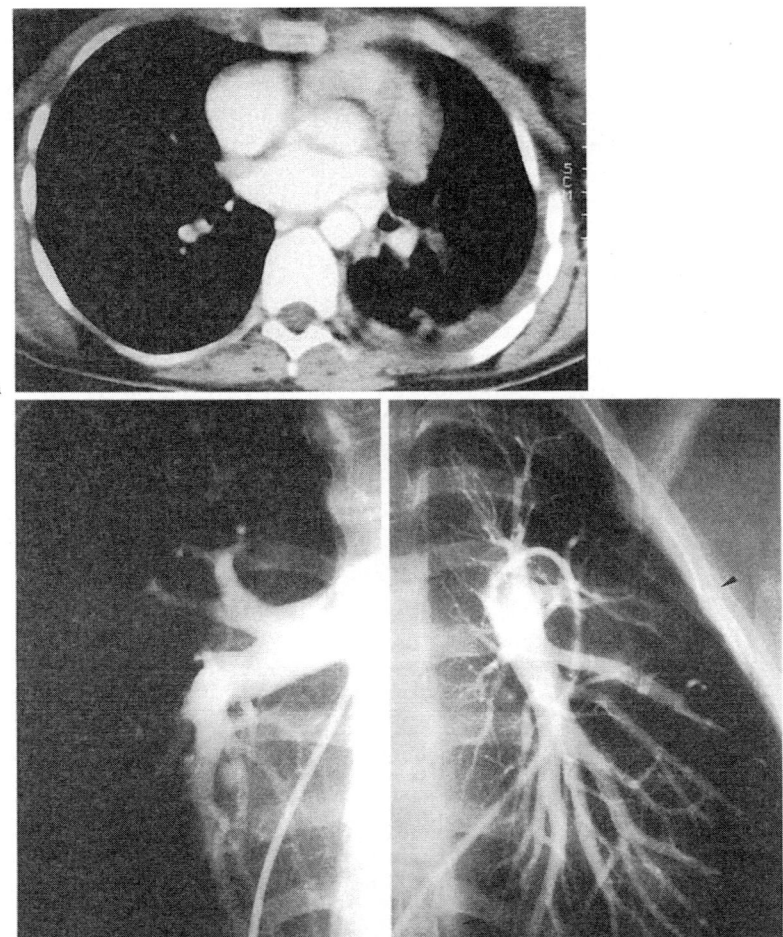

Fig. 10.13a–c. Images obtained in a 21-year-old woman with left-sided chest trauma and suspected pulmonary thromboembolism. **a** Spiral CT scan obtained at the level of the lower lobes (5-mm collimation; 5 mm/s table feed; 120 cc of 12% contrast material; 7 cc/s) shows hypoattenuating areas in the right lower lobe pulmonary artery (*arrows*) compared with the optimal contrast enhancement of the left lower lobe pulmonary artery (*arrow*). This asymmetry in arterial perfusion led to suspicion of right pulmonary thromboembolism. Left pleural effusion and posterior parenchymal consolidation are seen. **b,c** Right (**b**) and left (**c**) oblique pulmonary angiograms obtained 4 s after contrast material injection show no evidence of pulmonary embolism but marked perfusion asymmetry due to increased pulmonary vascular resistance in the left pulmonary arterial bed secondary to chest trauma. Note an anterior rib fracture (*arrowhead* in **c**) and left upper and lower lobe infiltrates and pleural effusion (*double arrowheads* in **c**). (From RÉMY-JARDIN et al. 1992)

overcome by their analysis on reformatted images obtained along the main axis of the vessels of interest.

When necessary, spiral volumetric CT enables multiplanar reformations (MPRs) by using data obtained from contiguous transverse CT scans in any anatomical plane, not only the coronal and sagittal planes. Vessels that are oriented in these planes can be imaged along their longitudinal axis, and this may help differentiate a filling defect due to an intraluminal thrombus from a narrowed central artery secondary to extrinsic hilar compression. In a recent study, we found that MPRs could be a useful complement to transverse CT scans in the diagnosis of pulmonary embolism (RÉMY-JARDIN et al. 1995b). Among 20 patients in whom acute central pulmonary embolism was confidently diagnosed on transverse CT scans, MPRs enabled a more precise assessment of the extent of thromboembolic disease in 13 (65%), either by excluding lobar and/or segmental emboli (11 patients) or by confirming additional central thrombi (two patients) (Fig. 10.14). When transverse

CT scans were normal except at the level of a few oblique arteries considered noninterpretable, MPRs enabled confident exclusion of central pulmonary embolism. This additional negative information provided by MPRs may help reduce the number of inconclusive CT examinations, a partial but relevant limitation of spiral CT in the depiction of acute central pulmonary embolism. However, we found no patients classified with normal CT examinations in whom the addition of MPRs to transverse CT scans enabled identification of pulmonary emboli.

From a practical point of view, MPRs of obliquely oriented arteries are generated from the initial data set without additional radiation exposure for the patient. As the aim of MPRs is to display a given vessel along its main axis, the adequate plane of reformation cannot be better selected than on the lateral view of the three-dimensional shaded surface display (3DSSD) of the ipsilateral pulmonary vasculature. The different steps of this procedure can be summarized as follows. From the initial data set, overlapped transverse images are first reconstructed using a 360°

linear interpolation algorithm as this yields MPRs of higher quality than are obtained with a 180° linear interpolation algorithm. From this volumetric data set a 3DSSD of the pulmonary vasculature is then generated after selection of a threshold value of −300 HU. This threshold enables visualization of the central pulmonary vessels (down to the segmental level) while eliminating peripheral pulmonary vasculature and bronchi. For each oblique artery of interest, the proper plane of reformation is selected by means of a localizing cursor positioned on the lateral view of the 3DSSD of the ipsilateral arterial tree. Then, the software reformats the data to display the selected plane of reformation (Fig. 10.15). The radiologist is able to interactively roam through the entire data set imaged along the selected plane of reformation. Such a real-time analysis of the 3D volume enables the user either to confirm the plane of reformation initially selected or to optimally update it to allow reformation of the artery of interest along its main axis. MPRs are generated exclusively at the level of lobar and/or segmental arteries considered

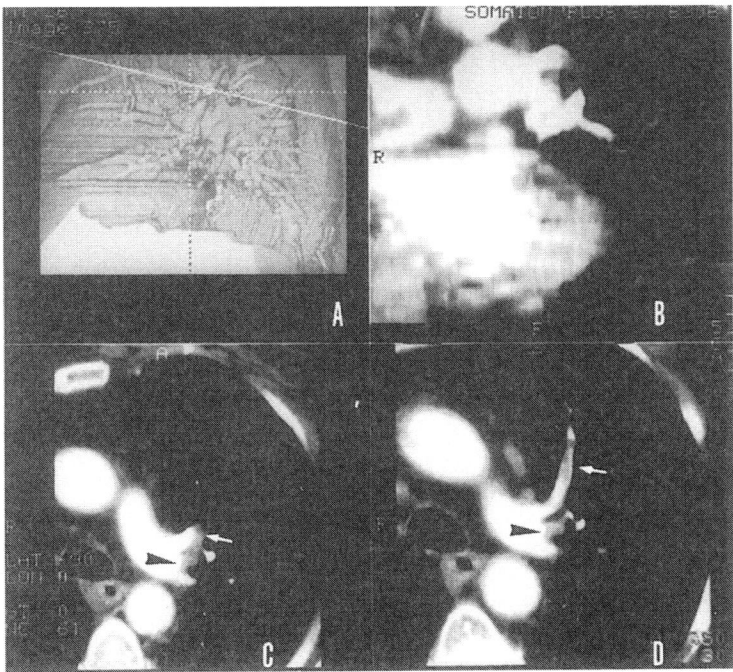

Fig. 10.14A–D. Spiral CT evaluation of a 69-year-old woman with unequivocal pulmonary emboli in the right and left lower lobe pulmonary arteries (20% ionic contrast material; 3-mm collimation; 6 mm/s table feed). **A** 3D shaded surface display of the left pulmonary vasculature; **B** coronal reformation; **C** transverse CT scan; **D** oblique transverse CT scan. The transverse CT scan (**C**) shows marginal areas of hypoattenuation lateral to LA2 (*arrow*) and along the lateral aspect of the left pulmonary arterial arch (*arrowhead*). Oblique transverse reformation (**D**) obtained along the main axis of LA2 shows multiple peripheral defects at the level of LA2 (*arrow*) not depicted on the transverse CT scan and a small lymph node between LA2 and LB2 (*arrowhead*). (From RÉMY-JARDIN et al. 1995b)

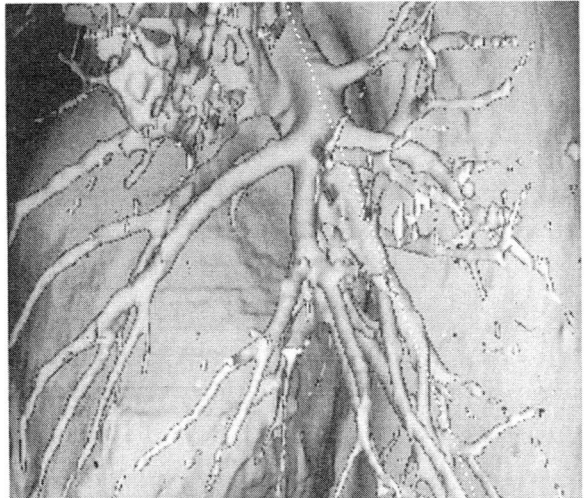

a

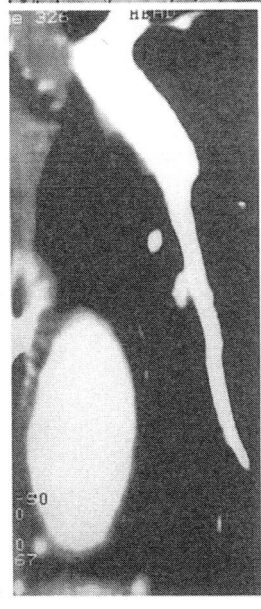

b

Fig. 10.15a,b. Spiral CT examination obtained in a 54-year-old woman (3-mm collimation; 5 mm/s table feed; 120 cc of 24% nonionic contrast agent; 5 cc/s). **a** Three-dimensional shaded surface display of the left pulmonary vasculature; lateral view. A plane of reformation is selected along the main axis of the posterior segmental artery of the left lower lobe. **b** Coronal oblique reformation enables visualization of the left interlobar pulmonary artery and the posterior segmental artery of the left lower lobe on a single image

nonanalyzable on transverse CT scans. Therefore, this additional procedure is responsible for a minimal increase in the duration of the overall procedure, 15 min on average. As recently pointed out by LA-CROSSE et al. (1995), there are several advantages in selecting the planes of reformation from a 3DSSD rather than from a transverse CT section. When the

reformation plane is defined through the drawing of a line on one of the transverse slices, the resulting MPR will be perpendicular to the transverse plane and parallel to the drawn line, thus allowing only single obliquity relative to the three fundamental planes. Moreover, while with this approach it usually proves difficult to achieve appropriate orientation relative to the more cranial or caudal parts of the structure to be imaged, both limitations are overcome if the MPRs are planned on the 3D virtual object itself.

As MPRs are known to be a helpful tool when looking at structures paralleling the transverse imaging plane or when reaching a tissue surface or interface, another potential application is the evaluation of chronic thromboembolic disease (Fig. 10.16). Evaluating the role of CT in the assessment of chronic pulmonary hypertension and its surgical operability, SCHWICKERT et al. (1994) reported false-negative results in detecting central thrombi with spiral CT. Among the 15 patients with inoperable thrombi on the basis of CT findings who underwent surgery, removable organized thrombi were found at surgery in 14. Thrombi missed on transverse CT images were either concentric and adherent to the arterial wall or located tangentially at the bottom or the roof of a vessel. Demonstration of thrombi in such locations should probably benefit from selective reformations. Another potential application of MPRs could be the demonstration of indirect signs of chronic thromboembolic pulmonary hypertension on oblique vessels. FALASCHI et al. (1992) reported that the A/B ratio, i.e., the ratio between the external diameter of a given pulmonary artery and the external diameter of the corresponding bronchus, is increased in most patients with chronic pulmonary hypertension, whereas it is equal to 1 in normal subjects in the supine position (WOODRING 1991). These authors pointed out that this ratio, measurable in most cases, had a low inter- and intraobserver variability that was almost completely limited to the lingular segments, which are known to be difficult to see in transverse sections. Therefore, the use of 2D images obtained in the equatorial diameter of a bronchus and its accompanying artery could also be proposed as a complementary tool in investigating CT features of chronic pulmonary hypertension.

10.6.5 Breathing Artifacts

The 10- to 20-s breath hold necessary for spiral CT remains a potential source of difficulty in severely tachypneic patients, who are usually instructed to breathe quietly during the examination. However, there are two main drawbacks of such breathing: (a) an inhomogeneous arterial opacification of the pulmonary arteries due to variations in pulmonary blood flow between inspiration and expiration, as further discussed below, and (b) changes in the orientation and diameter of the vessels. For vessels oriented along the z-axis, there are limited consequences due to scanning while the patient is breathing as the vascular sections will similarly occupy the entire width of the CT section whatever the respiratory phase. Conversely, vessels horizontally or obliquely oriented to the plane of the CT section will be observed with a slightly different orientation on successive images. As they will occupy variable portions of the section width in two successive scans, imaging of these vessels is likely to be associated with a partial volume effect. Consequently, any abruptly decreased attenuation at the level of a given arterial section between two contiguous sections should not be mistaken for an arterial filling defect (Fig. 10.17).

Owing to their relatively small diameter, the segmental arteries are particularly prone to these artifacts. GOODMAN et al. (1995) reported that, in one of 20 patients evaluated with spiral CT, a breathing artifact on two contiguous slices led to a false-positive diagnosis of an embolus in the posterobasal artery of the left lower lobe. In our clinical practice, we have observed these artifacts at the level of segmental arteries of the right middle lobe and/or lingula but also in the lower lobes. In tachypneic patients, we therefore usually consider spiral CT to be reliable only at the main and lobar arterial levels. Contrast-enhanced electron beam CT may offer a specific advantage with respect to the diagnosis of pulmonary embolism in this population. The 100-ms scanning time makes breath holding unnecessary, and there is minimal respiratory and cardiac motion artifact, as recently reported by TEIGEN et al. (1995). Although the radiologist will systematically consider this pitfall when interpreting the CT scans of a tachypneic patient, it may be more difficult to recognize it in cases of inadvertent breathing during the exposure. Such a possibility is usually raised by means of the identification of motion artifacts on lung images within the anatomical subvolume acquired during breathing.

10.7 Limitations of Spiral CT

Limitations inherent to suboptimal data acquisition should be considered transient as they will be re-duced as the experience of the radiologist with spiral CT angiography of pulmonary arteries increases. Apart from these, there are two main categories of limitations of spiral CT in the evaluation of pulmonary embolism which have to be taken into account: (a) those related to the patient's clinical status, and (b) those inherent to the CT technique.

10.7.1 Patient-Related Limitations

10.7.1.1 Disorders with Anatomical Shunts

10.7.1.1.1 Patent Foramen Ovale. A transient or permanent increase in pulmonary arterial pressure may be responsible for a right to left shunt through a patent foramen ovale which will result in a lower degree of pulmonary arterial enhancement on CT scans. This situation is suspected when a massive and early enhancement of the aorta is observed in conjunction with a faint pulmonary arterial opacification. Selection of a longer scan delay usually helps improve pulmonary arterial enhancement, thereby permitting the search for pulmonary arterial filling defects. We have observed a patient in whom systemic and pulmonary emboli were concomitantly demonstrated on enhanced spiral CT scans.

10.7.1.1.2 Left-to-right Shunts. There are acquired disorders which are associated with anatomical shunting from the systemic to the pulmonary circulation, and are thus responsible for anterograde or retrograde left-to-right shunt. This situation results in regional or unilateral changes in pulmonary blood flow, which is interrupted at the level of the anatomical communication between the systemic and the pulmonary circulation. The most common clinical situation is represented by patients with severe chronic inflammatory disease, particularly those with bronchiectasis, in whom prominent bronchopulmonary collateral circulation may develop and produce segmental retrograde flow. In these patients, nonvisualization of arteries or dilution defects may simulate emboli, as previously reported on pulmonary angiograms (BOOKSTEIN and SILVER 1974).

In patients with substantial regional variation in pulmonary blood flow, a long start delay (e.g., 15 s) and selection of a high-concentration, high-flow protocol can help suppress the focal hypoattenuation in the pulmonary arterial bed related to retrograde left-to-right shunting. These attempts are not always successful and this particular anatomical situation may lead to an inconclusive CT examination. However, one must keep in mind the fact that the difficulties in obtaining optimal enhancement of the pulmonary arterial vasculature on CT scans are similar to those encountered on unilateral angiograms, where poor opacification or pseudo-amputation is commonly seen. In most cases, hyperselective catheterization of the lobar or segmental arteries of this region is required to demonstrate their patency.

10.7.1.2 Obstruction of the Superior Vena Cava and Collaterals

Any acute or chronic obstruction of the systemic veins will be responsible for a delayed and suboptimal opacification of the pulmonary arteries. The way

to overcome this problem of arterial enhancement is to increase the start delay in order to allow enough contrast material to reach the pulmonary arteries at the time of scanning. Whereas this anatomical situation remains compatible with the detection of large central emboli, it usually precludes confident analysis of small emboli.

10.7.1.3 Severe Dyspnea

Scanning severely tachypneic patients represents a major limitation of spiral CT. Apart from the breathing artifacts previously quoted, this situation is usually associated with suboptimal quality of arterial opacification. The latter flaw is explained by respira-

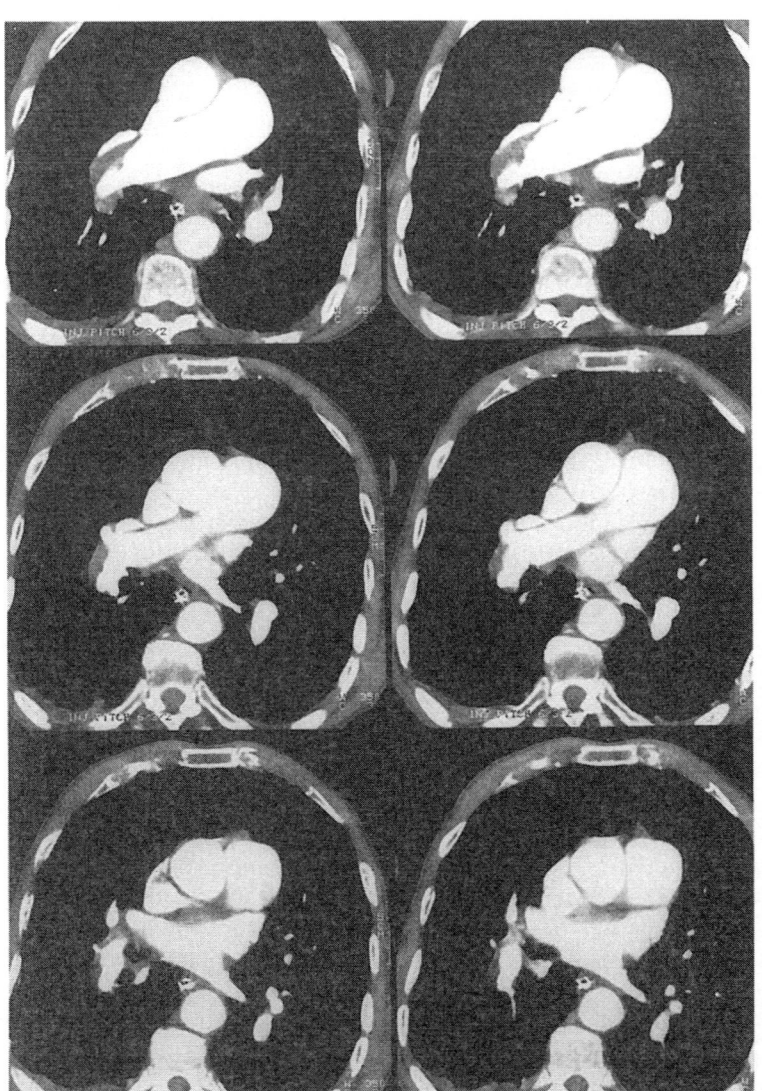

Fig. 10.16a,b. Spiral CT evaluation of a 53-year-old-male (inspiratory apnea; 24% ionic contrast material; 5 cc/s; 3-mm section thickness; 6 mm/s table feed). **a** Contiguous transverse CT sections show right-sided marginal filling defects with reduction in the arterial lumen. Note enlarged left pulmonary arterial branches suggestive of pulmonary hypertension. **b:** *B-1,* Three-dimensional shaded surface display of the left pulmonary arterial tree; *B-2,* coronal reformation; *B-3,* transverse CT section; *B-4,* oblique coronal image. Coronal oblique reformation (*B-4*) obtained along the main axis of the right interlobar pulmonary artery and RA10 enables analysis of the mural thrombus (*arrows*) in a single CT image

Fig. 10.16b

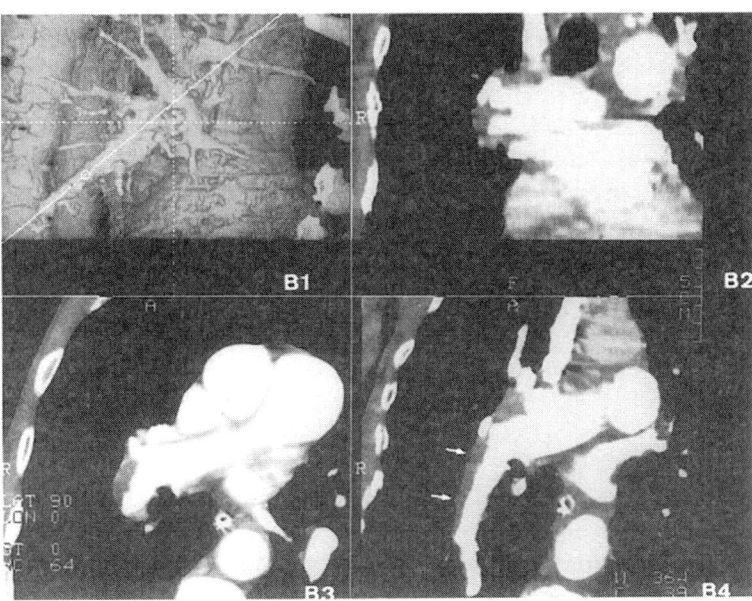

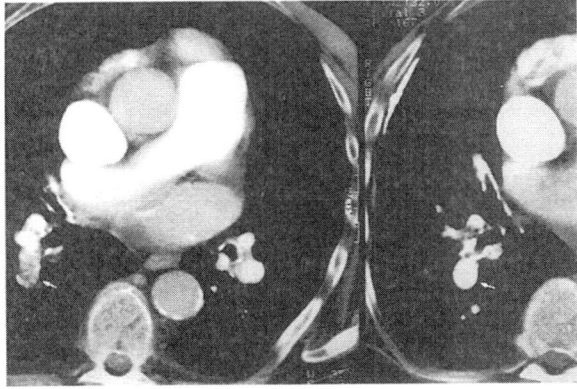

Fig. 10.17. Contiguous spiral CT scans (5-mm collimation; 5 mm/s table feed; 120 cc of 25% ionic contrast agent; 5 cc/s) obtained in a 69-year-old tachypneic patient at the level of the lower lobes. A hypoattenuated area is present at the level of the common trunk for the lateral and posterior segmental arteries of the right lower lobe (*arrow*), which is homogeneously enhanced 3 mm apart. A normal pulmonary angiogram confirmed that the hypoattenuated area corresponded to partial volume averaging at the level of the upper part of the common trunk in this tachypneic patient scanned during quiet breathing

tory-induced changes in pulmonary arterial flow (SOSTMAN et al. 1993a,b). Independent techniques have shown that, in conscious humans, the pulmonary blood flow increases during inspiration and decreases during expiration (GABE et al. 1969; VERMIERE and BUTLER 1968). These factors are likely to explain inhomogeneous arterial enhancement, which is often depicted in this population.

10.7.2 Limitations Inherent to the Technique

Several studies have emphasized that the spiral CT protocols currently used for detection of pulmonary embolism cannot reliably evaluate the subsegmental level. When considering exclusively larger arteries (i.e., main, lobar, and segmental arteries), GOODMAN et al. (1995) found that the sensitivity of spiral CT was 86% and the specificity was 92% whereas they were 63% and 89% respectively, when considering all vessels. Comparing spiral CT and digital angiography, SENAC et al. (1995) demonstrated the high diagnostic value of spiral CT in detecting acute central emboli (kappa coefficient = 1) whereas it was significantly reduced for emboli located below the segmental level (kappa coefficient = 0.28). Evaluating 60 patients for pulmonary embolism with electron-beam CT, TEIGEN et al. (1995) found no substantial difference in sensitivity and specificity when the central (i.e., main and lobar arteries) and peripheral (i.e., segmental and subsegmental arteries) were analyzed individually.

Owing to this limitation of spiral CT, it is of practical concern to be aware of the frequency and clinical significance of isolated subsegmental emboli in patients with acute pulmonary embolism. In a series of 20 patients, GOODMAN et al. (1995) reported that 4 for 11 patients (36%) with acute pulmonary embolism had subsegmental clots only. These authors found that the prevalence observed in their study was similar to that reported by OSER et al. (1994) on angiograms. In the latter study, 11 of 33 patients

(33%) with pulmonary angiograms had clots limited to the subsegmental level. However, the samples in both studies were small, and this may explain the difference in frequency as compared with recent reports by several authors (TEIGEN et al. 1995; RÉMY-JARDIN et al. 1995c). In three of the 60 patients evaluated by TEIGEN et al., a single embolus was seen in a distal segmental or subsegmental vessel, while in a fourth patient two subsegmental emboli were present (frequency of 6%). In a study group of 72 patients, we found isolated subsegmental clots in only four patients (5%) (RÉMY-JARDIN et al. 1995c). In the PIOPED study, 12 or 383 (3%) patients in whom pulmonary embolism was diagnosed had pulmonary embolism only in subsegmental and smaller vessels (P.D. STEIN and B.J. RELYA, personal communication based on unpublished data from PIOPED). Therefore, isolated peripheral clots appear to be an infrequent clinical situation whose diagnosis is beyond the scope of CT and requires pulmonary angiography.

The clinical significance of such small emboli remains controversial (GURNEY 1993; NOVELLINE et al. 1978). Some authors consider that tiny clots are from calf veins and do not require anticoagulation (MOSER 1990; GURNEY 1993; DALEN 1993). In the discordant cases reported by TEIGEN et al. (1995), duplex evaluation of the lower extremities was negative in all four cases, and the authors wondered whether these tiny emboli were responsible for the symptoms for which the patients were referred for pulmonary angiography. According to Goodman, most physicians think that small emboli must be considered the harbinger of future larger emboli and therefore are clinically significant (GOODMAN et al. 1995). In our clinical practice, isolated subsegmental clots have been found to be responsible for clinically acute pulmonary embolism in four patients with pre-existing bronchopulmonary disease (RÉMY-JARDIN et al. 1995c). In cases of severely reduced arterial perfusion due to underlying bronchopulmonary disease, occlusion of a few subsegmental branches previously perfusing the most "normal" part of the lung parenchyma may lead to respiratory failure. A rapid favorable outcome under anticoagulation in all cases supported this hypothesis. This clinical presentation could thus be considered specific to patients with preexisting impaired pulmonary arterial perfusion, namely the "pneumologist" form of acute pulmonary embolism. Conversely, in patients with no prior cardiac or pulmonary disease, isolated subsegmental clots are probably not clinically significant.

Recognition of peripheral emboli is difficult on transverse CT scans as subsegmental vessels cannot be reliably identified owing to their small diameter, short length, and frequent oblique orientation. However, one must bear it in mind that subsegmental emboli can be confidently demonstrated on CT scans inasmuch as pulmonary hypertension is present. In this anatomical situation, enlargement of proximal vessels also affects subsegmental arteries at the level of which endoluminal filling defects become easily detectable. It is important to emphasize that pulmonary angiography has been shown to have substantial variability in the detection of small peripheral emboli (STEIN et al. 1992; QUINN et al. 1987). The angiographers involved in the PIOPED study agreed on the presence of subsegmental pulmonary emboli only 66% of the time (STEIN et al. 1992). These data help to elucidate the current limitations in the accuracy of both CT and angiography in the depiction of subsegmental emboli.

10.8 Current Indications for Spiral CT

10.8.1 Diagnosis of Acute Pulmonary Thromboembolism

To date, standard pulmonary angiography is still considered the most specific and sensitive diagnostic procedure available for pulmonary embolism. However, the requirement of an experienced operator limits the study's availability and complications probably occur more frequently when the procedure is done by a nonexpert. Given the specific advantages of spiral CT angiography over conventional and/or digital angiography (Table 10.3), this technique can be considered a powerful imaging alternative for the detection of pulmonary emboli in second- to fourth-division pulmonary arteries (Fig. 10.6). Spiral CT represents a noninvasive and fast way to detect acute thromboembolic disease, avoiding the risks of catheterization inherent in angiographic procedures, including cardiac arrhythmia, cardiac perforation, endocardial and myocardial injury, and death (PIOPED Investigators 1990). This is of paramount importance for patients who are known to be at high risk for the complications of pulmonary angiography or for seriously ill patients. Owing to the size of emboli in patients with clinical evidence of massive pulmonary embolism, the initial diagnostic pulmonary angiography could also be replaced by contrast-enhanced spiral CT, as recently pointed out by

Table 10.3. Advantages of spiral CT angiography compared with conventional angiography in the evaluation of pulmonary vessels (modified from NAPEL 1995)

Conventional or digital pulmonary angiography	Spiral CT angiography
One view angle per contrast injection. Additional views require added x-ray exposure and contrast media. Hyperselective injections are sometimes necessary in patients with prior cardiopulmonary disease.	CT angiography acquires an entire volume of 3D data using a single injection of contrast agent. Thus, arbitrary views can be retrospectively targeted and reconstructed without the need for additional iodine or x-ray exposure.
Requires a technically and anatomically experienced angiographer; this limits the study's availability and its diagnostic value.	Requires basic technical and physiological background and precise anatomical knowledge; this limits only the study's diagnostic information.
Requires sophisticated equipment, exclusively dedicated to vascular studies, of limited diffusion.	Requires multipurpose equipment, of increasing accessibility.
Complications from angiography are operator-dependent: 0.5% mortality; 1% major and 5% minor complications.	Complications from CT angiography are non-operator-dependent; only minor complications are potentially observed with peripheral i.v. administration of contrast medium.
Close nursing; recovery period after the procedure owing to the arterial puncture (minimum of 6–8 h; sometimes an overnight hospital stay).	Peripheral i.v. injection: outpatient examination with minimal postprocedure observation required.
Diagnostic angiographic signs: 50% direct (i.e., pathognomonic); 50% indirect (i.e., prone to errors of interpretation).	Diagnostic signs: 100% direct (i.e., pathognomonic)
Unmodified technique over a number of years; low benefit from image digitalization owing to patients' clinical status sometimes aggravated by previous cardiopulmonary disease.	New technique; needs to be extensively evaluated; a 50–300 ms rotation time per slice, necessary for suppression of motion artifacts, seems accessible to electron-beam scanners but not to mechanical scanners.
Conventional angiography is a projection imaging technique that produces 2D images of 3D structures. Therefore, blood vessels and other structures that overlap in the direction of the projection may obscure the site of interest.	CT angiography is a 3D examination. Overlying structures may be eliminated by postprocessing.
Great intra- and interobservor variability in demonstrating subsegmental clots.	Subsegmental level beyond the scope of transverse CT imaging.
Angiography is an intraluminal technique and as such does not display mural abnormalities, making identification of mural defects difficult or impossible.	CT is a cross-sectional imaging modality that exhibits excellent soft tissue discrimination. As such, it has utility for depicting mural thrombus and calcifications.

CURTIN et al. (1994). It is interesting to note that similar percentages of technically inadequate examinations have been reported with spiral CT (4% of 75 spiral CT scans; major motion artifacts and/or poor arterial enhancement; RÉMY-JARDIN et al. 1995c) and angiography (3%; nondiagnostic angiograms; PIOPED Investigators 1990). Moreover, we found that 9% of CT scans were inconclusive, mainly due to inadequate analysis of oblique arteries, while insufficient visualization of pulmonary arteries has been reported up to 12% of completed angiograms (HULL et al. 1983). If spiral CT has the potential to replace pulmonary angiography as the initial screening test for central pulmonary embolism, the current limitations of this technique at the subsegmental level

explain why it cannot supplant pulmonary angiography as the definitive diagnostic imaging test.

More controversial is the current debate on the respective roles of spiral CT and ventilation-perfusion scanning as noninvasive screening procedures. In the PIOPED study, it was clearly demonstrated that the accuracy of ventilation-perfusion scans was high in two lung scan categories, namely the high-probability category and the normal or near-normal $\dot{V}/\dot{Q}$ scan, respectively seen in 13% and 14% of the study group (PIOPED Investigators 1990). Therefore, more than 60% of the patients entered in the PIOPED study were in nondiagnostic lung scan categories, i.e., the intermediate- and low-probability categories. This implies that the majority of patients undergoing a V̇/Q̇ scan will require an additional study to establish or exclude the diagnosis of pulmonary embolism. Moreover, if interobserver agreement in the PIOPED study was high for the normal and high-probability categories, there was disagreement between the initial two observers in 25%–30% of the ventilation-perfusion scans classified as intermediate or low probability. This was so despite the carefully defined criteria and pretrial practice aimed at reducing such variability. More recently, SOSTMAN et al. (1994) reported a better interobserver agreement when using the revised PIOPED criteria. However, these authors also pointed out that observers with less training and who have not interpreted many scans in consensus probably would not achieve these levels of agreement. These findings imply that the usual interpretation by single readers may not be as reliable as is assumed in clinical practice. Moreover, it has recently been suggested that the V̇/Q̇ scan does not accurately depict the distribution of large pulmonary emboli. In a study of the 185 perfusion defects seen on the V̇/Q̇ scans of 68 patients, only 16% of the defects were associated with angiographically proven pulmonary embolism (BRESLAW et al. 1992). Less than 30% of the segmental or larger V̇/Q̇ mismatches were associated with pulmonary embolism at angiography. Conversely, 43 segmental or larger pulmonary emboli found at angiography were not associated with significant V̇/Q̇ mismatches. The sensitivity and specificity of the V̇/Q̇ scan for determining the segmental location of PE were 42% and 78%, respectively. All these data suggest that there is a need for a noninvasive procedure with a greater sensitivity and specificity than that of V̇/Q̇ scan for the diagnosis of PE.

TEIGEN et al. (1995) were the first authors to compare the findings at V-P scanning, electron beam CT, and pulmonary angiography. Investigating a population of 38 patients, they demonstrated enhanced specificity and sensitivity with CT (i.e., sensitivity: 65%; specificity: 97%) as compared with V-P scanning (sensitivity: 20%; specificity: 52%) and concluded that CT appeared to offer an alternative to V-P scanning as a rapid noninvasive screening examination for the diagnosis of pulmonary embolism. In a study group of 25 patients, RÉMY-JARDIN et al. (1995c) found one patient with a negative V-P scan but abnormal spiral CT and angiographic examinations. These data contradict the usual statement according to which a normal lung perfusion scan provides virtual certainty that these is no pulmonary thromboembolic disease. However, they illustrate

that the major theoretical reasons for pulmonary embolism associated with a "normal" perfusion scan are central, nonobstructing, nonlateralized pulmonary embolism, or minimal defects on the scan that are not appreciated (SOSTMAN et al. 1986). If future studies confirm high sensitivity and accuracy of fast scanning techniques in diagnosing pulmonary thromboembolic disease, these techniques will probably replace ventilation-perfusion lung scanning as the initial screening test. In clinical practice, objective testing for venous thrombosis provides a practical alternative to performing any diagnostic procedure for pulmonary embolism. It is worthy of note that recent studies have demonstrated the effectiveness of spiral CT venography for the demonstration of deep venous thrombosis (STEHLING et al. 1994).

10.8.2 Evaluation of Patients with Chronic Thromboembolic Pulmonary Hypertension

The evaluation of patients with suspected chronic thromboembolic hypertension is the second indication for spiral CT, as a noninvasive means of diagnosis of chronic pulmonary embolism, and also as a complement to pulmonary angiography prior to surgery (SCHWICKERT et al. 1994; JAMALI et al. 1995). AUGER et al. (1992) have reported the angiographic pattern suggestive of chronic thromboembolic disease that is essential to make the correct diagnosis and to select patients in whom surgical removal of chronic thrombi from the main, lobar, and segmental pulmonary arteries is feasible. Although spiral CT is not as precise as angiography in the morphological analysis of the pulmonary arterial bed, it may assist in the analysis of central vascular irregularities secondary to organized thrombi, especially in arteries not adequately evaluated with selective pulmonary artery injections, and in the detection of associated acute pulmonary embolism in these patients. Evaluating 75 patients with CT (20 patients with conventional CT; 55 patients with spiral CT), SCHWICKERT et al. (1994) found that CT findings allowed confirmation of the diagnosis of chronic thromboembolism and ensured technical operability (sensitivity, 77%; specificity, 100%; overall accuracy, 80%) by means of direct visualization of thrombi in the central arteries of 53 patients. SENAC et al. (1995) found that spiral CT was more accurate than digital angiography for the diagnosis of chronic thromboembolic disease (kappa coefficient = 0.29). The superiority of spiral CT was related to the ability to demonstrate mural thrombi which were missed on pulmonary angiography owing to the regular and concentric narrowing of the arterial lumen. Due to the difficulty in analyzing oblique arteries, MPRs obtained at second intention should help improve depiction of indirect criteria of chronic pulmonary embolism (Fig. 10.8).

In the most recent study, by TEIGEN et al. (1995), 23 of the 60 patients evaluated had pulmonary embolism on angiograms. Among them, six patients had changes consistent with chronic thromboembolic disease and three patients had findings of both acute and chronic pulmonary embolism (TEIGEN et al. 1995). In two patients, weblike stenoses and occlusions were seen in segmental vessels on the pulmonary angiogram, consistent with chronic pulmonary embolism. Although subtle vascular changes were seen in one of these patients on the electron-beam CT scan, CT scans from both patients were prospec-

tively interpreted as negative for pulmonary embolism.

Apart from the evaluation of the pulmonary vasculature, an additional indication for spiral CT in this clinical setting could be the depiction of bronchial arteries. KAUCZOR et al. (1994) have reported that the CT depiction of bronchial arteries, dilatation, and tortuosity provides indicators for chronic thromboembolic pulmonary hypertension but cannot estimate its degree. They also found that dilated bronchial arteries are a significant predictor for survival of patients undergoing pulmonary thromboendarterectomy.

10.8.3 Follow-up of Patients Treated for Pulmonary Embolism

The third use of spiral CT is to monitor patients with documented central emboli. The course of the recanalization of the vascular bed and regression of peripheral attenuation changes may be followed with noninvasive spiral CT (RÉMY-JARDIN et al. 1992; TEIGEN et al. 1993) (Fig. 10.18). Given that thrombolytic therapy is effective when administered via a peripheral vein, CURTIN et al. (1994) have recently suggested that replacement of standard angiography with CT would further simplify both the diagnosis and the follow-up of patients with massive embolism, entirely obviating the need for pulmonary catheterization.

10.9 Conclusion

Because of its high sensitivity and specificity in the detection of pulmonary thromboembolism, spiral CT can be reliably used in patients with clinically suspected acute thromboembolism. The role of this technique as a screening test depends on the future development of this technology.

If accurate and noninvasive detection of pulmonary embolism is demonstrated to be feasible routinely, the indications for spiral CT may be expected to expand dramatically, probably to the point of replacing $\dot{V}/\dot{Q}$ scintigraphy totally, and pulmonary angiography partially.

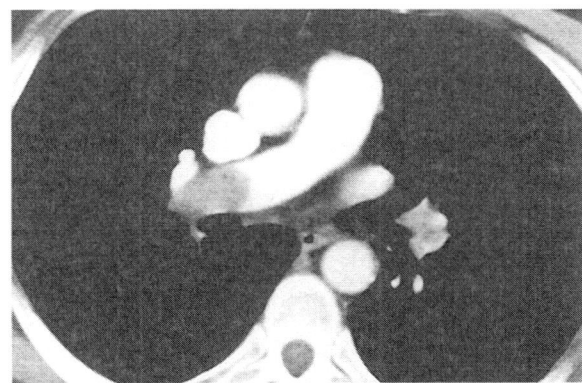
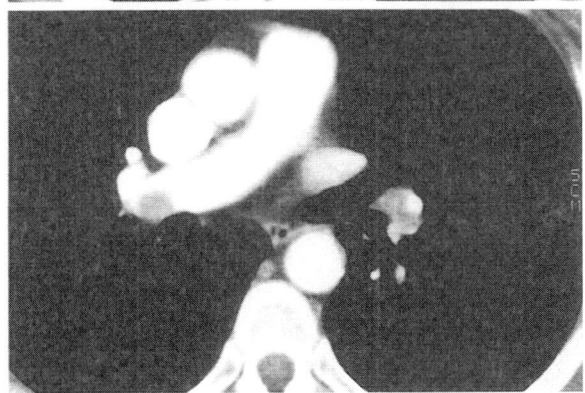

Fig. 10.18a,b. Spiral CT scans (5-mm collimation; 5 mm/s table feed) obtained in a 45-year-old man with dyspnea several weeks after heart trandsplantation (120 cc of 24% nonionic contrast agent; 5 cc/s; inspiratory apnea). **a** CT scan at the level of the bronchus intermedius reveals extensive clot within both interlobar arteries. **b** CT scan obtained at the same level as **a**, 48 h after the start of thrombolytic therapy. A considerable reduction is seen in the size of the right interlobar thrombus. Partial resolution of the left interlobar thrombus has occurred

References

Ashida C, Zerhouni EA, Fischman EK (1987) CT demonstration of prominent right hilar soft tissue collections. J Comput Assist Tomogr 11:57–59

Auger WR, Fedullo PF, Moser KM, Buchbinder M, Peterson KL (1992) Chronic major vessel thromboembolic pulmonary artery obstruction: appearance at angiography. Radiology 182:393–398

Blum AG, Delafau F, Grignon B et al. (1994) Spiral computed tomography versus pulmonary angiography in the diagnosis of acute massive pulmonary embolism. Am J Cardiol 74:96–98

Bookstein JJ, Silver TM (1974) The angiographic differential diagnosis of acute pulmonary embolism. Radiology 110: 25–33

Borrie J (1952) Primary carcinoma of the bronchus: prognosis following surgical resection. A clinicopathological study of 200 patients. Ann R Coll Surg Engl 10:165–186

Breatnach E, Stanley RJ (1984) CT diagnosis of segmental pulmonary artery embolus. J Comput Assist Tomogr 8:762–764

Breslaw BH, Dorfman GS, Noto RB et al. (1992) Ventilation/perfusion scanning for prediction of the location of pulmonary emboli: correlation with pulmonary angiographic findings. Radiology 185(P):180

Cauvain O, Rémy-Jardin M, Rémy J, Petyt L, Beregi JP, Steinling M, Duhamel A (1996) Tomodensitométrie par balayage spiralé volumique dans le diagnostic de l'embolie pulmonaire centrale. Rev Mal Resp 13:141–153

Chang CHJ, Zinn TW (1976) Roentgen recognition of enlarged lymph nodes: an antomical review. Radiology 120:291–296

Chintapelli K, Thorsen MK, Olson DL, Goodman LR, Gurney J (1988) Computed tomography of pulmonary thromboembolism and infarction. J Comput Assist Tomogr 12:553–559

Costello PH, Dupuy DE, Ecker CP, Tello R (1992) Spiral CT of the thorax with reduced volume of contrast material: a comparative study. Radiology 183:663–666

Curtin JJ, Mewissen MW, Crain MR, Lipchik RJ (1994) Postcontrast CT in the diagnosis and assessment of response to thrombolysis in massive pulmonary embolism. J Comput Assist Tomogr 18:133–135

Dalen JE (1993) When can treatment be withheld in patients with suspected pulmonary embolism? Commentary. Arch Intern Med 153:1415–1418

Di Carlo LA, Schiller NB, Herfkens RL, Brundage BH, Lipton MJ (1982) Noninvasive detection of proximal pulmonary artery thrombosis by two-dimensional echocardiography and computed tomography. Am Heart J 104:879–881

Falaschi F, Palla A, Formichi B et al. (1992) CT evaluation of chronic thromboembolic pulmonary hypertension. J Comput Assist Tomogr 16:897–903

Gabe IT, Gault JH, Ross JJ et al. (1969) Measurement of instantaneous blood flow velocity and pressure in conscious man with a catheter-tip velocity probe. Circulation 40:603–614

Geraghty JJ, Stanford W, Landas SK, Galvin JR (1992) Ultrafast computed tomography in experimental pulmonary embolism. Invest Radiol 27:60–63

Godwin JD, Webb WR, Gamsu G, Ovenfors CO (1980) Computed tomography of pulmonary embolism AJR 135:691–695

Goodman LR, Curtin JJ, Mewissen MW et al. (1995) Detection of pulmonary embolism in patients with unresolved clinical and scintigraphic diagnosis: helical CT versus angiography. AJR 164:1369–1374

Green JF (1977) Pressure-flow relationships of the pulmonary circulation. In: Green JF (ed) Mechanical concepts in cardiovascular and pulmonary physiology. Lea and Febiger, Philadelphia, pp 55–65

Gurney JW (1993) No fooling around: direct visualization of pulmonary embolism. Radiology 188:618–619

Hanson MW, Coleman RE (1989) Pulmonary nuclear medicine evaluation of thromboembolic disease. J Thorac Imaging 4:40–57

Howell JB, Permutt S, Proctor PF, Riley RL (1961) Effects of inflation of the lung on different parts of pulmonary vascular bed. J Appl Physiol 16:71–75

Hughes JM, Glazier JB, Maloney JE, West JB (1968) Effects of lung volume on the distribution of pulmonary blood flow in man. Respir Physiol 4:58–72

Hull RD, Hirsch J, Carter CJ et al. (1983) Pulmonary angiography, ventilation lung scanning, and venography for clinically suspected pulmonary embolism with abnormal perfusion lung scan. Ann Intern Med 98:891–899

Hull RD, Hirsch J, Carter CT et al. (1985) Diagnostic value of ventilation/perfusion lung scanning in patients with suspected pulmonary embolism. Chest 88:819–827

Jamali IN, McKay CR, Embrey RP, Galvin JR (1995) Electron beam computed tomography: use in pulmonary embolectomy. Ann Thorac Surg 59:1577–1579

Jardin M, Rémy J (1986) Bronchovascular segmental anatomy of the lower lobes: CT analysis. AJR 147:457–468

Kalebo P, Wallin J (1989) Computed tomography in massive pulmonary embolism. Acta Radiol 30:105–107

Kalender WA, Polacin A, Suss C (1994) A comparison of conventional and spiral CT: an experimental study on the detection of spherical lesions. J Comput Assist Tomogr 18:167–176

Kauczor HU, Schwickert HC, Mayer E, Schweden F, Schild HH, Thelen M (1994) Spiral CT of bronchial arteries in chronic thromboembolism. J Comput Assist Tomogr 1:855–861

King MA, Bergin CJ, Yeung DWC et al. (1994) Chronic pulmonary thromboembolism: detection of regional hypoperfusion with CT. Radiology 191:359–363

Lacrosse M, Trigaux JP, Van Beers BE, Weynants P (1995) 3D spiral CT of the tracheobronchial tree. J Comput Assist Tomogr 19:341–347

Loubeyre P, Revel D, Doueck P, Delignette A, Baldy C, Genin G, Amiel M (1994) Dynamic contrast-enhanced MR angiography of pulmonary embolism: comparison with pulmonary angiography. AJR 162:1035–1039

Moser KM (1990) Venous thromboembolism: state of the art. Am Rev Respir Dis 141:235–249

Nagaishi C (1972) Lymphatic system. In: Nagaishi C (ed) Functional anatomy and histology of the lung. University Park Press, Baltimore, pp 102–179

Napel SA (1995) Principles and techniques of 3D spiral CT angiography. In: Fischman EK, Jeffrey RB (eds) Spiral CT. Principles, techniques and clinical applications. Raven Press, New York, pp 167–182

Nohl HC (1972) An investigation of the anatomy of the lymphatic drainage of the lungs. Hunterian lecture. Ann R Coll Surg Engl 51:157–176

Novelline RA, Baltarowich OH, Athanasoulis CA, Waltman AC, Greenfield AJ, McKusick KA (1978) The clinical course of patients with suspected pulmonary embolism and a negative pulmonary arteriogram. Radiology 126:561–567

Osborne D, Vock P, Godwin JD, Silverman PM (1984) CT identification of bronchopulmonary segments: 50 normal subjects. AJR 142:47–52

Oser RF, Zuckerman DA, Guttierez FR, Brink JA (1994) Severity of pulmonary emboli at pulmonary angiography: implications for spiral and ultrafast CT (abstract). Radiology 193(P):352

Ovenfors CO, Batra P (1988) Diagnosis of peripheral pulmonary emboli by MR imaging: an experimental study in dogs. Magn Reson Imaging 6:487–491

Ovenfors CO, Godwin JD, Brito AC (1981) Diagnosis of peripheral emboli by computed tomography in the living dog. Radiology 141:519–523

PIOPED Investigators (1990) Value of the ventilation/perfusion scan in acute pulmonary embolism: results of the prospective investigation of pulmonary embolism diagnosis (PIOPED). JAMA 263:2753–2759

Polacin A, Kalender W, Marchal G (1992) Evaluation of section sensitivity profiles and image noise in spiral CT. Radiology 185:29–35

Porter J, Jick H (1977) Drug-related deaths among medical inpatients. JAMA 237:879–881

Quinn MF, Lundell CJ, Klotz TA et al. (1987) Reliability of selective pulmonary arteriography in the diagnosis of pulmonary embolism. AJR 149:469–471

Ralph DD (1994) Pulmonary embolism. The implications of prospective investigation of pulmonary embolism diagnosis. Radiol Clin North Am 32:679–687

Rémy-Jardin M, Deffontaines C, Rémy J (1991) Chest evaluation with spiral volumetric CT with single breath hold technique. Radiology 181(P):273

Rémy-Jardin M, Rémy J, Wattinne L, Giraud F (1992) Central pulmonary thromboembolism: diagnosis with spiral volumetric CT with the single breath hold technique. Comparison with pulmonary angiography. Radiology 185:381–387

Rémy-Jardin M, Duyck PH, Rémy J et al. (1995a) Spiral CT angiographic identification of hilar lymph nodes with pathologic-CT correlations. Radiology 196:387–394

Rémy-Jardin M, Rémy J, Cauvain O, Petyt L, Wannebroucq J, Beregi JP (1995b) Diagnosis of central pulmonary embolism with helical CT: role of two-dimensional multiplanar reformations. AJR 165:1131–1138

Rémy-Jardin M, Rémy J, Petyt L, Duhamel A, Marchandise X (1995c) Diagnosis of acute pulmonary embolism with spiral CT: comparison with pulmonary angiography and scintigraphy. Radiology 197(P):303

Riquet M (1992) Drainage lymphatique des segments pulmonaires chez le sujet adulte. Recherches basées sur 400 sujets. Thesis in Anatomy and Physiology, University of Paris V

Riquet M (1993) Anatomic basis of lymphatic spread from carcinoma of the lung to the mediastinum: surgical and prognostic implications. Surg Radiol Anat 15:1–7

Rouviere H (1929) Les vaisseaux lymphatiques des poumons et les ganglions viscéraux intrathoraciques. Ann Anat Pathol 6:113–158

Rubin GD, Jeffrey RB (1995) 3D Spiral CT angiography of the abdomen and thorax. In: Fischman EK, Jeffrey RB (eds) Spiral CT. Principles, techniques and clinical applications. Raven Press, New York, pp 183–195

Sagel SS, Greenspan RH (1970) Nonuniform pulmonary arterial perfusion. Pulmonary embolism. Radiology 99:541–548

Sarrazin R, Voog R, Dyon JF (1974) Contribution à l'étude des lymphatiques du poumon. Le Poumon et le Coeur 30:289–299

Schiebler ML, Holland GA, Hatabu H et al. (1993) Suspected pulmonary embolism: prospective evaluation with pulmonary MR angiography. Radiology 189:125–131

Schnyder P, Meuli R, Wicky S, Mayor B (1995) Injection techniques in helical CT of the chest. Eur Radiol (Suppl) 5:26

Schwickert HC, Schweden FJ, Schild HH et al. (1994) Pulmonary arteries and lung parenchyma in chronic pulmonary embolism: preoperative and postoperative CT findings. Radiology 191:351–357

Schwickert HC, Kauczor HE, Schweden FJ, Thelen M (1995) Mosaic oligemia in CT of patients with chronic pulmonary embolism: correlation with the diameter of the feeding pulmonary artery. Radiology 197(P):303

Senac JP, Verhnet H, Bousquet C et al. (1995) Embolie pulmonaire: apport de la tomodensitométrie hélicoïdale. J Radiol 76:339–345

Shah HR, Buckner B, Purcell GL, Walker CW (1989) Computed tomography and magnetic resonance imaging in the diagnosis of pulmonary thromboembolic disease. J Thorac Imaging 4:58–61

Silverman PM, Brown B, Wray H, Fox SH, Cooper C, Roberts S, Zeman RK (1995) Optimal contrast enhancement of the liver using helical (spiral) CT: value of Smartprep AJR 164:1169–1171

Sinner WN (1978) Computed tomographic patterns of pulmonary thromboembolism and infarction. J Comput Assist Tomogr 2:395–399

Sinner WN (1982) Computed tomography of pulmonary thromboembolism. Eur J Radiol 2:8–13

Sone S, Higashihara T, Morimoto S et al. (1983) CT anatomy of hilar lymphadenopathy. AJR 140:887–892

Sostman HD, Rapoport S, Gottschalk A, Greenspan RH (1986) Imaging of pulmonary embolism. Invest Radiol 21:443–454

Sostman HD, Debatin JF, Spritzer CE, Coleman RE, Grist TM, Mc Fall JR (1993a) MRI in venous thromboembolic disease. Eur Radiol 3:53–61

Sostman HD, MacFall JR, Foo TKF, Grist TM, Newman GE, Spritzer CE (1993b) Pulmonary arteries and veins. In: Potchen EJ, Haacke EM, Siebert JE, Gottschalk A (eds) Magnetic Resonance angiography: concepts and applications. Mosby, St. Louis, pp 546–572

Sostman HD, Coleman RE, Delong DM, Newman GE, Paine S (1994) Evaluation of the revised criteria for ventilation-perfusion scintigraphy in patients with suspected pulmonary embolism. Radiology 193:103–107

Spies WG, Burstein SP, Dillehay GL, Vogelzang RL, Spies SM (1986) Ventilation-perfusion scintigraphy in suspected pulmonary embolism: correlation with pulmonary angiography and refinement of criteria of interpretation. Radiology 159:383–390

Stanford W, Reiners TJ, Thompson BH, Landas SK, Galvin JR (1994) Contrast-enhanced thin slice ultrafast computed tomography for the detection of small pulmonary emboli: studies with autologous emboli in the pig. Invest Radiol 29:184–187

Stehling MK, Rosen MP, Weintrab J, Kim D, Raptopoulos V (1994) Spiral CT venography of the lower extremity. AJR 163:451–453

Stein PD, O'Connor JF, Dalen JE et al. (1967) The angiographic diagnosis of acute pulmonary embolism: evaluation of criteria. Am Heart J 73:730

Stein PD, Athanasoulis C, Alavi A et al. (1992) Complications and validity of pulmonary angiography in acute pulmonary embolism. Circulation 85:462–468

Stein PD, Henry JW, Gottschalk A (1993) Mismatched vascular defects. An easy alternative to mismatched segmental equivalent defects for the interpretation of ventilation/perfusion lung scans in pulmonary embolism. Chest 104:1468–1472

Tardivon AA, Musset D, Maitre S, Brenot F, Dartevelle PH, Simmonneau G, Labrune M (1993) Role of CT in chronic pulmonary embolism: comparison with pulmonary angiography. J Comput Assist Tomogr 17:345–351

Teigen CL, Maus TP, Sheedy PF II, Johnson CM, Stanson AW, Welch JJ (1993) Pulmonary embolism: diagnosis with electron beam CT. Radiology 188:839–845

Teigen CL, Maus TP, Sheedy PF II, Stanson AW, Johnson CM, Breen JF, McKusick MA (1995) Pulmonary embolism: diagnosis with contrast enhanced electron beam CT and comparison with pulmonary angiography. Radiology 194: 313–319

Van Rossum AB, Pattynama PM, Treurniet FE, Schpers R, Kieft GJ (1995) Spiral CT angiography for detection of pulmonary embolism: validation in 124 patients. Radiology 197(P):303

Vermiere P, Butler J (1968) Effect of respiration on pulmonary capillary blood flow in man. Circulation 22:299

Verschakelen JA, Vanwicijk E, Bogaert J, Baert AL (1993) Detection of unsuspected central pulmonary embolism with conventional contrast-enhanced CT. Radiology 188:847–850

White RD, Winkler ML, Higgins CB (1987) MR imaging of pulmonary arterial hypertension and pulmonary emboli. AJR 149:15–21

Woodard PK, Sostman HD, MacFall JR et al. (1995) Detection of pulmonary embolism: comparison of contrast-enhanced spiral CT and time-of-flight MR techniques. J Thorac Imaging 10:59–72

Woodring JH (1991) Pulmonary artery-bronchus ratios in patients with normal lungs, pulmonary plethora and congestive heart failure. Radiology 179:115–122

Worsley DF, Alasi A, Palevsky HI (1993) Role of radionuclide imaging in patients with suspected pulmonary embolism. Radiol Clin North Am 31:849–858

Yamashita H (1978) Anatomy of hilar lymph nodes. In: Yamashita H (ed) Roentgenologic anatomy of the lung. Thieme, Stuttgart, pp 31–34

11 Spiral CT Angiography of Pulmonary Vessels

J. RÉMY and M. RÉMY-JARDIN

CONTENTS

11.1 Introduction

Any technique that eliminates the artifacts from respiratory motion and optimizes intravenous contrast requirements is capable of replacing more invasive angiographic procedures. Minimal experience in spiral CT angiography is necessary to obtain a uniform and nearly constant opacification of intrathoracic vessels down to 2–3 mm in diameter with smaller volumes of contrast medium than those employed in conventional or digital routine angiography. A single breath hold of 15–20 s is easily obtained in most thoracic patients requiring a vascular study. Breath

holding at maximum inspiratory level is responsible for an increase in pulmonary vascular resistance. This explains why spiral CT angiography of the pulmonary vessels is of optimal contrast in 95% of patients, as a consequence of which spiral CT angiography of the chest is gaining widespread acceptance (NAIDICH 1994).

Due to the anatomical continuity of acquisition, high-quality multiplanar and three-dimensional images can be routinely obtained, and the radiologist has to be acquainted with these new modes of vessel visualization and to have the accompanying necessary basic knowledge in computer graphics.

The purpose of this chapter is to review the current indications for spiral CT angiography of the lung vessels. Unfortunately, this review is being written too soon in the users' experience to permit a rigorous comparative evaluation with both magnetic resonance angiography and transesophageal echocardiography. Further comparison between these modalities is mandatory and should be undertaken as soon as possible. The lack of numerous specific references to spiral CT articles in the bibliography of this chapter is hardly surprising. Although these references often refer to conventional or incremental CT, they can help the reader to extrapolate what could be achieved with spiral CT.

11.2 Pulmonary Arteriovenous Malformations

11.2.1 Clinical Signs

Pulmonary arteriovenous malformations (PAVMs) can be detected on clinical grounds and/or by familial screening in a population of patients with hereditary hemorrhagic telangiectasia (HHT). They can be incidentally discovered on the basis of morphological criteria as seen on chest x-ray, CT, magnetic resonance imaging (MRI), or pulmonary angiography.

Depending on the site of the rupture, massive hemoptysis, gaseous embolus, and hemothorax can

J. RÉMY, MD, Professor, Department of Radiology, Hospital Calmette, Boulevard Jules Leclerc, 59037 Lille Cedex, France
M. RÉMY-JARDIN, MD, PhD, Professor, Department of Radiology, Hospital Calmette, Boulevard Jules Leclerc, 59037 Lille Cedex, France

occur. FERENCE et al. (1994) reported these complications in 11 (8%) of 143 patients with HHT and PAVMs, including four men and seven women. Direct communication between a pulmonary artery and a pulmonary vein is responsible for a right to left shunt with hypoxemia, cyanosis, digital clubbing, and pulmonary bruit. Approximately two-thirds of the neurological symptoms in HHT are secondary to paradoxical embolism through PAVMs. This is one of the major reasons why a PAVM, whatever the circumstances of the diagnosis, must be detected, thereby avoiding the risks of a cerebral abscess or stroke. The majority of PAVMs, symptomatic or not, should be treated noninvasively. A decision between surgery and embolotherapy is required. Embolization or, more precisely, vaso-occlusion is the first treatment to be considered (ROBERTSON and ROBERTSON 1995).

11.2.2 Anatomical and Physiological Basis for Spiral CT Acquisition and Injection Techniques

Hypoxemia triggers polycythemia and a high cardiac output at rest and on exercise. It should be taken into account before the calculation of the amount of contrast medium, flow rate, and start delay required for the helical acquisition of the volume of interest. Breath hold at maximum inspiratory volume increases the pulmonary vascular resistance of the normal lung. The vascular resistance through PAVMs is lower than in the surrounding normal lung. Consequently, pulmonary blood flow and injected contrast medium are preferentially distributed toward the PAVMs. This steal effect generates a high flow through the PAVM and progressive enlargement of the feeding artery and draining vein. Conversely, the low flow through normal arterial branches is responsible for their decrease in size. This difference in diameter between normal and abnormal vessels is more striking in the subpleural parts of the lung than in the perihilar region. Thus, a tiny PAVM located subpleurally can be detected despite the absence of a large aneurysmal sac because its feeding artery and draining vein often have a diameter larger than the surrounding normal pulmonary vessels.

In close correlation with the vascular anatomy of the lung, the arterial pedicles of PAVMs of the apical part of the upper lobes are situated lateral to the draining veins. The arterial pedicles of PAVMs of the right middle lobe are superior to the draining veins.

The arterial pedicles of PAVMs located in the lower lobes are anterior, lateral, and posterior to the draining veins according to their anterior, lateral, and posterior segmental distribution. More than 80% of PAVMs are situated in the lung bases. This is probably correlated with the higher vascular pressures and the waterfall principle of the pulmonary perfusion when sitting and standing. The respiratory motions of the basal lung are very ample. As a consequence basal PAVMs can escape detection when an incremental discontinuous CT acquisition is performed, given the lack of reproducibility of the same inspiratory level at each breath hold.

11.2.3 Spiral CT Detection

Conventional CT has already proved useful and highly sensitive for the detection of PAVMs (RÉMY et al. 1992b) but it suffers from false-negative results due to variations in respiratory depth, partial volume averaging effects, and motion artifacts. Diaphragmatic motions of 10 cm maximum can occur between inspiration and expiration. These problems are completely overcome by using spiral CT within a single breath hold. In a group of 39 patients, a prospective study comparing conventional and spiral 10-mm slices without overlapping was undertaken (RÉMY-JARDIN et al. 1993). In this group of patients, CT was required for the pretherapeutic evaluation of solitary pulmonary nodules, metastases, and PAVMs. Despite the suboptimal acquisition and reconstruction protocol, 497 and 705 nodules were found with conventional and spiral CT, respectively. The mean number of nodules per patient was significantly higher with spiral CT (mean, 18 ± 4.5) than with conventional CT (mean ± SD, 12.6 ± 3.2). In comparison with conventional CT, spiral CT detected a greater number of nodules of less than 10 mm in diameter.

Technical refinements have recently been introduced by KALENDER et al. (1994). They demonstrated that the degradation of the slice sensitivity profile in spiral CT was outweighed by the images available for any table position in the volume of interest. They showed that images should be calculated at least in 2- to 3-mm increments for 5-mm collimation, or two to four images per nominal slice width. They emphasized that as the degree of degradation of the ideal rectangular shape is increased with the selected pitch, the contrast of every tiny lesion is reduced due to the partial volume effect. The only way of reducing this artifact, which may even lead to the disappearance of micronodules, is to calculate a large number of overlapping images, at least in the suspected areas, to decrease the computation time and increase the number of images generated. They also underlined that calculation of one image per slice width, as previously observed in a clinical study (RÉMY-JARDIN et al. 1993), compromises the inherent advantage of spiral CT.

Variable mode helical CT consists in using four helical acquisitions with 6-s delays and a biphasic injection of contrast medium (TOMIAK et al. 1995). The major disadvantage of this technique is the potential misregistration of adjacent spiral groups, leading to the risk of undetected PAVMs or to mistakes in the analysis of angioarchitecture.

A new reconstruction technique – the "sliding thin-slab maximum intensity projection" (STS-MIP) technique – has recently been published (NAPEL et al. 1993). It is generally applied at second intention after an initial screening scan, using 5- or 8-mm slice thickness with a pitch of 1 (5/5) or greater than 1 (16/8 or 12/8 or 8/5) according to the patient's size and ability to suspend respiration without discomfort. If a submillimetric lesion is suspected of being a tiny PAVM, a second acquisition is performed. A 1-, 2-, or 3-mm collimation is selected to scan the precisely defined volume of interest. A slab of three, five, and eight thin slices is performed and sliding into this subvolume is automatically or manually performed. On individual thin sections, vessels perpendicular and oblique to the plane of the CT section appear fragmented as rounded or elliptical structures. Their connection to the same vessel on other slices is not very obvious, particularly in the lung, where the vascular profusion is very dense. This vascular anatomy, difficult to comprehend from isolated transverse CT sections, is greatly improved when using STS-MIP, which computes overlapping MIPs of limited depth in order to improve vessel coherence. As previously pointed out (NAPEL et al. 1993), it represents a compromise between spatially paging up and down through the optimal volume and an MIP of the entirety of this acquired volume including more MIP artifacts and superimposed normal vessels not belonging to the malformation.

In contrast to what can be seen with solid organs, the high gradient of attenuation between the intraparenchymal vessels and the normal surrounding lung does not justify the systematic use of contrast material for diagnosis of PAVMs, in particular for tiny lesions. Consequently, one of the limitations of MIP (namely, the increase in mean background responsible for the potential loss of blood vessel defini-

tion) does not apply to STS-MIP of intrapulmonary microfistulas of 1 or 2 mm in diameter.

The potential detection power of CT, including conventional and spiral CT, was compared with unilateral pulmonry angiography by RÉMY et al. (1992b). Forty-two PAVMs (38.5%) were detected with CT only. This result indicates the superiority of CT over pulmonary angiography in the diagnosis of the tiniest vascular malformations. We can extrapolate that better results will be obtained with spiral CT, which is the only CT screening procedure expected to increase further the number of detected PAVMs.

Two-dimensional contrast echocardiography proved to be an excellent technique for the identification of a right-to-left shunt (BARZILAI et al. 1991). After an intravenous peripheral injection of agitated saline solution or of a mixture of saline solution and a small amount of air, microcavitations are seen in the left atrium with a delay time depending on the shunt localization (namely cardiac or pulmonary). However, attention must be drawn to the fact that a small bulla of air trapped in an angiographic catheter can be the source of EKG modifications during vasoocclusive treatment of a PAVM. Moreover, a transitory cerebral accident may occur following bubble contrast ultrasonography (RÉMY 1995, unpublished personal data). In addition, definite conclusions regarding the sensitivity of two-dimensional contrast echocardiography cannot be drawn from previous investigations because pulmonary angiography, until now the gold standard technique for the detection of PAVMs, is not always performed in patients with HHT and negative echocardiography. Moreover, this technique cannot determine the number of PAVMs, their location in the lung, or their size.

Very interesting publications have recently appeared concerning measurements of arterial oxygen saturation (SaO_2), estimation of the anatomical intrapulmonary shunt by measurements of arterial PaO_2 and hemoglobin after breathing of 100% oxygen for 15 min, and intravenous injection of technetium-99 m labelled albumin macroaggregates or microspheres (UEKI et al. 1994; WHYTE et al. 1992). Despite being able to detect and quantify right-to-left shunting, these techniques suffer from the same drawbacks as those cited for echocardiography. Consequently, they can be routinely used in HHT families for the detection of PAVMs (WHITE et al. 1992), but not for the detection and pretherapeutic evaluation of these malformations.

Magnetic resonance imaging using a combination of spin-echo, gradient recalled echo (GRE) cine, and 2D phase contrast cine sequences has recently been applied to the evaluation of PAVMs (SILVERMAN JM et al. 1994). In their discussion, the authors underlined as efficacious a noninvasive imaging modality able to visualize lesions greater than 2 cm in diameter as "PAVMs less than or equal to 2 cm in size usually do not lead to symptoms such as cerebral stroke or abscess." By contrast, WHITE and POLLAK (1994) stated that all PAVMs with a feeding artery measuring 3 mm or larger in diameter should be occluded because, in their experience, the arterial diameter through which a paradoxical embolus was able to pass and cause clinical stroke ranged from 2.9 to 4.6 mm. The smallest vascular malformation detected by SILVERMAN et al.'s MRI sequences was 1 cm.

11.2.4 Angioarchitecture

According to WHITE et al. (1983), there are two types of PAVMs. The simple type (80%) consists of a single feeding artery connected to the aneurysmal sac, which is drained by a single vein. From a therapeutic point of view, a PAVM draining into several veins should also be considered as a simple malformation when the endovascular treatment of such a malformation can be achieved by the occlusion of a single feeding artery, whether or not it divides into several smaller branches connected to the aneurysmal sac. A complex PAVM (20%) consists of two or more feeding arteries, their definitive number being optimally appreciated following successful cure by vasoocclusion. Surprisingly, the findings of HAITJEMA et al. (1995) were the reverse of those of WHITE et al.'s earlier study, since 20% of their PAVMs were simple while 80% were complex.

For diagnostic purposes, spiral CT of the entire thorax is performed, while for a pretherapeutic evaluation, a more sophisticated selective acquisition of the PAVM to be treated is performed, including the aneurysmal sac and vascular pedicles. The main technical aspects can be summarized as follows: The slice collimation depends on the location of the malformation: PAVMs with vertically oriented pedicles can require a collimation of up to 10 cm. Acquisitions can be obtained within a 22-s breath hold when choosing a 5-mm section thickness and a 5 mm/s table feed (i.e., a pitch of 1). The breath-hold duration or the slice thickness can be reduced when selecting a pitch of greater than 1. Despite the fact that it enables acquisition of a larger volume, a wider collimation should be avoided as it compromises spatial resolution. When a PAVM and its vascular

pedicles are horizontally oriented, 4–5 cm of the thorax is surveyed with a 2- to 3-mm collimation and a 2–3 mm/s table feed. This subvolume of interest is visualized and, on the transverse CT scans, a region of interest is traced over a representative single slice. The top of this region is selected so that the vessels of interest are situated within the center of the volume. From the CT data, an angiogram-like three-dimensional reformation can be obtained using surface and volumetric rendering techniques, generating shaded surface displays (3D-SSDs) and maximum intensity projections (MIPs) respectively. For 3D-SSDs, the thresholding segmentation is selected so that the unenhanced vascular malformation is depicted. The threshold values range from −600 to −700 HU.

In a group of a few PAVMs, 3D reformations of the malformations acquired with and without contrast medium were unable to show differences in angioarchitecture that could be taken into account in their management (Fig. 11.1). Should contrast medium be used, the thresholding segmentation has to be changed from −700 HU to +100 HU to +150 HU. The low vascular resistance of a PAVM enables its preferential enhancement at the expense of the surrounding normal pulmonary arterial branches. Small vessels in the acquired volume can be seen with apparent discontinuity in their course when too high a threshold is selected, which can create artificial holes, gaps, atresias, and stenoses. In such cases, an additional 3D display is systematically performed with a lower thresholding segmentation (−850 HU). This lower threshold markedly increases the profusion of vessels in the volume and creates a complex vascular background which may prevent optimal viewing of the malformation. This is the reason why a reconstruction with a lower threshold is not systematically performed but only when the cross-sectional images depict a small vessel suspected of participating in the PAVM. As previously pointed out, an MIP image can also be generated from the same data acquisition. Unless the cine loop technique is used, analysis of MIP images may be confusing since crossing and looping vessels are not correctly identified. In the pretherapeutic evaluation of PAVMs, 3D-SSDs with or without contrast medium seem to provide similar information to that obtained with 3D-MIPs with or without contrast medium (RÉMY, personal unpublished data).

The generated 3D images are oriented in the optimal viewing angles chosen according to the orientation of the pedicles and the superimpositions seen on

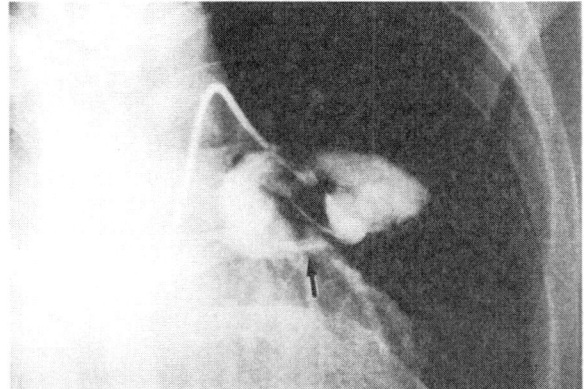
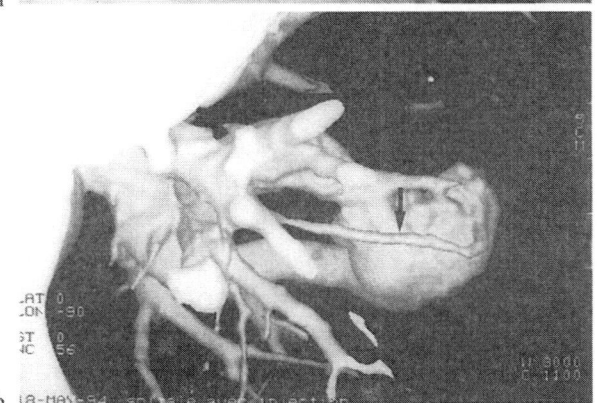
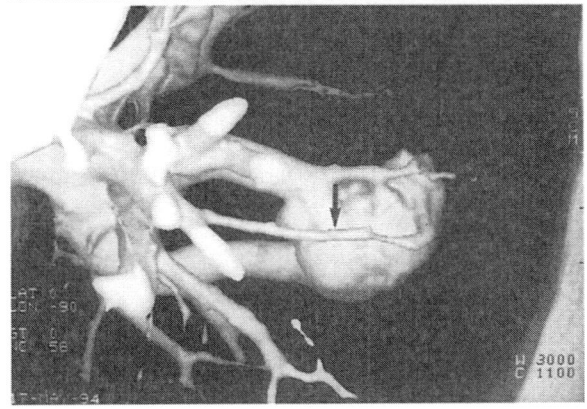

Fig. 11.1. PAVM of the anterobasal segment of the left lower lobe evaluated with hyperselective angiography (**a**) and 3D-SSD with (**b**) and without (**c**) contrast medium. (**b**: collimation, 3 mm; table feed, 5 mm/s; overlapping, 2 mm; 56 slices used for the reconstruction; 120 ml of a 240 mg/ml iodinated contrast agent; flow rate, 5 ml/s; 20-G needle in the antecubital vein; **c**: collimation, 3 mm; table feed, 3 mm/s; overlapping, 1 mm; 58 slices used for the reconstruction). According to its spatial position in the diseased volume, the small draining vein is better identified on the inferosuperior views of the 3D-SSDs (see *arrow* on **a–c**) than on the frontal view of the angiogram. No difference was observed between the 3D-SSD with (**b**) and that without (**c**) contrast medium, obtained with the same single thresholding segmentation (–400 HU)

the console. The superoinferior and inferosuperior viewing angles are the best for horizontally oriented PAVMs. For a vertically oriented PAVM the viewing angle depends on its situation: the posteroanterior view enables one to clearly depict a PAVM located in the posterobasal segments whereas the anteroposterior view is adopted for PAVMs situated in the anterobasal segments. When the angioarchitecture of a given PAVM cannot be confidently analyzed owing to the presence of numerous vessels located above or below the lesion of interest, one can stack a limited number of images in order to simplify the anatomical surroundings. However, such a simplification increases the risk of causing an artifactual reduction in the number of feeding arteries to be found and thus excluding an abnormal vessel.

In a group of patients previously reported (RÉMY et al. 1994), the value of 3D reconstructions and of pulmonary angiography was compared. As expected, it was found that unilateral and selective pulmonary angiography could still be considered the gold standard for the analysis of PAVM angioarchitecture. This technique does, however, suffer from several drawbacks: Whatever the viewing angle chosen, unilateral angiography is often unable to visualize tiny PAVMs owing to their superimposition on larger vessels. Conversely, too selective an injection can omit additional arteries. A prospective evaluation of spiral CT with an interpretation of the cross-sectional images alone depicted 87% of the PAVMs (RÉMY et al. 1994). A simultaneous analysis of transverse contiguous images and 3D reformations enables accurate evaluation of PAVM angioarchitecture in 95% of the cases. Both imaging modalities yield information which is not accessible with a single imaging modality.

A few limitations of 3D images can be encountered. A perihilar location of a malformation is quite rare, but when its vascular pedicles are as large as the surrounding normal arteries and veins, they can be hidden and attempts to suppress undesirable structures cannot be correctly handled by targeting a subvolume or by automatic volume editing. An inadequate selection of the volume of interest and/or of thresholding segmentation is easily avoided by a careful interpretation of the cross-sectional images. Regardless of the computed projection technique used, the individual slices represent the essential basis for interpretation. Insight into the MIP images is required to understand them. In this context it is strongly recommended that the reader turns to the book chapter by SIEBERT and ROSENBAUM (1993) on

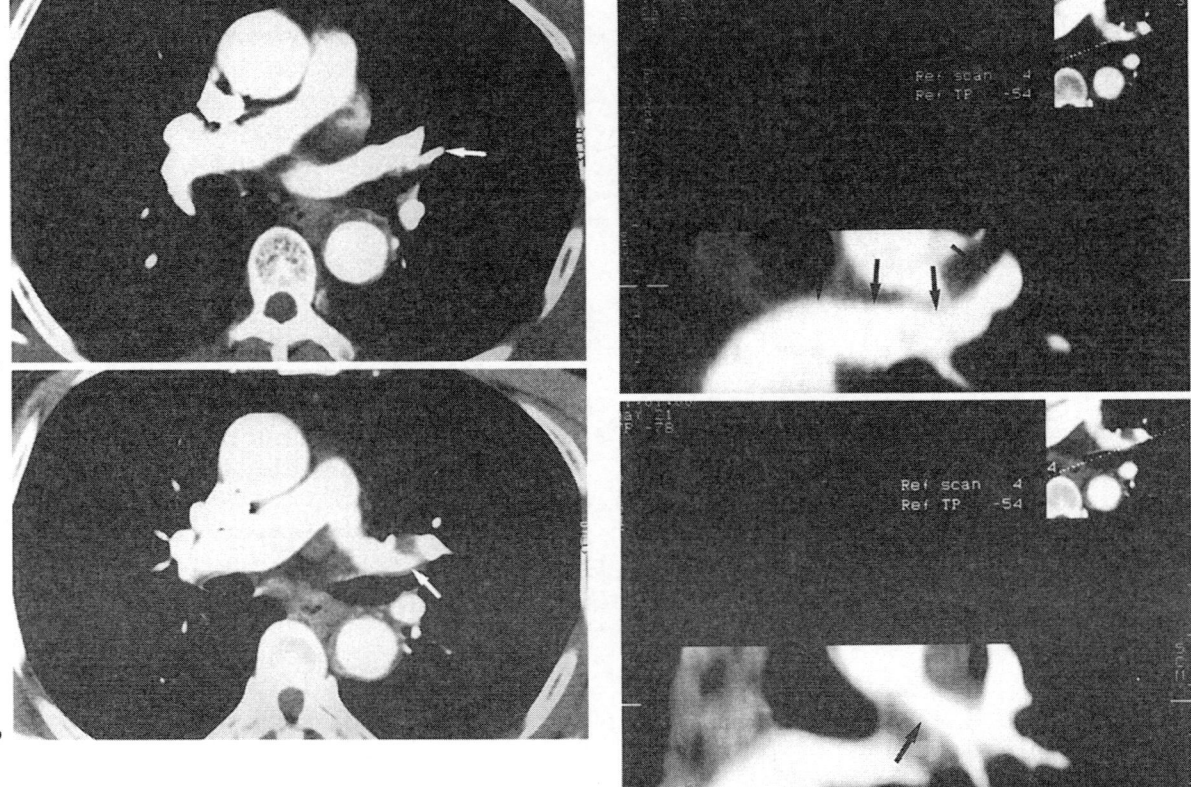

Fig. 11.2a–d. Preoperative spiral CT angiography of a right lower lobe bronchial carcinoma (collimation, 3 mm; table feed, 3 mm/s; overlapping, 1 mm; acquisition time, 12 s; 120 ml of a 300 mg/ml iodinated contrast agent; flow rate, 5 ml/s; start delay, 15 s; antecubital vein). The lingular artery (**a**, *arrow*) is seen emerging between the left superior pulmonary vein anteriorly and the left upper lobe bronchus posteriorly. Its origin from the concavity of the left pulmonary artery arch (**b**, *arrow*) is unusual. Oblique coronal reformats of the left hilum, parallel to the upper lobe bronchus, enable depiction of the relationships between the left superior pulmonary vein anteriorly (**c**, *arrows*) and the origin of the lingular artery posteriorly (**d**, *arrow*)

image presentation and postprocessing, in which the properties of MIP images are discussed.

Another interesting facet of spiral CT is the fascinating improvement that it makes possible in our knowledge of the vascular anatomy of the lung. The first step in this direction was the introduction of conventional CT, which led to an improvement in our knowledge of cross-sectional segmental anatomy (JARDIN and RÉMY 1986). Apart from the usual bronchovascular patterns, several variants have already been identified on transverse CT scans though they have not yet been extensively reviewed. As an example, difficulties in the selective catheterization of an ectopic artery can be predicted prior to the angiographic study on the basis of the information shown on transverse CT scans and multiplanar reformations (MPRs) (Fig. 11.2).

Some insights into the near future of 3D and 2D imaging can be applied to PAVMs. A volume of data can be used for the extraction of quantitative information. Recruitment of voxels after segmentation is a simple way to measure vascular sections and aneurysmal volume before and after endovascular treatment. As emphasized by ZONNEVELD (1994), segmentation is the logical successor to the classic volume calculation techniques. But, as previously underlined, the selection of a threshold affects the diameter of the resulting 3D object. Different windowing levels can also modify the diameter on axial slices. Therefore, when precise calculation of the diameter of a feeding artery is required in order to choose the optimal coil, these measurements must be regarded with extreme caution.

The data can be used for physical models. One of the latest developments is "stereolithography," which is mainly dedicated to rapid prototyping in industry. One can reasonably imagine a PAVM produced for surgical purposes or for medical students and resident teaching. Virtual endovascular navigation is also conceivable, as is endoscopic visualization of tubular organs (HAWKES et al. 1995).

11.2.5 Follow-up

Arterial blood gases, contrast echocardiography, microsphere scintigraphy, chest x-ray, and/or spiral CT of the chest are the most commonly used techniques in the posttherapeutic follow-up of PAVMs (WHITE and POLLACK 1994; WHITE 1992; WHYTE et al. 1992; UEKI et al. 1994; CHILVERS et al. 1990). Among these, only spiral CT follow-up will be of specific concern in the present chapter, where we shall consider the experience gathered in the follow-up of 102 PAVMs treated by endovascular coil deposition between 1979 and 1994 (RÉMY et al., personal unpublished data).

11.2.5.1 Acquisition Parameters

The follow-up of treated PAVMs entails a focal spiral CT acquisition with or without contrast medium injection. The acquisition parameters are similar to those applied before treatment and the injection techniques are similar to those used for spiral CT evaluation of pulmonary thromboembolic disease (see Chap. 10).

Several months after treatment, most treated PAVMs have completely collapsed (95/102 in our series). The aneurysmal sac is reduced to a micronodule. The pulmonary venous return is regularly reduced in diameter. The coils are responsible for minimal streak artifacts which do not compromise the quality of the reformatted images. The feeding artery has a tiny diameter above and beyond the scaffolded coils. It is not known how long it takes to reach this discrepancy in diameter, which may be expected to be proportionate to the reduction of flow through the feeding pedicle. This finding also emphasizes the inability of the coils to move belatedly (HAITJEMA et al. 1995).

11.2.5.2 Missed Feeding Artery

A PAVM considered to display simple angioarchitecture on the basis of angiographic and/or spiral CT angiographic data can prove to be a complex one. Such a discrepancy can be explained by the domination of a large feeding artery, which can cause a smaller arterial branch to be overlooked at the time of initial evaluation. In such instances, occlusion of the large feeding artery only results in a minimal aneurysal sac retraction. It is temporarily underperfused, it shrinks, and the draining vein or veins decrease in diameter. Further development of the previously undetectable arterial branch becomes evident. This sequence of events, also reported by HAITJEMA et al. (1995), depicts a particular association between a complete collapse of the feeding artery, a minimal aneurysmal collapse, and a persistent dilatation of the pulmonary venous return.

Very exceptionally, after a technically successful vaso-occlusion, delayed recanalization of the occluded pulmonary artery occurs (Rémy-Jardin et al. 1991b).

11.2.5.3 Systemic Collateral Supply to a Treated PAVM

Systemic collateral supply to a PAVM has been well known for a long time. Rarely, the systemic supply can be predominant and takes the place of the feeding pulmonary artery. When the pulmonary artery inflow is interrupted by vaso-occlusion, this systemic supply can develop. Such a sequence of morphological changes in the case of a treated PAVM was reported in one patient 3 years after a successful vaso-occlusion of a simple PAVM located in the inferior segment of the lingula (RÉMY et al. 1994). In comparison with the pretherapeutic CT evaluation, transverse CT scans and 3D reconstructions showed a dramatic reduction in the size of the feeding artery but persistence of a large draining vein and a minimally collapsed aneurysmal sac. Development of a preexisting or a posttreatment systemic supply to a vaso-occluded PAVM turns a right-to-left shunt into a left-to-right shunt. This is why arterial blood gas determination, contrast echocardiography, and microsphere scintigraphy cannot confidently assess the healing of a treated PAVM.

Approximately 10% of the patients treated have a self-limited pleural effusion which can be followed by pleural adhesions favoring a transpleural supply to the lung from systemic vessels. The same mechanism may be involved as a response to local resection (LAFFEY et al. 1985). Consequently, as much after partial surgery as after vaso-occlusion, the potential for development of systemic supply provides an argument for the pulmonary and systemic phases of spiral CT injection techniques.

11.2.5.4 Pulmonary Venous Reflux

After a pulmonary embolic event and in the case of persisting chronic embolic obstruction of a lobar artery, it is common to see a narrowing of the segmental and subsegmental arteries of the same lobe in conjunction with normal size and opacification of the corresponding intersegmental pulmonary veins. Two possible explanations can be given for these morphological findings: (a) the systemic circulation supplies the pulmonary arterial bed beyond the coils and drains into the pulmonary veins in a similar way to that frequently demonstrated in chronic thromboembolic disease; (b) there is retrograde opacification of the pulmonary veins from the left atrium, as previously observed on pulmonary angiograms. An experimental counterpart of the latter explanation was nicely demonstrated in a study in the goat by OBERMILLER et al. (1991), in which the excretion of an insoluble inert gas, introduced into the left atrium without bronchial or pulmonary blood flow, was measured during changes in lung volume and left atrial pressure. Spiral CT acquisition is performed at maximum lung volumes, and according to OBERMILLER et al.'s study, increased lung volumes augment effective reverse flow from the left atrium to the pulmonary capillaries. This supply explains why the lung does not suffer from ischemic damage when the pulmonary circulation is obstructed. Spiral CT and 3D CT angiography with contrast medium can demonstrate the sequence of events in pulmonary venous reflux, including a complete obstruction of the feeding artery, the absence of any additional pulmonary and/or systemic supply, and the reduction in size of both the aneurysmal sac and the draining vein.

11.2.5.5 Pleural and Parenchymal Changes

Pleural and parenchymal changes are not particularly relevant to spiral CT technology but they can be depicted on lung images which are generated from the same data set as is used for spiral CT angiography.

11.2.5.5.1 Parenchymal Changes. Within a few days to a few months, a pleuritic chest pain can reveal a pulmonary infarct ipsilateral to the arterial occlusion. The corresponding CT findings may consist of an area of ground glass attenuation, an airspace consolidation, or an excavated pulmonary nodule. These lesions are very often small, in correlation with the subsegmental or more distal deposition of the coils. Spiral CT acquisition can help one to follow the usual spontaneous healing of such parenchymal lesions. In asymptomatic patients, parenchymal abnormalities sometimes can be identified on follow-up CT scans. They have been described as segmental or subsegmental infiltrates and/or pleura-based nodules usually depicted distal to the PAVM (RÉMY-JARDIN et al. 1991b).

11.2.5.5.2 Pleural Changes. Pleural fluid, pleural thickening, and subpleural micronodules can appear.

11.3 Hemoptysis of Pulmonary Arterial Origin

Hemoptysis of pulmonary arterial origin is quite rare, representing approximately 5% of cases of bronchial bleeding treated by an endovascular approach. The mechanisms of bleeding have been demonstrated by pathological studies and angiographic findings (RÉMY et al. 1984). They are summarized in the following sections.

11.3.1 Bronchial Necrotizing Process

The necrotizing process of a bronchus can erode the accompanying pulmonary artery. It can be acute or chronic. Several examples of diseased bronchus perforating an initially normal pulmonary artery can be found in the literature. The prototype of a chronic disease is bronchial carcinoma, which can erode the pulmonary artery either because of its necrotizing potential or because of additional treatment-related necrotizing factors such as external or endobronchial radiation (KHANAVKAR et al. 1991).

Typical of an acute bronchial destructive process is invasive aspergillosis. The spectrum of this entity is expanding: one type is the well-known angio-invasive aspergillosis, and another is invasive aspergillosis of the airways based on identification of organisms located deeper than the basement membrane of bronchi or bronchioles (LOGAN et al. 1994).

The precise relationship between these two types has not yet been clearly defined. Different aspects of tracheobronchial aspergillosis have been reported depending on the depth of invasion of the bronchial wall (KRAMER et al. 1991; DENNING 1995). Surprisingly, there are numerous radiological descriptions of invasive aspergillosis (GEFTER 1992; BLUM et al. 1994) but few of them emphasize the potential value of spiral CT angiography in the therapeutic evaluation of *cavitating* invasive aspergillosis, which has become an increasingly frequent cause of mortality

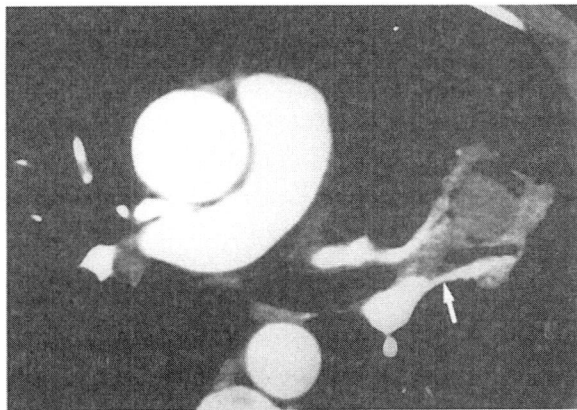

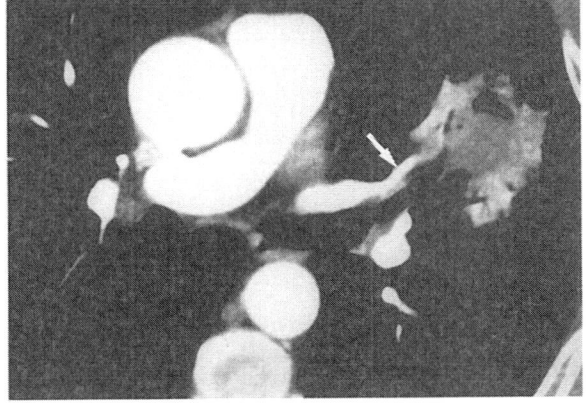

Fig. 11.3a,b. Invasive aspergillosis in an immunosuppressed leukemic patient (collimation, 3 mm; table feed, 5 mm/s; overlapping, 1 mm; 100 ml of a 240 mg/ml iodinated contrast agent injected via a central venous catheter; flow rate, 5 ml/s; start delay, 12 s). An excavated lesion is in close contact with the superior segmental lingular bronchus. The accompanying artery (**a**, *arrow*) courses along the posterior bronchial wall. The corresponding vein (**b**, *arrow*) is also in close contact with the cavity. Fiberoptic endoscopy performed during active hemoptysis showed the bleeding coming from the lingular bronchus. Due to the close contact between the cavity and the superior segmental lingular vein, embolization of the lingular artery was discounted and a left upper lobectomy was performed

in immunosuppressed hematological patients (Fig. 11.3). Once cavitation develops, the risk of massive hemoptysis arises (KIBBLER et al. 1988). Unfortunately, the precise mechanisms and origins of bleeding are seldom reviewed. YOUNG et al. (1992) postulated that bronchial bleeding could originate from intercostal arteries. GEFTER (1992) discusses the mycotic invasion and thrombosis of a pulmonary arterial branch which often occurs in association with the angioinvasive form of aspergillosis, and draws attention to large-vessel invasion by intravascular growth of hyphae affecting the aorta, the central pulmonary arteries, and even coronary arteries. A case of fatal hemorrhage during bronchoscopy in a patient with necrosis extending from the bronchus intermedius into the right pulmonary artery has been reported (BERLINGER and FREEMAN 1989). The authors emphasized the risk of misleading detection of endobronchial mycetomas "depending on the size of the interval between CT slices." Spiral CT angiography can be of value in the avoidance of endoscopic manipulation of suspected invasive aspergillosis of the airways in areas adjacent to vascular structures. In another patient, reported by KATZ et al. (1994), the extension of fungus through the wall of the descending aorta from a consolidation of the superior segment of the left lower lobe was responsible for death.

The crucial period of bleeding corresponds to the time immediately following recovery of granulocytes, especially the days following cavity and air crescent formation (ALBELDA et al. 1985). In bleeding patients or whenever the disease is focalized, a surgical therapeutic option can be discussed. Spiral CT can provide useful information by showing the location of the disease, the cavity size, and the vascular relationships of the cavities. This can help plan the surgical approach, which may consist of wedge resection, segmentectomy, lobectomy, or chest wall resection (TEMECK et al. 1994; ROBINSON et al. 1995).

11.3.2 Parenchymal Necrosis

Acute or chronic parenchymal necrosis can erode a neighboring pulmonary artery. Tuberculosis is the main cause of Rasmüssen's aneurysms. As previously emphasized, Rasmüssen's pseudo-aneurysms can receive simultaneous perfusion from a pulmonary artery and a bronchial artery (RÉMY et al. 1984). Multiple aneurysms are extremely rare (SANTELLI et al. 1994). Spiral CT angiography can demonstrate an enhancing mass adjacent to a pulmonary artery. Using 3D and multiplanar reformations, pretherapeutic evaluation of the lesion can obviate the need for more invasive pulmonary angiography before treatment. Any pulmonary abscess, whether acute or chronic, can also erode a pulmonary arterial branch and thus cause minor hemoptysis. Sometimes, patients can experience massive bleeding; this is mainly observed in cases of subacute and chronic cavities, as with tuberculosis. It should be emphasized that a lung abscess is a neglected cause of massive bleeding (PHILPOTT et al. 1993).

To summarize, in patients with tuberculosis, invasive mycoses, abscesses, or excavated lung carcinoma the vascular relationships of a cavity must be carefully investigated with spiral CT angiography, especially in the following three circumstances: (a) whenever an intracavitary mural nodule is detected, (b) in the presence of bronchial bleeding due to an erosive process in the lung parenchyma, whatever the amount of bleeding, and (c) when the cavity is in close contact with a vessel, such as a pulmonary artery or vein, or a mediastinal or chest wall vessel.

11.3.3 Perforation of a Pulmonary Artery

A perforating process of a pulmonary artery can erode an initially normal bronchus.

11.3.3.1 Mycotic Pulmonary Artery Aneurysms

Spiral CT angiography can play the same role as reported in PAVMs. Three-dimensional (3D) surface rendering reconstructions and 3D MIPs are able to identify precisely the relationships of the aneurysmal sac with the artery to be occluded (DONDELINGER et al. 1995), the number of aneurysms, the spatial orientation, and the diameter of the arteries before catheterization.

11.3.3.2 Behçet's Disease

The most common cause of vasculitides-related pulmonary artery aneurysms is Behçet's disease, which is characterized by periarterial or transmural lymphocytic plasma cells and neutrophilic infiltration, mucoid degeneration of the media, and intimal thickening of the larger elastic arteries. Pulmonary vascular involvement of Behçet's disease consists of thromboembolic complications, aneurysms, pulmonary infarcts, hemoptysis, and pulmonary hemorrhage (Do et al. 1990). Aneurysms and thrombotic complications can also occur at the site of venous or arterial puncture, leading one to avoid angiography whenever possible. Recently, TUNACI et al. (1995) have published a review article on thoracic involvement in this disease. The more invasive conventional or digital angiography, with the greater accompanying risks, can be avoided by using spiral CT angiography in the pretherapeutic evaluation and follow-up of pulmonary aneurysms and hemoptysis due to their rupture or fissuration. Additionally, MR angiography without the injection of contrast material can obviate the risk for thrombosis that accompanies a venous puncture. Spiral CT and/or MR angiography are also able to demonstrate involvement of other thoracic vessels, in particular the superior vena cava (AHN et al. 1995).

11.3.3.3 Takayasu's Disease

Takayasu's disease is an arteritis of unknown cause which commonly affects the pulmonary arteries. Using pulmonary angiography, YAMADA et al. (1992) found the upper lobe pulmonary branches to be more frequently involved than the lower lobe branches. The segmental and subsegmental arteries are the most frequent level of arterial involvement. Stenotic or occlusive lesions of the segmental arteries are supplied by collateral systemic arteries responsible for systemic-to-pulmonary artery shunts and enlargement of the pulmonary artery beyond its occlusion. These findings are explained by the development of vascular channels within the occluded pulmonary artery (the "vessel-in-vessel" appearance). Spiral CT is also able to suggest the presence of coronary artery-to-pulmonary artery collaterals by showing enlarged proximal coronary branches which are better identified on selective coronary angiograms (SHARMA et al. 1993). PARK et al. (1995) recently reported an interesting approach to the disease activity in the pulmonary artery and aortic walls using spiral CT angiography. Findings suggestive of active disease were early enhancement during the arterial phase, delayed mural enhancement, and an inner concentric, low-attenuation ring in the aorta and pulmonary artery. By contrast, lack of early and delayed mural enhancement, high mural attenuation on the pre-contrast images, and artery wall calcification were more likely to be seen in inactive disease. As with any other cause of proximal pulmonary artery stenosis, the broncho-arterial ratio is altered in Takayasu's disease, with diminutive pulmonary artery diameters beyond the occlusion.

11.4 Proximal Diseases of the Pulmonary Artery

11.4.1 Congenital diseases

11.4.1.1 Left Pulmonary Artery Sling

As described in the scimitar syndrome, the left pulmonary artery sling, sometimes called "origin of the left pulmonary artery from the right," should be regarded as a multiplanar anomaly as it requires multiple planes of reformation for an optimal pretherapeutic evaluation. Until now, the need for surgical repair has necessitated sophisticated diagnostic evaluation requiring: (a) a chest x-ray for the diagnosis of the ventilatory disturbances; (b) bronchoscopy and tracheobronchography for identification of compression and associated abnormalities; (c) barium swallow for depiction of an anterior esophageal indentation due to the intertracheo-esophageal course of the aberrant left pulmonary artery; (d) echocardiography, especially with color-flow Doppler studies, for demonstration of the anomalous origin of the left pulmonary artery; and (e) pulmonary angiography for the definitive preoperative diagnosis. In complete agreement with BACKER et al. (1992), we no longer believe that this angiography is necessary because of the precision of CT or MRI in establishing this diagnosis.

According to data reported from the analysis of dissected specimens, bronchograms or surgical findings, we can adopt WELLS' classification of this malformation into two types (WELLS et al. 1988): type 1 consists of a normal tracheobronchial pattern, while types 2A and 2B are associated with variable degrees of congenital tracheal stenosis in which the cartilages are complete. This is called the "napkin ring," and this anomaly was termed the "ring-sling complex" by BERDON et al. (1984). In types 2A and 2B, the tracheobronchial bifurcation represented by the bridging bronchus for the right lung and the normal left main bronchus is situated at an abnormally low level, on average at T6, and shows a larger angle of bifurcation than usual. This is called "pseudo-isomerism."

Spiral CT acquisition with the injection of contrast medium in a peripheral vein has the following advantages: Cross-sectional images are in the best orientation for depicting both the abnormal origin and the abnormal course of the left pulmonary artery. On a frontal pulmonary angiogram, the latter can be completely hidden behind the proximal part of the right pulmonary artery, thus explaining some angiographic mistakes (BACKER et al. 1992). Moreover, an overall understanding of the tracheobronchial tree can also be obtained from the spiral CT data set using a double thresholding segmentation. As recently emphasized by LACROSSE et al. (1995), multiplanar reformations from cross-sectional images, or preferably from 3D images, can demonstrate the tracheal lumen and the associated anomalies of the bronchial bifurcation.

According to the patient's age and condition, spiral CT acquisition can be performed with the patient under sedation or under general anesthesia with mask ventilation or tracheal intubation. This is the main drawback of this technique compared with electron beam CT (McCRAY et al. 1986). Despite this limitation, it must be pointed out that spiral CT can avoid endoscopy and tracheobronchography, which cannot be considered safe procedures in patients with compromised ventilation (SIEGEL et al. 1982). Rarely, left pulmonary artery sling is found in asymptomatic adults (PROCACCI et al. 1993), in whom it can mimic a mediastinal adenopathy.

11.4.1.2 Transposition of the Great Vessels

Surgically corrected transposition of the great vessels represents another entity in which spiral CT with 3D and multiplanar reformations is of paramount importance. A real anatomical repair of transposition of the great arteries consists in rerouting both the complete aortic root and the pulmonary artery trunk (BEX et al. 1980). This technique is also called the "arterial switch" and is performed in infancy.

After such a correction, the left main bronchus may be in close contact with the posterior aspect of the ascending aorta lying posterior to the pulmonary artery trunk. This unusual complication of the arterial switch can be demonstrated using spiral CT by means of spiral CT angiogram and, from the same data acquisition, spiral CT tracheobronchogram (Fig. 11.4). MRI is also able to show the great vessels, hyperinflation of the left lung field, and proximal obstruction of the left main bronchus in the anteroposterior direction (WORSEY et al. 1994).

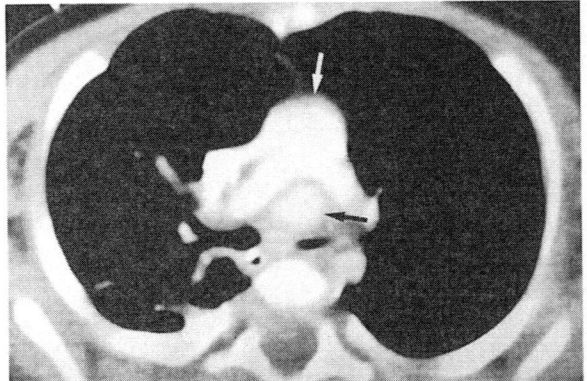

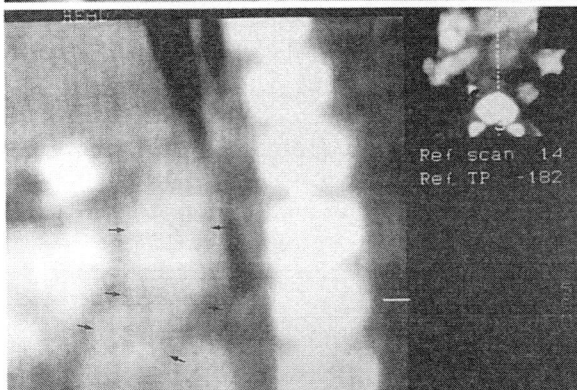

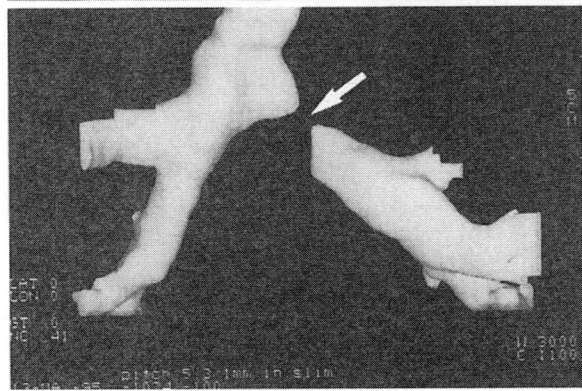

Fig. 11.4a–c. Spiral CT evaluation of a 3-month-old child operated on for a transposition of great vessels soon after birth. Chronic dyspnea and obstructive emphysema of the left lung led to an endoscopic diagnosis of external compression of the left main bronchus at its origin. Spiral CT angiography was performed under general anesthesia with endotracheal intubation (collimation, 3 mm; table feed, 5 mm; overlapping, 1 mm; manual injection of 20 ml of a 120 mg/ml iodinated contrast agent in a left arm vein). The suboptimal enhancement is explained by the low iodine concentration and the patient's tachycardia. **a** On the cross-sectional image, note the anterior location of the pulmonary artery trunk (*white arrow*) and the posterior location of the ascending aorta (*black arrow*), the latter being responsible for an anteroposterior compression of the proximal part of the left main bronchus. **b** The sagittal reformation depicts the poorly opacified ascending aorta (*arrows*). **c** From the same data acquisition, an anteroposterior 3D-SSD is generated using a double thresholding segmentation (−1024 HU; −100 HU), which allows optimal visualization of the tracheobronchial compression (*arrow*)

11.4.1.3 Occult Pulmonary Artery

It is preferable by far to use the term "occult pulmonary artery" rather than proximal "absence" of a pulmonary artery branch because, in the majority of cases, the so-called absent pulmonary artery does exist in the hilum and has to be found by noninvasive means. Whenever possible, spiral CT angiography should be used at first intention, owing to its ability to analyze the pulmonary parenchyma of both lungs. It is also able to estimate the importance and variable origins of the systemic collateral supply which develops from birth to adulthood and may become increasingly responsible for massive hemoptysis. Spiral CT angiography should replace the more invasive conventional or digital angiography in the majority of patients (CATALA et al. 1993).

Both the right occult pulmonary artery and the left occult pulmonary artery associated with a right aortic arch can present late in life, when they are not associated with congenital cardiac disease (Ko et al. 1990).

11.4.2 Acquired Diseases

11.4.2.1 Pulmonary Arterial Invasion from Bronchial Tumors

Precise staging is the key to rational management of bronchial tumors. This has been underlined by MILLER et al. (1992), who stated that "the benefit of resection, the surgical approach, the need for adjuvant therapy and the prognosis will all depend on the extent of the local invasion of a tumor." Until now, incremental CT has fallen short in predicting tumor extension in the mediastinum and the hilum. An improvement in CT-surgical correlations is expected with spiral CT using 3- to 5-mm thin sections routinely. Moreover, continuous acquisition of the volume of interest, optimally opacified, has already proven its utility. The CT findings can also be correlated with transesophageal ultrasonography, which seems to be very promising in defining the cardiovascular extent. From clinical experience, it is recommended that the enhanced spiral CT study of hila be performed after analysis of the noncontrast CT scans of the entire thorax, the latter being obtained by either the conventional or the spiral CT technique. Careful interpretation of these slices usually helps determine the most appropriate injection protocol, with special attention directed toward the concentration of the iodinated contrast agent and the optimal start delay (REMY et al. 1995, unpublished data). This chapter will be dedicated to the proximal pulmonary arteries. The venoatrial extension of bronchial tumors will be reviewed in Sect. 11.6.

Usual protocols involve a table feed of 5 mm/s and a 5-mm collimation (i.e., a pitch of 1:1). The choice of the interval of reconstruction for transverse CT scans depends on the expected utility of 3D and multiplanar reformations (MPRs). When 3D and MPRs are planned as a complement to transverse CT scans, 50% overlapping is recommended. From the level of the aorticopulmonary window to the level of the inferior pulmonary veins, the height of the acquired subvolume represents 10–12 cm. In the majority of preoperative oncological studies, no difficulties are encountered with regard to the 24-s breath-hold duration which is required to scan this subvolume with the pitch previously quoted. Administration via peripheral venous access of 120–140 ml of a 240–300 mg/ml iodinated contrast material with a flow rate of 5 cc/s and a start delay of 10 virtually guarantees optimal opacification not only of the me-

diastinal and hilar pulmonary arteries but also of the venoatrial confluence and the cardiac chambers.

Multiplanar reformations are nearly obtained in real time and may be useful in preoperative evaluation. Transaxial CT imaging is unable to precisely depict the vascular encasement whenever the interface between the vessel and the tumor or lymph nodes is horizontally oriented. Given the orientation of the upper and lower limits of the aorticopulmonary window, i.e., the concavity of the aortic arch and the convexity of the pulmonary artery trunk, respectively, one can understand why MPRs parallel to or perpendicular to the aorticopulmonary window are useful for the analysis of this anatomical region. Coronal reformations clearly depict the superior and inferior margins of the proximal right pulmonary artery. Sagittal or oblique sagittal reformations performed along the main axis of the left and right descending pulmonary arteries (Fig. 11.5) can easily demonstrate the length of extension in the perihilar areas. MPRs may show pulsation artifacts in the outlines of the ascending aorta, the pulmonary artery trunk, and the ventricles. By petrifying the invaded areas, hilar and mediastinal carcinomatous extension limits these artifacts. Other areas of the thorax having several horizontal interfaces, such as the thoracic outlet, the subcarinal region, and the peridiaphragmatic region, can also draw considerable benefit from the multiplanar capability of spiral CT.

Some specific indications for spiral CT angiography of the proximal pulmonary arterial tree will be reviewed according to some therapeutic options (SHIELDS 1993).

Central tumors may be resected by a sleeve lobectomy in conjunction with excision of the adjacent part of the main stem bronchus. The divided bronchus is repaired by an end-to-end anastomosis. Direct carcinomatous extension of the adjacent pulmonary artery may lead to modification of the initially planned surgical option and result in an additional angioplastic reconstruction of the artery or to pneumonectomy. The potential postoperative complications of a pulmonary artery anastomosis, such as anastomotic strictures and bronchoarterial fistula, have to be depicted and an accurate follow-up of the bronchial anastomosis must be obtained. Although resection of the great vessels and angioplastic procedures have long been employed, their operative mortality is high and long-term survival is poor (MILLER et al. 1992). The arch of the left pulmonary artery is in close contact with the upper lobe bron-

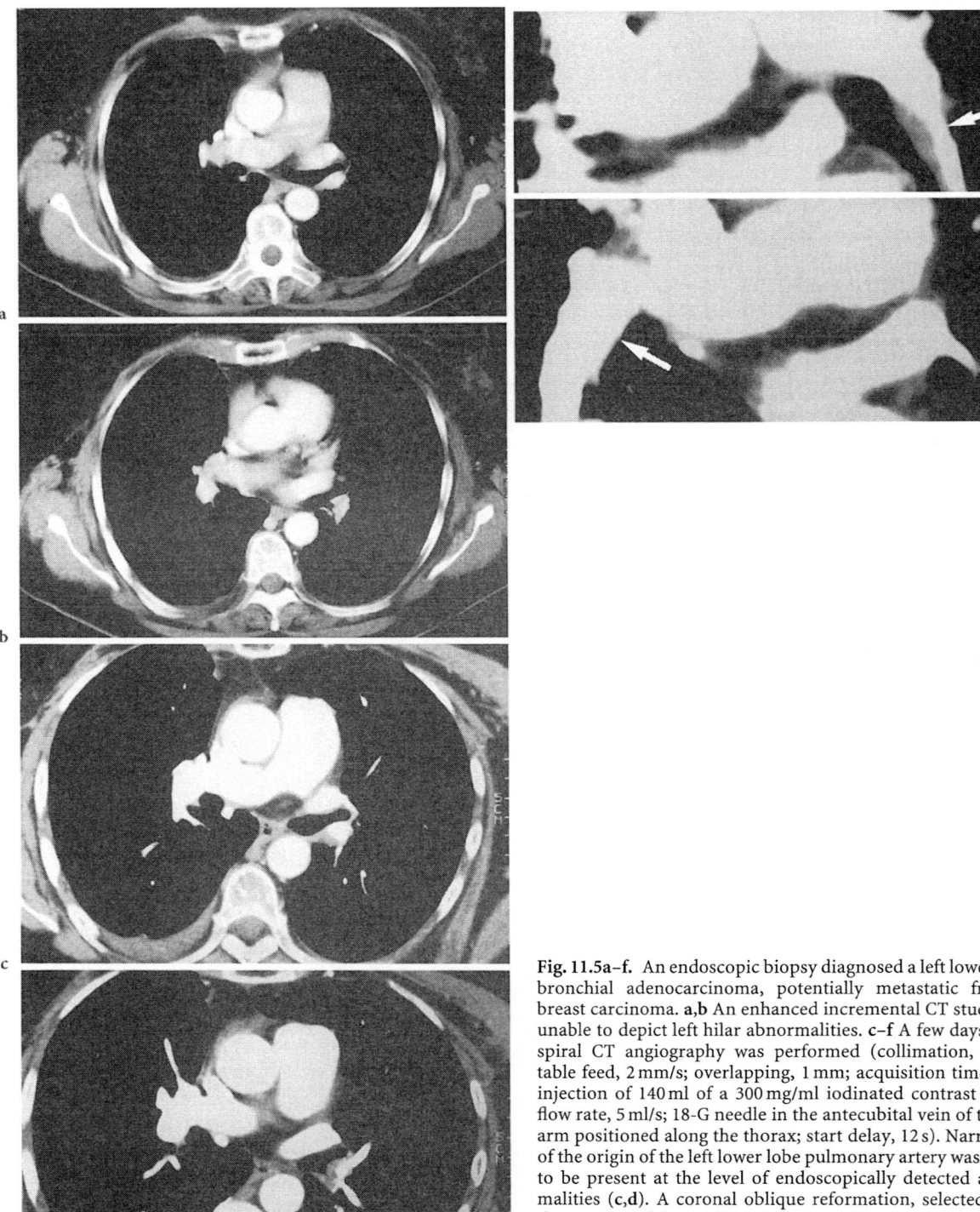

Fig. 11.5a–f. An endoscopic biopsy diagnosed a left lower lobe bronchial adenocarcinoma, potentially metastatic from a breast carcinoma. **a,b** An enhanced incremental CT study was unable to depict left hilar abnormalities. **c–f** A few days later, spiral CT angiography was performed (collimation, 2 mm; table feed, 2 mm/s; overlapping, 1 mm; acquisition time, 22 s; injection of 140 ml of a 300 mg/ml iodinated contrast agent; flow rate, 5 ml/s; 18-G needle in the antecubital vein of the left arm positioned along the thorax; start delay, 12 s). Narrowing of the origin of the left lower lobe pulmonary artery was found to be present at the level of endoscopically detected abnormalities (**c,d**). A coronal oblique reformation, selected from the 3D-SSD of the ipsilateral pulmonary vasculature, demonstrates the longitudinal narrowing of the left lower lobe pulmonary artery (**e**, *arrow*), which can be compared with the normal appearance of the right lower lobe pulmonary artery on a similar reformation (**f**, *arrow*)

chus. In READ et al.'s (1993) experience, this part of the left pulmonary artery is compromised by 14.4% of lesions, mainly T3N0–1 carcinomas otherwise suitable for left upper lobectomy. These data emphasize the imperative need to perfectly depict the left pulmonary arterial arch, which gives off from four to eight separate arteries to the left upper lobe. Most surgeons proceed to pneumonectomy once there is any vascular invasion but others, excluding tangential angioplasty or resection-anastomosis, strongly recommend interposition grafting (READ et al. 1993). A consequence of such a conservative procedure is that the blood flow to the lower lobe may be postoperatively jeopardized by end-to-end anastomosis stenosis. Here again, spiral CT angiography of the proximal left pulmonary artery using MPRs and simultaneous thresholding segmentation for renderings of both bronchial and vascular trees can play a role of the utmost importance pre- and postoperatively (MAGGI et al. 1993).

In the right lung, invasion of the interlobar portion of the pulmonary artery can necessitate a bilobectomy. A pneumonectomy can be enlarged to include the intrapericardial ligation of the pulmonary vessels. Consequently and whenever possible, vascular compression, infiltration, or invasion must be described in relation to the pericardium.

A hilar lymph node dissection can be influenced by the spiral CT findings. If an upper lobectomy is contemplated, lymph nodes smaller than 10 mm in diameter, outside the lobectomy field, can be discovered by their compression or invasion of the descending pulmonary artery (Fig. 11.5). They may remain unseen on an incremental CT scan because they hardly modify the external pulmonary artery morphology. For the same reason, mediastinaly lymph node imaging can also be improved by spiral CT angiography of the mediastinal vessels (REMY-JARDIN et al. 1995a).

Neoadjuvant chemotherapy has an initial response rate of approximately 50% and subsequent resection rates in the responders may approach 80%. Strictly comparative performances of spiral CT acquisition are mandatory before and after chemotherapy for a better estimation and, if necessary, quantification of response.

Roentgenographically occult squamous cell carcinoma involving mainstem bronchi and lobar bronchi can benefit from photodynamic therapy (CORTESE and EDELL 1993). These lesions may be extremely small and are very often beyond the limits of CT detection. But once they have been endoscopically detected and pathologically proven,

the two major tasks are to determine whether the lesion is limited to the bronchial wall and to eliminate N2 disease. Another point of interest is that, if there is an incomplete response after photodynamic therapy, the patient can undergo surgical resection. Spiral CT with thin sections and contrast medium can visualize the peribronchial tissues and play a role in the extrabronchial follow-up of the treated disease.

Use of a YAG laser with its tissue effects of photocoagulation and thermal necrosis, as well as endobronchial brachytherapy, may require optimal knowledge of the depth of the tumor to be treated. The prescribed treatment, high-dose or low-dose radiation techniques, can be planned on MPRs oriented perpendicularly to the long axis of the diseased bronchus so that the isodoses can be calculated. The optimal position of the iridium-192 line source can be virtually determined according to the localization of the surrounding vessels. Figure 1 from NORI et al. (1993) shows the transverse, coronal, and sagittal reconstructions of isodose distribution for endobronchial high-dose treatment. Fused images with MPRs and isodose calculations may be obtained once the high-activity source is in situ (certain anatomical factors can lead to placement of the source closer to the bronchial wall than originally planned). KHANAVKAR et al. (1991) pointed out that centrally located squamous cell carcinomas represent a predisposing factor to hemorrhage. They tried to identify patients at high risk of developing fatal hemoptysis after endobronchial brachytherapy and concluded that the following anatomical lesions represent risk factors: involvement of major arteries, significant bronchial wall destruction, and mediastinal invasion. Posttreatment necrotic cavitation of a tumor located a few millimeters from a major vessel can also be considered a potentially lethal situation. The preventive impact of spiral CT angiography should be seriously taken into account in the follow-up of this treatment as well as after vaso-occlusive therapy.

Whereas bronchial carcinoids can be highly vascular lesions, they may only be depicted with moderate homogeneous contrast enhancement on incremental CT (ABERLE et al. 1991). The transmural extension of this tumor can reach the peribronchial tissues and vessels as well as the adjacent pulmonary parenchyma. If an endobronchial biopsy is anticipated, the highly vascular component should be demonstrated to prevent any further hemorrhagic complications. A sleeve resection can be performed depending on the peribronchial extent. Both findings can be searched for on pulmonary and systemic spiral CT angiograms.

11.4.2.2 Lung Transplantation

Apart from the depiction of postoperative pleural and parenchymal changes (ENGELER 1995), spiral CT can be helpful in patients who have undergone lung transplantation, for the evaluation of anastomosis-related stenoses of the airways, arteries, and veins. This chapter will only review the potential applications of spiral CT in the follow-up of pulmonary arterial anastomosis. The frequency of pulmonary artery stenosis has recently been estimated by GRIFFITH et al. (1994), who observed obstructions in 5 of 60 single-lung recipients and in none of 74 double-lung transplantations. In one case, obstruction was associated with an intraluminal thrombus. The associa-

tion of systemic hypoxia, normal chest x-ray, and perfusion scan abnormalities represents an indication for spiral CT of the chest whenever the patient is able to support breath holding for a few seconds. It is not easy to make the differential diagnosis between a true stenosis and a distorted or kinked anastomosis resulting from excessive lengths of donor and recipient artery cuff. The latter can spontaneously improve over a follow-up period, in contrast to a true stenosis, which leads to a surgical revision or to endovascular procedures. Due to pulmonary-to-bronchial artery retrograde flow, pulmonary artery stenosis can compromise the bronchial anastomosis. In the absence of contraindications to contrast medium administration, a spiral CT study initially indicated for the follow-up of airway anastomosis can also allow evaluation of arterial and venous anastomoses. When the transplanted patient has to be treated by surgery, percutaneous angioplasty, and/or

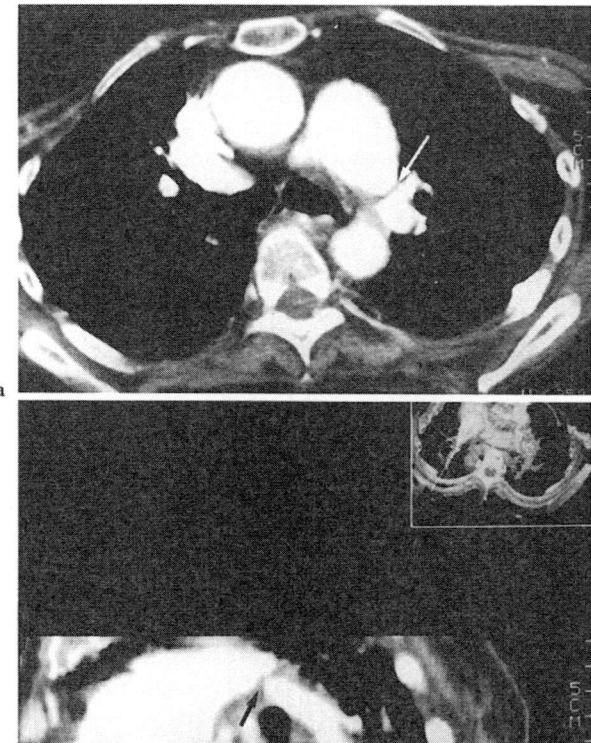

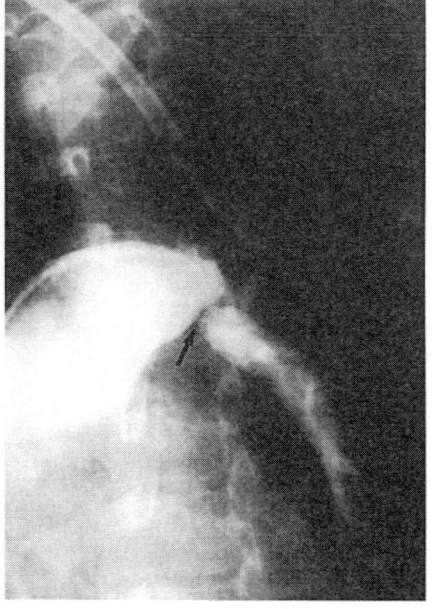

Fig. 11.6a–c. Spiral CT angiography performed 10 days after left lung transplantation in a hypoxemic patient with a normal chest radiograph. A postoperative perfusion lung scan showed that only 20% of the pulmonary blood flow was directed toward the transplanted lung (collimation, 3 mm; table feed, 5 mm/s; acquisition time, 14 s; overlapping, 1 mm; 120 ml of a 240 mg/ml iodinated contrast agent; flow rate, 4 ml/s; 22-G needle in an antecubital vein with the injected arm positioned along the thorax). An anastomotic stenosis of the left pulmonary artery is demonstrated on the transverse CT scan (**a**, *arrow*) and on the oblique coronal reformation (**b**, *arrow*), the latter being selected from the 3D-SSD of the ipsilateral pulmonary vasculature. Silmilar information is provided with the selective angiogram of the left pulmonary artery obtained in the same obliquity (**c**, *arrow*)

endoprosthesis (GAUBERT et al. 1993), the precise shape, site, and length of the stenosis can be better appreciated with 2D and 3D reformations as they permit unlimited viewing angles. Perfusion scan and spiral CT 3D angiography can also avoid the use of more invasive and repeated angiographic follow-ups (Fig. 11.6).

11.4.2.3 Primary Pulmonary Artery Sarcomas

Pulmonary artery sarcomas are exceedingly rare. A preoperative diagnosis is infrequent and a well-guided surgical intervention is unfortunately seldom performed. The feasibility of establishing this diagnosis depends on the tumor's behavior.

Primary pulmonary artery sarcomas are very often confused with acute and chronic thromboembolic disease. In this particular circumstance, the tumor grows inside the pulmonary arterial trunk and/or its proximal branches. This endovascular development can be unique or multicentric. The tumor itself can be seen as a floating mass corresponding to, or associated with, thrombus formation. The absence of predisposing factors for pulmonary embolism, the absence of "thrombus" dissolution despite anticoagulation, and atypical distribution of the filling defects as seen on 2D or Doppler ultrasonography, pulmonary angiography, MRI or CT, and V̊/Q̊ scanning should alert the radiologist (ENG and MURDAY 1992). Peripheral pulmonary infiltrates can correspond to pulmonary infarcts due to thrombi or embolization of tumor material from the original site.

The diagnosis can be strongly suspected when chest x-ray, CT, or MRI shows a lobulated and heterogeneous hilar mass originating from the pulmonary artery trunk or from the main right or left pulmonary arteries, which expands the artery (DELANY et al. 1993). Such polypoid intraluminal masses can be partly hemorrhagic, necrotic, and hypervascularized with enhancement on spiral CT scans or after administration of gadopentetate dimeglumine on T1-weighted MR images. This finding helps eliminate a thrombus and indicates a neoplastic process (BRESSLER and NELSON 1992). The pretherapeutic evaluation of this tumor can be performed with spiral CT, first during the passage of the contrast medium bolus, but also a few minutes later to search for contrast medium uptake by the tumor. In a minority of patients, the tumor arises from the right or left main pulmonary artery with or without contralateral spreading.

Direct transmural growth in the hilum, the mediastinum, the lung parenchyma, and the pericardium can occur. Such lesions can mimic a tumor from another origin, particularly a bronchial carcinoma invading the pulmonary artery. Extravascular infiltration and nodal invasion are also possible (KAUCZOR et al. 1994a). Osteo-, chondro-, and carcinosarcomas may exhibit osteoid and bone components (DELANY et al. 1993).

11.4.2.4 Postoperative Incidents, Accidents, and Follow-up

With precise knowledge of rearrangements of the pulmonary vascular pedicles after a lobectomy, the CT follow-up of patients with normal bronchial endocopy can be performed without administration of contrast material.

After pneumonectomy, a contrast-enhanced study is systematically recommended since, although it is infrequently noticed, the presence of a clot in a pulmonary artery stump is not that exceptional (TAKAHASHI et al. 1993). This is partly because carcinomatous patients are at high risk for an associated state of hypercoagulability and partly because there are anatomical factors which can account for the stasis of blood flow in the stump. After pneumonectomy, a right-sided stump is longer than a left-sided one, thus explaining the higher frequency of stump clots after right pneumonectomy. One patient observed by the authors had a left pulmonary arterial embolus and a large thrombus in his right stump several months after right pneumonectomy with no other origin for thrombosis. The stump clot may enlarge over time and has to be differentiated from tumor recurrence (TAKAHASHI et al. 1993).

The differential diagnosis of respiratory failure after pneumonectomy includes pulmonary edema, cardiac failure, infection, bronchospasm, and pulmonary emboli. Pulmonary emboli may be difficult to differentiate from the other causes (SATUR et al. 1991).

The postpneumonectomy syndrome is a rare complication of right pneumonectomy. Compression of the left main bronchus is due to rotation and displacement of the heart and vascular structures in the posterior right pleural space, thus causing bronchial compression between the aorta, the pulmonary artery, a vertebral body, and the ligamentum arteriosum (DOWNEY et al. 1994). The vascular relationships of the stenosed bronchus can be precisely

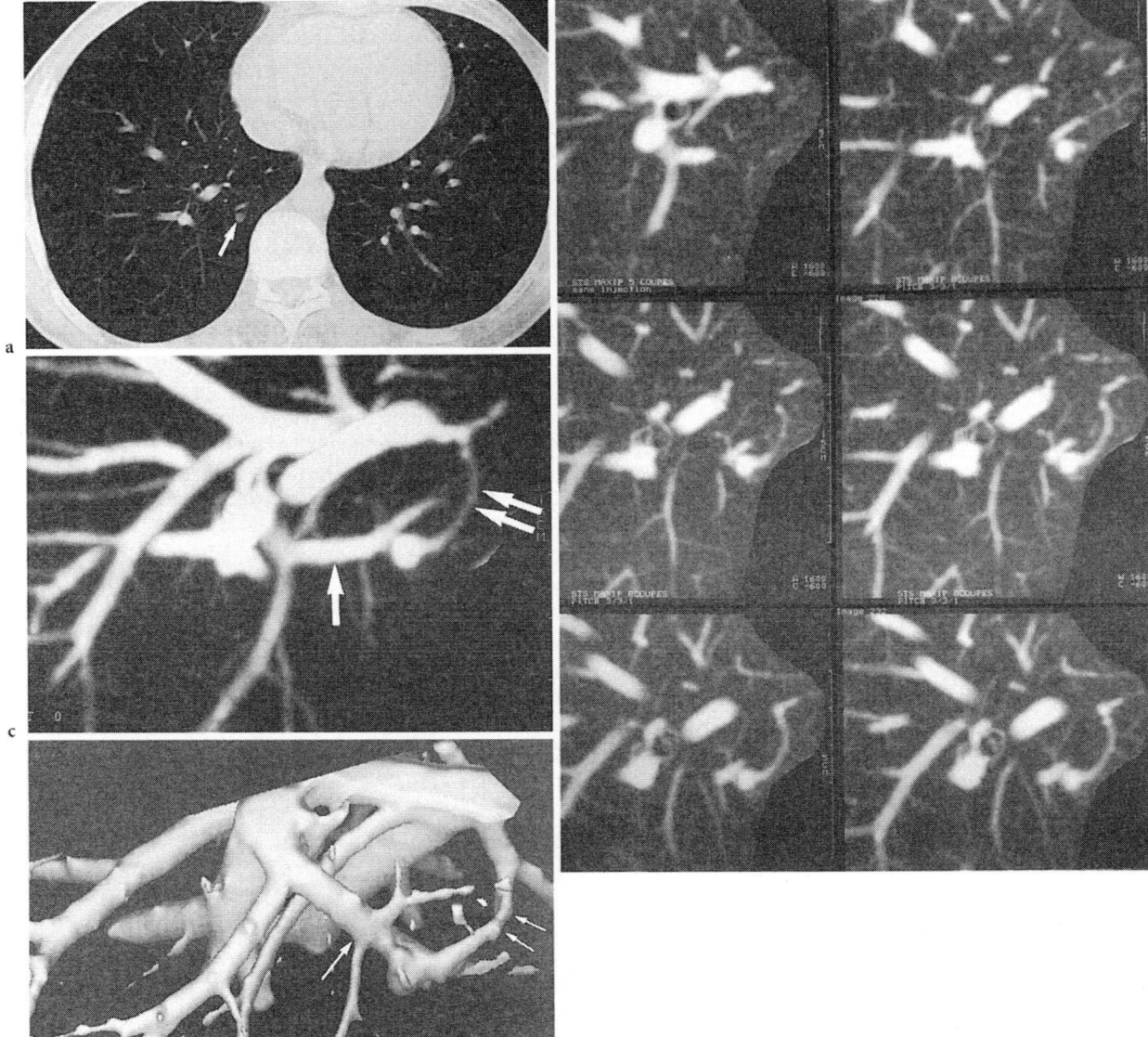

Fig. 11.7. a In the CT follow-up of a patient with a left lower lobe PAVM treated with coils, a micronodule was identified in the apical segment of the right lower lobe (*arrow*), and suspected to correspond to a tiny PAVM. A nonenhanced focal spiral CT acquisition was performed over a limited region of interest (collimation, 3 mm; pitch = 1; overlapping, 1 mm; acquisition time, 7 s). **b** Overlapping slabs of 8 mm thickness were generated according to the STS-MIP technique: owing to the respective orientations of the arterial and venous pedicles, it is impossible to image the complete malformation on a single slab. An MIP image of the acquired volume (**c**) and an SSD were obtained (**d**). The arterial pedicle (**c,d**, *single arrow*) originates from the posterobasal artery of the right lower lobe; note the right angle of this arterial origin and its small diameter (2–3 mm); the draining vein (**c,d**, *double arrow*) is horizontally oriented, ending in the right inferior pulmonary vein

depicted by performing MPRs along the bronchial axis.

The majority of cardiac herniations or torsions occur within hours after intrapericardial pneumonectomy; very rarely they occur after lobectomy including extensive pericardial resection (OHRI et al. 1992). This diagnosis might be greatly facilitated by spiral CT angiography, which could easily identify the cardiac torsion by means of the interventricular septal rotation.

A postoperative right-to-left shunt between the inferior vena cava and the left atrium through a patent foramen ovale might also be detected on spiral CT angiography with a lower leg injection.

In patients with a partial abnormal pulmonary venous return and a contralateral carcinoma, a minor left-to-right shunt can be turned into a major one after contralateral pneumonectomy. Consequently, it must be detected and imaged (BLACK et al. 1992).

11.5 Peripheral Diseases of the Pulmonary Artery

11.5.1 Techniques

As previously emphasized, the peripheral pulmonary vascular bed can be precisely depicted using a targeted subvolume and thin slices. For this purpose one may employ (a) a thin slab-maximum intensity projection (TS-MIP) with or without automatic sliding in the acquired volume or (b) targeted shaded surface displays (SSDs). These techniques are indicated in the morphological estimation of peripheral vessels anywhere within the lung.

11.5.2 Indications

Although the aforementioned techniques have not yet been fully evaluated, some potential indications can be suggested.

11.5.2.1 Microvascular Relationships of a Pulmonary Micronodule

Arteriovenous abnormalities may present as very small lesions looking like spider nevi. These submillimetric fistulas can be congenital or acquired, such as those detected in the hepatopulmonary syndrome. They can be better depicted using a focal thin slab reconstructed from thin slices (Fig. 11.7).

11.5.2.2 Microvascular Relationships of a Diffuse Micronodular Pattern

In patients suspected of suffering from pulmonary sarcoidosis, identification of a micronodular pattern and evaluation of its profusion are usually achieved by means of either thin or thick slices. On thin slices, peripheral pulmonary arteries and veins are multifragmented, slice by slice, and numerous vessels are not depicted in the nonacquired intervals of the lung. Conversely, in thick slices calculated with a high spatial frequency reconstruction kernel, the

distal vessels are correctly depicted but tiny micronodules are masked by the high amplitude volume averaging effect. An excellent compromise is the TS-MIP because: (a) it images submillimetric vessels over a longer length than on individual thin slices, (b) the contrast resolution is reinforced thanks to the MIP algorithm, (c) the background means is maintained at a minimal levels, and (d) there is no background enhancement in the absence of injected contrast medium. This technique permits demonstration of the perivascular distribution of the micronodules (Fig. 11.8) (see also Chap. 7).

11.5.2.3 Branching Pattern

Besides dichotomous branching, vessels may display a disproportionate mode of division. Dichotomous

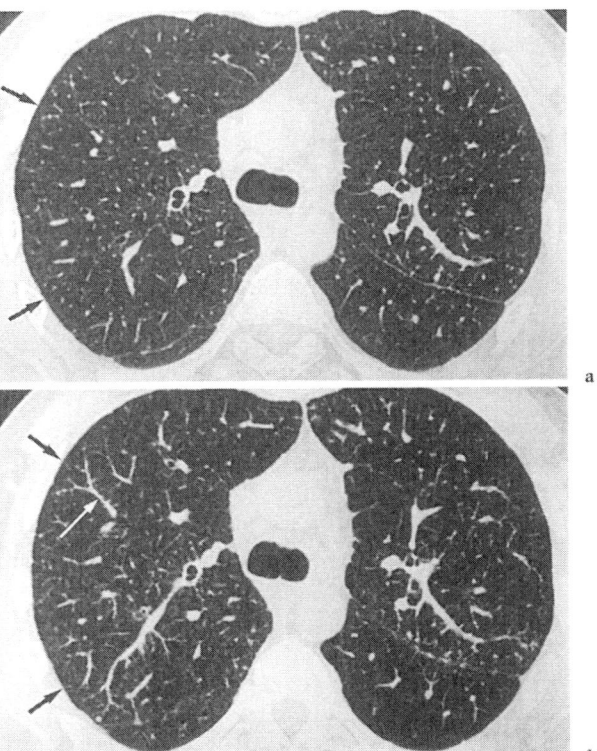

Fig. 11.8. a Suspicion of tiny parenchymal and subpleural micronodules (*between the two arrows*) on a transverse CT section obtained at the level of the upper lobes. After a focal unenhanced spiral CT acquisition (collimation, 1 mm; acquisition time, 10 s; no overlapping), overlapping 8-mm-thick slabs were generated according to the STS-MIP technique. One of these slabs (**b**) enables identification of a micronodular pattern predominantly distributed in the most peripheral lung (*between the two black arrows*). In addition, note the perivascular distribution of tiny lesions (*white arrow*) consistent with pulmonary sarcoidosis

branching consists in the division of a branch into two equal parts, both arising at an acute angle and having half the diameter of the original branch. The disproportionate mode consists in small branches arising at nearly a right angle from the native vessel and being of a smaller diameter than in the case of the usual dichotomous mode of bifurcation (Fig. 11.9). The importance of this asymmetric division mode, which is seen only on post-mortem injections and not on angiography, is not known.

11.5.2.4 Arteriolar and Venular Diameters

In the normal population, the diameters of pulmonary arteries and veins in the peripheral part of the lung are approximately equal. As in chronic thromboembolic disease, analysis of the flow-diameter relationship might represent an in vivo approach to the morphological changes in pulmonary hypertension. Thanks to the summation effect in the slab, some oblique pulmonary vessels can be seen in

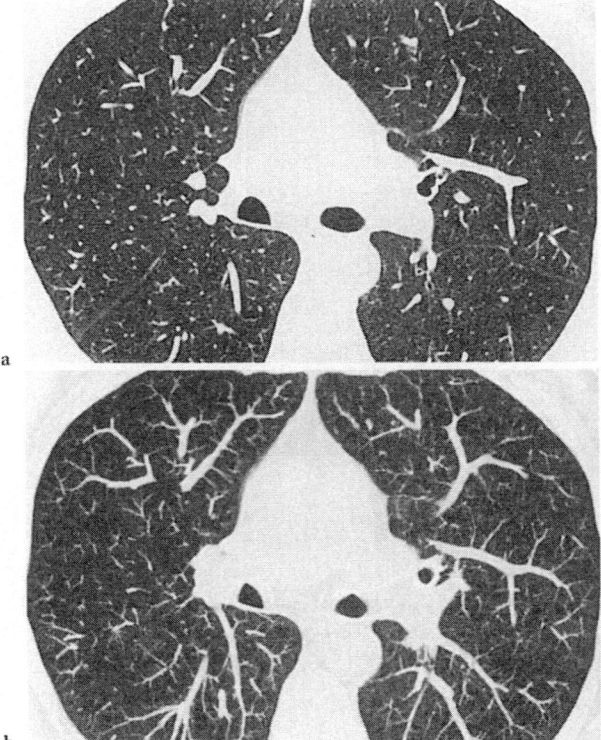

Fig. 11.9. Note the striking difference in the identification of supernumerary vessels between a 1-mm-thick section (**a**) and a 5-mm-thick slab (**b**) generated from a focal spiral CT acquisition according to the STS-MIP technique

their entirety between the hilum and the periphery. This enables easier distinction of arteries from veins.

11.5.2.5 Round Atelectasis

Any type of pleural inflammation reaction can lead to round atelectasis. Asbestosis is the principal cause today, and this diagnosis should be suspected when a peripheral nodule or mass is associated with signs of pleuritis and/or pleuroparenchymal changes related to asbestos.

Usually round atelectasis presents as a posterobasal, subpleural, round or lentiform lesion with some of the following features (TAYLOR 1988): (a) a peripheral location, with the mass being incompletely surrounded by the lung; (b) increased density of the mass at its periphery; (c) pleural thickening in the vicinity of the mass; (d) curving of vessels and bronchi toward the mass; and (e) presence of an air bronchogram within the mass. Correct diagnosis is very important, especially in asbestos-exposed patients owing to the increased incidence of mesothelioma and bronchogenic carcinoma in this population. Two main mechanisms are recognized to underlie round atelectasis: (a) pleural effusion or diffuse pleural thickening, and (b) thickening of the visceral pleura with progressive wrinkling and folding of the subpleural lung (HILLERDAL 1989). The lesion can be stable over time; however, it may progressively enlarge and then can be confused with a malignant tumor (VOISIN et al. 1995).

Use of the TS-MIP and SSDs with contrast medium and thin slices around the atelectatic lung has the following additional benefits:

1. There is very high contrast enhancement of round atelectasis. Such intense and homogeneous enhancement can help differentiate the atelectatic trapped lung from bronchial carcinoma or fibrosis, in which enhancement is usually poor (Fig. 11.10).

2. The vessels trapped in the atelectatic lung can be correctly opacified and enhanced by means of the maximum intensity projection principle, unless the parenchyma is too highly vascularized. The distortion and regular bending of these vessels can provide another argument against suspected carcinoma (Fig. 11.10).

3. On thick horizontal slices or on thin interspaced slices, the internal architecture of this atelectatic pseudo-tumor is not easy to analyze. With spiral CT, thin overlapped slices can show a large curved tongue of the neighboring pleural cavity with dense tissue or fluid invaginating into the underlying

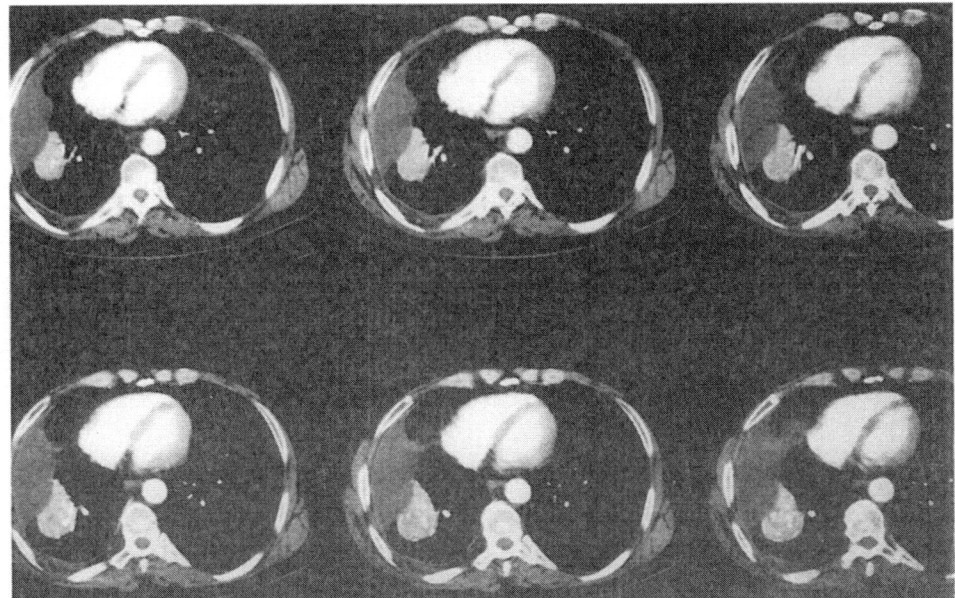

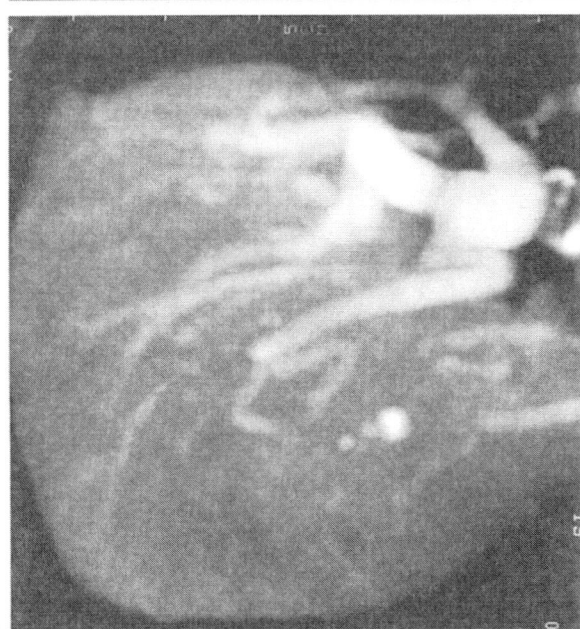

Fig. 11.10a,b. Enhanced spiral CT evaluation of a right lower lobe mass adjacent to a loculated pleural effusion (collimation, 3 mm; pitch of 1; overlapping, 1 mm; injection of 100 ml of a 300 mg/ml iodinated contrast agent at a flow rate of 5 ml/s in an antecubital vein). The lower lobe mass is highly hypervascularized (a). An MIP image (b) reveals distorted central and peripheral pulmonary vessels within the mass, which are easily identified despite enhancement of the surrounding atelectatic lung. In the clinical context of professional exposure to asbestos, these findings are highly suggestive of round atelectasis

lung parenchyma, in close correlation with the anatomical findings (REN et al. 1989).

4. By using MPRs from 3D-SSDs, it is possible to acquire images in multiple planes parallel to the converging vessels and bronchi.

According to McHUGH and BLAQUIERE (1989), when it is possible to identify the previously cited criteria on conventional and spiral CT examinations, further diagnostic evaluation is unnecessary. If most of the criteria are absent, cautious follow-up or percutaneous needle biopsy is recommended.

11.6 Diseases of the Pulmonary Veins

11.6.1 Congenital Diseases

Congenital anomalies of the pulmonary venous return can be conveniently classified into three categories. The *first category* comprises abnormal pulmonary venous drainage into the systemic veins. From a radiological viewpoint, this first category of congenital anomalies can be subdivided into: (a) abnormal venous connections without an abnormal course in the lung, and (b) abnormal venous connections associated with an abnormal course in the lung, the latter group usually being easier to diagnose on chest x-rays than the former. The *second category* of congenital anomalies of the pulmonary venous return comprises an abnormal venous route without an abnormal connection. The *third category* is represented by abnormal venous diameters, including varices and stenoses.

11.6.1.1 Abnormal Venous Drainage Without an Abnormal Course in the Lung

11.6.1.1.1 Partial Anomalous Pulmonary Venous Drainage of the Left Upper Lobe in a Vertical Vein.
This is reported to be one of the commonest types of abnormal pulmonary venous drainage. It runs the risk of being confounded with two other anomalies including a vertical vein on the left border of the mediastinum, namely a left superior vena cava ending in the coronary sinus, and a left superior vena cava draining into the left atrium. These differential diagnoses can be easily discounted with spiral CT and specific injection techniques. In the case of a left superior vena cava draining into either the coronary sinus or the left atrium, the systemic venous flow is directed superoinferiorly, in the usual direction. Opacification of this abnormal vein is obtained with a very low concentration of iodinated contrast material, injected at a slow flow rate into the left arm positioned alongside the thorax to avoid the risk of obstruction at the thoracic inlet. An 8%–12% iodine concentration and a flow rate of 2cc/s are usually optimal technical parameters because the contrast medium is directed primarily toward the left superior vena cava owing to the absence or the small size of the left innominate vein. The start delay between injection and acquisition is short, usually 5 s. In the case of partial anomalous venous return of the left upper lobe in a vertical vein, the blood flow is directed inferosuperiorly, partially draining the left upper lobe venous blood into the origin of the left innominate vein (Fig. 11.11). Owing to the reversed flow, the vertical vein cannot be opacified using the aforementioned technique as the small and slow bolus would be diluted in the left innominate vein. Consequently, the optimal injection technique employs a high iodine concentration, e.g., 300mg/ml, a flow rate of 5cc/s, and a minimum start delay of 12–15 s. As previously suggested, the most appropriate injection protocol can only be selected once the morphological criteria are identified on precontrast scans. In the case of partial anomalous venous return in the vertical vein, its connection with the origin of the vertical vein is easily identified. Consequently, the rest of the normally positioned left superior pulmonary vein anterior to the left upper lobe bronchus is depicted as a small structure or is absent. The left innominate vein draining the left subclavian vein, the left internal jugular vein, and the vertical vein is normal or slightly dilated. The coronary sinus is normal. When it is associated with a septal defect, obstructive airway disease, or any other cause of restriction of the vascular bed, a left-to-right shunt due to the ectopic drainage of a part of the left upper lobe can be responsible for some dilatation of intraparenchymal vessels (DILLON and CAMPUTARO 1993).

If the left superior vena cava drains into the coronary sinus or the left atrium, the left innominate vein is absent or small, and the confluence of the left upper lobe pulmonary venous tributaries in the vertical vein does not exist. The left upper pulmonary vein has a normal size. If drainage is into the coronary sinus, the latter is dilated, whereas it is of normal size when drainage is into the left atrium.

It is thus evident that precise analysis of relevant morphological features on precontrast CT slices and physiologically adapted injection techniques constitute the state-of-the-art approach for these three diagnoses. Moreover, multiplanar reformations and 3D images can elucidate further the course of the abnormal vessels. When isolated, the degree of the left-to-right shunt is equal to or less than 25% of the cardiac output and is compatible with a normal life. However, this acceptable hemodynamic condition can decompensate after contralateral surgery and can become a major left-to-right shunt, almost 50% of the cardiac output, after a right pneumonectomy (BLACK et al. 1992). Consequently, when routinely using preoperative CT of the thorax it is important to bear in mind the surgical importance of an unsuspected partial anomalous drainage of the left superior pulmonary vein into the left innominate vein whenever the patient is a candidate for right lung surgery. Depending on the importance of the lung volume to be resected, the anomalous vein may be preventively reimplanted into the left atrial appendage.

11.6.1.1.2 Partial Anomalous Pulmonary Venous Drainage of the Right Upper Lobe to the Right Superior Vena Cava.
The diagnosis of partial anomalous pulmonary venous return to the right superior vena cava or the azygos arch can be made on incremental

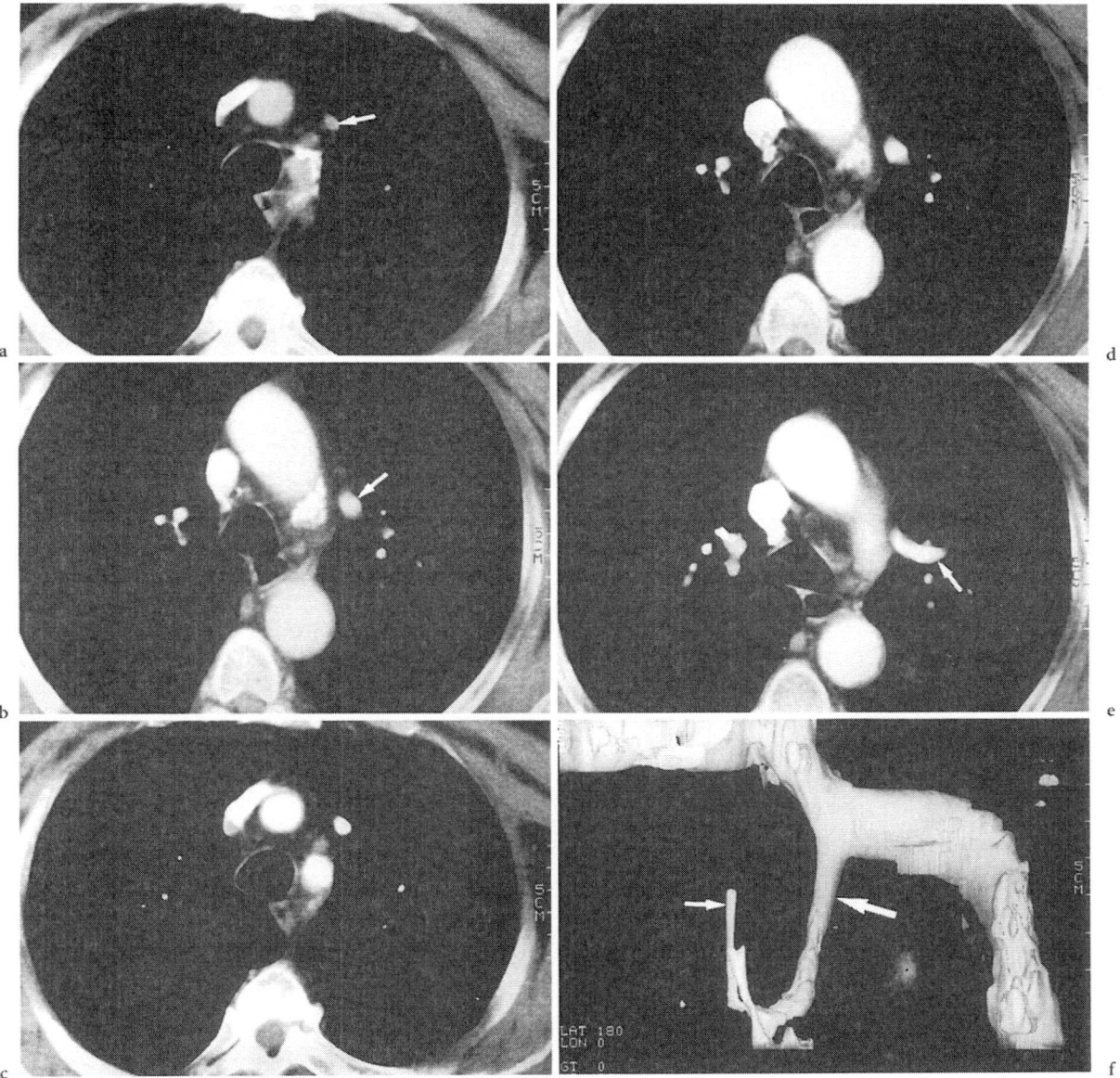

Fig. 11.11a–f. Spiral CT examination indicated for the suspicion of a left superior vena cava in a patient with obstructive airway disease (5-mm collimation; table feed, 5 mm/s). **a,b** A first injection of contrast medium in the antecubital vein of the left arm (80 ml of a 120 mg/ml iodinated contrast material; flow rate, 3 ml/s; start delay, 5 s; superoinferior acquisition) allows optimal opacification of the left innominate vein and of the superior vena cava but the left vertical vein is not opacified (**a**, *arrow*); at a slightly lower level, a poorly enhanced vascular shadow is present (**b**, *arrow*). **c–e** A second injection is performed using 120 ml of a 300 mg/ml iodinated contrast agent, administered at a rate of 5 ml/s with a start delay of 15 s with an inferosuperior acquisition. A highly enhanced left vertical vein (**c**) and its afferents is shown (**d,e**, *arrow*). **f** A 3D reformat of the systemic veins (posteroanterior viewing angle) provides an overall understanding of this anomaly: there is partial anomalous pulmonary venous drainage (*small arrow*) of the left upper lobe in a vertical vein (*large arrow*)

CT (POSNIAK et al. 1993; THORSEN et al. 1990). Cross-sectional images, without contrast enhancement, show right dilated pulmonary veins in close contact with the superior vena cava and/or the terminal portion of the azygos arch. As previously pointed out with regard to the left superior pulmonary vein, the expected normal part in the hilum and near the left atrium is not found or is too small. The diagnosis is easily confirmed with spiral CT angiography. But, optimally, the contrast injection should be performed in the inferior vena cava in order to avoid simultaneous opacification of the pulmonary venous return and of the superior vena cava from an injected arm.

11.6.1.2 Abnormal Venous Drainage with an Abnormal Route in the Lung

In the majority of patients, a partial or total pulmonary anomalous venous return of the right lung, usually into the inferior vena cava or the right atrium, is easily diagnosed on a chest x-ray providing that the right lung is not too hypoplastic. The abnormal vein can be an isolated finding or may be associated with other anomalies, gathered under the term "scimitar syndrome" or "scimitar spectrum." This syndrome includes:

1. Abnormal lobation of the right lung, justifying the term "congenital veno-lobar syndrome" or "hypogenetic right lung syndrome."
2. Mediastinal shift to the right; the term "dextrocardia" should be avoided since the cardiac apex still points to the left (PARTRIDGE et al. 1988).
3. Other abnormalities: congenital cardiac disease, most often atrial septal defect.
4. Bronchial cysts or diverticula; accessory diaphragm and right cupola defects.
5. Horseshoe lung (FREEDOM et al. 1986); abnormal systemic vascular supply of the right lung, sometimes including the scimitar syndrome in the "sequestration spectrum."

The abnormal right pulmonary vein drains the right lung or only one portion of it into the inferior vena cava just above or below the diaphragm, looking like a Turkish sword. It receives the abnormal systemic arterial supply, which triggers an additional more or less severe left-to-right shunt. It can be stenosed at its implantation in the inferior vena cava.

Like the retrotracheal left pulmonary artery, the scimitar syndrome can be considered a multiplanar anomaly. It requires 3D reformations with or without contrast medium to provide a global view of the entire abnormal vein (Fig. 11.12) as well as high-resolution CT sections dedicated to the analysis of fine detail, such as septal lines when the abnormal pulmonary venous return is obstructed. In the context of a preoperative evaluation, the pseudo-fissural line corresponding to the close contact between the right lung herniated behind the heart (horseshoe lung) and the left lung also needs thin slices. 3D reformations of the tracheobronchial tree are useful for

an easier description of the abnormal right bronchial tree, and 3D reformations of the abnormal systemic artery or arteries require good opacification. These vessels can be identified by their spontaneous high contrast if the right lower lobe has a normal attenuation. However, their subdiaphragmatic origin and course is only clearly seen with contrast medium.

When surgery is needed, noninvasive follow-up after reimplantation of the abnormal vein in the left atrium can also require spiral CT angiography, especially when postoperative obstruction to the reimplanted abnormal pulmonary venous return in itself represents a further indication for pneumonectomy (SCHRAMEL et al. 1995).

11.6.1.3 Abnormal Route Without an Abnormal Connection

Three-dimensional reconstructions with or without contrast medium can help differentiate between some variants of the scimitar syndrome. In a first variation, the anomalous vein courses down to the diaphragm and drains simultaneously into the inferior vena cava and the left atrium. Surgical ligation of the part draining into the inferior vena cava may be required for rerouting of the venous return toward the left atrium. In another variant, despite a scimitar-like course in the lung, the vein normally enters the left atrium without any connection with the inferior vena cava (TAKEDA et al. 1994). Sometimes, this entity is called "pseudo-scimitar syndrome." However, there may be a more important overlap between scimitar and pseudoscimitar syndromes as the latter can also include a hypoplastic right lung and an abnormal systemic arterial supply (CUKIER et al. 1994).

Other ectopic venous routes can mimic a partial anomalous pulmonary venous return and can also be associated with dextroposition of the heart and hypoplasia of the right lung (REY et al. 1986). Whenever patients are asymptomatic without any cardiac hemodynamic alterations, pulmonary angiography must be considered disproportionate and 3D CT angiography or MR angiography should be the first investigation to be envisaged.

11.6.2 Acquired Diseases

Acquired diseases of the large pulmonary veins are rather rare. Here, discussion will be limited to the venoatrial extension of bronchial carcinoma and to postoperative venous thrombosis.

Apart from an outside to inside extension progressively invading and obstructing a pulmonary vein, another mode of extension for primary or secondary tumors of the lung consists in using a pulmonary vein as a channel for extension and in secondarily invading the left atrium through it. The most common tumor able to invade the left atrium in this way is bronchogenic carcinoma. However, similar extension has also been reported with metastatic carcinoma and pulmonary sarcoma of the lung. A preoperative diagnosis is imperative since intraoperatively dislodging a macroscopic tumoral thrombus from the pulmonary vein can be fatal or give rise to multiple systemic tumor emboli (SPENCER et al. 1993). In patients with large central carcinomas in contact with one or several major pulmonary veins, a preoperative transthoracic or transesophageal echocardiogram and spiral CT angiography are recommended, because a carcinomatous thrombus of a pulmonary vein may go unnoticed at surgery and be dislodged during surgical manipulations. The CT signs of venous invasion are those of a pulmonary veno-obstructive syndrome including pulmonary edema and hemorrhage, pul-

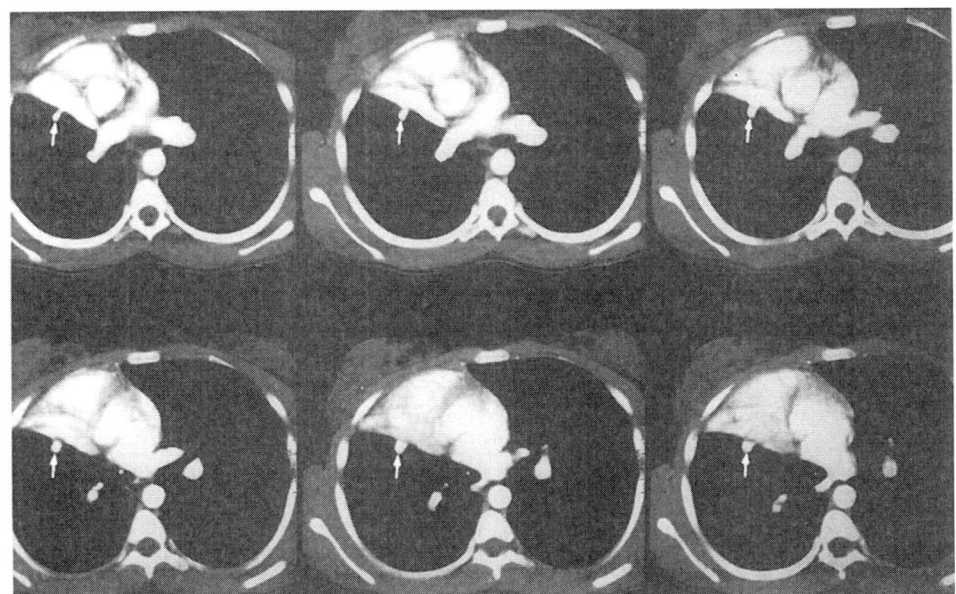

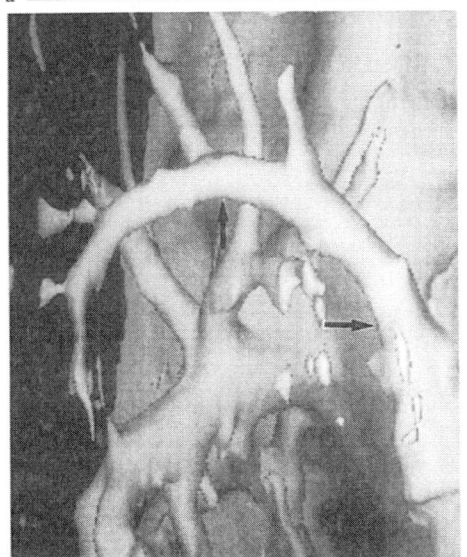

Fig. 11.12a,b. Spiral CT evaluation of a 13-year-old child with a small right lung incidentally found in the follow-up of respiratory infections (collimation, 5 mm; pitch of 1; overlapping, 2 mm). The cross-sectional images viewed at lung window settings (not shown) depicted an abnormal lobation of the right lung and a horseshoe lung. a Spiral CT angiography of the pulmonary vessels shows a large vessel running close to the right heart border in a vertical direction (*arrow*). b A 3D-SSD of the right lung helps in the recognition of the abnormal vein with a first horizontal portion running over the hilum (*vertical arrow*) and a second vertical portion (*horizontal arrow*)

monary venous infarct, interlobular septal thickening, increased bronchial wall thickening, and pleural effusion. Spiral CT angiography can additionally show a massive enlargement in diameter of the invaded vein with an absence of opacification or a more or less important filling defect of the adjacent part of the left atrium. The focal increase in pulmonary vascular resistance can also explain the absence or late opacification of the pulmonary arterial bed in the veno-obstructed area and, later, an unusual optimal opacification of this arterial network due to pulmonary arterial stasis. On incremental CT, a space-occupying lesion in the left atrium could be easily missed on an insufficiently contrast-enhanced CT scan (Koo et al. 1984).

Proximal pulmonary veno-occlusive disease has also been reported secondary to a tumor extending from the left atrium into pulmonary veins, or secondary to the reimplantation of pulmonary veins in the left atrium (Matsumoto et al. 1987; Van Son et al. 1995).

After lobectomy or bilobectomy, an acute episode of dyspnea with or without thoracic pain and hemoptysis, a complete consolidation of the remaining lobe, a reduction in the hematocrit and no flow on the lung perfusion scan can have two main causes: lobar torsion or pulmonary vein obstruction due to torsion, angulation, or thrombosis. A venous obstruction can be seen after a middle lobectomy alone or middle and lower lobectomy because ligation of the lowermost one or two branches of the superior pulmonary vein can traumatize this large remaining vein (Hovaguimian et al. 1991). Spiral CT angiography, performed after endobronchial endoscopy excluding a lobar torsion, can show the normal postoperative pulmonary artery anatomy and the absence of a venous phase. If the patient is not operated on for this complication, the development of a venous collateral bronchial and nonbronchial systemic supply to this persisting venous obstruction can be expected through the bronchial veins, the chest wall veins, and the azygos-hemiazygos system.

11.7 Systemic Arterial Supply to the Lung

The abnormal systemic circulation to the lung can have a developmental or an acquired origin. The multiple possibilities for normal and abnormal systemic arterial supply to the lung include the bronchial arteries and the nonbronchial systemic arteries. In addition to these two common origins, congenital cardiac disease, congenital lung disease, and anomalous systemic arterial supply to normal lung can involve the abnormal persistence of primitive postbranchial arteries, also called major aorto-pulmonary arteries (Ellis 1991). Obviously, it is largely beyond the scope of this chapter to review the clinical impact of spiral CT angiography of these numerous abnormal systemic arteries to the lung. We are going to limit this review to bronchopulmonary sequestration and to a few commonly hypervascularized acquired diseases of the lung.

Whatever the disease, the acquisition and injection techniques differ from what is usually selected for pulmonary arterial indications. Thin slices, e.g., 1–3 mm, are very often required for correct fitting to the small size of the systemic arteries. They are reconstructed at 1-mm intervals. Moreover, administration of a highly concentrated contrast medium, i.e., 300 mg/ml, at a flow rate of 4 or 5 ml/s is also recommended to obtain adequate enhancement of these small vessels. The time delay between injection and acquisition is about 20 s in order to enable the contrast material to reach the systemic circulation at the time of scanning. 3D-SSD with a single thresholding segmentation is usually performed using bony structures, i.e., the sternum, ribs, and vertebral bodies, as anatomical references for better understanding of the anatomy of the abnormal systemic arteries. Whenever necessary, the bony structures will be removed to provide an exclusive 3D reformation of the systemic arteries.

It could be very useful to apply the current work in progress dedicated to the CT approach for transvenous coronary arteriography to the pulmonary systemic arteries. Adequate opacification of the coronary arteries can be achieved following a right-sided injection of contrast material (Thomas et al. 1995) and, in addition, most of the systemic arteries are spared from the cardiogenic through-plane motion.

11.7.1 Bronchopulmonary Sequestration

Nonbronchial systemic arteries of congenital origin or major aorto-pulmonary arteries are commonly found in intra- and extralobar sequestrations. The large systemic artery is unique in 80%–85% of the cases and multiple in the remainder. In both extralobar and intralobar types of bronchopulmonary sequestrations and associated derivatives, the abnormal vessel averages 6–7 mm in diameter and, most often, arises from the lower thoracic or upper abdominal aorta. In 25% of the cases, bronchopulmonary sequestrations receive their blood supply from the subclavian, intercostal pulmonary, pericardiacophrenic, innominate, internal thoracic, celiac, gastric, splenic, or renal arteries (SAVIC et al. 1979). Other origins are possible, for instance the coronary arteries (SILVERMAN et al. 1994). These ectopic origins of a systemic supply to the lung can also be observed in cases of so-called acquired sequestrations. In this group of patients, a congenital origin of the disease cannot be established and an acquired cause can be neither proven nor discarded. Asymptomatic patients suspected of having a pulmonary sequestration should benefit from spiral CT angiography, which is very often able to replace the more invasive thoracoabdominal aortography. This

minimally invasive way of delineating abnormal vascular anatomy can help select the best therapeutic option in order to prevent a dramatic outcome (RUBIN et al. 1994).

By performing two consecutive scans, one in the craniocaudal direction and the other in the inverted direction with a short interscan delay, dual-volume imaging can be performed. It is thus possible to examine the suspected area first in a pulmonary arterial phase and then in a systemic phase, allowing a much better utilization of the contrast medium bolus. To date, this technique has not been evaluated in the pretherapeutic management of pulmonary sequestrations but it has the potential to become the gold standard technique in patients in whom pulmonary and systemic angiographic examinations are required (MATA et al. 1991). As there is a considerable

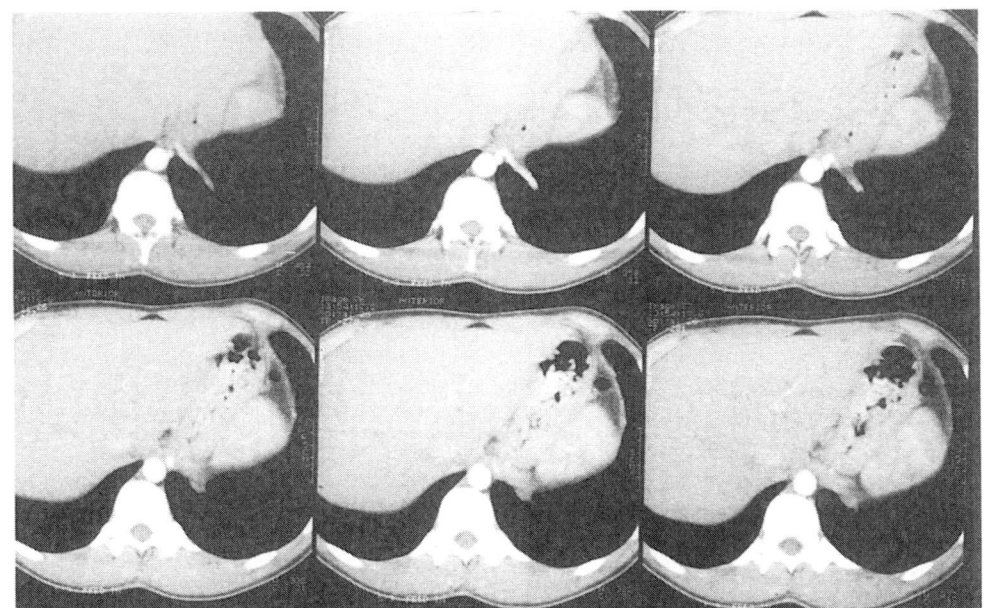

a

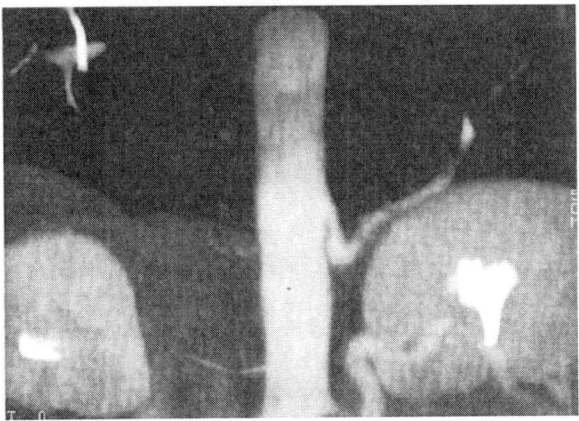

b

Fig. 11.13a,b. Spiral CT evaluation in a 17-year-old man indicated for clinical and radiological suspicion of bronchopulmonary sequestration (collimation, 3 mm; table feed, 5 mm/s; overlapping, 1 mm; acquisition time, 26 s; injection of 120 ml of a 300 mg/ml iodinated contrast agent via a 20-G needle inserted into an antecubital vein of the left arm; start delay, 15 s). **a** A small artery emerges from the left lateral wall of the descending anorta and runs into the left pulmonary ligament. **b** The ascending course of the abnormal systemic artery is clearly demonstrated on the MIP image, thus obviating the need for a thoracoabdominal aortogram. An adequate selection of the viewing angle for the MIP image precludes any misinterpretation of the arterial pathway, thus definitely excluding any subdiaphragmatic course of the abnormal artery

overlap between the development anomalies that may be associated with the scimitar syndrome, the "sequestration spectrum," and the right dysmorphic lung, a complete angiographic study is mandatory, even in asymptomatic patients, provided it is not invasive (CUKIER et al. 1994). At one end of the sequestration spectrum, a systemic supply to normal basal segments, more often of the left lung, can be found. In this situation also, spiral CT has the potential to become the gold standard diagnostic technique as a single spiral acquisition may demonstrate the normal appearance of the lung and the bronchial tree, the absence of an accompanying interlobar artery, and an abnormal dilated systemic artery taking the place of the pulmonary artery along the basal segmental bronchi and their branches. Multiplanar reformations and 3D imaging dedicated to the pulmonary artery, the systemic artery, the bronchial tree, and the pulmonary venous return may help provide additional information in comparison with conventional CT (KUROSAKI et al. 1993) (Fig. 11.13).

11.7.2 Acquired Systemic Supply to the Lung

11.7.2.1 Pretherapeutic Evaluation of Intracavitary Aspergilloma

Massive bleeding is responsible for the very high operative mortality associated with pulmonary resection of pulmonary mycetoma, which has been estimated to vary between 7% and 34% (NIWA et al. 1995). Transthoracic drainage may also be responsible for massive bleeding. The main cause of development of the fungus ball is the presence of cavitary tuberculosis, usually located in the posterior and apical segments of the upper lobes. Consequently, two types of abnormal systemic supply can be found. The ipsilateral bronchial artery usually supplies the hilar part of the cavity whereas transpleural nonbronchial systemic arteries supply its peripheral component. Spiral CT angiography may be useful in imaging abnormally enlarged collaterals of the subclavian artery. Such enlargement of these arteries can require surgical ligation or embolization in the operating room prior to the resection or to the transthoracic drainage and instillation of amphotericin in the cavity (NIWA et al. 1995). Spiral CT angiography should be performed in every case of intracavitary aspergilloma before percutaneous or surgical treatment, both of which are at high risk of massive iatrogenic bleeding (Fig. 11.14).

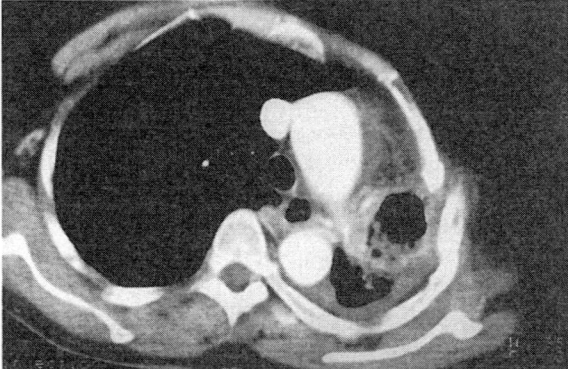

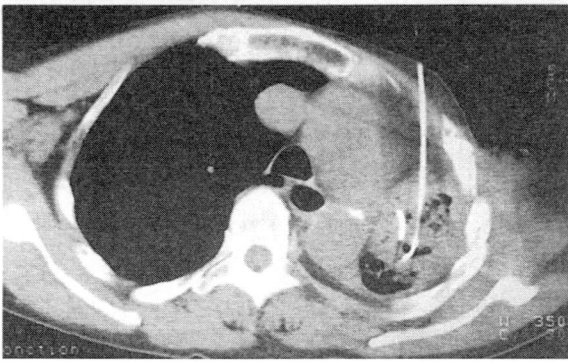

Fig. 11.14a,b. Spiral CT evaluation of an intracavitary aspergilloma located in the apical segment of the left lower lobe, several years after left upper lobectomy and prior to transthoracic drainage of the cavity (collimation, 5 mm; table feed, 5 mm/s; overlapping, 2 mm; acquisition time, 18 s; region of interest; from the subclavian area to the left hilum; 120 ml of a 300 mg/ml iodinated contrast agent injected at 5 ml/s in an antecubital vein; start delay, 18 s). a Bronchial hypervascularization surrounding the internal border of the cavity in close correlation with the angiographic findings. The absence of any other abnormal systemic artery allowed an anterior thoracic approach (b) (in correlation with intercostal and internal thoracic angiograms, not shown)

11.7.2.2 Diseases Known to Be Responsible for Systemic Hypervascularization and with a Possible Vascular Shadow

In various pathological conditions such as pulmonary artery or venous obstructions, chronic inflammatory disease of the lung, bronchi, and pleura, and neoplasms, the bronchial arterial blood flow can be dramatically increased. One of the commonest diseases responsible for the chronic and propressive development of profuse bronchial arterial supply to the lung is bronchiectasis. In a study of 260 patients treated by embolization for hemoptysis, bronchiectasis was found to represent the third most common cause of recurrent bronchial bleeding (RÉMY et al. 1992a). The pretherapeutic CT evaluation of

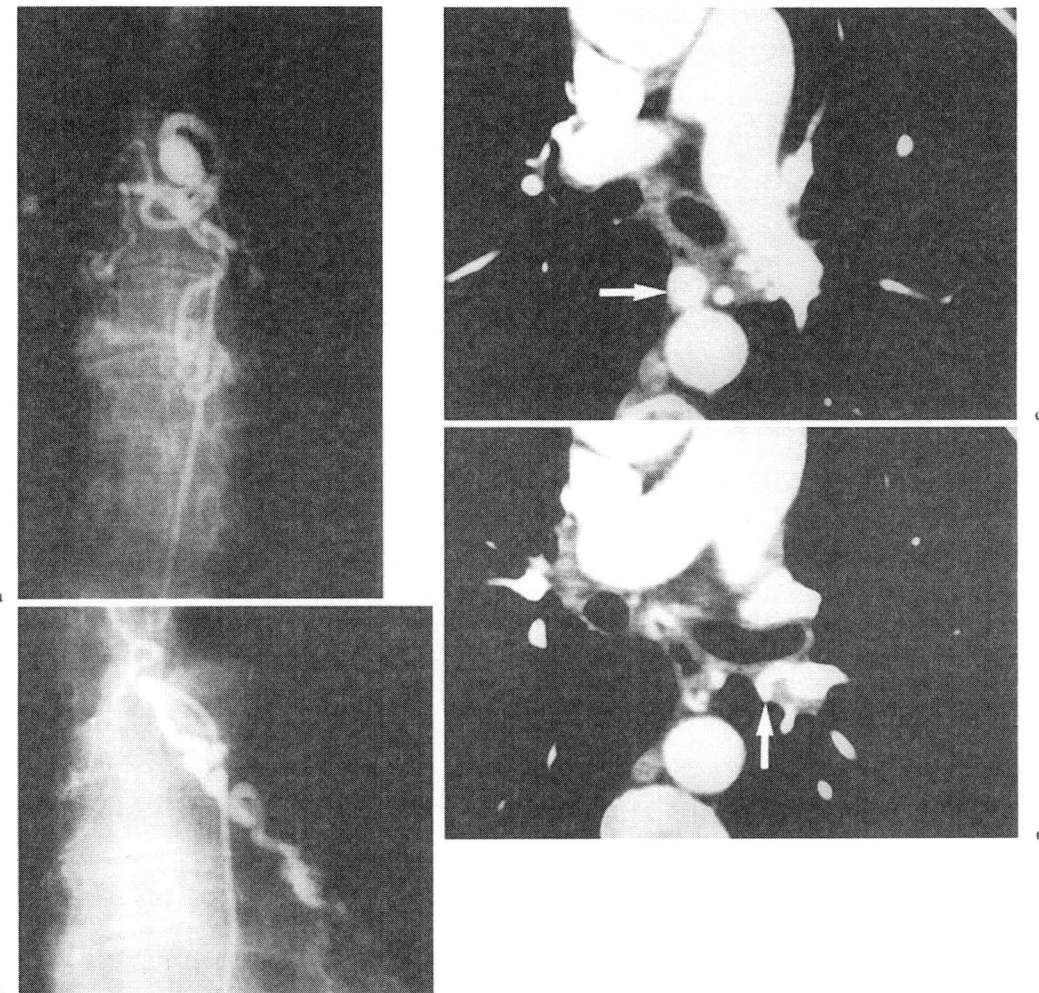

Fig. 11.15a–d. Spiral CT evaluation of bronchial arteries in a 54-year-old patient with bilateral bronchiectasis and a previous history of surgery and embolization procedures for recurrent massive hemoptysis. **a,b** Frontal views of bronchial artery angiograms showing a proximal aneurysm of the common trunk for the right and left lung (**a**) and a large left descending bronchial artery (**b**). **c,d** Spiral CT scans obtained 8 years after the angiograms for the follow-up of the bronchial aneurysm (collimation, 2 mm; table feed, 2 mm; overlapping, 1 mm; ac-quisition time, 16 s; 120 ml of a 300 mg/ml iodinated contrast agent injected at a rate of 5 ml/s in the left antecubital vein with the injected arm positioned along the thorax). There is optimal enhancement of the bronchial artery aneurysm, which is seen in a preaortic and retroesophageal location (**c**, *arrow*). Note the increased diameter and the tortuous course of the left bronchial artery along the internal border of the left lower lobe pulmonary artery (**d**, *arrow*)

bronchiectasis is usually performed with thin and noninjected spaced slices. This rule does have a few exceptions, however, one of them being when an abnormal shadow is suspected of being of vascular origin. Bronchial artery aneurysm is reportedly rare, but this rarity may be due to the usual absence of diagnosis when the aneurysm is asymptomatic or responsible for an idiopathic hemomediastinum. An abnormal opacity in the mediastinum anywhere along the course of the bronchial arteries should be investigated by means of spiral CT angiography (REMY-JARDIN et al. 1991a) (Fig. 11.15).

11.7.2.3 Hemoptysis Topographically Proven by Endoscopy but of Indeterminate Diagnosis

Spiral CT angiography can be helpful in two circumstances. First, it can show an artery of abnormal origin and course, and help to locate it on subsequent

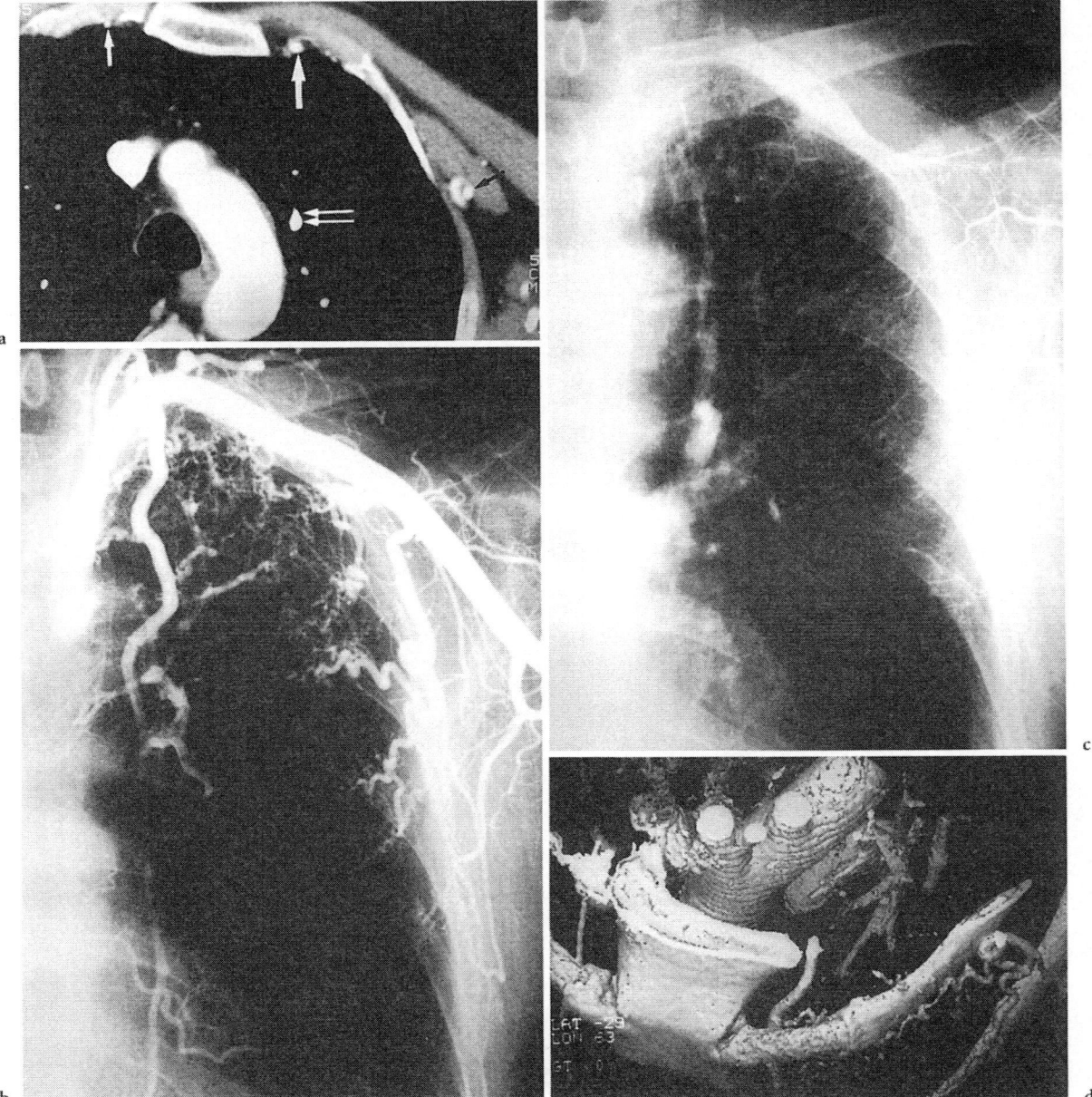

Fig. 11.16a–d. CT and angiographic evaluation for a continuous murmur over the left anterior chest wall several months after partical pleurectomy for bullous disease. **a,d** Spiral CT angiography of the upper part of the thorax (collimation, 3 mm; table feed, 3 mm/s; overlapping, 1 mm; 120 ml of a 300 mg/ml iodinated contrast medium injected at rate of 5 ml/s; right antecubital vein with the injected arm positioned along the thorax; acquisition time, 20 s; start delay, 20 s). In comparison with the right one (**a**, *small white arrow*), the proximal part of the left internal thoracic artery is dilated (**a**, *large white arrow*). Another arterial branch, running along the left lateral chest wall in contact with the posterior aspect of the pectoralis minor muscle (**a**, *black arrow*), is also dilated. There is dilatation of a left anterior intercostal artery. Among well-enhanced pulmonary vessels, note the presence of a larger branch (**a**, *double white arrow*) shown to correspond to a branch of the left superior pulmonary vein on the lung window settings (not shown). **b,c** Subsequent angiography of left subclavian and axillary arteries confirms the CT data. The 3D-SSD (**d**) confirms the abnormal dilatation of the left internal thoracic artery (thresholding segmentation: 100 HU). Some dilated left anterior intercostal arteries are also seen

selective angiography or at surgery. Second, approximately 5% of patients treated with embolization have either a diffuse and moderate or a focal area of bronchial hypervascularization without known bronchial or parenchymal disease, or, exceptionally, a bronchial artery aneurysm bulging in the bronchial lumen and pulsating on endoscopy. Some of these lesions can be compared with Dieulafoy's disease of the gastric and, less frequently, the intestinal arteries (SWEERTS et al. 1995). They can be depicted on spiral CT angiography sharply oriented by means of previous endoscopy. Spiral CT angiography may also avoid dangerous endobronchial biopsy of these vascular lesions (REMY et al. 1992).

11.7.2.4 Chronic Thromboembolic Disease

As expected, after chronic pulmonary artery occlusion the bronchial blood flow has been shown to dramatically increase. Using a section thickness of 4 mm, a table feed of 6 mm/s, a reconstruction increment of 3 or 4 mm, and a 100-ml intravenous bolus of a 300 mg/ml contrast medium at a flow rate of 2–3 ml/s, KAUCZOR et al. (1994b) detected bronchial arteries in 77% of patients with pulmonary hypertension and in 30% of patients without pulmonary hypertension. The mean proximal diameter was 1.5 mm in the first group, compared with 0.9 mm in the second group. According to these authors, the CT depiction of bronchial arteries represents a significant criterion for the suspicion of chronic thromboembolic pulmonary hypertension.

11.7.2.5 Bruit and Hyperemia over the Chest Wall

In addition to hemoptysis, inflammatory, neoplastic, postoperative, and traumatic processes may be the source of hypervascularization of the chest wall with a bruit or a shunt increasing the risk of heart failure (HUANG et al. 1995) or hemorrhage. The systemic origin of a shunt can be localized using minimally invasive techniques such as technetium-99m-labelled radionuclide enhanced angiography, pulmonary perfusion scintigraphy, Doppler ultrasonography of the chest wall, and spiral CT systemic angiography (Fig. 11.16). Some infectious processes of the chest wall can be intensely hypervascularized, including actinomycosis and bacillary angiomatosis (COCHE et al. 1995). Aspergillosis can erode the chest wall vessels. Primary and secondary hypervascularized tumors of the chest wall or ribs, such as angiosarcoma, hemangiopericytoma, and epithelioid hemangioma, can display intense contrast enhancement from the systemic arteries of the pleural or the chest wall. Their follow-up after chemotherapy or embolization can be achieved noninvasively with spiral CT.

References

Aberle DR, Brown K, Young DA, Batra P, Steckel RJ (1991) Imaging techniques in the evaluation of tracheobronchial neoplasms. Chest 99:211–215

Ahn JM, Im JG, Ryoo JW et al. (1995) Thoracic manifestations of Behçet syndrome: radiographic and CT findings in nine patients. Radiology 194:199–203

Albelda SM, Talbot GH, Gerson SL, Miller WT, Cassileth PA (1985) Pulmonary cavitation and massive hemoptysis in invasive pulmonary aspergillosis. Am Rev Respir Dis 131:115–120

Backer CL, Idriss FS, Holinger LD, Mavroudis C (1992) Pulmonary artery sling. Results of surgical repair in infancy. J Thorac Cardiovasc Surg 103:683–691

Barzilai B, Waggoner AD, Spessert C, Picus D, Goodenberger D (1991) Two-dimensional contrast echocardiography in the detection and follow-up of congenital pulmonary arteriovenous malformations. Am J Cardiol 68:1507–1510

Berdon WE, Baker DH, Wung JT et al. (1984) Complete cartilage-ring tracheal stenosis associated with anomalous left pulmonary artery: the ring-sling complex. Radiology 152:57–64

Berlinger NT, Freeman TJ (1989) Acute airway obstruction due to necrotizing tracheobronchial aspergillosis in immunocompromised patients: a new clinical entity. Ann Otol Rhinol Laryngol 98:718–720

Bex JP, Lecompte Y, Baillot F, Hazan E (1980) Anatomical correction of transposition of the great arteries. Ann Thorac Surg 29:86–88

Black MD, Shamji FM, Goldstein W, Sachs HJ (1992) Pulmonary resection and contralateral anomalous venous drainage: a lethal combination. Ann Thorac Surg 53:689–691

Blum U, Windfuhr M, Buitrago-Tellez C, Sigmund G, Herbst EW, Langer M (1994) Invasive pulmonary aspergillosis. MRI, CT, and plain radiographic findings and their contribution for early diagnosis. Chest 106:1156–1161

Bressler EL, Nelson JM (1992) Primary pulmonary artery sarcoma: diagnosis with CT, MR imaging, and transthoracic needle biopsy. AJR 159:702–704

Catala FJ, Marti-Bonmati L, Morales-Marin P (1993) Proximal absence of the right pulmonary artery in the adult: computed tomography and magnetic resonance findings. J Thorac Imaging 8:244–247

Chilvers ER, Whyte MKB, Jackson JE, Allison DJ, Hughes JMB (1990) Effect of percutaneous transcatheter embolization on pulmonary function, right-to-left shunt, and arterial oxygenation in patients with pulmonary arteriovenous malformations. Am Rev Respir Dis 142:420–425

Coche E, Beigelman C, Lucidarme O, Finet JF, Bakdach H, Grenier P (1995) Thoracic bacillary angiomatosis in a patient with AIDS. AJR 165:56–58

Cortese DA, Edell ES (1993) Role of phototherapy, laser therapy, brachytherapy and prosthetic stents in the management of lung cancer. Clin Chest Med 14:149–159

Cukier A, Kavakama J, Teixeira LR, Terra-Filho M, Vargas FS (1994) Scimitar sign with normal pulmonary venous drainage and systemic arterial supply. Scimitar syndrome or bronchopulmonary sequestration? Chest 105:294–295

Delany SG, Doyle TCA, Bunton RW, Hung NA, Joblin LU, Taylor DR (1993) Pulmonary artery sarcoma mimicking pulmonary embolism. Chest 103:1631–1633

Denning DW (1995) Commentary: unusual manifestations of aspergillosis. Thorax 50:812–813

Dillon EH, Camputaro C (1993) Partial anomalous pulmonary venous drainage of the left upper lobe vs duplication of the superior vena cava: distinction based on CT findings. AJR 160:375–379

Do P, Rémy-Jardin M, Lemonnier P et al. (1990) Pulmonary artery aneurysms in Behçet's disease: successful treatment with vaso-occlusion. J Intervent Radiol 5:91–93

Dondelinger RF, Vanderschelden P, Capasso P, Trotteur G (1995) Spiral CT applied to interventional procedures. JBR-BTR 78:118–125

Downey RJ, Trastek VF, Clay RP (1994) Right pneumonectomy syndrome: surgical correction with expandable implants. J Thorac Cardiovasc Surg 107:953–955

Ellis K (1991) Developmental abnormalities in the systemic blood supply to the lungs. AJR 156:669–679

Eng J, Murday AJ (1992) Leiomyosarcoma of the pulmonary artery. Ann Thorac Surg 53:905–906

Engeler CE (1995) Heart-lung and lung transplantation. Radiol Clin North Am 33:559–580

Ference BA, Shannon TM, White RI, Zawin M, Burdge CM (1994) Life-threatening pulmonary hemorrhage with pulmonary arteriovenous malformations and hereditary hemorrhagic telangiectasia. Chest 106:1387–1390

Freedom RM, Burrows PE, Moes CAF (1986) "Horseshoe" lung: report of five new cases. AJR 146:211–215

Gaubert JY, Moulin G, Thomas P, Reynaud-Gaubert M, Noirclerc M, Bartoli JM (1993) Anastomotic stenosis of the left pulmonary artery after lung transplantation: treatment by percutaneous placement of an endoprosthesis. AJR 161:947–949

Gefter WB (1992) The spectrum of pulmonary aspergillosis. J Thorac Imaging 7:56–74

Griffith BP, Magee MJ, Gonzalez IF et al. (1994) Anastomotic pitfalls in lung transplantation. J Thorac Cardiovasc Surg 107:743–754

Haitjema TJ, Overtoom TTC, Westermann CJJ, Lammers JWJ (1995) Embolisation of pulmonary arteriovenous malformations: results and follow up in 32 patients. Thorax 50:719–723

Hawkes DJ, Ruff CF, Studholme C, Edwards PJ, Wong WL, Padhani A (1995) Three-dimensional multimodal imaging in image-guided interventions. Semin Intervent Radiol 12:63–74

Hillerdal G (1989) Rounded atelectasis. Clinical experience with 74 patients. Chest 95:836–841

Hovaguimian H, Morris JF, Gately HL, Floten HS (1991) Pulmonary vein thrombosis following bilobectomy. Chest 99:1515–1516

Huang CL, Kitano M, Shindo T, Nagasawa M (1995) Systemic artery-to-pulmonary artery shunt after using an omental pedicle flap. Ann Thorac Surg 59:993–995

Jardin M, Rémy J (1986) Segmental bronchovascular anatomy of the lower lobes: CT analysis. AJR 147:457–468

Kalender WA, Polacin A, Suss C (1994) A comparison of conventional and spiral CT: an experimental study on the de-

tection of spherical lesions. J Comput Assist Tomogr 18:167–176

Katz JF, Yassa NA, Bhan I, Bankoff MS (1994) Invasive aspergillosis involving the thoracic aorta: CT appearance. AJR 163:817–819

Kauczor HU, Schwickert HC, Mayer E, Kersjes W, Moll R, Schweden F (1994a) Pulmonary artery sarcoma mimicking chronic thromboembolic disease: computed tomography and magnetic resonance imaging findings. Cardiovasc Intervent Radiol 17:185–189

Kauczor HU, Schwickert HC, Mayer E, Schweden F, Schild HH, Thelen M (1994b) Spiral CT of bronchial arteries in chronic thromboembolism. J Comput Assist Tomogr 18:855–861

Khanavkar B, Stern P, Alberti W, Nakhosteen JA (1991) Complications associated with brachytherapy alone or with laser in lung cancer. Chest 99:1062–1065

Kibbler CC, Milkins SR, Bhamra A, Spiteri MA, Noone P, Prentice HG (1988) Apparent pulmonary mycetoma following invasive aspergillosis in neutropenic patients. Thorax 43:108–112

Ko T, Gatz MG, Reisz GR (1990) Congenital unilateral absence of a pulmonary artery: a report of two adult cases. Am Rev Respir Dis 141:795–798

Koo BC, Woldenberg LS, Kim KT (1984) Pulmonary vein tumor thrombosis and left atrial extension in lung carcinoma. J Comput Assist Tomogr 8:331–336

Kramer MR, Denning DW, Marshall SE et al. (1991) Ulcerative tracheobronchitis after lung transplantation. Am Rev Respir Dis 144:552–556

Kurosaki Y, Kurosaki A, Irimoto M, Kuramoto K, Itai Y (1993) Systemic arterial supply to normal basal segments of left lower lobe: CT findings. J Comput Assist Tomogr 17:857–861

Lacrosse M, Trigaux JP, Van Beers BE, Weynants P (1995) 3D spiral CT of the tracheobronchial tree. J Comput Assist Tomogr 19:341–347

Laffey KJ, Thomashow B, Jaretzki A, Martin EC (1985) Systemic supply to a pulmonary arteriovenous malformation: a relative contraindication to surgery. AJR 145:720–722

Logan PM, Primack SL, Miller RR, Müller NL (1994) Invasive aspergillosis of the airways: radiographic, CT, and pathologic findings. Radiology 193:383–388

Maggi G, Casadio C, Pischedda F, Cianci R, Ruffini E, Filosso P (1993) Bronchoplastic and angioplastic techniques in the treatment of bronchogenic carcinoma. Ann Thorac Surg 55:1501–1507

Mata JM, Caceres J, Lucaya X (1991) CT diagnosis of isolated systemic supply to the lung: a congenital bronchopulmonary vascular malformation. Eur J Radiol 13:138–142

Matsumoto AH, Parker LA, Delany DJ (1987) CT demonstration of central pulmonary venous and arterial occlusive diseases. J Comput Assist Tomogr 11:640–644

Mazzucco A, Luciani GB, Bertolini P, Faggian G, Morand G, Ghimenton C (1994) Primary leiomyosarcoma of the pulmonary artery: diagnostic and surgical implications. Ann Thorac Surg 57:222–225

McCray P, Grandgeorge S, Smith W, Wagener J, Frey E (1986) Cine CT diagnosis of pulmonary artery sling. Pediatr Radiol 16:508–510

McHugh K, Blaquiere RM (1989) CT features of rounded atelectasis. AJR 153:257–260

Miller JD, Gorenstein LA, Patterson GA (1992) Staging: the key to rational management of lung cancer. Ann Thorac Surg 53:170–178

Naidich DP (1994) Helical computed tomography of the thorax. Clinical applications. Radiol Clin North Am 32:759–774

Napel S, Rubin GD, Jeffrey RB (1993) STS-MIP: a new reconstruction technique for CT of the chest. J Comput Assist Tomogr 17:832–838

Niwa H, Yamakawa Y, Fukai I, Kiriyama M, Kobayashi Y, Masaoka A (1995) Subclavian artery branch ligation reduces hemorrhage during resection of pulmonary aspergilloma. Ann Thorac Surg 59:1234–1235

Nori D, Allison R, Kaplan B, Samala E, Osian A, Karbowitz S (1993) High dose-rate intraluminal irradiation in bronchogenic carcinoma. Chest 104:1006–1011

Obermiller T, Lakshminarayan S, Willoughby S, Mendenhall J, Butler J (1991) Influence of lung volume and left atrial pressure on reverse pulmonary venous blood flow. J Appl Physiol 70:447–453

Ohri SK, Siddiqui AA, Townsend ER (1992) Cardiac torsion after lobectomy with partial pericardectomy. Ann Thorac Surg 53:703–705

Okada K, Okada M, Yamamoto S, Mukai T, Tsukube T, Matsuda H, Okada M (1993) Successful resection of a recurrent leiomyosarcoma of the pulmonary trunk. Ann Thorac Surg 55:1009–1012

Padhani AR, Fishman EK (1995) Spiral CT evaluation of lung cancer. In: Fischman EK, Jeffrey RB (eds) Spiral CT: principles, techniques and clinical applications. Raven Press, New York, p 131

Park JH, Chung JW, Im JG, Kim SK, Park YB, Han MC (1995) Takayasu arteritis: evaluation of mural changes in the aorta and pulmonary artery with CT angiography. Radiology 196:89–93

Partridge JB, Osborne JM, Slaughter RE (1988) Scimitar et cetera – the dysmorphic right lung. Clin Radiol 39:11–19

Philpott NJ, Woodhead MA, Wilson AG, Millard FJC (1993) Lung abscess: a neglected cause of life threatening haemoptysis. Thorax 48:674–675

Posniak HV, Dudiak CM, Olson MC (1993) Computed tomography diagnosis of partial anomalous pulmonary venous drainage. Cardiovasc Intervent Radiol 16:319–320

Procacci C, Residori E, Bertocco M, Di Benedetto P, Andreis IAB, D'Attoma N (1993) Left pulmonary artery sling in the adult: case report and review of the literature. Cardiovasc Intervent Radiol 16:388–391

Read RC, Ziomek S, Ranval TJ, Eidt JF, Gocio JC, Schaefer RF (1993) Pulmonary artery sleeve resection for abutting left upper lobe lesions. Ann Thorac Surg 55:850–854

Rémy J, Lemaitre L, Lafitte JJ, Vilain MO, Saint Michel J, Steenhouwer F (1984) Massive hemoptysis of pulmonary arterial origin: diagnosis and treatment. AJR 143:963–969

Rémy J, Rémy-Jardin M, Voisin C (1992a) Endovascular management of bronchial bleeding. In: Butler J (ed) The bronchial circulation. Lung biology in health and disease. Dekker, New York

Rémy J, Rémy-Jardin M, Wattinne L, Deffontaine C (1992b) Pulmonary arteriovenous malformations: evaluation with CT of the chest before and after treatment. Radiology 182:802–816

Rémy J, Rémy-Jardin M, Giraud F, Wattinne L (1994) Angioarchitecture of pulmonary arteriovenous malformations: clinical utility of three-dimensional helical CT. Radiology 191:657–664

Rémy-Jardin M, Rémy J, Ramon P, Fellous G (1991a) Mediastinal bronchial artery aneurysm: dynamic computed tomography appearance. Cardiovasc Intervent Radiol 14:118–120

Rémy-Jardin M, Wattinne L, Rémy J (1991b) Transcatheter occlusion of pulmonary arterial circulation and collateral supply: failures, incidents, and complications. Radiology 180:699–705

Rémy-Jardin M, Rémy J, Giraud F, Marquette CH (1993) Pulmonary nodules: detection with thick-section spiral CT versus conventional CT. Radiology 187:513–520

Rémy-Jardin M, Duyck P, Rémy J et al. (1995a) Hilar lymph nodes: identification with spiral CT and histologic correlation. Radiology 196:387–394

Rémy-Jardin M, Rémy J, Petyt L, Duhamel A (1995b) Sliding thin slab-maximum intensity projection (STS-MIP) in diffuse infiltrative lung disease: clinical value in detection of mild micronodular pattern. Radiology 197(P):404

Ren H, Hruban RH, Kuhlman JE, Fishman EK, Wheeler PS, Zerhouni EA, Hutchins GM (1989) Computed tomography of rounded atelectasis. J Comput Assist Tomogr 12:1031–1034

Rey C, Vaksmann G, Francart CH (1986) Anomalous unilateral single pulmonary vein mimicking partial anomalous pulmonary venous return. Cathet Cardiovasc Diagn 12:330–333

Robertson RJH, Robertson IR (1995) Pulmonary arteriovenous malformations. Thorax 50:707–708

Robinson LA, Reed EC, Galbraith TA, Alonso A, Moulton AL, Fleming WH (1995) Pulmonary resection for invasive aspergillus infections in immunocompromised patients. J Thorac Cardiovasc Surg 109:1182–1197

Rubin EM, Garcia H, Horowitz MD, Guerra JJ (1994) Fatal massive hemoptysis secondary to intralobar sequestration. Chest 106:954–955

Santelli ED, Katz DS, Goldschmidt AM, Thomas HA (1994) Embolization of multiple Rasmussen aneurysms as a treatment of hemoptysis. Radiology 193:396–398

Satur CHR, Robertson RH, Da Costa PE, Saunders NR, Walker DR (1991) Multiple pulmonary microemboli complicating pneumonectomy. Ann Thorac Surg 52:122–126

Savic B, Birtel FJ, Tholen W, Funcke HD, Knoche R (1979) Lung sequestration: report of seven cases and review of 540 published cases. Thorax 34:96–101

Schiller VL, Gray RK (1994) Causes of clot in the pulmonary artery after pneumonectomy. AJR 163:744–745

Schramel FMNH, Westerman CJJ, Knaepen PJ, Van den Bosch JMM (1995) The scimitar syndrome: clinical spectrum and surgical treatment. Eur Respir J 8:196–201

Sharma S, Talwa KK, Rajani M (1993) Coronary artery to pulmonary artery collaterals in nonspecific aortoarteritis involving the pulmonary arteries. Cardiovasc Intervent Radiol 16:111–113

Shields TW (1993) Surgical therapy for carcinoma of the lung. Clin Chest Med 14:121–147

Siebert JE, Rosenbaum TL (1993) Image presentation and post-processing. In: Potchen EJ, Haacke EM, Siebert JE, Gottschalk A (eds) Magnetic resonance angiography: concepts and applications. Mosby, St. Louis, pp 220–245

Siegel J, Shackelford GD, McAlister WH (1982) Tracheobronchography in the evaluation of anomalous left pulmonary artery. Pediatr Radiol 12:235–238

Silverman JM, Julien PJ, Herfkens RJ, Pelc NJ (1994) Magnetic resonance imaging evaluation of pulmonary vascular malformations. Chest 106:1333–1338

Silverman ME, White CS, Ziskind AA (1994) Pulmonary sequestration receiving arterial supply from the left circumflex coronary artery. Chest 106:948–949

Spencer DD, Garza JL, Walker WA (1993) Multiple tumor emboli after pneumonectomy. Ann Thorac Surg 55:169–171

Sweerts M, Nicholson AG, Goldstraw P, Corrin B (1995) Dieulafoy's disease of the bronchus. Thorax 50:697–698

Takahashi T, Yokoi K, Mori K, Miyazawa N (1993) Clot in the pulmonary artery after pneumonectomy. AJR 161:1110–1110

Takeda S, Imachi T, Arimitsu K, Minami M, Hayakawa M (1994) Two cases of scimitar variant. Chest 105:292–293

Taylor PM (1988) Dynamic contrast enhancement of asbestos-related pulmonary pseudotumours. Br J Radiol 61:1070–1072

Temeck BK, Venzon DJ, Moskaluk CA, Pass HI (1994) Thoracotomy for pulmonary mycoses in non-HIV-immunosuppressed patients. Ann Thorac Surg 58:333–338

Thomas PJ, McCollough CH, Ritman EL (1995) An electron-beam CT approach for transvenous coronary arteriography. J Comput Assist Tomogr 19:383–389

Thorsen MK, Erickson SJ, Mewissen MW, Youker JE (1990) CT and MRI imaging of partial anomalous pulmonary venous return to the azygos vein. J Comput Assist Tomogr 14:1007–1009

Tomiak MM, Foley WD, Jacobson DR (1995) Variable-mode helical CT: imaging protocols. AJR 164:1525–1531

Tunaci A, Berkmen YM, Gökmen E (1995) Thoracic involvement in Behçet's disease: pathologic, clinical, and imaging features. AJR 164:51–56

Ueki J, Hughes JMB, Peters AM et al. (1994) Oxygen and ^{99m}Tc-MAA shunt estimations in patients with pulmonary arteriovenous malformations: effects of changes in posture and lung volume. Thorax 49:327–331

Van Son JAM, Danielson GK, Puga FJ, Edwards WD, Driscoll DJ (1995) Repair of congenital and acquired pulmonary vein stenosis. Ann Thorac Surg 60:144–150

Voisin CH, Fisekci F, Voisin Saltiel S, Ameille J, Brochard P, Pairon JC (1995) Asbestos-related rounded atelectasis. Radiologic and mineralogic data in 23 cases. Chest 107:477–481

Wells TR, Gwinn JL, Landing BH, Stanley P (1988) Reconsideration of the anatomy of sling left pulmonary artery: the association of one form with bridging bronchus and imperforate anus. Anatomic and diagnostic aspects. J Pediatr Surg 23:892–898

White RI (1992) Pulmonary arteriovenous malformations: how do we diagnose them and why is it important to do so? Radiology 182:633–635

White RI, Pollak JS (1994) Pulmonary arteriovenous malformations: diagnosis with three-dimensional helical CT. A breakthrough without contrast media. Radiology 191:613–614

White RI, Mitchell SE, Barth KH, Kaufman SL, Kadir S, Chang R, Terry PB (1983) Angioarchitecture of pulmonary arteriovenous malformations: an important consideration before embolotherapy. AJR 140:681–686

White RI, Lynch-Nyhan A, Terry P et al. (1988) Pulmonary arteriovenous malformations: techniques and long-term outcome of embolotherapy. Radiology 169:663–669

Whyte MKB, Peters AM, Hughes JMB, Henderson BL, Bellingan GJ, Jackson JE, Chilvers ER (1992) Quantification of right to left shunt at rest and during exercise in patients with pulmonary arteriovenous malformations. Thorax 47:790–796

Worsey J, Pham SM, Newman B, Park SC, Del Nido PJ (1994) Left main bronchus compression after arterial switch for transposition. Ann Thorac Surg 57:1320–1322

Yamada I, Shibuya H, Matsubara O, Umehara I, Makino T, Numano F, Suzuki S (1992) Pulmonary artery disease in Takayasu's arteritis: angiographic findings. AJR 159:263–269

Young VK, Maghur HA, Luke DA, McGovern EM (1992) Operation for cavitating invasive pulmonary aspergillosis in immunocompromised patients. Ann Thorac Surg 53:621–624

Zonneveld FW (1994) A decade of clinical three-dimensional imaging: a review. III. Image analysis and interaction, display options, and physical models. Invest Radiol 29:716–725

12 Spiral CT of the Superior Vena Cava

C.J. Herold, A.A. Bankier, and D. Fleischmann

CONTENTS

12.1 Introduction

The advent of spiral CT has revolutionized our approach to the assessment of chest disorders, not only in terms of examination technique but also in the detection and characterization of thoracic pathology. Moreover, the inherent advantages of the method, including the ability to perform single breathhold studies, the optimal use of contrast material, continuous data acquistion, and the possibilities of three-dimensional imaging have provided new clinical applications, particularly in the evaluation of vas-

C.J. Herold, MD, Department of Radiology, University of Vienna, Währinger Gürtel 18–20, 1090 Vienna, Austria
A.A. Bankier, MD, Department of Radiology, University of Vienna, Währinger Gürtel 18–20, 1090 Vienna, Austria
D. Fleischmann, MD, Department of Radiology, University of Vienna, Währinger Gürtel 18–20, 1090 Vienna, Austria

cular abnormalities. Spiral CT angiography, which includes the option to reformat any desirable imaging plane, is now viewed as a valuable alternative to established vascular imaging methods such as conventional angiography, phlebography, or recently, magnetic resonance (MR) angiography.

Spiral CT angiography is an exquisite method for the assessment of the superior vena cava (SVC). The SVC can be affected by disorders such as thrombosis or displacement, compression, or occlusion secondary to tumors of the mediastinum or the adjacent lung. Because the SVC serves as the main pathway for contrast media import into the vascular system, SVC abnormalities are routinely depicted on contrast-enhanced CT scans of the thorax. However, in some cases, the detection and especially the characterization of SVC abnormalities may require a tailored methodological approach, i.e., a modification of the examination technique routinely used for the evaluation of the thorax.

In this chapter, we will provide information on the anatomic and physiologic basis of helical SVC imaging, touch upon the examination technique and technical problems inherent to SVC imaging, and discuss the use of this innovative method for the evaluation of specific disorders. We will also attempt to characterize the role of spiral CT angiography in relation to other imaging methods such as venography and MR angiography.

12.2 Anatomical and Physiological Considerations Relevant to Spiral CT of the SVC

The SVC is designed to carry blood from the head, the upper extremities, and the upper parts of the thorax to the right atrium of the heart. From its origin at the confluence of the left and the right brachiocephalic vein, the SVC arches slightly forward and courses caudally across the anterior mediastinum (Fig. 12.1) to empty into the superior orifice of the right atrium. Along its way through the thorax the

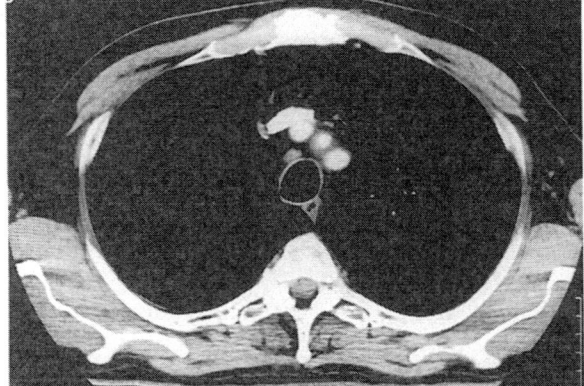

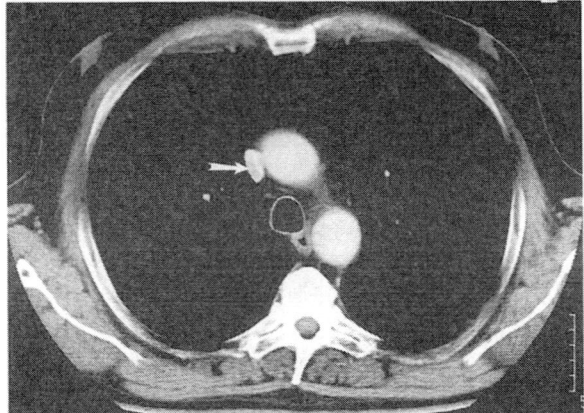

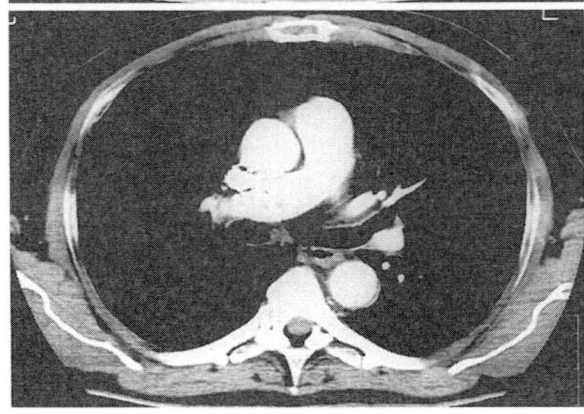

Fig. 12.1a–c. Anatomic correlates of the SVC. The SVC originates from the confluence of the left and right brachiocephalic veins (**a**) and descends downward through the right mediastinum, forming its right-hand border (**b,c**). The SVC has a close anatomic relationship to the ascending aorta, the right pulmonary artery, the right paratracheal space, and the right parietal pleura. For more details see text. Regarding the anatomic relationship of the SVC to other structures, see also all other figures. Note the pseudo-filling defect in the SVC due to an inflow phenomenon from unopacified blood (**b**, *arrow*)

only vessel discharging into the SVC is the azygos vein.

From its origin at the confluence of the right and the left brachiocephalic vein to its end at the orifice of the right atrium, the SVC has a total length of 6.5–8 cm. Because it is partially covered by the pericardium, the SVC can be divided into a larger extrapericardial portion and a smaller intrapericardial portion.

The extrapericardial portion accounts for two-thirds of the vessel's course and has an average length of 4–5 cm. Because of the oblique orientation of the pericardium, the extrapericardial portion of the SVC extends more caudally on its right lateral than on its left lateral margin. Due to the close anatomic relationship to numerous mediastinal structures as well as the pleura and lung, the extrapericardial portion of the SVC is exposed to any changes that result from disorders in this region.

The extrapericardial portion of the SVC is in contact *at the left* with the cranial part of the ascending aorta, from which it is separated by a narrow interstitial space. Owing to this intimate relationship, disorders of the ascending aorta, such as aneurysms, result in a displacement of the SVC mostly to the right. *At the right* the SVC adjoins the right phrenic nerve, which courses caudally, together with the right superior pericardiophrenic artery and vein, between the SVC and the parietal pleural layer. The vessel's close anatomic vicinity to the pleura and the lung makes it vulnerable to infiltration, compression, or displacement by bronchogenic tumors. *At the ventral aspect* the SVC is in contact with the costomediastinal pleural sac, with the anterior border of the right lung, with the right paratracheal lymph nodes, and with the right aspect of the thymus. Thus, the SVC is exposed to tumors arising in the thymic space, such as thymomas, lymphomas, or germ cell neoplasms. Finally, *at the dorsal aspect* the SVC borders the right pre- and paratracheal space, the anterior wall of the right pulmonary artery, and the cranial parts of the right pulmonary hilum. Here, the azygos vein arching cranially and ventrally empties into the dorsal part of the SVC. Space-occupying lesions in the right paratracheal space as well as massive dilatation of the right pulmonary artery can result in an anterior diplacement of the SVC (Fig. 12.2).

The intrapericardial portion of the SVC accounts for approximately one-third of the vessel's course and, from the penetration into the pericardium to the orifice of the right atrium, has a length of 2.5–3 cm. The pericardium circumferentially covers only three-quarters of the SVC, and this pericardial wrap-

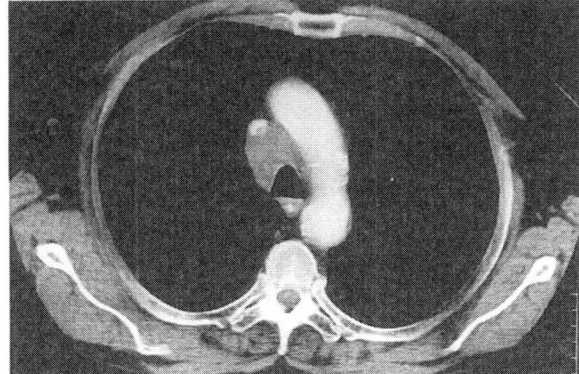

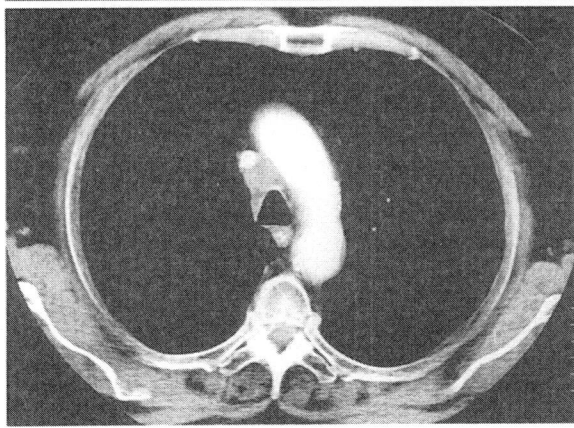

Fig. 12.2a,b. Effect of a space-occupying lesion in the right para- and pretracheal space on the SVC. **a** A small cell bronchogenic carcinoma is present in the right para- and pretracheal space, displacing and obstructing the SVC. Following chemotherapy, a decrease in tumor size can be observed (**b**), allowing the SVC to return to a nearly normal position and lumen

ping is more extensive ventrally and on the left than laterally and on the right. The intrapericardial portion of the SVC is in contact (a) *at the right*, with the pericardium, which separates the SVC from the phrenic nerve and the right superior pericardiophrenic artery and vein; (b) *at the left*, with the right orifice of the transverse sinus of the pericardium, which separates the SVC from the ascending aorta; (c) *at the ventral aspect*, with the right cardiac auricle; and (d) *at the dorsal aspect*, with the anterior part of the right superior pulmonary vein, from which it is separated by a small pericardial diverticulum. Compared to the extrapericardial portion of the SVC, the intrapericardial part can be regarded as somewhat more protected against the effects of space-occupying lesions of the mediastinum. It may, however, be affected by pericardial lesions as well as by enlargement of the right auricle and the right superior pulmonary vein.

The circular orifice of the SVC has a diameter of 2–2.5 cm and carries no valvular structures. At the level of the sinoatrial node the cranial part of the cardiac crista terminalis delimits the anatomic border between the SVC and the right atrium.

Due to its perpendicular axis with respect to the transaxial scan plane, the SVC has an oval or round configuration on CT sections (HEITZMANN 1988; GODWIN and CHEN 1986; WECHSLER et al. 1988; WEBB et al. 1982; PROTO 1987) (Fig. 12.1, 12.3). On CT scans of normal individuals the diameter of the SVC should be one-third to two-thirds that of the simultaneously depicted ascending aorta (GUTHANER et al. 1979). Care must be exercised, however, when evaluating the shape and the caliber of the SVC on CT because both its shape and its caliber can be subject to a large spectrum of varia-

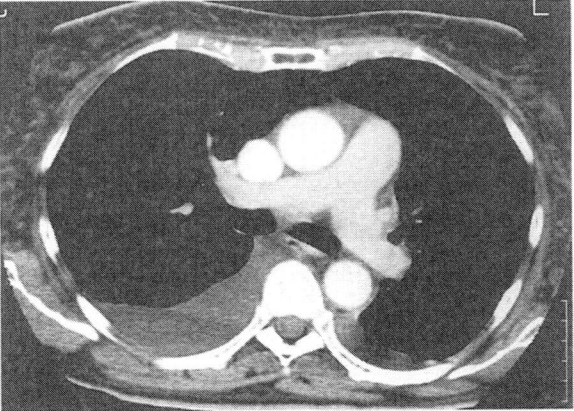

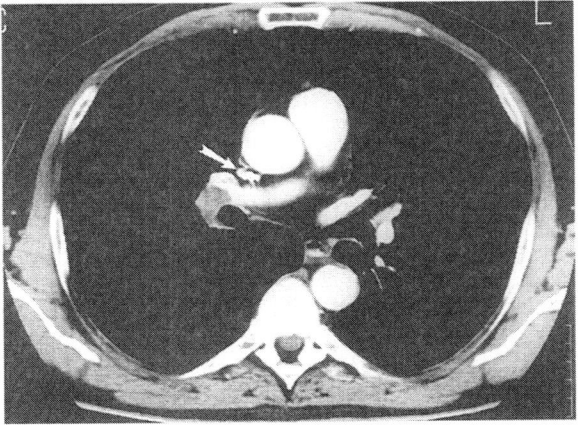

Fig. 12.3a,b. Variation in the appearance of the SVC due to different pathophysiologic conditions. **a** A dilated SVC is seen in a patient with combined left and right heart failure (compare with the normal appearance of the SVC in Fig. 12.1). Note also the soft tissue edema. The patient shown in **b** suffers from dehydration resulting in a slit-like appearance of the SVC (*arrow*). The soft tissue density lesion in the right hilum represents a bronchogenic carcinoma

tions under physiologic and pathologic conditions. Physiologic conditions that may alter the appearance of the SVC include forced expiration, forced inspiration, recumbency, pregnancy, and postoperative conditions. Pathologic conditions that may influence the appearance of the SVC include overhydration, dehydration, increased central venous pressure, emphysema, mediastinal fibrosis, and mediastinal or pulmonary neoplasms. Generally speaking, conditions resulting in increased intrathoracic pressure and/or decreased intravascular pressure (e.g., forced expiration, dehydration) will decrease the caliber of the SVC; the vessel may then appear flattened (Fig. 12.3). Conversely, conditions resulting in decreased intrathoracic pressure and/or increased intravascular pressure (e.g., forced inspiration, overhydration, increased central venous pressure) will increase the caliber of the SVC (Heitzmann 1988; Baron et al. 1981; Herman et al. 1994; Webb et al. 1982; Proto 1987; Godwin and Chen 1986) (Fig. 12.3). Moreover, both the shape and the caliber of the SVC may be subject to physiologic variations with age. As the great arterial vessels become ectatic in later life, the SVC is frequently displaced further into the right lung by the dilated and tortuous ascending aorta that lies medial to it.

Various radiographic signs that should help to distinguish pathologic from physiologic alterations of the SVC have been extensively described (Tocino and Watanabe 1986). It is important to be aware of the factors that could potentially influence the shape and caliber of the SVC because these factors can be helpful in elucidating unexpected or contradictory images of the SVC on CT.

12.3 Technical Considerations Relevant to Spiral CT of the SVC

In spiral CT imaging of the body, the SVC normally serves as the channel through which contrast medium is imported. To achieve adequate opacification of vascular and parenchymal structures, large amounts of iodine must be injected per unit of time, which provides a markedly dense opacification of the SVC. Thus, despite the excellent visualization of most mediastinal and thoracic vessels in contrast-enhanced spiral CT applications, the SVC often represents a source of artifacts. These artifacts not only may hinder assessment of the SVC but also can obscure neighboring structures that are of clinical interest.

A working knowledge of the dynamics of contrast enhancement in the SVC and an understanding of artifacts inherent to the CT image generation process can help to select appropriate contrast delivery techniques for optimal visualization of the SVC, as well as for other thoracic vessels. In the following section, we will discuss some of the technical parameters relevant to high-quality examinations of the SVC.

12.3.1 Dynamics of Bolus Contrast Injection

When contrast is injected via an antecubital vein, an increase in density in the SVC can be measured after an interval of a few seconds (2.5–5.5 s; phase 0) (Fig. 12.4). The attenuation values within the vessel then rapidly increase (phase I) until a plateau phase (phase II) is reached. In the ideal plateau phase there

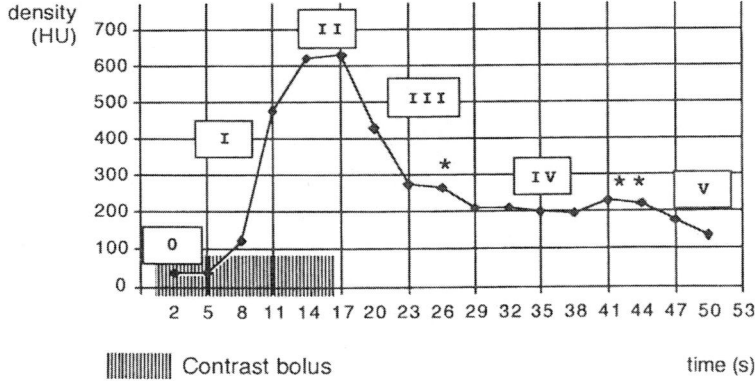

Fig. 12.4. Time-density curve from a single-slice dynamic CT study of the SVC following automated injection of 40 ml of iodinated contrast (300 mg I/ml) at a flow rate of 2.5 ml/s. ROI placement in the SVC was at the level of the pulmonary arter- ies. 0–V, Phases 0–V; see text for details; *, recirculation from the brain; **, recirculation from the inferior vena cava/renal veins

is a constant proportion of inflowing iodine to flowing blood within the measured volume (ROI area × slice thickness). Thus, the maximum enhancement in the initial plateau phase is primarily dependent on the amount of iodine per unit of time injected (mg I/s) and thus may be triggered by either changing the flow rate or the iodine concentration of the agent.

If the contrast bolus is sufficiently long, a further increase in density occurs when injected contrast mixes with "preopacified" blood that already contains iodine molecules. This "preopacified" blood first appears in the SVC approximately 20 s after the initial contrast injection [corresponding to the transit time required by an antecubitally injected bolus to reach the jugular veins (NAIDICH et al. 1991)], which is predominantly attributable to blood from the brain, where the intact blood-brain barrier does not allow iodine molecules to be distributed to the extravascular space. Another short increase in density may be observed approximately another 20 s later (40 s after contrast injection), which is most probably due to recirculating blood from the inferior vena cava and renal veins. Both events can be registered in time-density curves of the SVC on dynamic nonincremental studies after injection of a short (16 s) bolus of contrast (Fig. 12.4)

The flow rate of the injected volume (regardless of its iodine concentration) influences contrast dynamics in that larger volumes are forwarded faster in the venous system and thus arrive a little earlier at the ROI in the SVC. Another consideration with flow rates is that low flow–high concentration protocols probably lead to more marked density differences within the inhomogeneously mixing opacified and nonopacified blood, resulting in more pronounced streak artifacts.

Almost immediately after cessation of contrast injection, density values decrease rapidly (phase III) as no more iodine is added to preopacified blood flowing through the SVC (Fig. 12.4). When the length of the contrast injection does not exceed 1 min (which is usually the case for thoracic spiral CT applications), and thus no equilibrium between intravascular and extravascular iodine concentrations has yet evolved, a more shallow decrease (phase IV) in density may be seen subsequently. This shallow decrease is caused by ongoing distribution of the iodine molecules to the comparatively large extravascular space. As soon as an intra-/extravascular equilibrium is reached, a further decrease in density (phase V) is primarily caused by renal excretion of contrast material (ONO et al. 1980; GARDEUR et al. 1980). The density levels of phases IV and V depend primarily on

the total amount of iodine administered and its relation to individual extracellular fluid volume and thus are inversely related to body weight.

12.3.2 Artifacts and Pitfalls

Artifacts are frequently seen on spiral CT scans of the SVC. Because they are a major source of misinterpretation, it is important to be familiar with the phenomena potentially leading to false-positive or false-negative results. Most commonly, diagnostic pitfalls are due to streak artifacts and, second, due to flow phenomena.

12.3.2.1 Streak Artifacts

Streak artifacts arising from the densely opacified SVC as well as other high-density structures, such as indwelling catheters or pacemaker wires, are a well-recognized problem in contrast-enhanced thoracic spiral CT. Such artifacts may obscure clinically relevant abnormalities in the SVC and, because they extend beyond the limits of this vessel, also in the adjacent mediastinal structures (Fig. 12.5). In addition, they may mimic abnormalities such as "pseudothrombi" in the SVC and the right pulmonary artery (Fig. 12.5). These filling defects are particularly disturbing because they may render a conclusive diagnosis of the presence or absence of pulmonary emboli impossible. Thus, it is important to be familiar with the technical background in order to interpret these artifacts, and with the basic strategies employed to curb them.

Artifacts inherent to the CT imaging process arise because of geometric inconsistencies in the view data (JOSEPH 1981). If a single ray sample is grossly different from its neighboring ray samples (as in the case of marked density differences within or at the edge of the enhanced SVC), this will give rise to a streak on back-projection and in the final image. Likewise, if one of the views that are used to reconstruct a single image is grossly different from neighboring views, streaks will also occur. The latter may be the case when there is rapid motion (in the range of cardiac pulsation) of a high-contrast edge (SVC) during data acquisiton, but also with smoother motion that can lead to inconsistencies between the first and last views used to reconstruct an image.

In a preliminary series of four patients who underwent single-slice dynamic CT at the level of the SVC (17 scans/patient, obtained within 1 min) prior

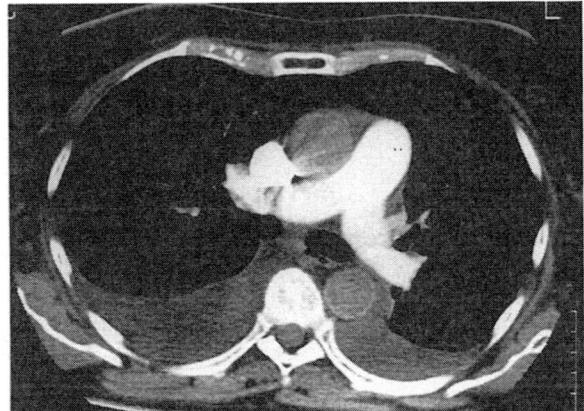

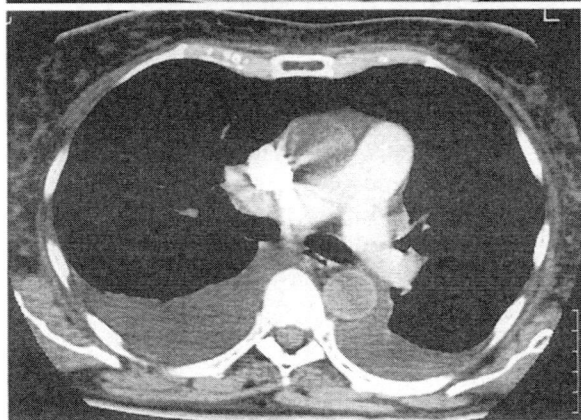

Fig. 12.5a,b. Marked streak artifacts arising from the densely opacified SVC. On consecutive slices at 11 s (**a**) and 14 s (**b**) after the beginning of contrast injection, streaks appear in different locations and orientations on both images despite only a minor change in the density of the SVC (478 HU in **a** versus 501 HU in **b**). Streak artifacts may render the assessment of adjacent strictures difficult and result in "pseudo thrombi" in the right pulmonary artery (**a**)

to spiral CT studies of the pulmonary arteries in our institution, we did not observe relevant streak artifacts arising from the SVC when density values in the SVC were less than 200 Hounsfield units (HU). In the majority of those images in which attenuation values of the SVC exceeded 250 HU, streak artifacts were present. Artifacts were more prominent when opacified and nonopacified blood was inhomogeneously distributed in the SVC. In the latter case, streaks arose not only from the edges of the SVC but also from central parts of the vessel.

It is interesting that streak artifacts appeared neither in exactly the same location nor in the same orientation on consecutive slices even if the attenuation values remained practically unchanged in the SVC (Fig. 12.5). The primary explanation for this is

probably the fact that the thin-walled SVC is never motionless within the time needed for the acquisition of an image, and the velocity and direction of motion are unlikely to be identical in different time windows of data acquisition.

In principle, streak artifacts can be avoided by the use of a lower concentration of contrast medium (150 mg iodine/ml) and/or by performing a delayed second helical CT scan in the redistribution phase in which the opacification of the SVC is generally very homogeneous (Fig. 12.6). Alternatively, spiral CT allows the reconstruction of axial slices from the volumetric data set at arbitrary table positions and thus at arbitrary time windows (KALENDER et al. 1990) with artifacts in different positions and different orientations on each of the reconstructed axial slices.

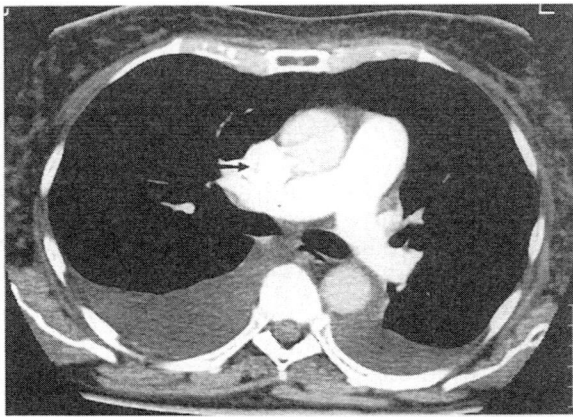

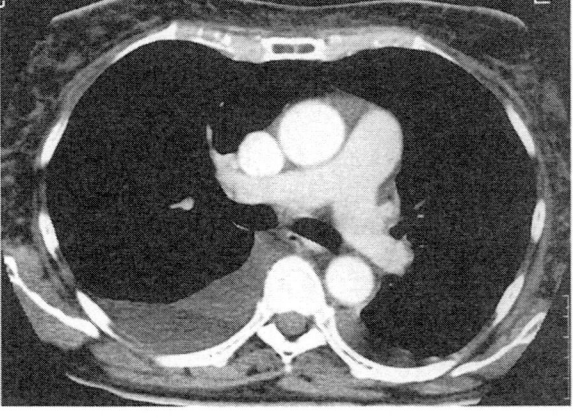

Fig. 12.6a,b. Inflow artifact in the SVC (same patient as shown in Figs. 12.3a and 12.5). **a** A pseudo-thrombus is displayed in the SVC (*arrow*) due to inflow of nonopacified blood from the azygos vein (time after initiation of contrast injection: 26 s; density in SVC: 268 HU). Note that mild streak artifacts occur not only from the edges of the SVC but also from contrast differences within the vessel itself. **b** Homogeneous opacification (196 HU) of the SVC in the redistribution phase (phase IV, at 35 s p.i.) can be seen

Thus, the use of overlapping reconstruction increases the probability that the particular structure of interest, e.g., the aorta or pulmonary artery, is not obscured by streaks on some of the reconstructed slices.

12.3.2.2 Flow-Related Artifacts

The second major source of of potentially confusing artifacts that can cause misinterpretation are flow phenomena (GODWIN and WEBB 1982). Flow artifacts may arise from (a) inhomogeneous distribution of the contrast medium in the bloodstream, especially when power injectors are used, and (b) inflow phenomena due to unenhanced blood from the brachiocephalic, jugular, or azygos vein. In both cases, nonopacified blood intermingles with contrast-enhanced blood, resulting in an inhomogeneous distribution with layering or swirling of contrast material, or displacement of contrast material to the periphery of the SVC due to laminar flow. The inhomogeneous opacification of the SVC may produce a variety of intraluminal pseudo-filling defects (GODWIN and WEBB 1982) which are indistinguishable from a floating thrombus on a single or even multiple sections (Figs. 12.1, 12.6). Nevertheless, differentiation of these artifacts from true thrombi is frequently possible by analyzing a cohort of images. Also, performing a delayed second helical CT scan in the redistribution phase, in which the opacification of the SVC is generally very homogeneous, or a follow-up study is usually helpful.

12.4 Practical Recommendations for the Assessment of the SVC

Optimal visualization of the SVC requires the use of intravenous contrast. A nonenhanced sequence or a number of nonenhanced slices prior to a contrast-enhanced spiral CT study, however, may provide helpful information in individual cases. Despite the fact that there is no consensus concerning the means of achieving optimal visualization of various mediastinal vessels (VERSCHAKELEN 1995), we can provide some basic recommendations about scanning procedures for spiral CT of the SVC that have proved useful in clinical practice.

For a tailored approach to the evaluation of the SVC, scanning should not be started during excessive opacification of the SVC but, rather, after the end of the contrast injection phase (scan delay: 55–80 s). We

have now started to use an intermediate-volume (80–120 ml, 300 mg I/ml), low-flow (1.5 ml/s) protocol which results in higher plasma iodine concentrations in the equilibrium phase compared with high-flow studies (ONO et al. 1980). This technique provides good opacification of all mediastinal vessels and allows adequate lesion enhancement. Scanning should be started immediately (when scanning from caudal to cranial) or 5 s after (when scanning from cranial to caudal) cessation of contrast injection.

If a high grade of vascular opacification in mediastinal vessels other than the SVC or the assessment of nonvascular structures in the mediastinum or upper abdomen is of particular interest, one may use a *double helix protocol* with an initial large-volume/high-flow sequence (100–150 ml, 300 mg I/ml, 2.5–3.5 ml/s), followed by an interscan delay of 10–15 s and then by another spiral CT acquisition through the upper mediastinum in the equilibrium phase (Fig. 12.6). If contrast dynamics are unpredictable, as in the case of known thrombosis of the SVC or in patients with cardiac failure, or when a different injection site (e.g., lower extremity) has to be used, a dynamic nonincremental sequence with a limited amount of contrast prior to the spiral CT sequence may help to design the best study protocol.

Beam collimation in spiral CT sequences of the SVC (5–10 mm) and pitch (1–1.5) are adjusted to the total study volume of interest. We normally use reconstruction intervals of one-half to four-fifths of beam collimation (50%–80% overlap). When streak artifacts excessively impair image quality, we retrospectively reconstruct more overlapping slices from the raw data to increase the diagnostic accuracy of the study.

To evaluate more complex vascular or perivascular abnormalities, simple multiplanar reformatting (Fig. 12.7) and/or cinematic viewing ("cine-mode") may be helpful. In addition, CT angiography, using maximum intensity projection or surface shading techniques, can be used to provide accessory information (RUBIN et al. 1994). Finally, volume rendering techniques with interactive real-time rendering now provide a unique ability to interactively render diagnostically useful images of the vasculature (JOHNSON P.T., personal communication, 1995).

12.5 Congenital Anomalies of the SVC

In view of the complex embryogenesis of the venous system, the relative frequency of congenital anoma-

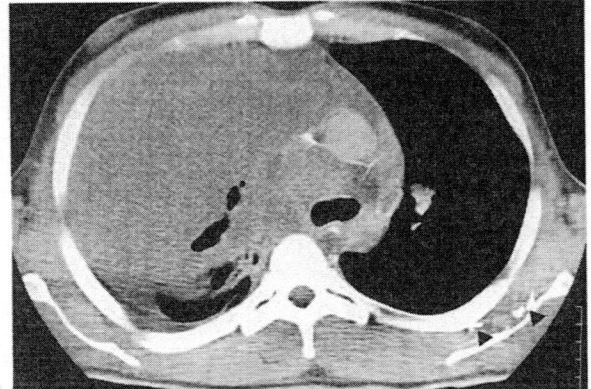

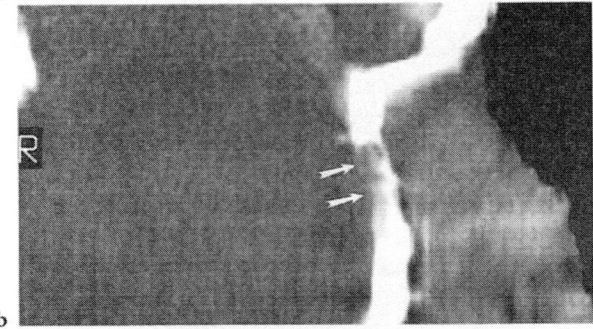

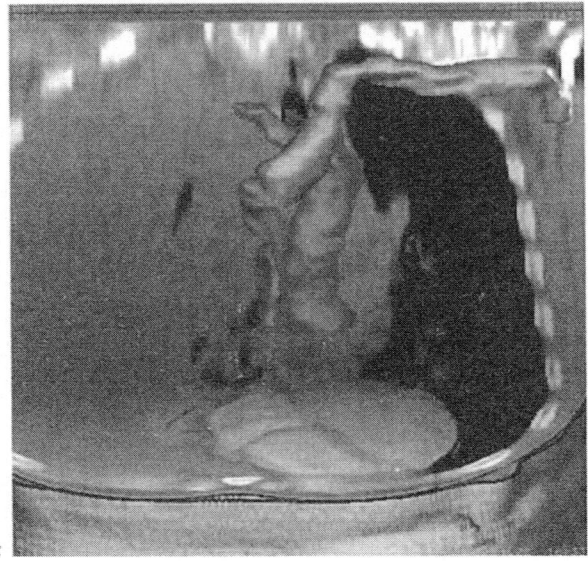

Fig. 12.7a–c. Value of multiplanar reformatting and 3D reconstruction in the assessment of SVC obstruction. Spiral CT scans through the upper mediastinum in a patient with small cell lung cancer demonstrates a large mediastinal mass displacing but also invading the SVC. Note unilateral venous collaterals in the parascapular space (*arrowheads*). Whereas the invasion is not well appreciated on the axial spiral CT scan (**a**), it is nicely demonstrated on a reformatted coronal image (**b**, *arrows*). 3D reconstruction provides a plastic impression of the pathoanatomic situation but fails to depict the invasion (**c**)

lies of large systemic veins is not surprising. Since such abnormal venous channels almost always empty into other systemic veins, they rarely cause clinically apparent functional changes. Therefore, congenital abnormalities are usually discovered incidentally during the course of radiographic or angiographic procedures, or at postmortem examinations (HEITZMANN 1988; BARON et al. 1981; WINTER 1954). It is interesting that most congenital malformations of the SVC occur in its inferior aspect. Four major distinct types of anomalies occur in or affect the SVC: (a) the persistent left SVC; (b) azygos and hemiazygos continuation of the inferior vena cava; (c) total anomalous pulmonary venous connection to the left SVC; and (d) the anomalous left brachiocephalic vein. In the following, we describe these major disorders and the role of CT imaging in their detection and diagnosis.

12.5.1 Persistent Left SVC

In 0.3%–0.5% of the healthy population and in 4.4%–12.9% of those with congenital heart disease, a persistent left SVC is present (WINTER 1954; CORMIER et al. 1989; CHA and KHOURY 1972). This anomaly results from failure of obliteration of the left common cardinal vein during fetal development (WINTER 1954). On CT scans, the diagnosis of a persistent left SVC usually poses no problem provided the reader is aware of the abnormality and contrast material is injected into the left cubital or forearm veins (WEBB et al. 1982; HUGGINS et al. 1982; CORMIER et al. 1989). The left SVC originates from the junction of the left jugular and subclavian veins and travels vertically through the left mediastinum, passing anterior to the left main bronchus before joining the left coronary sinus along a course ordinarily occupied by the ligament and vein of Marshall (GUTHANER et al. 1979; BARON et al. 1981; BUIRSKI et al. 1986) (Fig. 12.8). From this point the blood flows into the right atrium through the coronary sinus (which is significantly larger than normal because of the increased blood flow) while the right SVC drains into the right atrium. A persistent left SVC may be seen in the absence or presence of a normal right SVC.

Multiplanar reformatting provides an excellent possibility to create venography-like images and thus helps the radiologist or the clinician to aid in the diagnosis of the abnormality. It may also allow differentiation of a persistent left SVC from partial anomalous venous drainage of the left upper lobe

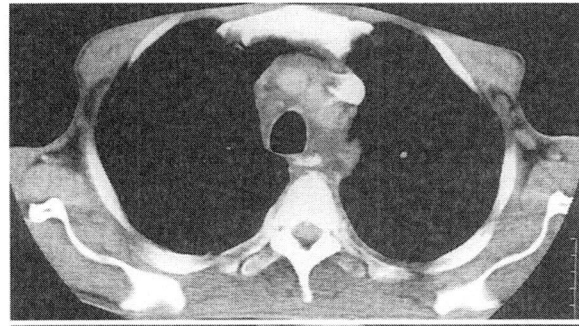
a
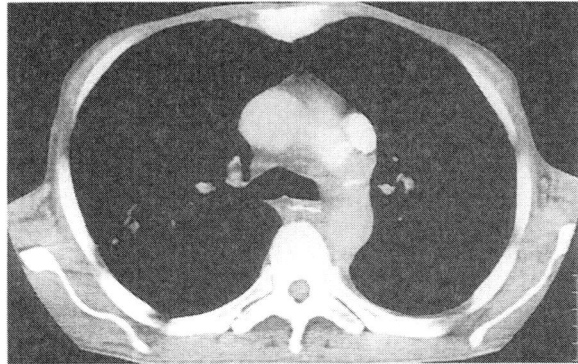
b
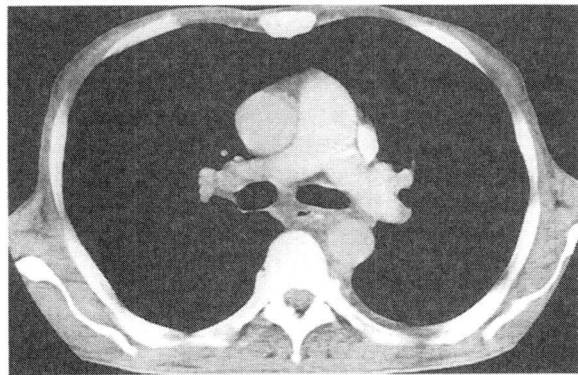
c
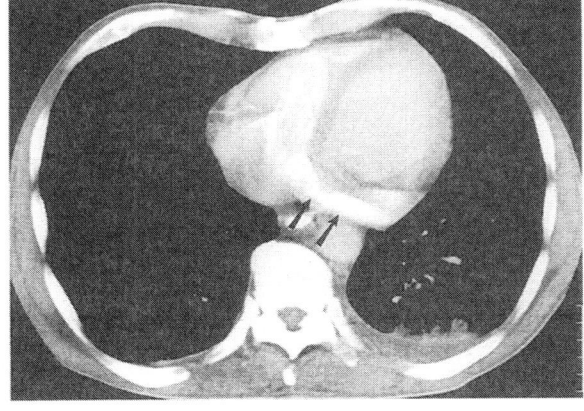
d

Fig. 12.8a–d. Spiral CT demonstration of a persistent left SVC. The left SVC can be nicely seen on spiral CT scans traveling through the left mediastinum and draining into the right atrium via the coronary sinus (*arrows*)

(DILLON and CAMPUTARO 1993). On unenhanced scans a persistent left SVC may, however, be confused with mediastinal lymphadenopathy if the full course of the vessel is not appreciated (HUGGINS et al. 1982; WEBB et al. 1982).

12.5.2 Azygos and Hemiazygos Continuation of the Inferior Vena Cava

Azygos and hemiazygos continuation of the inferior vena cava (IVC) derives from failure of the infrahepatic segment of the IVC to achieve patency. In this case, the intermediate segment of the supracardinal veins will join the IVC to the azygos or hemiazygos system. On spiral CT scans, azygos connection and hemiazygos continuation of the IVC with azygos connection may demonstrate similar findings in the region of the azygocaval junction. Due to increased blood flow, the ascending azygos vein, the azygos arch, and the distal SVC are dilated (DUDIAK et al. 1989). At a lower level, in cases of azygos continuation, the dilated vein is seen in a normal position slightly right of the midline in front of the vertebral spine. In hemiazygos continuation of the IVC with azygos connection, the dilated hemiazygos vein lies posterior to the aorta and left of the spine. If the hemiazygos continuation fails to reach azygos connection, the dilated vein remains on the left and drains into the dilated left superior intercostal vein or persistent left SVC. These associated abnormalities, as well as others such as polysplenia and congenital heart disease, should be searched for on spiral CT scans.

12.5.3 Total Anomalous Pulmonary Venous Connection to the Left SVC

Total anomalous pulmonary venous connection to the left SVC is the most frequent type of anomalous pulmonary venous connection (GUTHANER et al. 1979; HEITZMANN 1988). In this type of anomaly, the right pulmonary veins converge to form a single vessel that runs behind a small left atrium to join the left pulmonary veins. From the junction of the right and left pulmonary vein a large single vessel representing a persistence of the distal left SVC carries the pulmonary venous blood by way of a dilated left brachiocephalic vein and the right SVC to the right atrium. Frequently, an atrial septal defect or, more commonly, a widely patent foramen ovale is present. In this case, tremendous right atrial and right ventricular enlargement develop early and rapidly (GUTHANER et al. 1979; BUIRSKI et al. 1986).

Spiral CT easily depicts the venous vascular, cardiac, and parenchymal anomalies seen in this disorder. Because of the complex anatomic situation, multiplanar reformatting, particularly in a coronal plane, as well as CT angiography with volume rendering may be helpful in the diagnosis of this disorder. In addition, spiral CT can also visualize changes in the lung parenchyma due to increased pulmonary blood flow.

12.5.4 Anomalous Left Brachiocephalic Vein

It is suggested that the incidence of an anomalous left brachiocephalic vein is approximately 0.2%. This abnormality has no functional significance; however, cardiac catheterization or transvenous pacemaker placement may be technically difficult when a left arm approach is used (KIM et al. 1994). Whereas the normal brachiocephalic vein embryologically results from a connection between the left and the right anterior cardinal veins, the abnormal brachiocephalic vein enters the right SVC below and behind the aortic arch, below the entrance of the azygos vein, and thus represents a connection between the left anterior cardinal vein and the right common cardinal vein.

The anomalous left brachiocephalic vein is usually not visible on plain radiographs but spiral CT accurately depicts this abnormality (KIM et al. 1994). Multiplanar reconstruction of spiral CT data may enhance the prompt recognition of this condition (KIM et al. 1994).

12.6 Specific Abnormalities of the SVC

Spiral CT angiography with its rapid scan times, its volumetric data acquisition, and its multiplanar reformatting capabilities has rapidly emerged as an attractive technique for the assessment of specific abnormalities of the SVC. With the exception of extremely rare cases of idiopathic aneurysms of the SVC (MONCADA et al. 1985), most disorders involving the SVC present with displacement, obstruction, or occlusion of the vessel. Space-occupying lesions in the immediate vicinity of the SVC tend to compress or displace this thin-walled low-pressure structure. Thrombosis due to tumorous disorders or indwelling catheters may completely occlude the SVC lumen. When the venous flow in the SVC is significantly compromised, signs and symptoms of the so-called

superior vena cava syndrome may become apparent, particularly if the azygos vein is also obstructed. In cases where the SVC obstruction develops slowly and continuously, the recruitment of venous collaterals may prevent the development of the SVC syndrome.

12.6.1 The Superior Vena Cava Syndrome

Obstruction or occlusion of the SVC, resulting from extrinsic compression or intrinsic thrombosis, may produce a distinct constellation of clinical symptoms, the so-called superior vena cava syndrome. The latter is characterized by a variety of clinical signs triggered by proximal venous hypertension, including (a) severe headaches, (b) cyanosis of the face and conjunctivae, (c) edema, plethora, and suffusions of the head, neck, and arms, (d) dilatation of the veins of the head, neck, and the thoracic inlet, and (e) visible collaterals along the chest wall.

In patients with SVC syndrome, the role of spiral CT imaging resides in the clarification of the signs and severity of venous obstruction, the demonstration of sufficient collateralization, and the detection of vessels accessible to cannulation. In patients with clinically apparent SVC syndrome, the spiral CT examination technique should be tailored to the evaluation of the SVC (see Sect. 12.4). In the following, we will discuss specific abnormalities causing SVC syndrome.

12.6.2 Thrombosis of the SVC

Thrombosis of the SVC is a well-known phenomenon which may appear due to malignant tumors or is observed as a complication of central venous catheters and pacemakers. In malignant disorders, tumors obstructing or occluding the SVC may trigger partial or complete secondary venous thrombosis (EDWARDS et al. 1992). In addition, tumors of the lung, the mediastinum, or the thyroid gland may invade adjacent venous structures with centripedal intravascular tumor growth that results in partial or complete obstruction of the SVC (NIEDERLE et al. 1990; KOROBKIN and CASANO 1989) (Fig. 12.9).

With the widespread use of central venous catheters, catheter-related thrombosis is observed with increasing frequency. Prospective series have demonstrated partial or complete central venous thrombosis by venography in 28%–54% of all patients with central venous catheters (LOWELL and

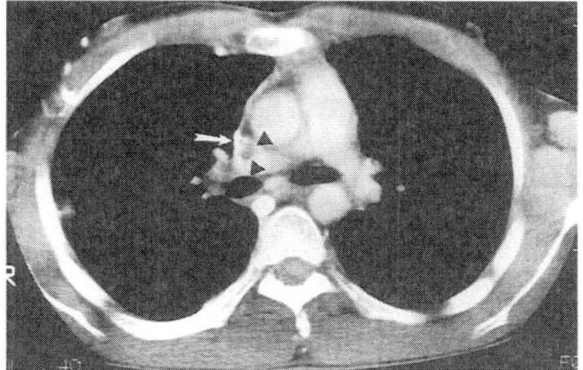

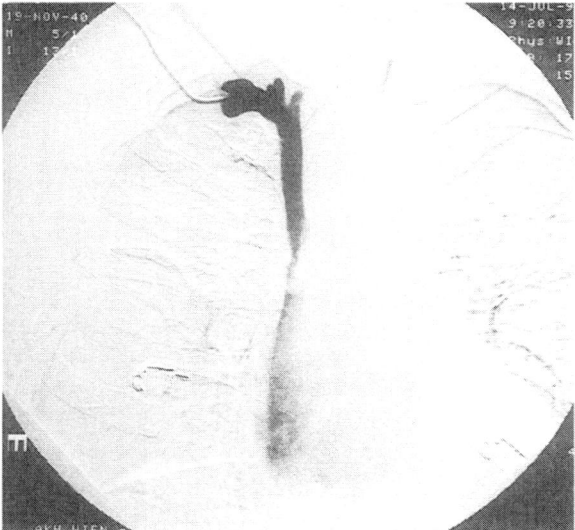

Fig. 12.9a,b. Spiral CT scan of a large tumor thrombus in the SVC in a patient with thyroid cancer. Spiral CT through the upper mediastinum shows a large filling defect in the anterior portion of the SVC (a). Note also multiple lymph nodes in the upper mediastinum and a small filling defect in a left upper lobe artery representing a fresh embolus. During surgical removal of the primary tumor, a large tumor thrombus extending into the SVC was simultaneously resected (b)

BOTHE 1991). Therefore, one must be aware that any indwelling catheter may harbor a potentially significant thrombus.

On spiral CT, catheter-related thrombi (especially when small) can easily be missed because of potentially severe streak artifacts arising from the indwelling catheter. If visible, thrombi present as a mass-like or sheath-like lesion surrounding the distal part and/or tip of the indwelling catheter which partially or completely obstructs the SVC lumen. Often, apposition of thrombotic material leads to growth of the thrombus which may extend into the distal SVC or the right atrium. It is of note that thrombi may persist in the SVC after removal of the catheter (Fig. 12.10). These "leftover" thrombi

present as wall-adherent masses or central filling defects, the latter indicating the presence of a floating component of the thrombus. Gas bubbles within the thrombus may indicate its septic nature (MORI et al. 1990).

If central venous thrombosis is suspected clinically, bilateral injection of low osmolarity contrast media is advantageous to demonstrate the site and extent of the thrombus, to demonstrate venous collateral pathways, and to avoid misinterpretation due to flow artifacts. In cases where the catheter-induced thrombosis incompletely obstructs the lumen of the SVC, the clinical presentation may be silent. In such

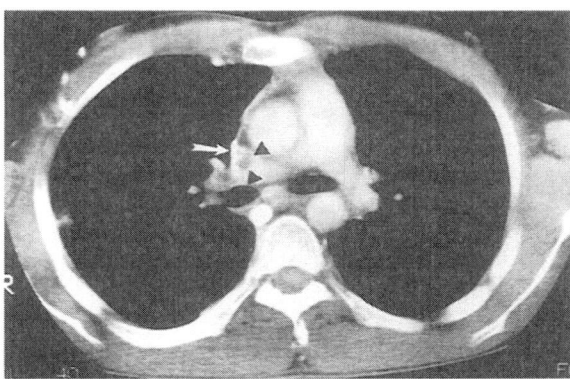

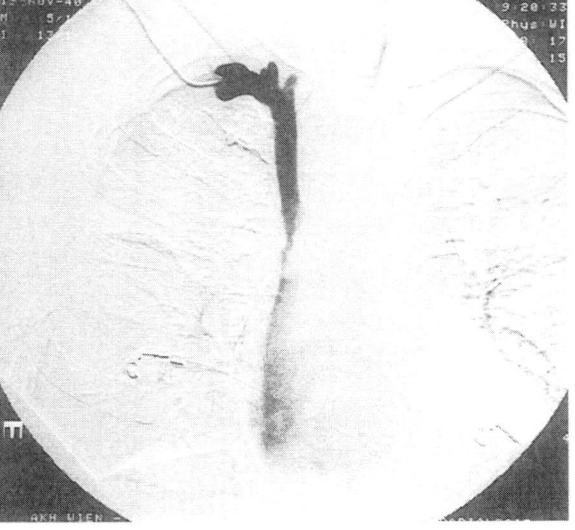

Fig. 12.10a,b. Catheter-related thrombosis of the SVC. a There is marginal contrast enhancement of the SVC (arrow) while the lumen is subtotally occluded by a large clot (arrowheads). Note contrast enhancement of the subcutaneous, lateral thoracic, and internal mammary veins representing collateral circulation. The early venogram (b), performed 1 week prior to the spiral CT scan of the same patient, demonstrates the marked obstruction but fails to depict the underlying cause. The catheter in this patient was removed prior to the radiologic examinations

patients, the central venous catheter may be used for the injection of contrast material. Therefore, the SVC proximal to the tip of the indwelling catheter may not be opacified and the thrombus surrounding the tip or distal part of the indwelling catheter can easily be missed during a spiral CT examination. Consequently, a double helix study through the upper mediastinum is recommended to overcome this problem. Multiplanar reformatting and cine-viewing may be extremely helpful in the evaluation and diagnosis of SVC thrombosis. Coronal, sagittal, and curved reconstructed images generate a phlebographic impression of the SVC and its tributaries and serve as a useful aid in interpretation and diagnosis. Also, CT angiography with volume rendering (KUSZYK et al. 1995) may be helpful in the diagnosis of partial or complete thrombosis as well as in the demonstration of collateralization (TELLO et al.

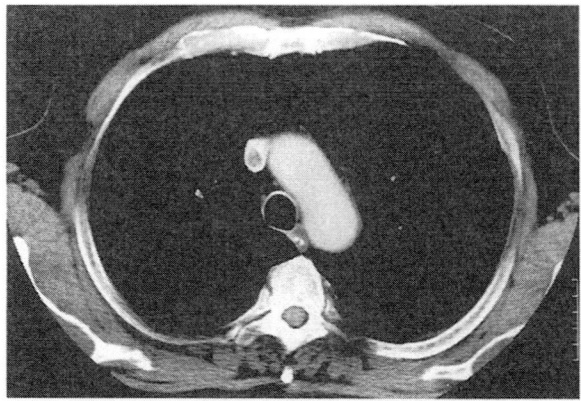

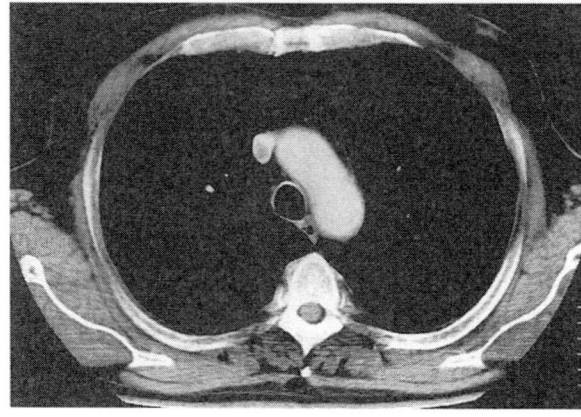

Fig. 12.11a,b. Value of follow-up contrast-enhanced spiral CT scan in the diagnosis of SVC thrombosis in a clinically silent patient after removal of a central venous catheter. **a** A central filling defect is present in the SVC, surrounded by contrast-enhanced blood. To differentiate a flow phenomenon from a floating thrombus, the patient was brought back to the CT unit. A repeated spiral CT scans confirmed the presence of SVC thrombosis (**b**)

1993). Finally, in cases where differentiation of thrombi from flow phenomena is difficult, a follow-up study will help to elucidate the problem (Fig. 12.11).

12.6.3 Displacement, Obstruction, and Occlusion of the SVC

Displacement, obstruction, and occlusion of the SVC may occur secondary to malignant or benign disorders. The vast majority of cases of SVC obstruction are due to malignant processes (YEDLICKA et al. 1989; SHIMM et al. 1981). Benign entities, including fibrosing mediastinitis, aortic aneurysms, abscesses, and bronchogenic cysts, once the leading cause of SVC displacement or obstruction, now play a minor role because of the increase in malignant processes (PEREZ et al. 1978; PARISH et al. 1981; BANKOFF et al. 1985). Displacement of the SVC without major compression or occlusion may occur in all of the above disorders but also commonly in patients with large mediastinal goiters (VERLOOY et al. 1994).

The most common neoplasm leading to SVC obstruction or occlusion is bronchogenic carcinoma. LOCHRIDGE et al. (1979) reported that of patients with malignant SVC obstruction, 82% had bronchogenic carcinoma, 12% had lymphoma, and 6% had metastatic disease. In patients with bronchogenic carcinoma, compromised SVC flow may be based on obstruction or occlusion due to expansive tumor growth, and also because of direct tumor infiltration. In our experience, it is frequently impossible to differentiate between external tumor compression and direct infiltration, particularly in large mass lesions. This is however, a moot issue in patients with SVC syndrome, since extensive infiltration of the mediastinum by bronchogenic carcinoma represents unresectable T4 status and alternative therapeutic strategies have to be used in these patients.

On spiral CT scans, SVC obstruction is characterized by concentric or eccentric luminal narrowing, primarily depending upon the location, size, and biological behavior of the underlying process (Figs. 12.2, 12.7, 12.9, 12.12, 12.13). Because the SVC is a thin-walled low-pressure structure, even small lesions can cause considerable SVC stenosis (Fig. 12.13). Benign mediastinal processes, such as aortic aneurysms or large mediastinal goiters, tend to cause SVC displacement with a varying degree of SVC obstruction. In such cases, the SVC appears as a narrow, slit-like structure with an eccentric location with respect to the underlying space-occupying lesion.

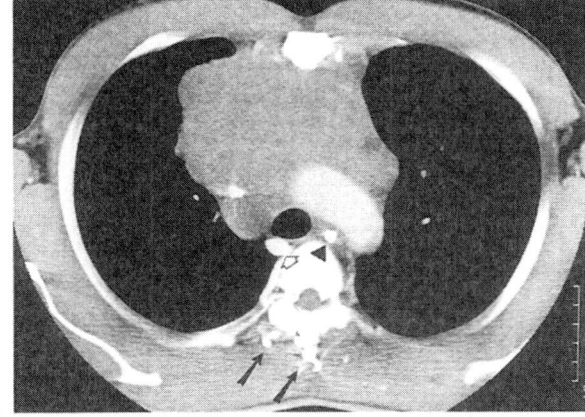

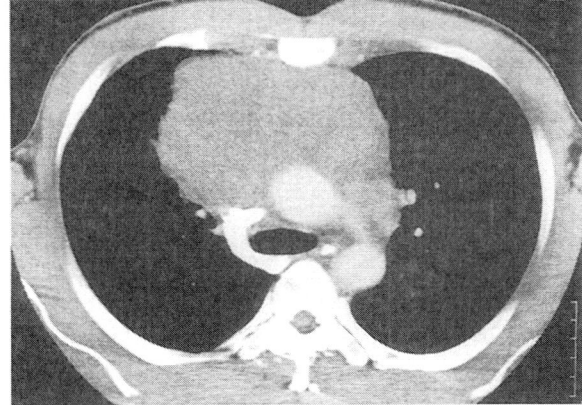

Fig. 12.12a,b. SVC obstruction and venous collateralization in a patient with non-Hodgkin's lymphoma and SVC syndrome. Spiral CT scan (**a**) demonstrates a large mediastinal mass with displacement and obstruction of the SVC. SVC flow obstruction is confirmed by the presence of multiple venous collateral channels in the paravertebral venous network (*arrows*) as well as in the azygos (*open arrow*) and hemiazygos (*arrowhead*) system. In **b**, the dilated azygos arch is opacified

Spiral CT angiography is an ideal method to evaluate displacement, compression, and occlusion of the SVC (with or without SVC syndrome) as well as the site and etiology of obstruction. Optimal vascular opacification delineates the SVC even in cases of severe vascular compromise and minimal residual lumen. In such cases, spiral CT venography may be superior to MR angiography, which generally does not provide similar spatial resolution (Fig. 12.13). In addition, spiral CT allows the evaluation of the underlying abnormality and thus helps to determine the cause of vascular obstruction. In such cases, staging of the malignancy can be performed without additional diagnostic efforts. Thus, spiral CT helps in the evaluation of surgical options and interventional procedures such as the implementation of stents, in planning radiation therapy and in the assessment of

effects of therapy (Fig. 12.2). Consequently, radiologists, radiation therapists, and surgeons routinely benefit from this attractive methodology.

12.6.4 Collateral Pathways of Venous Circulation

Spiral CT is not only a valuable method to assess abnormalities of the SVC, but also an excellent method to demonstrate venous collateral pathways (Figs. 12.7, 12.10, 12.12, 12.13). In most cases, opacification of collateral venous channels indicates compromised venous flow due to thrombosis, occlusion, or severe compression of the SVC or of the

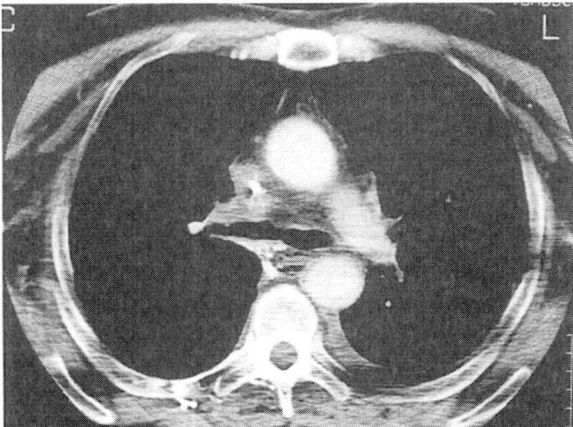

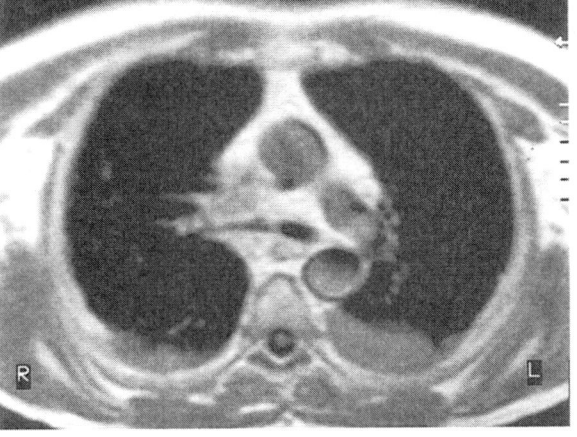

Fig. 12.13a,b. Marked obstruction of the SVC due to a small central bronchogenic carcinoma. Spiral CT (**a**) scans through the upper mediastinum show a somewhat small ill-defined soft tissue mass in the right tracheobronchial angle extending to the right mediastinum and encasing and severely obstructing the SVC. On spiral CT, residual flow of contrast-enhanced blood can be clearly seen. In contrast, a T1-weighted MR scan of the same patient performed 2 days prior to the spiral CT examination shows the primary tumor but does not allow a definite diagnosis regarding the patency of the SVC (**b**)

more proximal central vessels such as the brachio-cephalic veins.

The typical collateral pathways of venous circulation between the superior and inferior vena cava include the azygos-hemiazygos system (Fig. 12.12), the paravertebral venous network (Fig. 12.12), the internal mammary route (Fig. 12.10), and lateral thoracic (Fig. 12.10) as well as thoracoepigastric veins. In addition, accessory collateral routes in cases of SVC obstruction frequently involve the venous plexus around the shoulder and in the parascapular region (Fig. 12.7), the anterior cervical veins, and subcutaneous venous networks (ENGEL et al. 1983) (Fig. 12.10). Finally, the left and right superior intercostal veins connect with all major collateral pathways.

It is important to be aware of the fact that azygos vein opacification is not a reliable indicator of collateralization. The azygos vein may opacify retrogradely, especially in cases of elevated right heart pressure due to congestive heart failure or constrictive pericarditis (SMATHERS et al. 1982) but also in normal individuals (ENGEL et al. 1983). Other veins potentially opacifying in patients without central venous obstruction include the internal jugular, internal mammary, and right superior intercostal veins. Thus, the opacification of collateral pathways is, as a sole symptom, not sufficient to diagnose SVC flow obstruction (KIM et al. 1993). Consequently, the clinical significance of venous collateral opacification on spiral CT scans must be seen in conjunction with the presence of SVC obstruction and the clinical symptomatology of the SVC syndrome.

In general, the demonstration of collateral vessels is a good indicator of flow obstruction in the SVC or in more proximal central veins, particularly in the presence of clinical symptoms. KIM et al. (1993) have demonstrated that the presence of collateral vessels on CT scans is a highly accurate predictor of the clinical SVC syndrome with a sensitivity of 96% and a specificity of 92%. Among 23 patients who had signs and symptoms of SVC syndrome, 22 had collateral vessels on CT scans. Of 24 patients without signs or symptoms of SVC syndrome, only two had collateral vessels on CT scans (KIM et al. 1993). Thus, venous collateral pathways probably represent a significant morphologic correlate for clinical symptoms that indicate SVC obstruction.

Continuing debate exists about the correlation between the demonstration of collateral pathways on CT and the severity of SVC stenosis. Whereas GÖRICH et al. (1988) have shown that venous collaterals appear only in patients with a significantly narrowed SVC lumen, TRIGAUX and co-authors found no interdependence between these two parameters (TRIGAUX and VAN BEERS 1990). These divergent results may reflect the fact that bilateral contrast injection was not used in TRIGAUX et al.'s study. It is important to emphasize that in the majority of patients, collaterals are unilateral (TATU et al. 1985) and thus can be missed at contralateral contrast injection. Thus, as mentioned above, bilateral contrast injection is useful to detect venous collateral circulation in spiral CT examinations of patients with suspected SVC obstruction.

12.6.5 Central Venous Aneurysms

Venous aneurysms are rare disorders and may occur secondary to hereditary venous wall weakness, aneurysmal expansion of a vein by thrombus or a neoplasm, longstanding increased intraluminal venous pressure, or excessive blood flow (MONCADA et al. 1985). Spiral CT angiography is an ideal tool to demonstrate the potentially complex anatomy in the area of the aneurysm and to separate associated abnormalities such as tumor or thrombus from the flowing contrast-enhanced blood. Thus, spiral CT angiography is superior to conventional phlebography, which allows only a one-dimensional indirect approach to the vascular abnormality. Catheter phlebography is not advisable because of the potential danger of iatrogenic rupture of the aneurysmal wall.

12.7 The Role of Spiral CT Versus Other Imaging Modalities

Compared with other methods, spiral CT angiography has gained a pivotal role in the evaluation of SVC disorders. Spiral CT angiography, because of its optimal contrast enhancement of the SVC and its multiplanar imaging capabilities, provides more comprehensive information on central venous anatomy and pathology than catheter venography, which has long been regarded as the standard procedure to diagnose central venous abnormalities. In a review of cases of SVC syndrome, SCHWARTZ et al. (1986) have found venography to be of limited value in the management of SVC obstruction in comparison to CT. This was due to the observation that venography could only confirm the clinical diagnosis of SVC obstruction, but, in contrast to CT, would not provide additional insights into the nature of the underlying abnormality. Spiral CT angiography affords information on both the presence and the cause of a vascular abnormality (Fig. 12.10) and, because of multiplanar reformatting and the use of volume rendering techniques, produces venography-like images from the same data set.

Within the past few years, duplex Doppler and color Doppler ultrasonography have played an increasing role in the diagnosis of disorders affecting the central venous system, particularly in the evaluation of central venous thrombosis (BAXTER et al. 1991). These methods, however, are largely limited to the subclavian and brachiocephalic veins and rarely help to visualize the SVC. Conversely, spiral CT not only provides a global view of the entire venous system within the thorax, including the SVC, but also gives information on possibly associated arterial or nonvascular abnormalities.

Magnetic resonance angiography is now advocated as an accurate technique for the evaluation of the central venous system, including the SVC (FINN et al. 1993; FUJIMOTO et al. 1992). MR angiography allows noninvasive 3D angiography and thus facilitates interpretation of complex vascular pathology. Limitations of this technique, however, include low spatial resolution, the unpredictability of flow effects on spin-echo MR (Fig. 12.13), the insensitivity of gradient-echo images to in-plane flow, and the problems of imaging in the presence of indwelling catheters. Apart from these problems, scanner availability, high cost, and long scan times offset the advantages of this method. In comparison, spiral CT angiography is already widely available, relatively cheap, very fast, relatively noninvasive, and accurate. The possibilities of performing multiplanar reformatting, 3D reconstruction (KATZ et al. 1995), and CT angiography with volume rendering (JOHNSON, P.T. personal communication 1995) have largely outweighed the advantages of MR angiography. Thus, spiral CT angiography has gained important ground in the noninvasive evaluation of the central venous system in the chest. At this point in time, both CT and MR angiography provide similar diagnostic information on vascular abnormalities in the chest (KHIMJI and ZEISS 1992; MEIER et al. 1993). Mostly for practical reasons, spiral CT angiography can currently be regarded as a standard procedure for the evaluation of central venous disorders including the SVC.

12.8 Conclusion

The SVC may be affected by a variety of disorders that commonly cause obstruction of venous flow.

Contrast-enhanced spiral CT is an excellent method to evaluate these processes because it demonstrates not only the vascular abnormality but also the underlying pathology. Although in the vast majority of cases SVC disorders are easily depicted on spiral CT scans, a knowledge of the anatomy and physiology and an understanding of the dynamics of contrast enhancement and fundamental aspects of artifact generation help to enhance the diagnostic abilities of the observer and avoid misinterpretation. In most instances, axial scans are sufficient to allow proper analysis of an abnormality. In selected cases, however, the performance of spiral CT angiography may be substantially enhanced by multiplanar reformatting and volume rendering. Spiral CT is a valuable alternative to conventional venography, particularly when evaluating the cause of SVC obstruction. Compared to MR angiography, spiral CT angiography involves the use of contrast media and ionizing radiation, but it is already widely available, faster, more cost-effective, and probably as accurate. Technical advances, such as the introduction of subsecond image reconstruction and the increased development of postprocessing tools, will undoubtedly further enhance the role of spiral CT in the assessment of central venous disorders.

References

Bankoff MS, Daly BDT, Johnson HA, Carter BL (1985) Bronchogenic cyst causing superior vena cava obstruction: CT appearance. J Comput Assist Tomogr 9:951–952

Baron RL, Gutierrez FR, Sagel SS, Levitt RG, McKnight RC (1981) CT of anomalies of the mediastinal vessels. AJR 137:571–576

Baxter GM, Kincaid W, Jeffrey RF et al. (1991) Comparison of colour Doppler ultrasound with venography in the diagnosis of axillary and subclavian vein thrombosis. Br J Radiol 64:777–781

Buirski G, Jordan SC, Joffe HS et al. (1986) Superior vena caval abnormalities: their occurrence rate, associated cardiac abnormalities and angiographic classification in a paediatric population with congenital heart disease. Clin Radiol 37:131–138

Cha EM, Khoury GH (1972) Persistent left superior vena cava: radiologic and clinical significance. Radiology 103:375–381

Cormier MG, Yedlicka JW, Gray RJ et al. (1989) Congenital anomalies of the superior vena cava: a CT study. Semin Roentgenol 24:77–83

Dillon EH, Camputaro C (1993) Partial anomalous pulmonary venous drainage of the left upper lobe vs duplication of the superior vena cava: distinction based on CT findings. AJR 160:375–379

Dudiak CM, Olson MC, Posniak HV (1989) Abnormalities of the azygos system: CT evaluation. Semin Roentgenol 24:47–55

Edwards RD, Cassidy J, Taylor A (1992) Case report: superior vena cava obstruction complicated by central venous thrombosis – treatment with thrombolysis and gianturco-Z stents. Clin Radiol 45:278–280

Engel IA, Auh YH, Rubenstein WA et al. (1983) CT diagnosis of mediastinal and thoracic inlet venous obstruction. AJR 141:521–526

Finn JP, Zisk JHS, Edelman RR et al. (1993) Central venous occlusion: MR angiography. Radiology 187:245–251

Fujimoto K, Abe T, Kumabe T et al. (1992) Anomalous left brachiocephalic vein: MR demonstration. AJR 159:479–480

Furuta S, Zuguchi M, Takahashi S (1994) Diverticulum of the superior vena cava. AJR 162:233

Gardeur D, Lautrou J, Millard JC et al. (1980) Pharmacokinetics of contrast media: experimental results in dog and man with CT implications. J Comput Assist Tomogr 4:178–185

Godwin JD, Chen JTT (1986) Thoracic venous anatomy. AJR 147:674–684

Godwin JD, Webb WR (1982) Contrast-related flow phenomena mimicking pathology on thoracic computed tomography. J Comput Assist Tomogr 6:460–464

Görich VJ, Flentje M, Gückel F, Beyer-Enke SA, van Kaick G (1988) Computertomographische Darstellung von Kollateralbahnen bei Stenosen großer Mediastinalvenen. Fortschr Röntgenstr 148:560–565

Guthaner DF, Wexler L, Harell G (1979) CT demonstration of cardiac structures. AJR 133:75–81

Hasan F, Glesson F, Lock MR et al. (1992) Diverticulum of the inferior vena cava. J Vasc Surg 15:578–580

Hayward I, Forrest JV, Sagel SS (1989) Hemiazygos vein aneurysm: CT documentation. J Comput Assist Tomogr 13:1072–1074

Heitzmann ER (1988) The mediastinum-radiologic correlations with anatomy and pathology, 2nd edn. Springer, Berlin Heidelberg New York

Herman SJ, Winton TL, Weisbrod GL et al. (1994) Mediastinal invasion by bronchogenic carcinoma: CT signs. Radiology 190:841–846

Huggins TJ, Lesar ML, Friedman AC et al. (1982) CT appearance of persistent left superior vena cava. J Comput Assist Tomogr 6:294–297

Joseph PM (1981) Artifacts in computed tomography. In: Newton TH, Potts DG (eds) Radiology of the skull and brain: technical aspects of computed tomography. Mosby, St. Louis

Kalender WA, Seissler W, Klotz E (1990) Spiral volumetric CT with single-breath-hold technique, continuous transport, and continuous scanner rotation. Radiology 176:181–183

Katz M, Konen E, Rozenman J et al. (1995) Spiral CT and 3D image reconstruction of vascular rings and associated tracheobronchial anomalies. J Comput Assist Tomogr 19:564–568

Khimji T, Zeiss J (1992) MRI versus CT and US in the evaluation of a patient presenting with superior vena cava syndrome. Clin Imaging 16:269–271

Kim HJ, Kim HS, Chung SH (1993) CT diagnosis of superior vena cava syndrome: importance of collateral vessels. AJR 161:539–542

Kim HJ, Kim HS, Lee G (1994) Anomalous left brachiocephalic vein: spiral CT and angiographic findings. J Comput Assist Tomogr 18:872–875

Korobkin M, Casano VA (1989) Intracaval and intracardiac extension of malignant thymoma: CT diagnosis. J Comput Assist Tomogr 13:348–350

Kuszyk BS, Heath DG, Ney DR et al. (1995) CT angiography with volume rendering: imaging findings. AJR 165:445–448

Lochridge SK, Knibble WP, Doty DB (1979) Obstruction of the superior vena cava. Surgery 85:14–24

Lowell JA, Bothe A Jr (1991) Venous access. Surg Clin North Am 127:1225–1248

Meier RA, Marianacci EB, Costello P et al. (1993) 3D image reconstruction of right subclavian artery aneurysms. J Comput Assist Tomogr 17:887–890

Moncada R, Cardella R, Demos TC et al. (1984) Evaluation of superior vena cava syndrome by axial CT and CT phlebography. AJR 143:731–736

Moncada R, Demos TC, Marsan R et al. (1985) CT diagnosis of idiopathic aneurysms of the thoracic systemic veins. J Comput Assist Tomogr 9:305–309

Mori H, Fukuda T, Isomoto I, Maeda H, Hayashi K (1990) CT diagnosis of catheter-induced septic thrombus of vena cava. J Comput Assist Tomogr 14:236–238

Naidich DP, Zerhouni EA, Siegelman SS (1991) Principles and techniques of thoracic CT and MR. In: Naidich DP, Zerhouni EA, Siegelman SS (eds) Computed tomography and magnetic resonance of the thorax, 2nd edn. Raven Press, New York

Niederle B, Hausmaninger C, Kretschmer G, Polterauer P, Neuhold N, Mirza DF, Roka R (1990) Intraatrial extension of thyroid cancer: technique and results of a radical surgical approach. Surgery 108:951–957

Ono N, Martinez CR, Fara JW et al. (1980) Diatrizoate distribution as a function of administration rate and time following intravenous injection. J Comput Assist Tomogr 4:174–177

Parish JM, Marschke RF Jr, Dines DE, Lee RE (1981) Etiologic considerations in superior vena cava syndrome. Mayo Clin Proc 56:407–413

Perez CA, Presant CA, Van Amburg AL (1978) Management of superior vena cava syndrome. Semin Oncol 5:123–134

Proto AV (1987) Mediastinal anatomy: emphasis on conventional images with anatomic and computed tomography correlations. J Thorac Imag 2:1–48

Rubin G, Dake M, Napel S (1994) Spiral CT of renal artery stenosis: comparison of three-dimensional rendering techniques. Radiology 190:181–189

Schwartz EE, Goodman RL, Haskin ME (1986) Role of CT scanning in the superior vena cava syndrome. Am J Clin Oncol 9:71–78

Shimm DS, Logue GL, Rigsby LC (1981) Evaluating the superior vena cava syndrome. JAMA 245:951–953

Smathers RL, Buschi AJ, Pope TL Jr, Brenbridge AN, Williamson BR (1982) The azygous arch: normal and pathologic CT appearance. AJR 139:477–483

Tatu WF, Winzelberg GG, Boller M, Wholey MH (1985) Computed tomographic evaluation of compression of the superior vena cava and its tributaries. Cardiovasc Intervent Radiol 8:89–99

Tello R, Scholz E, Finn JP, Costello P (1993) Subclavian vein thrombosis detected with spiral CT and three-dimensional reconstruction. AJR 160:33–34

Tocino IM, Watanabe A (1986) Impending catheter perforation of superior vena cava: radiographic recognition. AJR 146:487–490

Trigaux JP, Van Beers B (1990) Thoracic collateral venous channels: normal and pathologic CT findings. J Comput Assist Tomogr 14:769–773

Verlooy H, Monteyne R, Noyen J, Coolen J (1994) Superior vena cava syndrome due to a substernal nontoxic goiter. Clin Nucl Med 19:353–355

Verschakelen JA (1995) Acquisition and injection techniques. In: State-of-the-art Symposium: spiral CT of the chest; European Congress of Radiology 1995. Eur Radiol 5(a):158

Webb WR, Gamsu G, Speckman JM et al. (1982) Computed tomographic demonstration of mediastinal venous anomalies. AJR 139:157–161

Wechsler RJ, Steiner RM, Kinori I (1988) Monitoring the monitors: the radiology of thoracic catheters, wires, and tubes. Semin Roentgenol 23:61–84

Winter FS (1954) Persistent left superior vena cava. Survey of world literature and report of thirty additional cases. Angiology 5:90–132

Yedlicka JW, Schultz K, Moncada R, Flisak M (1989) CT findings in superior vena cava obstruction. Semin Roentgenol 24:84–90

13 Spiral CT of the Thoracic Aorta and Its Branches

P. COSTELLO

CONTENTS

13.1 Introduction

Because of the rapid scan time of spiral CT, a complete data set of the entire thorax is acquired during a single breath-hold. Respiratory motion is eliminated and the short scan time enables studies to be performed during the arterial phase of intravenous contrast injection. As little as 60 ml of 60% contrast material can produce aortic enhancement similar to conventional CT using twice the amount of contrast material (COSTELLO et al. 1992a). Not only can studies be performed more quickly than with conventional CT, but a more detailed study of the thoracic aorta and its branches is produced. Spiral CT's unique processing capabilities allow three-dimensional renderings to be made, producing studies that simulate conventional arteriography. Shaded surface displays, maximum intensity projection (MIP), and multi or curved planar reformations can be generated from the spiral CT data set. Each of these rendering techniques has unique advantages and limitations, as discussed in Chap. 5 by Dr. G.D. Rubin.

P. COSTELLO, MD, Senior Director, Radiology, The Queen Elizabeth Hospital, 28 Woodville Road, Woodville, 5011 S. Australia

13.2 Technique

Prior to a thoracic spiral CT study it is important that the volume of interest be localized on a noncontrast study, enabling one to limit the region scanned. Noncontrast scans are obtained with 10-mm collimation at 2-cm intervals through the thorax. This is followed by breath-hold coaching for 30 s since respiratory motion can produce misregistration problems. Occasionally a 40-s breath-hold scan, at a lower mAs, is used in thinner, younger patients.

Contrast is delivered via an intravenous injection using an 18 or occasionally a 20 gauge antecubital vein catheter. A test bolus is initially performed so that the contrast timing is precise. Twenty milliliters is injected at 4 ml/s and 10 s after the initial injection has begun, single-level images are obtained at 2 s apart through the proximal descending aorta using low mA technique. A time-density curve is generated to determine the appropriate scan delay, with a range of 10–25 s for the thoracic aorta.

Using the time delay determined by the test scan, 100–140 ml of contrast at a concentration of 300 mg iodine/ml is delivered at 3–4 ml/s. Nonionic contrast is used exclusively in order to avoid the discomforts of heat, nausea, and vomiting associated with ionic agents. We prefer to inject via the right antecubital vein since the great vessel origins are not obscured by contrast filling the left innominate vein.

Collimation is chosen so that the minimal value selected allows a spiral scan pitch of less than 2. With a pitch of 2 and a collimation of 3 mm it is possible to cover a volume of 18 cm using 6 mm/s table feed, which, in most patients, will allow for a study of the entire thoracic aorta. With newer CT systems, a 40-s exposure with 24 cm of coverage is possible. Overlapping sections generated at 2-mm increments produce smoother three-dimensional and multiplanar renderings and reduce partial volume effects with improved small vessel visualization. Not all axial images are filmed but they can be viewed consecutively in a cine loop presentation. For patients in whom pathologies extend into the abdomen (e.g., aortic dissection) collimation may be increased to 4 or 5 mm with 8 or 10 mm/s table feed to provide a longer range of coverage. In the future, improvements in x-ray tube heat loading will make it easier to study the entire aorta during single contrast bolus at 3-mm collimation.

If there are limitations to the amount of intravenous contrast that can be used because of renal disease or for patients in whom three-dimensional imaging is considered unnecessary, alternative protocols can be employed. We recommend starting scans 2 cm above the aortic arch with 8-mm collimation and 8–10 mm/s table feed. Between 80 and 100 ml of contrast (300 mg I/ml) is infused at 2 ml/s with a 20-s delay to spiral scan. Images may be reconstructed at 5-mm intervals.

13.3 Atherosclerotic Aortic Aneurysms

Aneurysms due to atherosclerosis are almost always located in the distal arch or descending thoracic aorta. Patients remain asymptomatic until the aneurysm attains a sufficient size to compress surrounding structures or undergoes rupture. Since the descending thoracic aorta is not surrounded by solid viscera, aneurysms may attain a large size before becoming symptomatic. The left recurrent laryngeal nerve arising from the vagus nerve wraps around the ligamentum arteriosum; stretching or compression of this nerve can cause vocal cord paresis or paralysis with hoarseness. Occasionally the left mainstem bronchus is compressed by large aneurysms, causing wheezing, recurrent infections, or even collapse of the left lower lobe or left lung. Rupture of an aneurysm usually occurs into the pleural cavity and patients are unlikely to survive. Aneurysms may also erode into the adjacent viscera such as the pulmonary parenchyma, bronchi, or esophagus.

The CT findings of aneurysm include localized dilatation of the aorta, intraluminal thrombus (85%), calcification in the aortic wall, and secondary compressive effects (MACHIDA and TASAKA 1980; GODWIN et al. 1980) (Fig. 13.1). Unlike angiography, CT detects calcification with a high degree of sensitivity, showing its relationship to the aortic wall. Aneurysms can be either fusiform and generalized or localized and saccular. The decision to perform surgery is influenced by aneurysm size and shape. Saccular aneurysms in particular and aneurysms measuring greater than 6 cm in diameter are considered more likely to undergo rupture (WHITE et al. 1986).

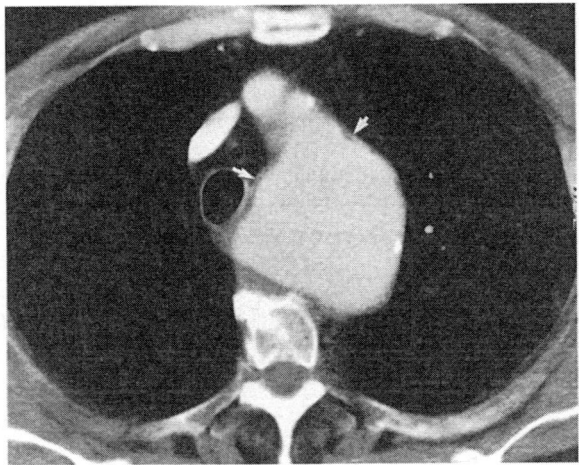

Fig. 13.1. Arch aneurysm; 65-year-old woman with a 7.5-cm aortic arch aneurysm. Transverse CT section at the level of the arch; 8-mm collimation with a pitch of 1; 60 ml of contrast (300 mg I/ml) infused at 2 ml/s. There is a small amount of mural thrombus (*arrows*) and aortic wall calcification. (From COSTELLO et al. 1992b)

CT clearly demonstrates the secondary effects of an aneurysm on surrounding structures including compression of the left main bronchus, left pulmonary artery, and adjacent mediastinal structures (Fig. 13.2).

Thoracic aortic aneurysms grow faster than abdominal aortic aneurysms, with aortic arch aneurysms expanding most rapidly. A thoracic aneurysm grows at 0.42 cm per year representing a 9% per year growth rate (HIROSE et al. 1992). According to Laplace's law, the larger the diameter of an aneurysm, the faster its growth rate will be if pressure remains constant. A rapidly increasing size of an aneurysm is worrisome for impending rupture. CT can demonstrate the actual rupture itself or high-attenuation periaortic hematoma representing a leak (Fig. 13.3). Blood within the pleural space may be of high attenuation but occasionally pleural fluid may be serosanguinous and therefore of low attenuation.

13.3.1 Advantages of Spiral CT

In order to distinguish an atherosclerotic aneurysm from aortic dissection, the location of calcification needs to be precisely defined. Where the aorta crosses the scan plane transversely, as in the arch or with tortuous descending aortic aneurysms, it can be difficult to distinguish the relationship between intimal calcification and thrombus due to volume averaging of conventional CT (GODWIN et al. 1982;

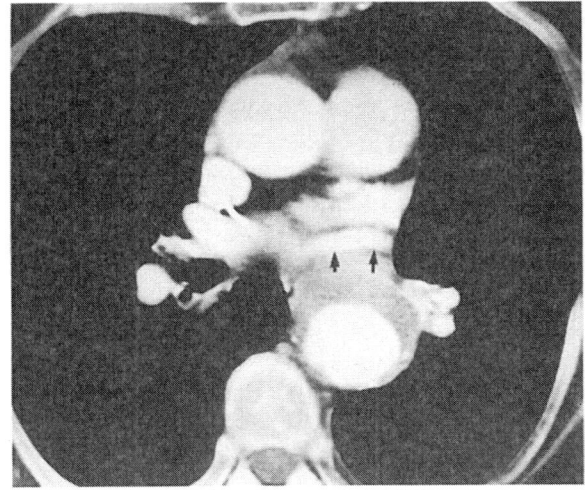
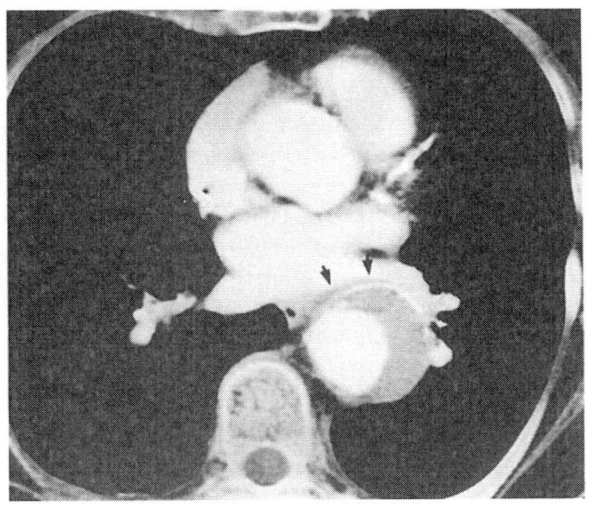

Fig. 13.2a,b. Descending thoracic aortic aneurysm; 100 ml of contrast (300 mg I/ml) infused at 3 ml/s; 5-mm collimation with pitch of 1.5. **a** A partially thrombosed descending thoracic aortic aneurysm compresses the pulmonary veins (*ar*-*rows*). **b** There is clear separation of mural calcification from luminal thrombus and compression of the left atrium (*arrows*). (From COSTELLO et al. 1992b)

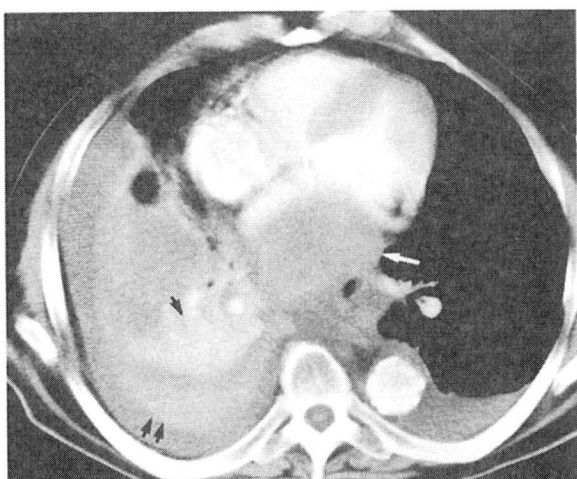
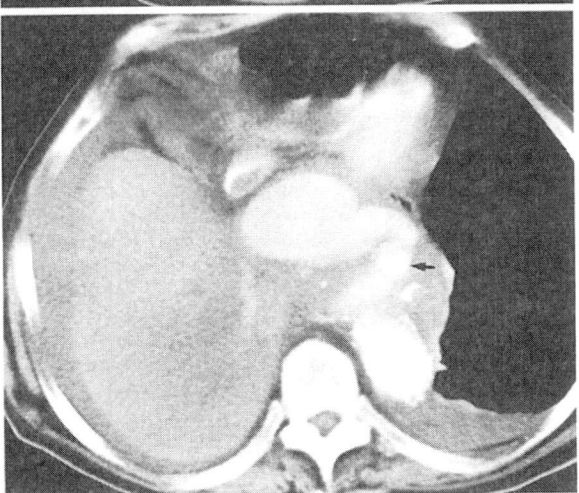
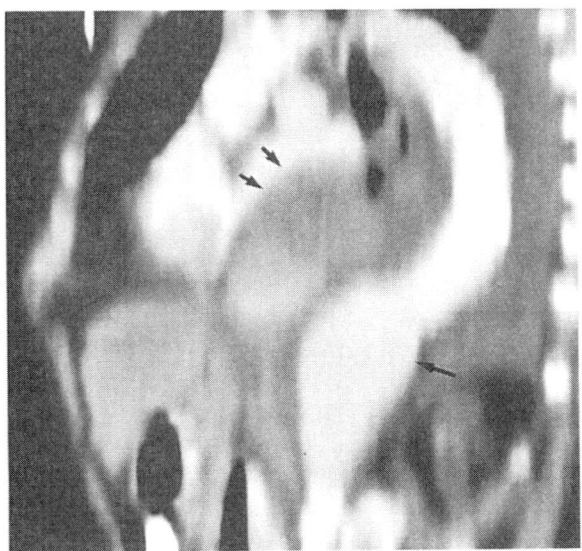

Fig. 13.3a–c. Aoritc aneurysm rupture; 65-year-old male with chest pain and hypotension. **a** CT section through the level of the left atrium demonstrates a soft tissue density compressing the left atrium (*white arrows*) with right lower lobe atelectasis (*arrow*) and high attenuation blood in the pleural space (*ar*-*rows*). The soft tissue mass represents thrombus surrounding the rupturing aneurysm. **b** Transverse CT section 3 cm inferiorly shows the neck (*arrow*) of the aneurysm with rupture into the right pleural space. **c** Paraxial reformat through the descending aorta shows a large aneurysm of the descending aorta (*arrow*) undergoing rupture into the right pleural space. The left atrium is compressed (*arrows*) by hematoma. (From COSTELLO et al. 1992b)

GODWIN 1990). Sometimes intimal calcification in the aortic arch appears to be abnormally separated from the aortic wall, suggesting a dissection. This volume averaging phenomenon of thick-slice conventional CT can be eliminated by spiral CT and reconstruction of overlapping sections (ZEMAN et al. 1994). Spiral CT also eliminates the need for repeat thin sections through levels susceptible to volume averaging artifacts. Unfortunately not all calcification lies within the intima since dystrophic calcification can occur on a mural thrombus and therefore can be separated from the aortic wall (HEIBERG et al. 1985; TORRES et al. 1988).

Aneurysms arising adjacent to the great vessels or the inferolateral aspect of the arch near the ligamentum arteriosum need to be clearly defined to determine what type of surgical procedure should be performed (HARDER et al. 1987). The relationship between aortic aneurysms and branch vessels is hard to define because of volume averaging on thick-slice conventional CT. For this reason catheter angiography is usually performed preoperatively in these patients. Spiral CT can eliminate the need for angiography in such patients by overlapping section analysis, and more importantly, multiplanar reconstructions and three-dimensional renderings (Fig. 13.4). Shaded surface displays show the relationship between aneurysms and great vessels more readily than MIP images. MIP displays can show the differences in attenuation values of calcification, thrombus and contrast, but depth relationships are only apparent when images are viewed in a cine loop presentation. The ability to rotate images in an interactive real-time format allows the surgeon to determine precise relationships between these aneurysms and adjacent aortic branches.

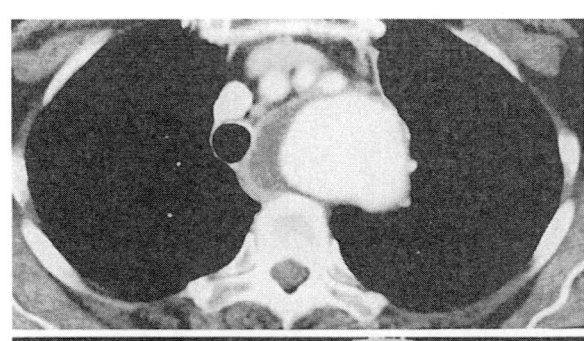

a

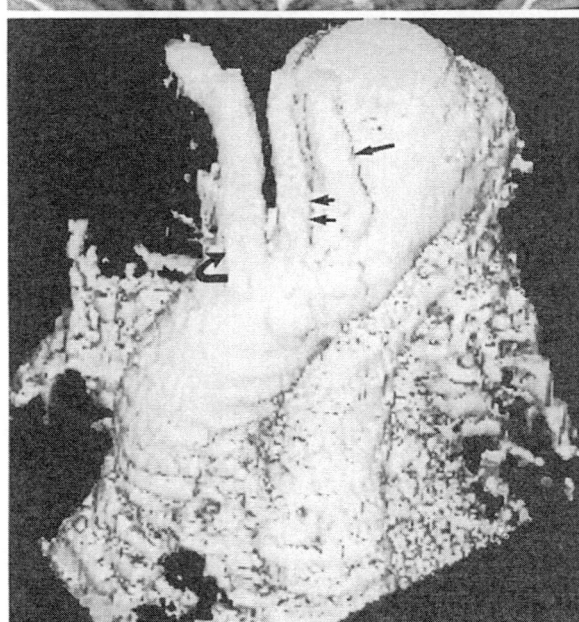

b

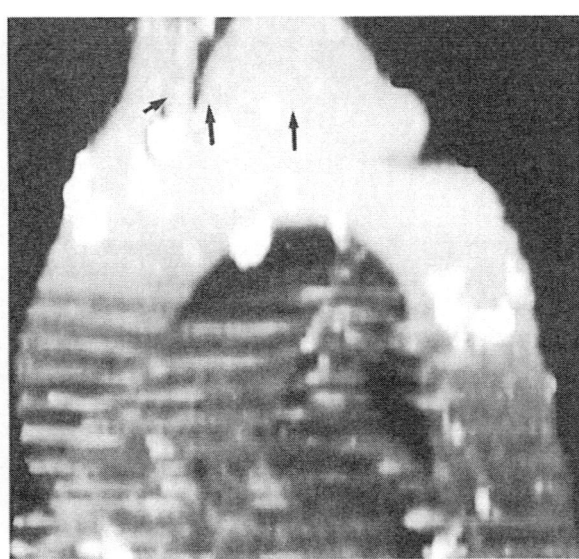

c

Fig. 13.4a–c. Aortic arch aneurysm; 120 ml of contrast (300 ml I/ml) infused at 4 ml/s; 3-mm collimation with a pitch of 2. **a** Transverse CT section through a partially thrombosed aortic arch aneurysm adjacent to the origin of the great vessels. **b** Shaded surface display viewed anteriorly reveals the origins of the left subclavian (*single arrow*), left carotid (*double arrow*), and innominate (*curved arrow*) arteries separate from the atherosclerotic aneurysm. **c** MIP image viewed laterally reveals the focal aortic arch aneurysm (*arrows*) adjacent to the origin of the left subclavian artery (*small arrow*). (From COSTELLO 1994)

13.3.2 Differential Diagnosis

Many aortic aneurysms are initially diagnosed as mediastinal masses on plain films. CT is an essential requirement before biopsy or surgery of any mediastinal mass. The ability to scan during the arterial phase is a major advantage of spiral CT over conventional CT. Without a good contrast bolus a thrombosed saccular aneurysm may be misdiagnosed as a mediastinal mass or centrally located carcinoma (Figs. 13.5–13.7). In these patients it is imperative to look for irregularity of the aortic wall representing ulceration at the site of aneurysm formation (Fig. 13.8). Subtle irregularities of the aortic wall at the site of aneurysm formation are easily detected on spiral CT by analysis of overlapping

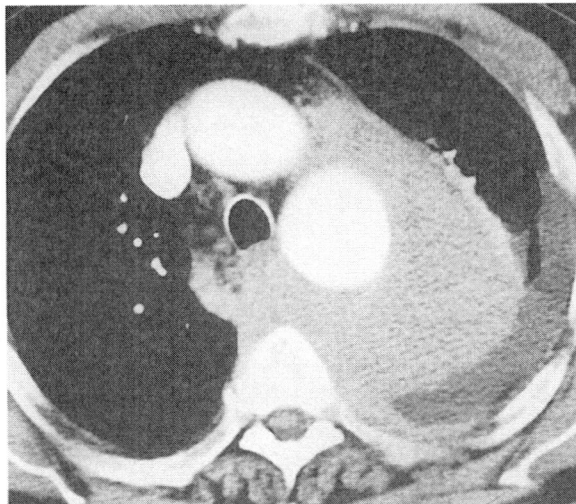

Fig. 13.5. Non-Hodgkin's lymphoma; 100 ml contrast (300 mg I/ml) infused at 3 ml/s; 8-mm collimation with a pitch of 1. CT section just above the carina reveals a soft tissue density surrounding the aorta and displacing it anteriorly. The soft tissue density simulates a thrombosed aortic aneurysm but represents a mass diagnosed as intermediate-grade non-Hodgkin's lymphoma

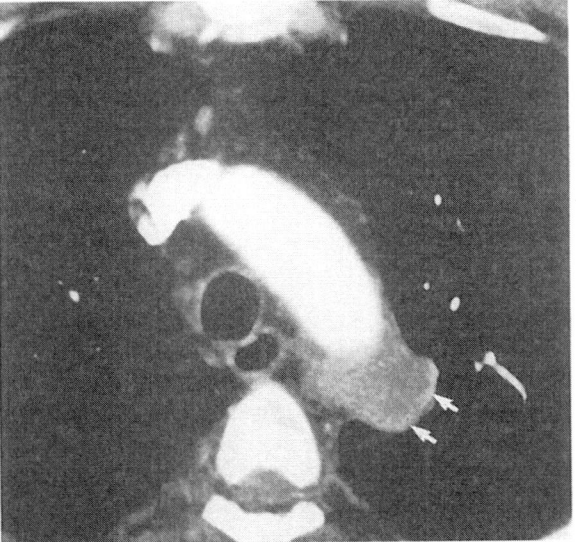

a

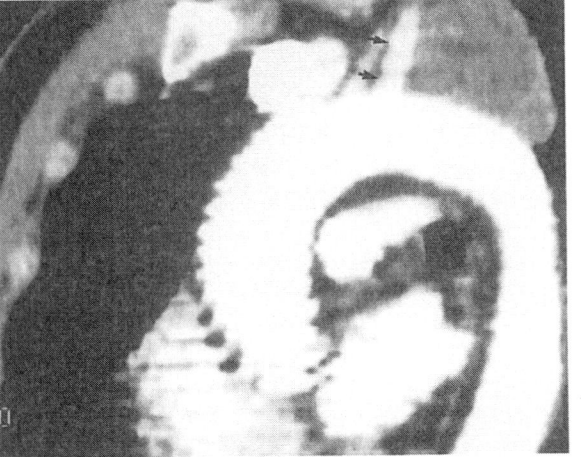

b

Fig. 13.7a,b. Carcinoma of the lung simulation aortic aneurysm; 100 ml contrast (300 mg I/ml) infused at 3 ml/s; 3-mm collimation with a pitch of 2. **a** Transverse CT section through the aortic arch reveals a mass on the surface of the aorta (*arrows*). **b** Sagittal reconstruction reveals the mass on the surface of the aorta extending around the origin of the left subclavian artery (*arrows*). This represents a carcinoma of the lung simulating a focal aortic aneurysm on plain radiographs

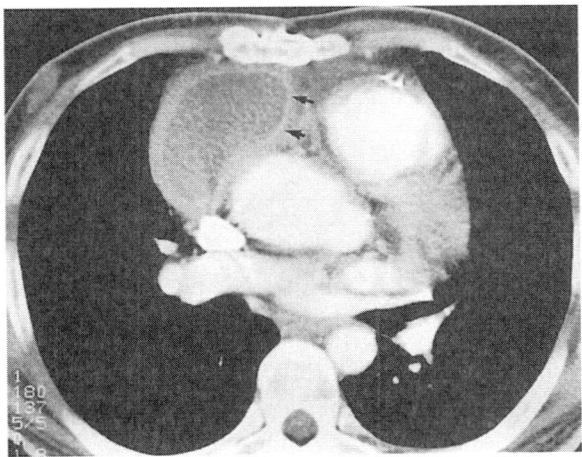

Fig. 13.6. Mediastinal seroma; 60 ml contrast (300 mg I/ml) infused at 2 ml/s; 8-mm collimation with a pitch of 1. Transverse section through the ascending aorta reveals a hypovascular soft tissue density lying anterior to the ascending aorta (*arrows*) with central low density and peripheral higher attenuation. It represents a post coronary artery bypass graft mediastinal seroma

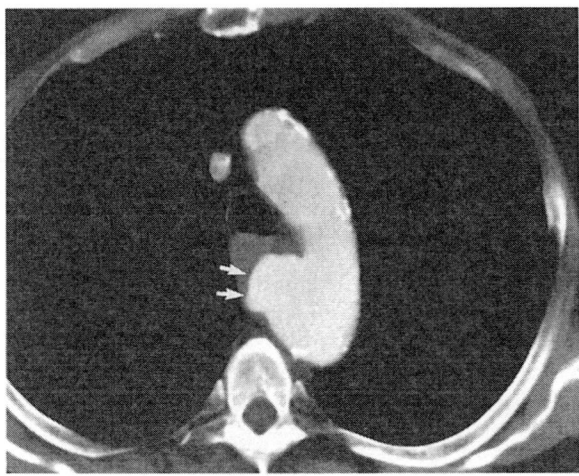

Fig. 13.8. Aortic aneurysm in a 59-year-old man with a "mediastinal mass" shown on chest x-ray. Sixty milliliters of contrast (300 mg I/ml) infused at 2 ml/s; 8-mm collimation with a pitch of 1. CT section shows an atherosclerotic aneurysm of the proximal descending aorta bulging into the mediastinum posterior to the trachea (*arrows*)

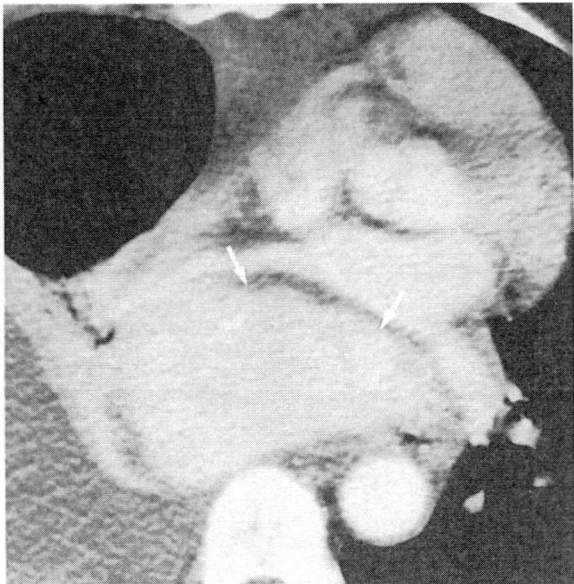

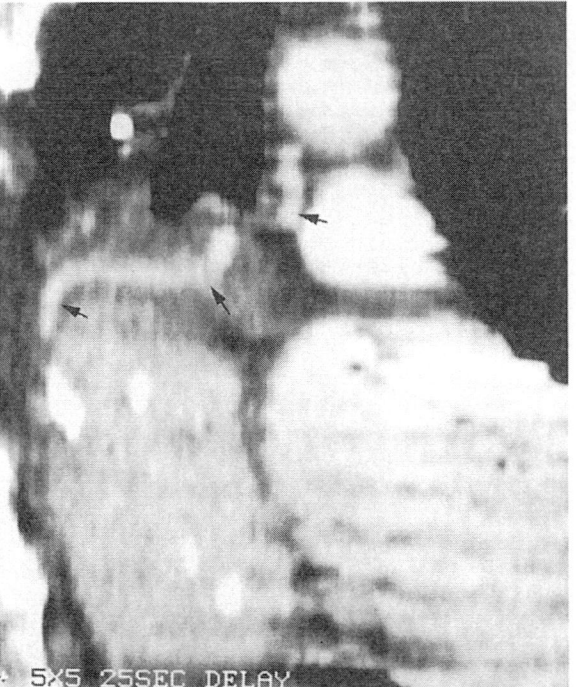

Fig. 13.9a,b. Castleman's disease; 100 ml contrast (300 mg I/ ml) infused at 3 ml/s; 5-mm collimation with a pitch of 1; reconstructed at 1 mm. **a** CT section through the level of the left atrium shows a very vascular mass (*arrows*) compressing the left atrium. **b** Curved planar reformat through the mass reveals a hypertrophied bronchial artery (*arrows*) supplying the mass. (From Costello 1995)

sections with a densely opacified aorta. Not only can aneurysms be distinguished from mediastinal masses but the vascularity of mediastinal masses can be determined. The blood supply of vascular mediastinal masses, such as Castleman's disease (Fig. 13.9), can be shown on multiplanar reconstructions, eliminating the need for catheter angiography.

13.4 Acute Aortic Dissection

Acute aortic dissection is the most common life-threatening disease affecting the aorta, and has a dramatic onset and rapid course (Hirst et al. 1958). Over the past 15 years, cross-sectional imaging has become critical for its detection, replacing angiography in most hospitals. For untreated patients, the mortality is approximately 70% in the first 2 weeks and up to 90% after 3 months (Wheat et al. 1965). Therapeutic advances have resulted in contemporary 30-day survival rates of 80%–90% (Miller 1983; DeBakey et al. 1982; Miller et al. 1984; Crawford et al. 1988, 1989; Wheat 1987; Reul et al. 1975) and overall 5- and 10-year survival rates of 57%–66% and 32%–44% with treatment (Miller 1983; DeBakey et al. 1982; Crawford et al. 1988). Given these impressive data, it is important that radiologists understand the advantages and limitations of spiral CT from the perspective of a cardiovascular surgeon.

The widely used Stanford classification of dissection designates type A proximal dissections as those involving the ascending aorta with or without involvement of the descending thoracic aorta and type

B as disease involving the descending thoracic aorta. Of all dissections, 60% are type A and 40% are type B (HIRST et al. 1958). With type A dissections, the intimal tear can be located anywhere in the aorta, with 89% in the ascending aorta and the rest in the arch (7%) (HAVERICH et al. 1985) or descending aorta (4%). Type B dissections usually begin 2–5 cm distal to the origin of the left subclavian artery and rarely extend retrograde into the ascending aorta. Information required by both the medical and the surgical team includes a confirmation of the diagnosis of dissection, determination of ascending aortic involvement, and finally any abnormal anatomical variations.

Both the site of tear and the extent of involvement are principal determinants of the patient's course, prognosis, and treatment. Type A dissections require immediate surgical intervention once the patient's condition has stabilized. The purpose of a repair is to prevent rupture into the pericardium, which is the cause of 90% of deaths due to ascending aortic dissections (MITCHELL 1993). A graft is positioned into the ascending aorta just above the coronary arteries and the false lumen is obliterated with the graft sewn distally into the single new lumen. The aortic valve may occasionally need replacement, and, if there is coronary artery involvement (more commonly on the right), they also are bypassed. Survival rates of 90% are possible with surgical repair of ascending aorta (MITCHELL 1993). Medical therapy is the initial treatment for type B aortic dissection and surgery is reserved for when failure occurs (20%) as shown by persistent symptoms. Surgery is indicated if there is progression of dissection with the development of visceral, renal, or peripheral ischemia or formation of an aneurysm of the false lumen.

Two mechanisms may explain the development of acute aortic dissection. In most cases, the primary event is an intimal tear and a hematoma propagates along the aortic wall. In other cases the primary event is a rupture of the vasa vasorum in the aortic wall without an initial intimal rupture (GODWIN et al. 1982). Patients who are predisposed to dissection include those with hypertension, connective tissue disorders such as Marfan syndrome, cystic medial necrosis, Ehlers-Danlos syndrome, and Turner syndrome. Pregnancy, aortic stenosis, and coarctation of the aorta are additional risk factors.

Chest radiographic findings suggestive of acute dissection include progressive aortic enlargement on serial films, a double contour of the aortic arch, and displacement of intimal calcification of more than 6 mm (CHEN 1990). One prospective study showed that signs suggestive of dissection were detected in only 25% of patients with proved aortic dissection (LUKER et al. 1994). In the same patients a retrospective review of chest radiographs showed detectable abnormalities in 48% of patients. Apparent displacement of intimal calcification may be a projectional artifact with calcification in the anterior part of the aortic arch overlying the descending aorta. Even normal aortic arch configuration, seen in 25% of patients with dissection, does not exclude the presence of a dissection (DEMOS et al. 1989).

Computerized tomography was first described in 1979 as a noninvasive method for diagnosing aortic dissection (HARRIS et al. 1979). Since that time it has replaced angiography as the primary method for diagnosis in most institutions. Its first use was limited by x-ray tube heat loading considerations and early techniques involved three scan levels with separate bolus contrast injections. Differential opacification of the true and false lumen could be identified but distal extent was not always determined by this technique. More rapid scan times associated with spiral CT allow imaging of the entire thoracic and abdominal aorta during a single injection of contrast material (COSTELLO et al. 1992b). In addition, the dense aortic opacification achieved with spiral CT results in images of high quality which markedly enhance our diagnostic capabilities.

Precontrast scans are important in the diagnosis of acute dissections since nonenhanced CT sections may show displacement of intimal calcifications or a high attenuation aortic wall containing fresh hemorrhage (Fig. 13.10). Fresh hematomas may occur in as many as 44% of acute dissections and do not occur in uncomplicated chronic dissections (HEIBERG et al. 1985). In some cases, a hematoma may be the only sign of an aortic dissection and probably reflects clotting of the false channel occurring when there is no reentry site in the intima to permit blood flow. GODWIN (1990) described this to be a nonclassic dissection. An intramural hematoma representing aortic dissection without intimal rupture (YAMADA et al. 1988) may resolve on serial scans (Fig. 13.11), whereas in other patients it evolves into a classic dissection with an intimal flap and a double lumen. Dissection with rupture probably represents an early or incomplete form of dissection and may or may not progress and likely results from rupture of the vasa vasorum.

The classical features of acute dissection on CT are an intimal flap and false lumen, seen in approximately 70% of patients (VASILE et al. 1986). Demonstration of an intimal flap is conclusive evidence of

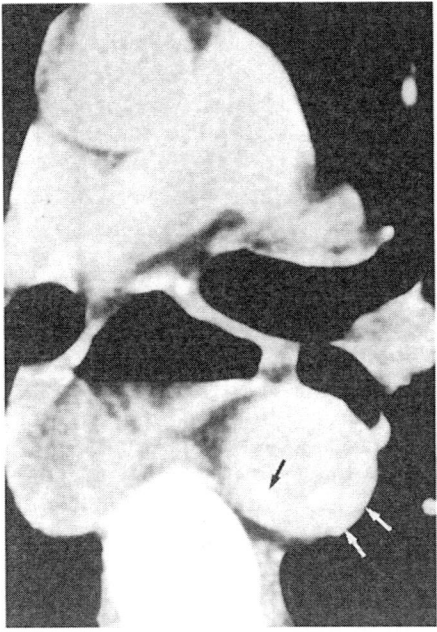

Fig. 13.10. Aortic dissection – precontrast CT. CT section through the mid thorax reveals a high attenuation ring in the descending aorta (*white arrows*) with displaced intimal calcification (*black arrow*). This represents intramural hematoma from an acute dissection

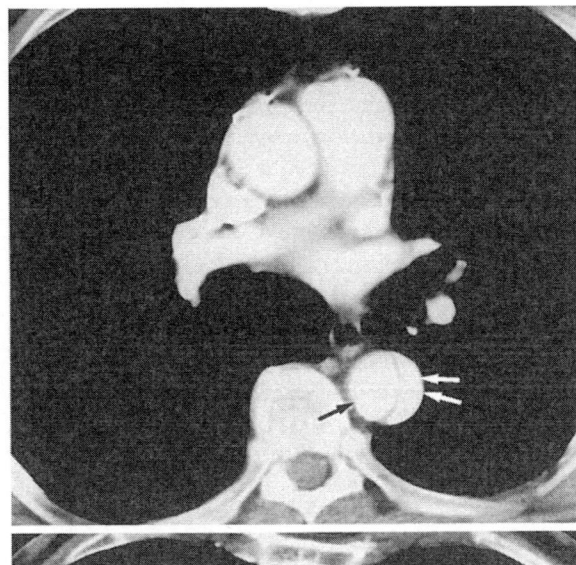

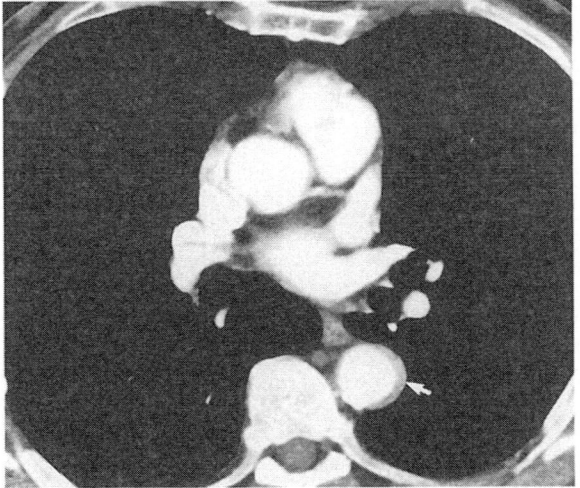

Fig. 13.11a,b. Aortic dissection; 100 ml contrast (300 mg I/ml) infused at 3 ml/s; 3-mm collimation with a pitch of 2. Sections through the descending aorta. **a** A retrograde dissection at the time of transfemoral cardiac catheterization with clear separation of the true lumen (*black arrow*) and false lumen (*white arrows*). **b** At 24h the dissection shows healing with only a small mural hematoma noted (*arrow*)

dissection (Figs. 13.12–13.14). When the wall of the aorta dissects, residual strands of tissue either bridging the dissection or with one end free in the bloodstream have been shown in the false lumen in up to 80% of surgical or autopsy specimens (WILLIAMS et al. 1994). These strands, termed aortic "cobwebs," are an absolute marker for the false lumen not occurring in the true lumen (Fig. 13.15). Aortic cobwebs most likely represent residual ribbons of media that have been incompletely sheared from the aortic wall during the process of dissection. Aortic cobwebs, best seen on magnetic resonance imaging (MRI), can be appreciated on spiral CT and are probably responsible for the "Mercedes-Benz sign" of the triple-barreled aortic dissections (SHIN et al. 1988). Recently introduced interventional techniques for treating aortic dissection require precise localization of the true and the false lumen. Angioplasty with or without stent placement to relieve compression of branch vessels and fenestration of the dissected septum to provide local flow between the true and the false lumen require precise orientation as to the true and false channels (WALKER et al. 1993; WILLIAMS et al. 1990).

Secondary findings associated with dissection include displacement of intimal calcifications, seen in 17% of cases, and a hematoma or thrombus in the wall of the aorta. High-attenuation material in the aortic wall, periaortic tissues, or pericardium is likewise suggestive of dissection but can also occur with rupture of an atherosclerotic aneurysm. Associated findings seen on CT not diagnostic of a dissection include variable amounts of intraluminal thrombus, dilatation of the aorta with compression of the true lumen, irregular contour of the contrast-filled portion of the aorta, disparate sizes of the ascending and descending limbs of the aorta, and pleural or pericardial effusion. Ischemia or infarction of organs sup-

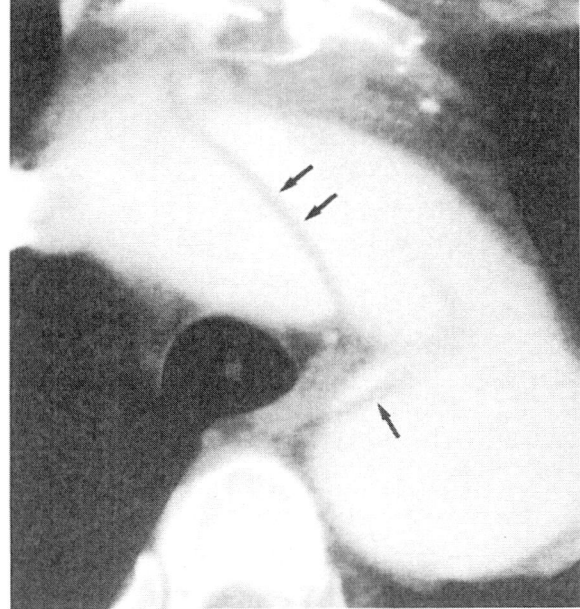

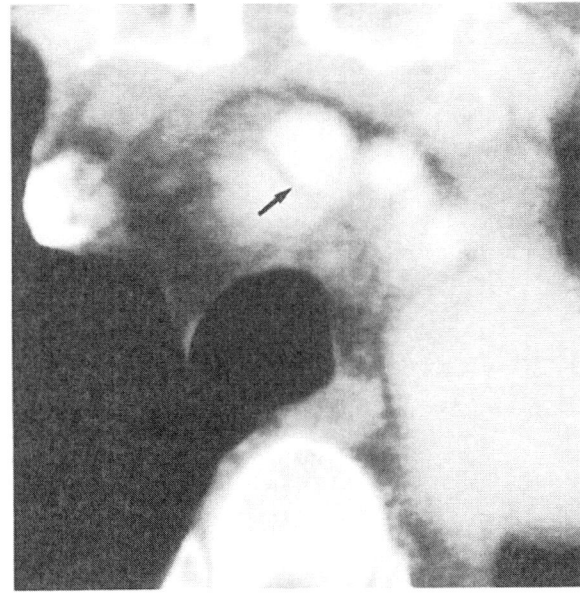

Fig. 13.12a,b. Type A aortic dissection; 60 ml contrast (300 mg I/ml) infused at 2 ml/s; 8-mm collimation with a pitch of 1. **a** An intimal flap is noted in the ascending (*double arrows*) and descending (*single arrow*) aortas. **b** The intimal flap extends into the right innominate artery (*arrow*). (From COSTELLO et al. 1992b)

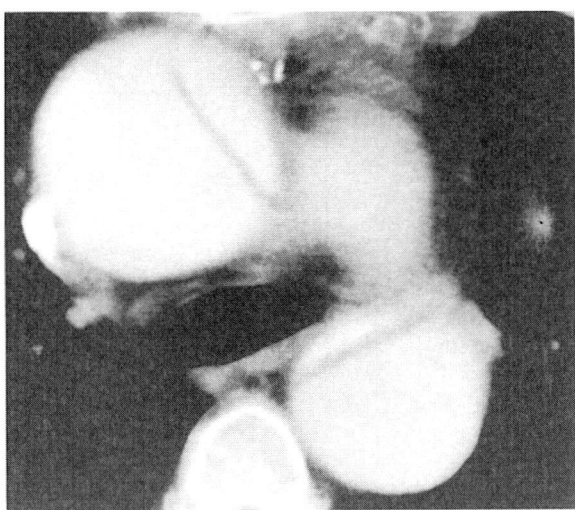

Fig. 13.13. Type A aortic dissection. (Same technique as Fig. 13.12.) An intimal flap is present in both the ascending and the descending aorta. (From COSTELLO et al. 1992b)

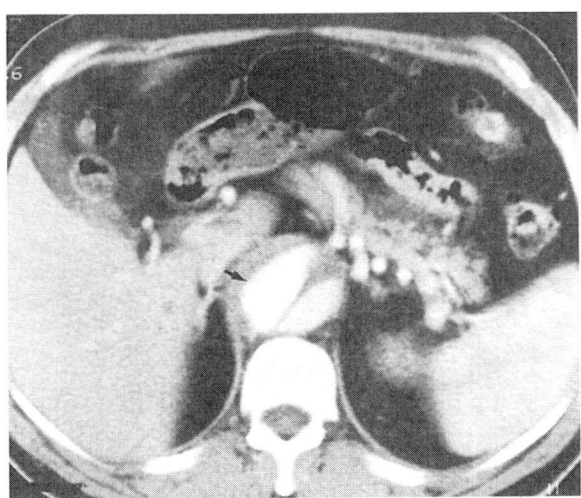

Fig. 13.14. Type B aortic dissection at the level of the celiac axis reveals and the true lumen lies to the right of midline (*arrow*). One hundred milliliters of contrast (300 mg I/ml) infused at 3 ml/s; 8-mm collimation with a pitch of 1. (From COSTELLO et al. 1992b)

plied by branch vessels from the false lumen are important secondary findings.

Computerized tomography is a rapid, relatively noninvasive and readily available method for evaluation of acute aortic dissection with a diagnostic accuracy of 88%–100% (THORSEN et al. 1985; MONCADA et al. 1981; THORSEN et al. 1983; VASILE et al. 1986; WHITE et al. 1986; LAAS et al. 1987). A recent study by NIENABER et al. in 1993 reported a sensitivity of 93.8% and a specificity of 87.1% using nonspiral CT. Pitfalls that arise with conventional CT scanning are reduced by the use of spiral CT (Fig. 13.16). Insufficient opacification of the aorta was common with the longer scan times and slower contrast injection rates of nonspiral CT, causing a failure to identify intimal flaps. Streak artifacts from patient motion and high attenuation contrast material in the superior vena

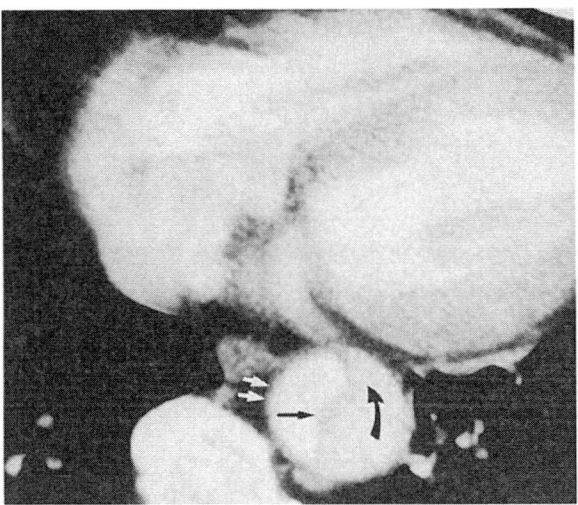

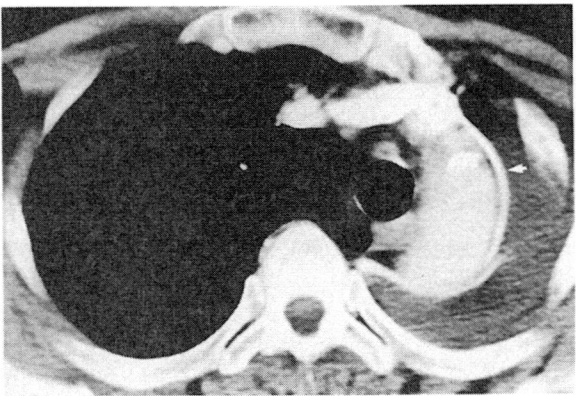

Fig. 13.16. Left superior intercostal vein simulating aortic dissection. (Same technique as Fig. 13.14.) The left superior intercostal vein lies (*arrow*) on the surface of the proximal descending aorta and is clearly separated from the aortic arch as a denser structure draining into the left innominate vein

Fig. 13.15. Type B aortic dissection; aortic cobweb. (Same technique as Fig. 13.14.) CT section through the descending aorta shows the true lumen is denser and lies medially (*double arrows*). Adjacent to the intimal flap (*single arrow*) is another linear density extending through the false lumen (*curved arrows*) representing an aortic cobweb. This aortic cobweb is a marker of the false lumen

cava can simulate intimal flaps. The intimal flap may be made less conspicuous by atypical configurations of the flap, such as with a short dissection which has multiple false channels in which the flaps are complex or aortic anomalies (FISHER et al. 1994).

13.4.1 Advantages of Spiral CT

Spiral CT offers many advantages when imaging patients suspected of arotic dissection. Arterial phase imaging makes recognition of intimal flaps, aortic cobwebs, branch vessel involvement, and reentry sites easier. Reconstruction of overlapping images reduces the effects of partial voluming and improves the quality of multiplanar and three-dimensional renderings. Multiplanar images are done first since they are less time consuming than three-dimensional images (Fig. 13.17). Both techniques are better able to depict the relationship of intimal flaps to the great vessels than transverse images alone (ZEMAN et al. 1995). Curved planar reformats can be reconstructed to show the intimal flap, false channel, and hematoma extension better than catheter angiography. When both channels fill with contrast, a denser true lumen is shown, separated from the less dense false lumen on MIP displays. Our vascular surgeons prefer the angiographic-like renditions of these three-dimensional displays and are often will-

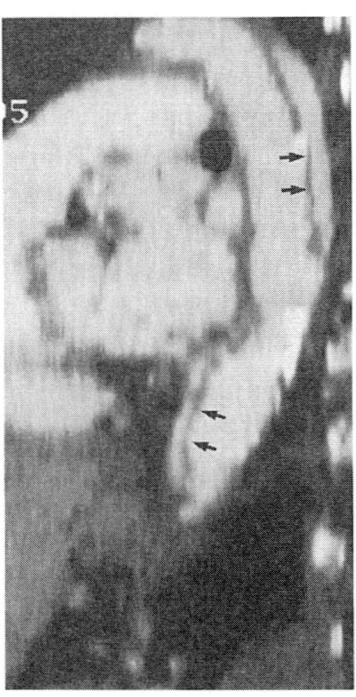

Fig. 13.17. Acute aortic dissection – paraxial reformat. CT data acquired during 100 ml infusion at 3 ml/s; 5-mm collimation. pitch 2, and reconstructions at 2 mm. The intimal flap separating the true and false lumens spirals from a posterior to an anterior location (*arrows*)

ing to perform surgery without confirmatory angiography (Fig. 13.18).

Spiral CT is associated with a unique artifact in the ascending aorta which can mimic arotic dissection (BURNS et al. 1991). It results from expansion and contraction of the ascending aorta seen more with heart rates averaging between 0.6 and 1/s (1.0–

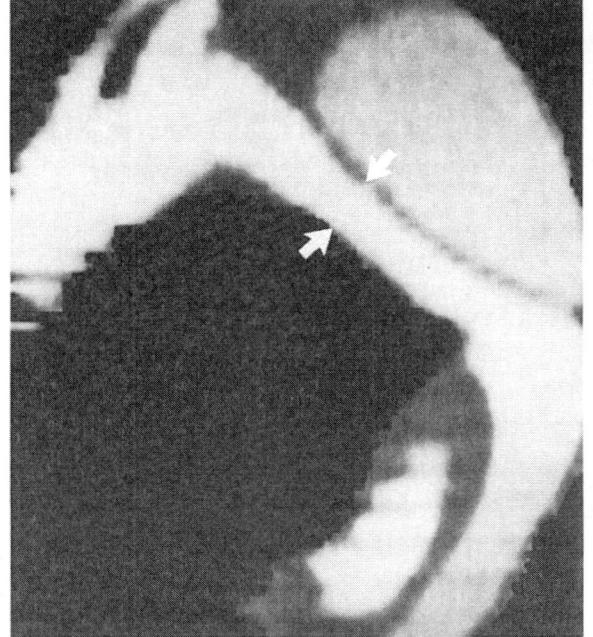

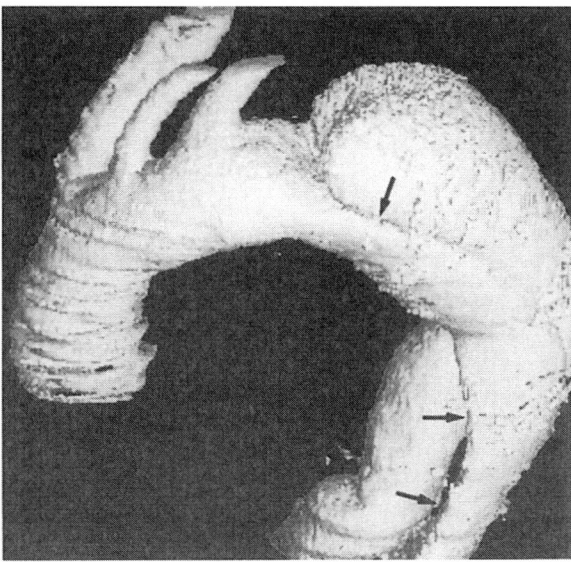

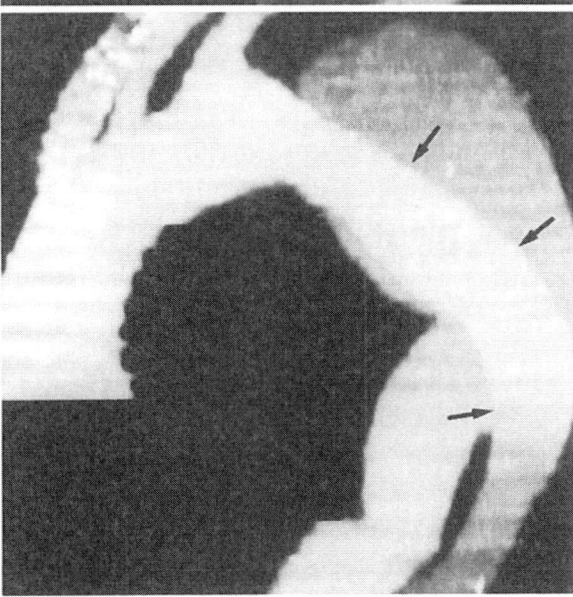

Fig. 13.18a–c. Type B aortic dissection; 120 ml contrast (300 mg I/ml) injected at 4 ml/s; 3-mm collimation with a pitch of 2; 2-mm reconstruction intervals. **a** Sagittal reconstruction shows the true lumen (*white arrows*) compressed by the larger, less dense false lumen. **b** Shaded surface display viewed laterally shows the relationship between the false lumen and the true lumen with visualization of the intimal flap (*arrows*). There is no discrimination of the attenuation differences between the true and false lumens. **c** Maximum intensity display viewed laterally of a type B aortic dissection. The compressed true lumen (*arrows*) is denser than the false lumen and is separated from it by an intimal flap

1.6 H2) (SILVERMAN et al. 1995) (Fig. 13.19). Reconstruction of partial scans can reduce or eliminate this artifact but images are noisy (POSNIAK et al. 1993); however, the technique is useful in problematic cases.

13.4.2 Complications

Rupture, which usually occurs from the right lateral wall of the ascending aorta, can result in death. Acute pericardial tamponade may cause hemopericardium

and rupture of the arch results in a mediastinal hematoma. Rupture of the descending aorta results in bleeding into the left pleural space (ROBERTS 1981). Aortic insufficiency from proximal extension of a dissection undermining the aortic valve can cause acute cardiac decompensation (DOROGHAZI et al. 1984). Branch involvement with extension into the coronary arteries, aortic arch branches, spinal artery, or visceral branches of the abdominal aorta produces a variety of clinical syndromes such as acute neurological events, including paraplegia or paraparesis, or vascular events. Vascular presentations include

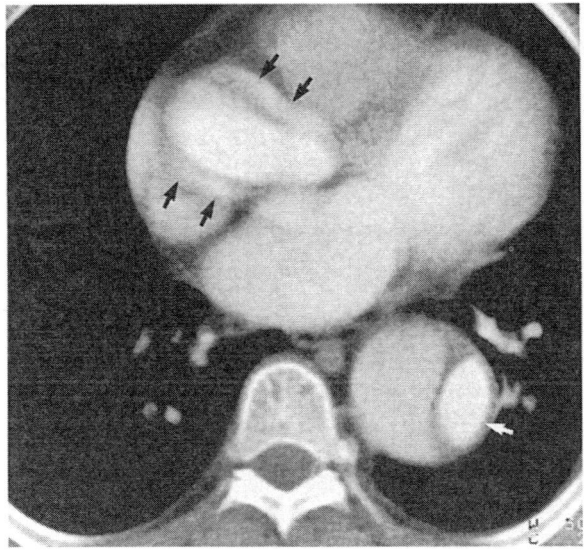

Fig. 13.19. Type B aortic dissection. (Same technique as Fig. 13.14.) A denser true lumen lying laterally (*arrow*) is compressed by the false lumen and separated from it by an intimal flap. Note a pulsation artifact of the ascending aorta at the level of the aortic valve (*arrows*)

shortness of breath from aortic insufficiency, pericardial tamponade, obstruction of the pulmonary artery or superior vena cava, myocardial infarction, and mesenteric or renal infarction (CHARNSANGAVEJ 1979).

13.4.3 Comparison with Other Imaging Modalities

Since the introduction of cross-sectional imaging, aortography has been shown to be less sensitive for detection of dissection than was once thought. Although angiography has a high degree of accuracy, false-negative results do occur (ERBEL et al. 1990). The false lumen may not be opacified if it is thrombosed or if the catheter tip is distal to the site of intimal tear (SANDERS 1990). If both the true and false lumens opacify simultaneously, an intimal falp may not be opacified. The advantages of aortography include its ability to consistently demonstrate the major aortic branches and coronary artery involvement and to make possible evaluation of the aortic valve.

Magnetic resonance imaging (MRI) can provide similar information to CT without the need for intravenous contrast medium. It has a reported accuracy of 83%–100% (AMPARO et al. 1985; SPRITZER et al. 1989; GLAZER et al. 1985). Major advantages of MRI include an ability to show the aorta in multiple

planes and to provide functional data on blood flow. Problems related to MRI of acute dissection include a heterogeneous signal intensity in the false lumen representing slow flow or thrombus or both. A thrombosed false lumen can be difficult to differentiate from an aortic aneurysm or mural thrombus. Patient motion, irregular respirations or poor ECG gating limit MR image quality. Many life support and monitoring devices essential to patients with acute dissection cannot be brought into an MRI facility. These problems combined with the long imaging time, possibly 30–60 min, limit MRI's role for many acutely ill patients suspected of acute dissection.

Transesophageal echocardiography (TEE) combined with transthoracic echocardiography has a sensitivity of 98% and specificity of 99% for acute aortic dissection (BALLAL et al. 1991). These studies take less than 20 min and can be performed in the emergency room or intensive care unit, precluding movement of critically ill patients. Ninety-eight percent of patients can tolerate esophageal intubation with only minimal sedation and TEE is excellent in depicting the intimal flap entry sites into the false lumen, thrombi, pericardial effusion, aortic valve, and the entire heart. It is extremely useful in detecting cardiac complications of dissection such as aortic regurgitation, pericardial effusion, and myocardial ischemia.

The final choice of an imaging modality for acute aortic dissection depends upon the speed with which

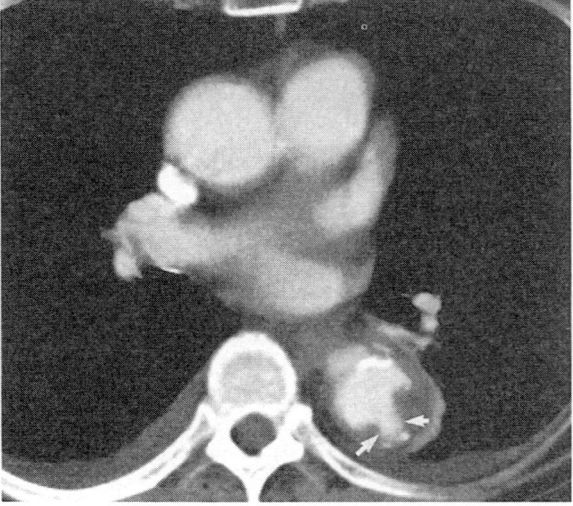

Fig. 13.20. Penetrating aortic ulcer in a 73-year-old woman with severe back pain. Sixty milliliters of contrast (300 mg I/ml) infused at 2 ml/s; 8-mm collimation with a pitch of 1. A penetrating aortic ulcer is demonstrated (*arrows*) in the descending thoracic aorta with pleural fluid. (From COSTELLO et al. 1992b)

the study can be performed and interpreted in a particular hospital environment. In most hospitals, spiral CT or transesophageal echocardiography are the imaging modalities of choice. MRI is a strong second but is not always available in the acute setting and is more often useful for the follow-up of chronic dissections.

13.5 Penetrating Atherosclerotic Ulcers of the Aorta

Penetrating atherosclerotic ulcer of the aorta was first described by STANSON et al. in 1986 as a distinct pathological entity that clinically mimics classic aortic dissection. Penetrating atherosclerotic ulcers usu-

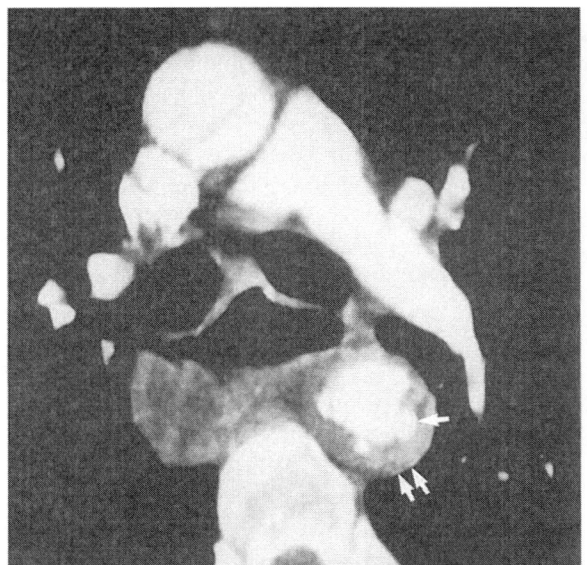

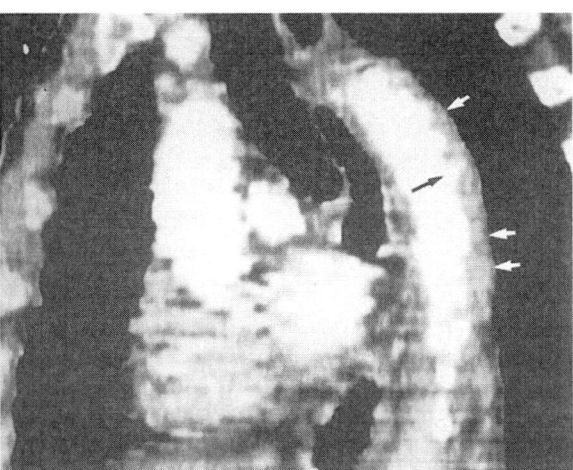

a

b

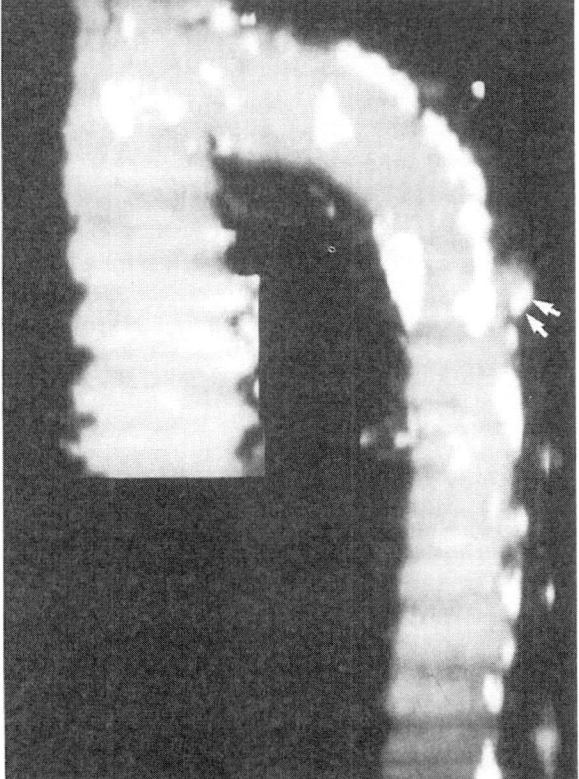

c

Fig. 13.21a–c. Penetrating aortic ulcer in a 64-year-old male with severe back pain and hypertension. One hundred and twenty milliliters of contrast (300 mg I/ml) injected at 4 ml/s; 3-mm collimation with a pitch of 2; 2-mm reconstruction intervals. a Note an ulcer in the proximal descending aorta (*arrow*) with intramural hematoma (*arrows*). b Oblique sagittal reconstruction through the aorta reveals the extent of the intramural hematoma (*white arrows*) and the penetrating aortic ulcer (*black arrow*). c MIP viewed laterally reveals an extensively calcified atherosclerotic aorta with visualization of the penetrating aortic ulcer (*double arrows*). This projection does not demonstrate intramural hematoma

ally occur in elderly, hypertensive (87%) individuals with severe atherosclerotic disease (KAZEROONI et al. 1992). Patients may be asymptomatic or present with chest or back pain (81%) (KAZEROONI et al. 1992). An ulcerated plaque erodes the internal elastic lamina and penetrates the media of the aortic wall, allowing blood to dissect. If the hematoma is not confined by adventitia it will eventually lead to aortic rupture.

Findings of CT are those of an intramural hematoma clearly defined as subintimal by the presence of displaced intimal calcifications, which are seen in 81% of patients (KAZEROONI et al. 1992; TISANDO et al. 1980; WELCH et al. 1990; COOKE et al. 1988). The aortic wall can be thickened or enhanced in up to 37% of patients and pleural fluid collections occur in 44%. CT demonstrates a focal ulceration in 94% of patients located predominantly in the middle to distal third of the descending thoracic aorta (Figs. 13.20, 13.21). Rarely, multiple ulcers are present in the same individual and both shallow and large penetrating ulcers may develop.

It is clinically important to separate penetrating aortic ulcer from aortic dissection since surgery is more extensive with penetrating ulcers. A longer aortic interposition graft for the very friable aorta is necessary for repair of a penetrating ulcer. More limited resection and grafting are performed with the intimal tears of type B dissections (STANSON et al. 1986; COOKE et al. 1988). Most patients are treated conservatively initially with antihypertensive therapy. Medical therapy may be effective, but if patients become hemodynamically unstable or experience persistent or recurrent chest or back pain, surgical intervention becomes necessary.

High false-negative diagnosis rates were observed using nonspiral CT techiques because of lack of contrast or suboptimal aortic enhancement (HARRIS et al. 1994). Spiral CT provides the ideal imaging method to assess patients with penetrating aortic ulcers. By timing the contrast delivery through the diseased segment of the aorta, a high degree of enhancement allows visualization of the aortic wall ulcer and intramural hematoma.

The multiplanar imaging capabilities of spiral CT clearly demonstrate the extent of the aortic wall ulceration and hematoma propagation. These images can provide surgeons with a road map to the length of aorta needing graft replacement. Conventional angiography may demonstrate aortic ulceration but does not define the extent of hematoma dissection.

Up to 50% of patients with atherosclerotic ulcers develop saccular aneurysms with a longer follow-up interval associated with a greater likelihood of progression to aneurysm. Of patients followed conservatively for a mean of 4.6 years, an average growth rate to saccular aneurysms of 7.2% per year was noted (HARRIS et al. 1994). Concentric aortic dilatation and loss of definition of an ulcer crater are the first signs of aneurysm formation. Once focal periaortic adventitial bulging begins, progressive enlargement of the ulcer to a saccular aneurysm occurs in all individuals. Progression to aneurysm development is a slow process with a low incidence of aortic rupture or other life-threatening complications. Therefore, immediate aortic repair is not mandatory in all patients, particularly in those with advanced age or poor general health who have associated high morbidity and mortality rates for surgical resection.

13.6 Thoracic Aortic Trauma

Controversy still exists regarding the role of CT in patients suffering thoracic trauma. It was initially assumed that the presence of a mediastinal hematoma would be an accurate predictor of aortic laceration (MIRVIS et al. 1987; MORGAN et al. 1992; RAPTOPOULOS et al. 1992; RICHARDSON et al. 1991; NAKAJIMA et al. 1992; KAWADA et al. 1990; MADAYAG et al. 1991). Those patients with mediastinal blood will have aortic rupture 25% of the time as compared to a 5%–20% incidence of rupture in patients who have angiograms prior to CT evaluation (BROOKS et al. 1989; MIRVIS et al. 1987; RAPTOPOULOS et al. 1992; RICHARDSON et al. 1991; NAKAJIMA et al. 1992; ISHIKAWA et al. 1989). By using CT to detect mediastinal hematoma it was thought that the number of negative angiograms could be reduced. However, a small percentage of patients have aortic or great vessel injury without a mediastinal hematoma and false-negative CT studies have been reported with aortic rupture, subclavian artery rupture, and vertebral artery rupture (BROOKS et al. 1989; MILLER et al. 1989; HEIBERG et al. 1983; MIRVIS et al. 1987; MORGAN et al. 1992; RAPTOPOULOS et al. 1992; RICHARDSON et al. 1992; NAKAJIMA et al. 1992; FENNER et al. 1990). Because of these problems it is recommended that CT be reserved for patients who are clinically stable and in whom the likelihood of aortic injury is relatively low. Those patients who have a strong suspicion of aortic trauma based on clinical signs and clear-cut evidence of mediastinal hematoma on chest x-ray should go directly to conventional catheter angiography.

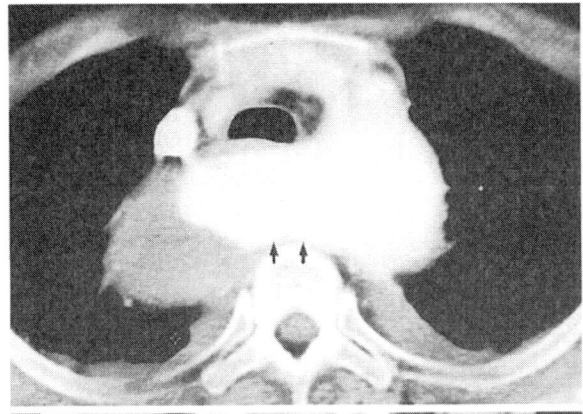

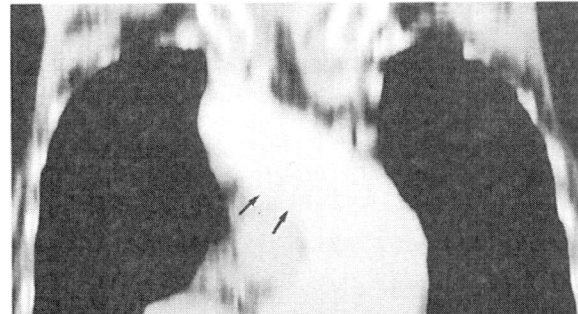

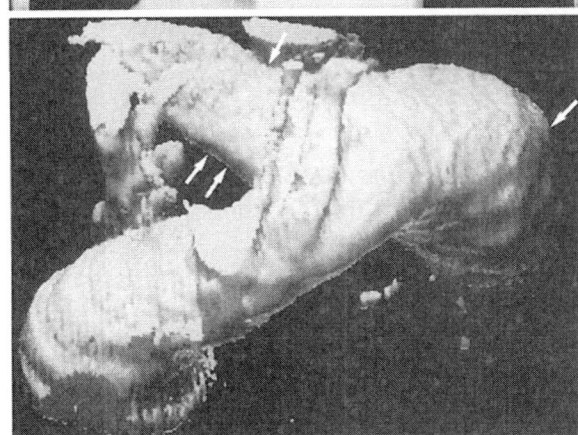

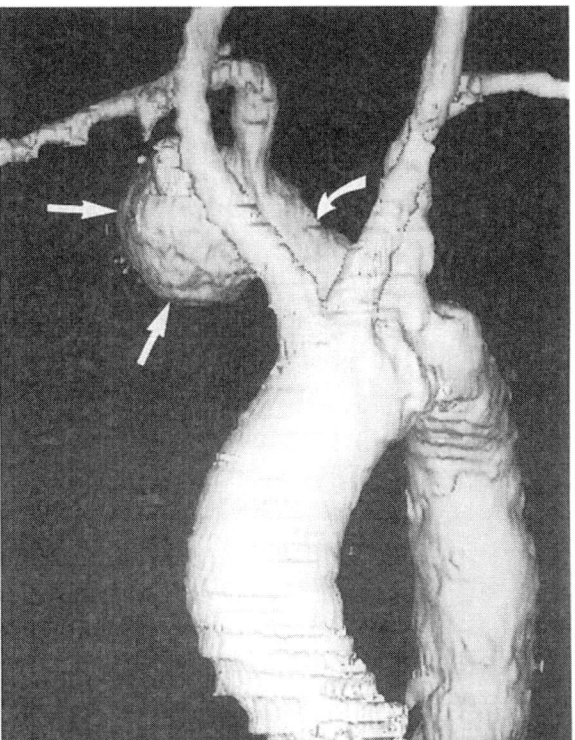

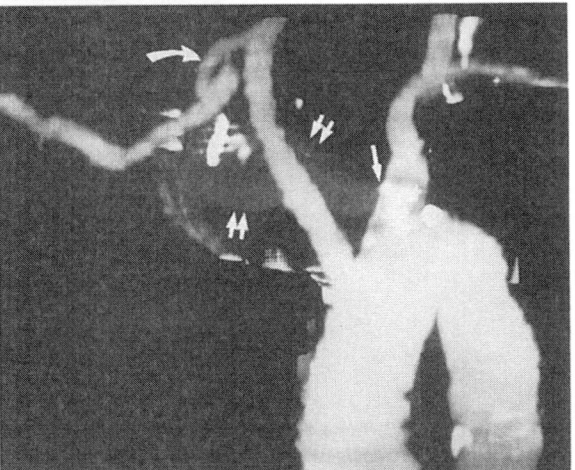

Fig. 13.22a–c. Aberrant right subclavian artery aneurysm. (Same technique as Fig. 13.21.) **a** Transverse CT section just above the aortic arch reveals a partially thrombosed, aberrant right subclavian artery aneurysm posterior to the trachea (*arrows*). **b** Coronal section through the descending aorta reveals an aneurysm of the descending aorta and an aberrant right subclavian artery aneurysm (*arrows*) crossing posterior to the esophagus and trachea. **c** Shaded surface display of the aberrant right subclavian artery aneurysm (*arrows*) originating from the proximal descending aorta (*arrow*). (From COSTELLO 1995)

Fig. 13.23a,b. (Same technique as Fig. 13.21.) **a** Aberrant right subclavian artery aneurysm. Three-dimenstional shaded surface display reveals an aberrant right subclavian artery (*curved arrow*) with a focal aneurysm 5 cm in diameter (*arrows*). **b** Postoperative aberrant right subclavian artery aneurysm repair. Appearance 6 months following ligation of an aberrant right subclavian artery and a right carotid to the right subclavian artery bypass graft. The patient presented with a further widening of the mediastinum. Maximum intensity display reveals contrast filling the original aberrant right subclavian artery aneurysm (*double arrows*) through an anastomotic breakdown (*single arrows*). The right carotid to right subclavian artery graft is patent (*curved arrow*)

The rapid scan time of spiral CT is beneficial in patients who are critically ill and undergoing abdominal, thoracic, and head or spine CT studies. When contrast is administered, the direct signs of aortic rupture such as false aneurysm, irregularity of the aortic contour, and visualization of an intimal flap may be more precisely delineated by dense vascular opacification. Theoretically thin-section spiral CT with overlapping sections maight be able to detect aortic lacerations in the absence of a

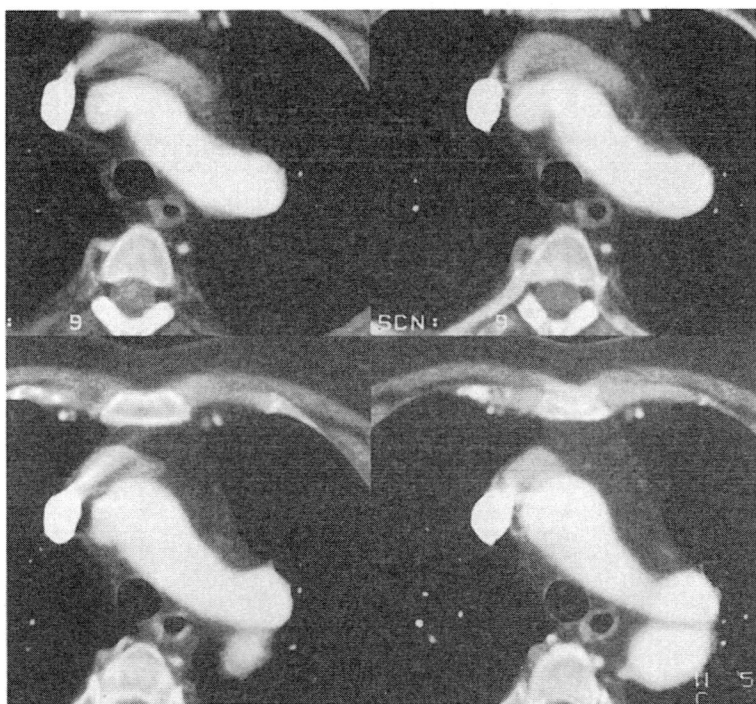

Fig. 13.24a,b. Pseudocoarctation of the aorta. (Same technique as in Fig. 13.21.) a Transverse section through the aortic reveals a tortuous course to the proximal descending aorta. b Shaded surface display reveals a very tortuous aorta, kinked at the level of the ligamentum arteriosum (*arrows*). The left subclavian artery and descending aorta are aneurysmally dilated. c Maximum intensity projection image clearly demonstrates the pseudocoarctation (*arrows*), dilated descending aorta, and left subclavian arteries

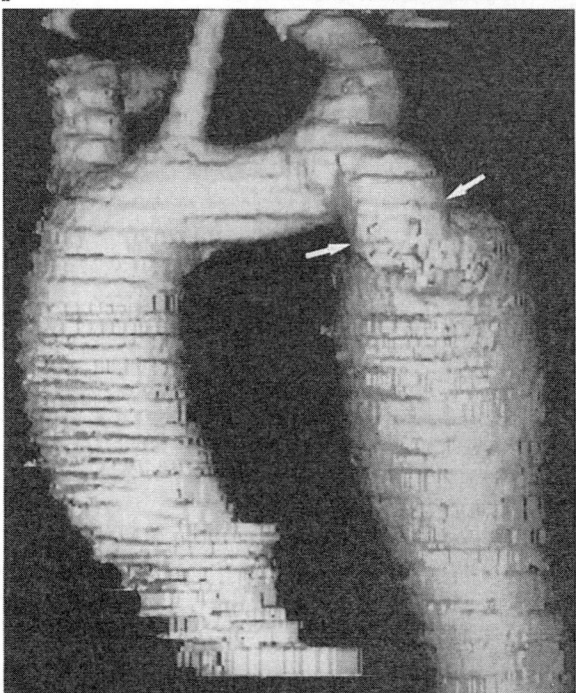

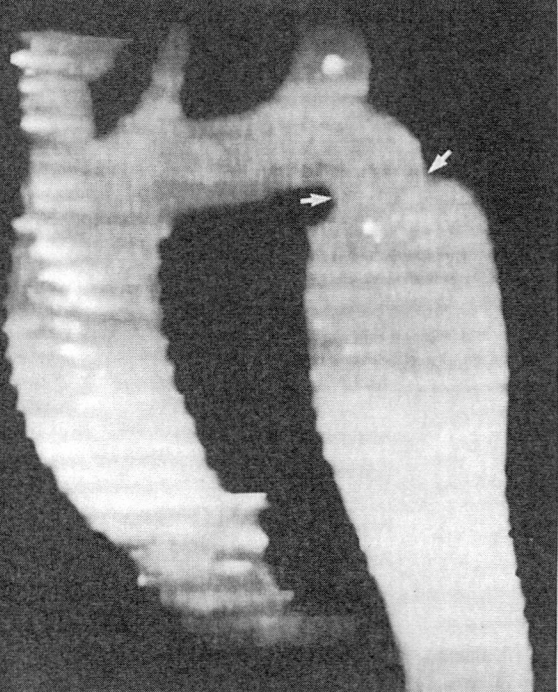

mediastinal hematoma. The adjunctive value of sagittal, coronal, oblique, and three-dimensional reconstructions may allow CT to approach the sensitivity of angiography. Although the false-negative rate for CT in the diagnosis of aortic laceration appears to be low (1%–6%), further studies will be needed comparing spiral CT with conventional angiography.

13.7 Mediastinal Vascular Abnormalities

An aberrant right subclavian artery is the most common congenital anomaly of the aorta, occurring in less than 1% of the population. The anomalous right subclavian artery arises as the last branch of the distal part of the aortic arch and crosses the mediastinum obliquely from left to right behind the esophagus. It may be dilated as its origin and can become aneurysmal focally or diffusely. Spiral CT with three-dimensional reconstructions provides excellent anatomical depiction of the origin of the vessel and its relationship to the aortic arch and other vessels (MEIER et al. 1993) (Fig. 13.22). It is used instead of angiography to plan surgical resection of the aneurysm and postoperatively for patient follow-up (Fig. 13.23).

The two most common right-sided aortic arch anomalies can be demonstrated by spiral CT. A right aortic arch with an aberrant left subclavian artery is rarely associated with congenital heart disease. By contrast, a right-sided aortic arch with mirror image branching has a high incidence of associated congenital heart disease, especially tetralogy of Fallot and truncus arteriosus.

Computerized tomography can demonstrate the aortic deformity at the site of coarctation but MRI is more often used, particularly in the pediatric age group.

Pseudocoarctation or kinking of the aortic arch in the region of the ligamentum arteriosum can be mistaken for true coarctation or a mediastinal mass. The aortic arch is abnormally high and as it descends, curves anteriorly, kinks, and courses posteriorly to its normal position (Fig. 13.24).

13.8 Pulmonary Sequestration

Intralobar pulmonary sequestration derives its arterial supply most commonly from the descending thoracic aorta or occasionally from the abdominal aorta or one of its branches. Contrast-enhanced CT

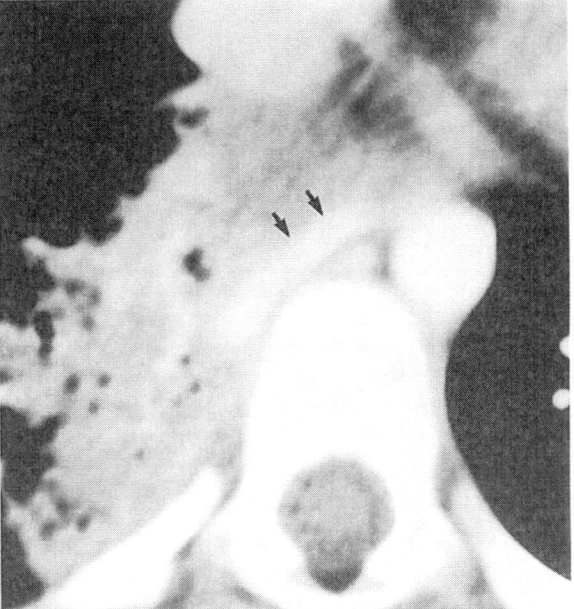
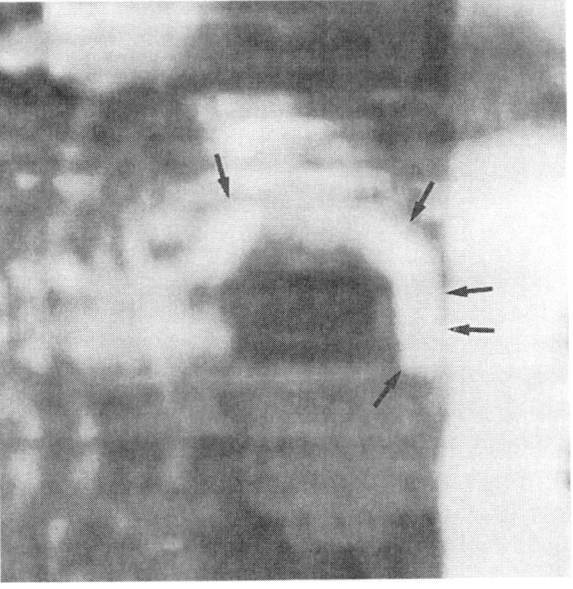

Fig. 13.25a,b. Pulmonary sequestration in a 7-year-old male with a focal area of increased density in the right lower lobe. **a** Contrast-enhanced transverse CT at the level of T9 reveals an enlarged artery (*arrows*) supplying the abnormality of the right lower lobe. **b** MIP image viewed frontally reveals that the right lower lobe is supplied by an artery originating from the celiac axis (*arrows*). Diagnosis was an intralobar pulmonary sequestration. (Courtesy of Dr. S. Kramer, Philadelphia)

studies can demonstrate the anomalous systemic arterial supply to the aberrant lung tissue, so that angiography is no longer necessary prior to surgery. (Fig. 13.25).

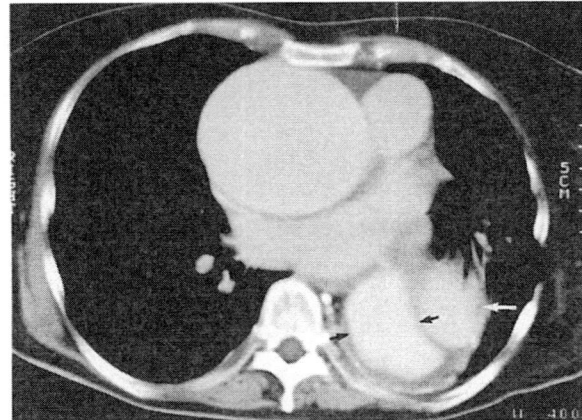

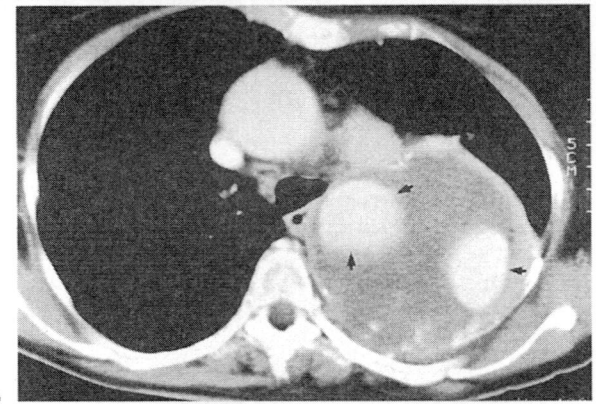

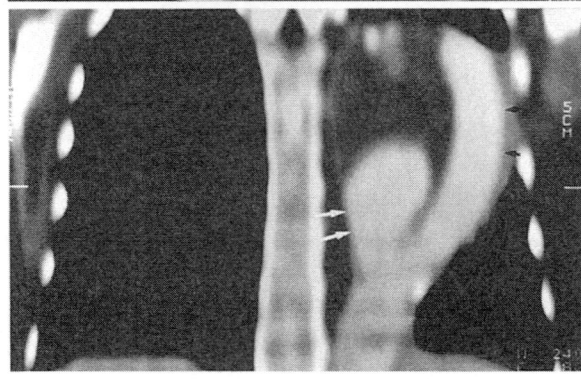

13.9 Postoperative Evaluation

Patients who have undergone aortic surgery or by-pass graft procedures can be easily evaluated with CT angiography (RUBIN et al. 1993; TELLO et al. 1993). Complications of the graft site such as infection, stenosis, or aneurysms at the anastomosis can be demonstrated (Fig. 13.26).

Aortic aneurysms can be treated by transluminal placement of stainless steel stents covered with either Dacron or polytetrafluoroethylene graft material. Spiral CT provides measurements from which the prosthesis can be customized to the patient. Following stent deployment, CT is used to assess the position and expansion of the stent, formation of neointimal hyperplasia, and aneurysm occlusion (RUBIN et al. 1994).

Spiral CT has been used in the assessment of patients who underwent coronary artery bypass grafts (TELLO et al. 1993). It can establish graft patency with a sensitivity of 85.7% and 100% specificity compared to angiography. Thin incremental sections combined with three-dimensional reconstructions provide an elegant, noninvasive way of demonstrating the course and patency of grafts. Three-dimensional reconstructions enhance clinical acceptance and assist

Fig. 13.26a–c. Fifty-nine-year-old woman with respiratory infections and collapse of the left lower lobe. The descending aorta had been replaced 5 years previously with a Teflon graft from the left subclavian artery origin to the distal thoracic aorta. The mediastinum had widened further over the intervening 4 years. **a** CT section at the level of the right pulmonary artery shows contrast filling two ovoid structures. Contrast material opacifies the graft laterally (*white arrow*) whereas medially contrast (*black arrows*) opacifies a partially clot filled aneurysm. **b** CT section through the proximal descending aorta reveals the graft laterally (*single arrow*) and the original aneurysm opacifying (*double arrows*) with contrast material. **c** Coronal reconstruction through the tube graft (*arrows*) with opacification of the original aneurysm through distal anastomotic breakdown (*white arrows*)

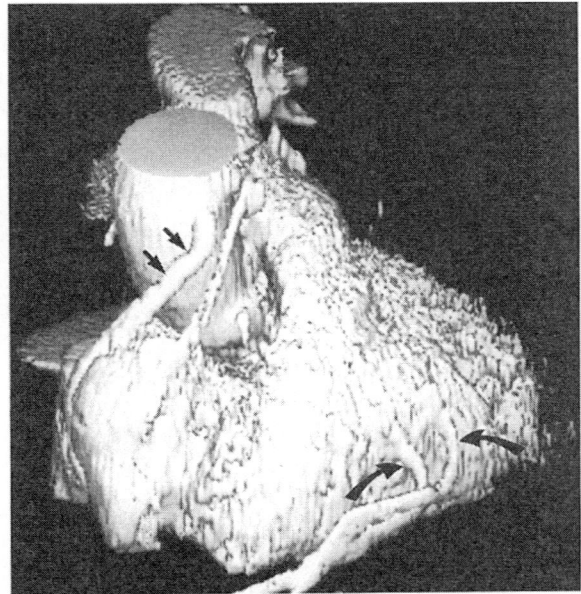

Fig. 13.27. Coronary artery bypass graft; 80 ml contrast (300 mg I/ml) infused at 3 ml/s and 5-mm collimation with a pitch of 1; reconstructions at 1 mm. Shaded surface display of the ascending aorta revealing a patent saphenous vein graft to the right coronary artery (*arrows*). Note the external pacer leads (*curved arrows*)

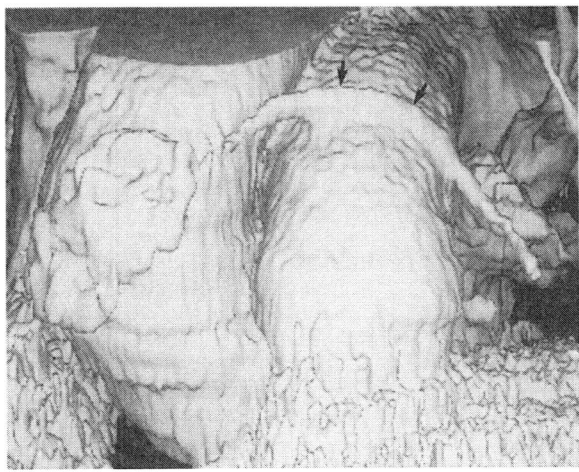

Fig. 13.28. Coronary artery bypass graft. (Same technique as Fig. 13.27.) Shaded surface display of the ascending aorta reveals a cranial loop of the left saphenous vein graft (*arrows*) in its course to the left anterior descending coronary artery. Transverse CT sections were initially interpreted as two patent vein grafts due to the tortuous course of this graft

in the evaluation of tortuous grafts, which, on conventional CT studies, may give the appearance of two grafts rather than a single graft (Figs. 13.27, 13.28).

References

Amparo EG, Higgins CB, Hricak H, Sollitto R (1985) Aortic dissection: magnetic resonance imaging. Radiology 155: 339–406

Ballal RS, Nanda NC, Gatewood R et al. (1991) Usefulness of transesophageal echocardiography in assessment of aortic dissection. Circulation 84:1903–1914

Brooks AP, Olson LK, Shackford SR (1989) Computed tomography in the diagnosis of traumatic rupture of the thoracic aorta. Clin Radiol 40:133–138

Burns MA, Molina PL, Gutierrez FR, Sagel SS (1991) Motion artifact simulating aortic dissection on CT. AJR 157:465–467

Charnsangavej C (1979) Occlusion of the right pulmonary artery by acute dissecting aortic aneurysm. AJR 132:274–276

Chen JTT (1990) Plain radiographic evaluation of the aorta. J Thorac Imaging 5:1–17

Cooke JP, Kazmier FJ, Orszulak TA (1988) The penetrating aortic ulcer: pathologic manifestations, diagnosis, and management. Mayo Clin Proc 63:718–725

Costello P (1994) Thoracic helical CT. Radiographics 14:913–918

Costello P (1995) Thoracic imaging with spiral CT. In: Fishman EK, Jeffrey RB Jr (eds) Spiral CT: principles, techniques and clinical applications. Raven Press, New York

Costello P, Dupuy DE, Ecker CP, Tello R (1992a) Spiral CT of the thorax with reduced volume of contrast material: a comparative study. Radiology 183:663–666

Costello P, Ecker CP, Tello R, Hartnell G (1992b) Assessment of the thoracic aorta by spiral CT. AJR 158:1127–1130

Crawford ES, Swensson LG, Coselli JS, Safi HJ, Hess KR (1988) Aortic dissection and dissection aortic aneurysms. Ann Surg 208:254–273

Crawford ES, Swensson LG, Coselli JS, Safi HJ, Hess KR (1989) Surgical treatment of aneurysm and/or dissection of the ascending aorta, transverse aortic arch and ascending aorta and transverse aortic arch. J Thorac Cardiovasc Surg 98:659–674

DeBakey ME, McCollum H, Crawford ES et al. (1982) Dissection and dissecting aneurysms of the aorta: twenty-year follow-up of five hundred twenty-seven patients treated surgically. Surgery 92:1118–1134

Demos TC, Posniak HV, Marsan RE (1989) CT of aortic dissection. Semin Roentgenol 24:22–37

Doroghazi RM, Slater EE, DeSanctis RW, Buckley MJ, Austen WG, Rosenthal S (1984) Long-term survival of patients with treated aortic dissections. J Am Coll Cardiol 3:1026–1034

Erbel R, Daniel W, Visser C et al. (1990) Echocardiography in the diagnosis of aortic dissection. Lancet I:457–460

Fenner MN, Fisher KS, Sergel NL et al. (1990) Evaluation of possible traumatic thoracic aortic injury using aortography and CT. Am Surg 56:497–499

Fisher ER, Stern EJ, Godwin JD, Otto CM, Johnson JA (1994) Acute aortic dissection: typical and atypical imaging features. Radiographics 14:1263–1271

Glazer HS, Gutierrez FR, Levitt RG, Lee JKT, Murphy WA (1985) The thoracic aorta studied by MR imaging. Radiology 157:149–155

Godwin JD (1990) Conventional CT of the aorta. J Thorac Imaging 5:18–31

Godwin JD, Herfkens RL, Skioldebrand CG, Federle MP, Lipton MJ (1980) Evaluation of dissections and aneurysms of the thoracic aorta by conventional and dynamic CT scanning. Radiology 136:125–133

Godwin JD, Breiman RS, Speckman JM (1982) Problems and pitfalls in the evaluation of thoracic aortic dissection by computed tomography. J Comput Assist Tomogr 6:750–756

Harder T, Nicolas V, Steudel A, Orrelano L (1987) Radiological diagnosis of the thoracic aortic aneurysm. Thorac Cardiovasc Surg 35:122–125

Harris JA, Bis KG, Glover JL, Bendick PJ et al. (1994) Penetrating atherosclerotic ulcers of the aorta. J Vasc Surg 19:90–99

Harris RD, Usselman JA, Vint VC, Warmath MA (1979) Computerized tomographic diagnosis of aneurysms of the thoracic aorta. Comput Tomogr 3:81–91

Haverich A, Miller DC, Scott WC et al. (1985) Acute and chronic aortic dissections – determinants of long-term outcome for operative survivors. Circulation 72(Suppl 2):22–34

Heiberg E, Wolverson MK, Sundaram M et al. (1983) CT in the aortic trauma. AJR 140:1119–1124

Heiberg E, Wolverson MK, Sundaram M, Shields JB (1985) CT characteristics of aortic atherosclerotic aneurysm versus aortic dissection. J Comput Assist Tomogr 9:78–83

Hirose Y, Hamada S, Takamiya M et al. (1992) Aortic aneurysms: growth rates measured with CT. Radiology 185:249–252

Hirst AE Jr, Johns VJ Jr, Kime SW Jr (1958) Dissecting aneurysm of the aorta: a review of 505 cases. Medicine 37:217–279

Ishikawa T, Nakajuma Y, Kaji T (1989) The role of CT in traumatic rupture of the thoracic aorta and its proximal branches. Semin Roentgenol 24:38–46

Kawada T, Mieda T, Abe H et al. (1990) Surgical experience with traumatic rupture of the thoracic aorta. J Cardiovasc Surg 31:359–363

Kazerooni EA, Bree RL, Williams DM (1992) Penetrating atherosclerotic ulcers of the descending thoracic aorta: evaluation with CT and distinction from aortic dissection. Radiology 183:759–765

Laas J, Schluter G, Daniel W, Hendrick PH, Haverich A (1987) Acute type-A dissection of the aorta: which diagnostic modes remain for surgical indication? Eur J Cardiothorac Surg 1:169–172

Luker GD, Glazer HS, Eagar G, Gutierrez R, Sagel SS (1994) Aortic dissection: effect of prospective chest radiographic diagnosis on delay to definitive diagnosis. Radiology 193:813–819

Machida K, Tasaka A (1980) CT patterns of mural thrombus in aortic aneurysms. J Comput Assist Tomogr 4:840–842

Madayag MA, Kirshenbaum KJ, Madimpalli SR, et al. (1991) Thoracic aortic trauma role of dynamic CT. Cardiovasc Radiol 179:853–855

Meier RA, Marianacci EB, Costello P, Fitzpatrick PJ, Hartnell GG (1993) 3D image reconstruction of right subclavian artery aneurysms. J Comput Assist Tomogr 17:887–890

Miller DC (1983) Surgical management of aortic dissections: indications, perioperative management, and long-term results. In: Doroghazi RM, Slater EE (eds) Aortic dissection. McGraw-Hill, New York, pp 193–243

Miller DC, Mitchell RC, Oyer PE, Stinson EB, Jamieson SW, Shumway NE (1984) Independent determinants of operative mortality for patients with aortic dissections. Circulation 70(Suppl I):153–164

Miller FB, Richardson D, Thomas HA et al. (1989) Role of CT in diagnosis of major arterial injury after blunt thoracic trauma. Surgery 106:596–603

Mirvis SE, Kostrubiak I, Whitley NO, et al. (1987) Role of CT in excluding major arterial injury after blunt thoracic trauma. AJR 149:601–605

Mitchell RS (1993) Thoracic aortic aneurysms. In: Greenfield LJ, Mulholland MW, Oldham KT, Zelenock GB (eds) Surgery: scientific principles and practice. Lippincott, Philadelphia, pp 1690–1706

Moncada R, Churchill R, Reynes C et al. (1981) Diagnosis of dissecting aortic aneurysm by computed tomography. Lancet I:238–241

Morgan PW, Goodman LR, Aprahamian C et al. (1992) Evaluation of traumatic aortic injury: does dynamic contrast-enhanced CT play a role? Radiology 182:661–666

Nakajima Y, Kurihara Y, Galvin J et al. (1992) Diagnosis of traumatic aortic rupture: utility of CT screening. Scientific Paper. 78th Scientific Assembly and Annual Meeting, RSNA, Chicago. Radiology 185(P) (Suppl)

Nienaber CA, von Kodolitsch Y, Nichols V et al. (1993) The diagnosis of thoracic aortic dissection by noninvasive imaging procedures. N Engl J Med 328:1–9

Posniak MV, Olson MC, Demos TC (1993) Aortic motion artifact simulation dissection on CT scars: elimination with reconstructive segmented images. AJR 161:557–558

Raptopoulos V, Sheiman RG, Phillips DA et al. (1992) Traumatic aortic tear: screening with chest CT. Radiology 182:667–673

Reul GL, Cooley DA, Hallman GL, Reddy SB, Kyger ER, Wukasch DC (1975) Dissecting aneurysm of the descending aorta. Arch Surg 110:632–640

Richardson P, Mirvis SE, Scorpio R et al. (1991) Value of CT in determining the need for angiography when findings of mediastinal hemorrhage on chest radiographs are equivocal. AJR 156:273–279

Roberts WC (1981) Aortic dissection anatomy, consequences, and causes. Am Heart J 101:195–214

Rubin GD, Walker PJ, Dake MD et al. (1993) 3D spiral CT angiography: an alternative imaging modality for the abdominal aorta and its branches. J Vasc Surg 18:656–666

Rubin GD, Dake MD, Semba CP, Napel SA, Jeffrey RB (1994) Helical CT angiography for evaluation of endovascular intervention (abstr). Radiology 193(P):379–380

Sanders C (1990) Current role of conventional and digital aortography in the diagnosis of aortic disease. J Thorac Imaging 5:48–59

Shin MS, Zorn GL, Ho KJ (1988) Computed tomography manifestation of a triple-barreled aortic dissection: the Mercedes-Benz mark sign. J Comput Tomogr 12:140–143

Silverman PM, Cooper CJ, Weltman DJ, Zeman RK (1995) Helical CT: practical considerations and potential pitfalls. Radiographics 15:25–36

Spritzer CE, Blinder RA (1989) Vascular applications of magnetic resonance imaging. Magn Reson Q 5:205–227

Stanson AM, Kazmier FJ, Hollier LH et al. (1986) Penetrating atherosclerotic ulcers of the thoracic aorta: natural history and clinicopathologic correlations. Ann Vasc Surg 1:15–23

Tello R, Costello P, Ecker C, Hartnell G (1993) Spiral CT evaluation of coronary artery bypass graft patency. J Comput Assist Tomogr 17:253–259

Thorsen MK, San Dretto MA, Lawson TL, Foley WD, Smith DF, Berland LL (1983) Dissecting aortic aneurysms: accuracy of computed tomographic diagnosis. Radiology 148:773–777

Thorsen MK, Lawson TL, Foley WD (1985) CT of aortic dissections. Crit Rev Diagn Imaging 26:291–324

Tisnado J, Cho S, Beachley MC, Vines FS (1980) Ulcerlike projections: a precursor angiographic sign to thoracic aortic dissection. Am J Roentgenol 135:719–722

Torres WE, Maurer DE, Steinberg HV et al. (1988) CT of aortic aneurysms: the distinction between mural and thrombus calcification. AJR 150:1317–1319

Vasile N, Mathieu D, Keita K, Lellouche D, Bloch G, Cachera JP (1986) Computed tomography of thoracic aortic dissection: accuracy and pitfalls. J Comput Assist Tomogr 10:211–215

Walker PJ, Dake MD, Mitchell RS, Miller DC (1993) The use of endovascular techniques for the treatment of complications of aortic dissection. J Vasc Surg 18:1042–1051

Welch TJ, Stanson AW, Sheedy PF, Johnson CM, McKusick MA (1990) Radiologic evaluation of penetrating atherosclerotic ulcer. Radiographics 10:675–685

Wheat MW Jr (1987) Acute dissection of the aorta. Cardiovasc Clin 17:241–262

Wheat MW Jr, Palmer RF, Bartley TD, Steelman RC (1965) Treatment of dissecting aneurysms of the aorta without surgery. J Thorac Cardiovasc Surg 50:364–373

White RD, Lipton MJ, Higgins CB et al. (1986) Noninvasive evaluation of suspected thoracic aortic disease by contrast-enhanced computed tomography. Am J Cardiol 57:282–290

Williams DM, Brothers TE, Messina LM (1990) Relief of mesenteric ischemia in type III aortic dissection with percutaneous fenestration of the aortic septum. Radiology 174:450–452

Williams DM, Joshi A, Dake MD, Deeb GM, Miller C, Abrams GD (1994) Aortic cobwebs: an anatomic marker identifying the false lumen in aortic dissection – imaging and pathologic correlation. Radiology 190:167–174

Yamada T, Tada S, Harada J (1988) Aortic dissection without intimal rupture: diagnosis with MR imaging and CT. Radiology 168:347–352

Zeman RK, Silverman PM, Berman PH et al. (1994) Abdominal aortic aneurysms: evaluation with variable-collimation helical CT and overlapping reconstruction. Radiology 193: 555–560

Zeman RK, Berman PM, Silverman PM et al. (1995) Diagnosis of aortic dissection: value of helical CT with multiplanar reformation and three-dimensional rendering. AJR 164: 1375–1380

14 Spiral CT of the Chest: Diaphragm, Chest Wall, and Pleura

J.A. VERSCHAKELEN

CONTENTS

14.1 Diaphragm

14.1.1 Introduction

The diaphragm is a thin, flat musculotendinous structure that separates the thoracic cavity from the abdominal cavity and, being a respiratory muscle, has an important role in respiration.

Although diseases of the diaphragm itself are relatively infrequent, knowledge of the radiographic appearance of the diaphragm and of the peridiaphragmatic region is mandatory. It is important to differentiate between pathology originating from the diaphragm itself and pathological processes located immediately above or below the diaphragm. Since diaphragmatic disease is often benign, it is also important to be able to differentiate between abnormalities that have no clinical relevance and abnormalities that need further exploration.

Unfortunately, radiology of the diaphragm is difficult (PANICEK et al. 1988; TARVER et al. 1989), in part because many diaphragmatic and also peridiaphragmatic abnormalities are obscure clinically, but also and mainly because there is no

J.A. VERSCHAKELEN, MD, Department of Radiology, University Hospitals K.U. Leuven, Herestraat 49, 3000 Leuven, Belgium

imaging technique that can clearly and entirely visualize the diaphragm. Moreover the radiological appearance of the diaphragm is variable since it depends on the function and integrity of the diaphragmatic muscle and since it is related to the thoracic and abdominal volumes and contents and to the motion of the rib cage and abdomen.

Although we usually speak of the top of the opaque abdominal mass (usually composed of liver, spleen, stomach, and colon) as being the diaphragm on a conventional chest film, the diaphragmatic muscle as such is only visible when air is present above and below it.

Ultrasonography (PERY et al. 1984; LEWANDOWSKI and WINSBERG 1983; OYEN et al. 1984; VERSCHAKELEN et al. 1989b), computerized tomography (CT) (GALE 1986; KLEINMAN and RAPTOPOULOS 1985; SHIN and BERLAND 1985), and magnetic resonance imaging (MRI) (YAMASHITA et al. 1993) are the only imaging modalities that can visualize the diaphragm itself, although visualization is usually partial and dependent on the presence of pleural disease when using ultrasonography (VERSCHAKELEN et al. 1989b) and on the presence of subdiaphragmatic fat when using CT and MRI (GALE 1986; KLEINMAN and RAPTOPOULOS 1985). Despite the fact that CT has a better spatial resolution than MRI, the latter technique has a major advantage over CT in that it is able to image the diaphragm in imaging planes other than the axial plane. Visualization of the diaphragm in the sagittal and frontal planes is indeed often helpful in the study of diaphragmatic and especially of peridiaphragmatic disease (BRINK et al. 1994). Since the introduction of spiral CT, it has become possible to obtain high-quality multiplanar and even 3D reconstructions of the diaphragmatic area. Moreover, the ability to perform image acquisition during one breath-hold allows elimination of respiratory misregistration artifacts; this improves image quality and also makes it possible to visualize the diaphragm at different levels of respiration.

14.1.2 Acquisition and Injection Techniques

Since high detail is necessary to identify the diaphragm correctly and since spiral CT is often performed to achieve high-quality reformations, a scanning protocol should be chosen that offers the highest image quality (BRINK et al. 1994). A small collimation (2–5 mm) and a pitch of 1 are preferred. In most cases this is possible since the scanning volume is relatively small. When the scanning volume is too large, the pitch can be increased but, in order to avoid an important reduction in resolution, it should not exceed 1.5. This problem can also be solved by performing multiple spiral scans, although final interpretation of scans and reformatting can be impaired by differences in lung volume and position of the diaphragm during these scans. Thin interval reconstructions (1–3 mm) with high overlap also improve image quality.

The administration of contrast is not necessary in every patient. Contrast is given in order to better locate or identify peridiaphragmatic masses and abnormalities. The diaphragm itself does not show marked enhancement and its visualization depends more on the presence or absence of subdiaphragmatic fat. In order to achieve good opacification of atelectatic lung tissue or lung tumor adjacent to the diaphragm and good enhancement of the liver, a long scan delay (45–60 s) is preferred. The administration of oral contrast can be necessary when there is suspicion of herniated bowel or stomach.

14.1.3 Normal CT Appearance

On CT scans the costal part of the diaphragm can be visible as a soft tissue stripe between the fat below and the aerated lung above (Fig. 14.1). The diaphragm is not visible when it is tangential to the scanning plane or when there is no fat separating it from soft tissue structures such as the liver, spleen, stomach, or colon (GALE 1986; KLEINMAN and RAPTOPOULOS 1985). Spiral CT-generated multiplanar reconstructions can resolve to a certain degree the first of these problems but good visualization of the diaphragm is only achieved when enough fat separates it from adjacent tissue even when high-detail reformations are available. In some cases it is possible with CT to differentiate between the muscular part of the diaphragm and the central tendon. The muscular part presents as a double line representing the muscle layers while the central tendon presents as a single line (see Fig. 14.13). Unlike

with ultrasonography, pleural disease does not need to be present in order to differentiate between these two parts of the diaphragm (VERSCHAKELEN et al. 1989b). The diaphragm can appear nodular because of the visualization of hypertrophic muscular bundles.

In most patients the diaphragmatic crura can be easily recognized on both axial and reformatted images. In most cases they appear as smooth linear opacities originating from the central tendon and oriented downward, parallel and lateral to the aorta (Fig. 14.2). They usually appear smooth but can have a nodular appearance (CASKEY et al. 1989). These pseudo-tumors increase in number and severity with age. Defects in the crura can also be present and are more frequently seen in older patients and patients with emphysema (CASKEY et al. 1989).

14.1.4 Pathology of the Diaphragm

14.1.4.1 Diaphragmatic Hernia

Bochdalek's hernia, Morgagni's hernia, and hiatus hernia are the most frequently occurring herniations of the diaphragm.

Large Bochdalek's hernias usually become evident in the neonatal period because they cause respiratory symptoms (SNYDER and GREANY 1965). Small Bochdalek's hernias, however, only rarely produce symptoms and are often an incidental finding in adults (GALE 1985; WILBUR et al. 1994). They are usually without any clinical importance but they should be differentiated from diaphragmatic and peridiaphragmatic masses. These hernias often first present in the same way as tumors do: a single focal bulge on the diaphragmatic contour. However, such a finding is very suggestive for Bochdalek's hernia when the patient has no symptoms and when the bulge is centered approximately 4–5 cm anterior to either posterior diaphragmatic insertion. CT can make the diagnosis in cases of doubt (GALE 1985). The hernia presents as a soft tissue or fatty mass abutting the surface of the posteromedial aspect of either hemidiaphragm. This mass is in continuity with subdiaphragmatic structures through a diaphragmatic defect presenting as a discontinuity of the soft tissue line of the diaphragm. The fact that the defect is located in the posteromedial aspect of the diaphragm usually renders it visible on axial scans. In some cases, sagittal reformations yield additional information because the diaphragmatic stripe is better identified (YAMANA and OHBA 1994). Also, 3D

Fig. 14.1. Spiral CT of the diaphragm: frontal (**a**) and sagittal (**b**) reconstructions. The costal part of the diaphragm is visible as a thin line between the fat below and the lung above. However, when there is no fat separating the diaphragm from the liver, the stomach, or the heart, the diaphragm is not visible. CT protocol: collimation 5 mm, table increment 5 mm, reconstruction interval for frontal and sagittal reformation 1 mm. Breath-hold at functional residual capacity (FRC)

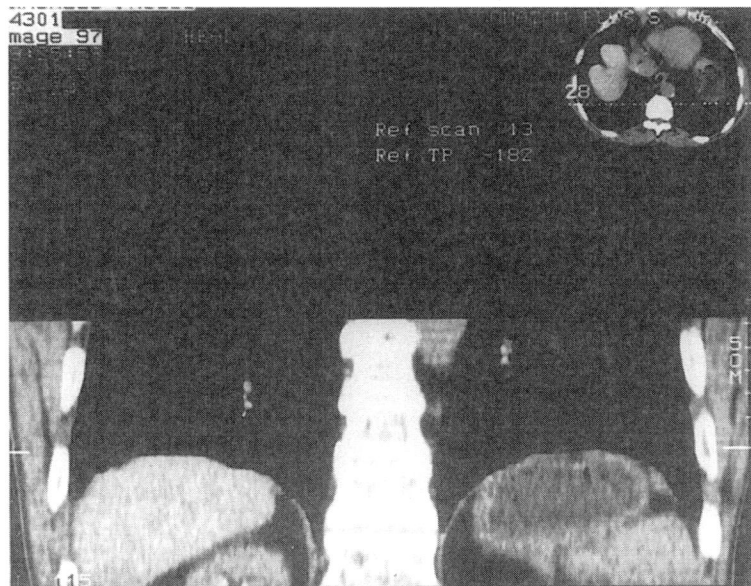

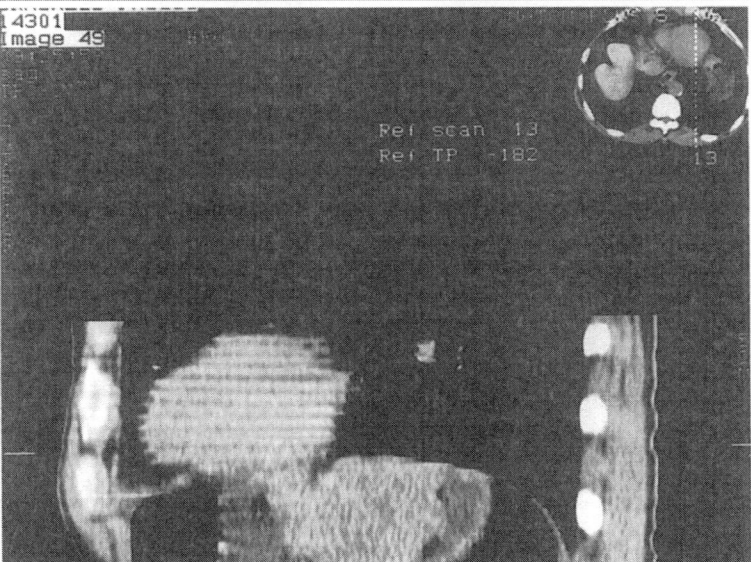

imaging can be useful for stereographic demonstration of the hernia (YAMANA and OHBA 1994).

The incidence of Morgagni's hernia detected in the neonatal period because of symptoms is low. In older children and adults, Morgagni's hernia is often an incidental finding. Although the weak area at the fibrotendinous elements between the costal and the crural part of the diaphragm is congenital, Morgagni's hernia can be acquired. Increase in abdominal pressure due to severe effort, trauma, or obesity is probably responsible (PARIS et al. 1973; THOMAS and CLITHEROW 1977; WILBUR et al. 1994).

When bowel is herniated to the chest, the diagnosis usually can be made with conventional chest film and barium studies. Herniated liver or fat can be identified with CT. Because there is very often fat above and below the diaphragm in that area, the diaphragmatic defect is frequently visible on axial scans or on sagittal and frontal reformations.

The diagnosis of hiatus hernia can be made on conventional PA chest films, but its presence is usually confirmed by a barium study. Hiatus hernias are often an incidental finding on CT. Spiral CT with multiplanar reconstructions can be helpful in some selected cases, by better demonstrating the exact position of the diaphragm (BOGAERT et al. 1995) (Fig. 14.3).

14.1.4.2 Traumatic Diaphragmatic Rupture

Blunt trauma and penetrating wounds of the chest are the most frequent causes of traumatic diaphragmatic rupture. In blunt trauma the tear is left sided in 70%–90% of all cases (DEE 1992). This is probably

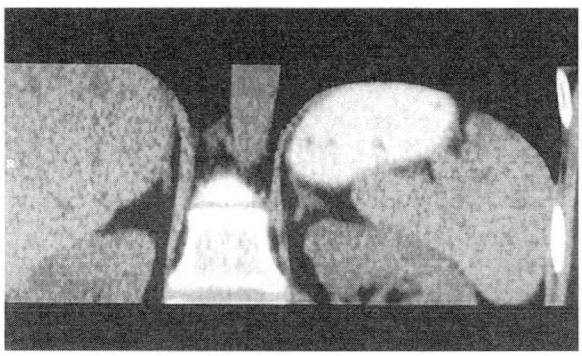

Fig. 14.2. Spiral CT of the diaphragm: frontal reconstruction. The diaphragmatic crura are visible as smooth linear opacities originating from the central tendon and oriented downward, parallel to the vertebral column. CT protocol: collimation 5 mm, table increment 5 mm, reconstruction interval for frontal and sagittal reformation 1 mm. Breath-hold at FRC

due to the protective function of the liver (VAN DAELE et al. 1987; FATAAR et al. 1979). Injuries from penetrating wounds may be found in any area of the diaphragm (COTTER and TYNDAL 1986).

Although in the majority of patients with diaphragmatic rupture, abnormalities are demonstrated on the chest radiograph at the time of the injury, diagnosis is made in only 17%–40% of the cases. Aspecific clinical symptoms and radiographic findings are responsible for the fact that the diagnosis is often not achieved until up to 3 years after the injury, when patients present with symptoms of bowel herniation (CARTER et al. 1951; HEIBERG et al. 1980).

There is disagreement in the literature about the use of CT in the diagnosis. Several case reports have demonstrated that traumatic diaphragmatic rupture can be identified by CT (HEIBERG et al. 1980; GURNEY et al. 1985; DEMOS et al. 1989; HOLLAND and QUINT 1991). However, in a series of seven patients reported by GELMAN et al. (1991), only in one patient was the correct diagnosis made by CT. On the other hand, WORTHY et al. (1995) identified diagnostic features with CT in 9 out of 11 patients. This contradiction is not surprising since, as discussed previously, it is often difficult to identify the diaphragm on CT scan, especially when it is immediately adjacent to abdominal organs. CT is generally more diagnostic when herniated abdominal organs or bowel can be demonstrated and less diagnostic when there is a small tear without herniation of abdominal content.

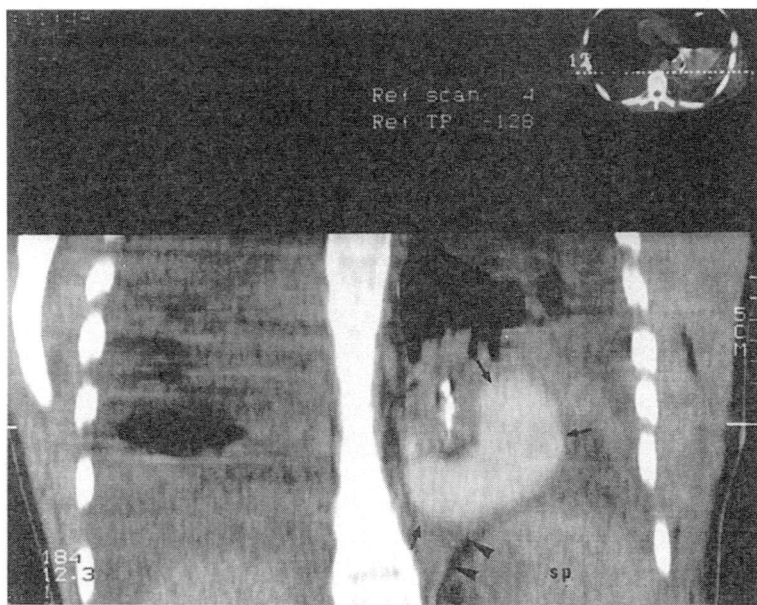

Fig. 14.3. Intrathoracic gastric herniation 1 week after fundoplication with antireflux procedure. The contrast-filled stomach (*arrows*) is clearly located above the left hemidiaphragm (*arrowheads*). Note the normal position of the spleen (*sp*). CT protocol: collimation 5 mm, table increment 8 mm, reconstruction interval for frontal reformation 1 mm. Breath-hold at FRC. Oral contrast

CT signs of diaphragmatic rupture are: discontinuity of the diaphragm, herniation of abdominal organs, stomach, or bowel, and constriction of the stomach or bowel (collar sign) (GURNEY et al. 1985; NAIDICH et al. 1991). Although not yet proven, it can be expected that spiral CT with multiplanar reformations will improve diagnostic accuracy. Also, the use of thin-section CT (2–5 mm) may help to identify small diaphragmatic defects.

14.1.4.3 Tumors of the Diaphragm

Tumors of the diaphragm are rare lesions which are often difficult to assess and classify both clinically and roentgenographically (ANDERSON and FORREST 1973). Malignant tumors are more frequent than benign tumors and can be primary or secondary (TARVER et al. 1989; ANDERSON and FORREST 1973). Benign tumors (lipomas, fibromas, angiofibromas, neurofibromas, and neurolemmomas) (Fig. 14.4) are mostly asymptomatic and often found at post-mortem examination (ANDERSON and FORREST 1973; SCHWARTZ and WECHSLER 1989). Cysts of the diaphragm can be acquired or congenital. Acquired cysts include simple cysts, fibrous lined cysts, and post-traumatic cysts. Congenital cysts include teratoid cysts, mesothelial lined cysts, and those of pulmonary origin which histologically resemble bronchogenic cysts or sequestrations. Hydatid disease and tuberculosis rarely may cause inflammatory tumors of the diaphragm (ANDERSON and FORREST 1973; SCHWARTZ and WECHSLER 1989) (Fig. 14.4). The majority of the primary malignant tumors are of fibrous origin (fibrosarcoma, fibromyosarcoma, fibro-angio-endothelioma) or are undifferentiated sarcomas (ANDERSON and FORREST 1973; SCHWARTZ and WECHSLER 1989). In contrast with benign tumors, malignant tumors usually induce symptoms (pleuritic chest pain, pain referred to the epigastrium) and are often associated with pleural effusion. Secondary malignant tumors are mostly due to direct invasion from adjacent lesions originating from the lung, the stomach, the pancreas, the adrenals, the colon, or the liver (ANDERSON and FORREST 1973; SCHWARTZ and WECHSLER 1989). Metastatic implants are rare and only found in cases of widely disseminated disease. Thin-section spiral CT performed during one breath-hold and multiplanar reformations generated from spiral CT data allow a better delineation of the diaphragm and of the relationship between the mass and the diaphragmatic muscle. Even when the diaphragmatic muscle

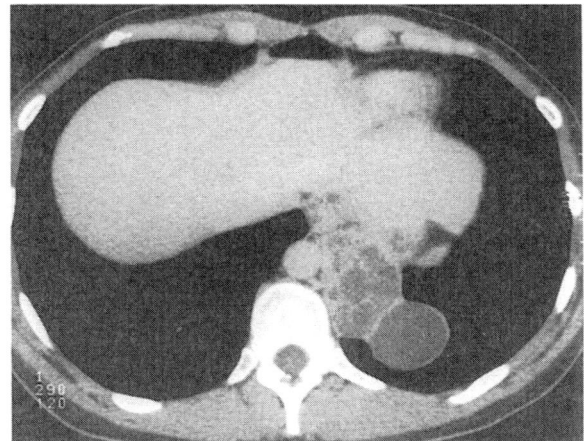

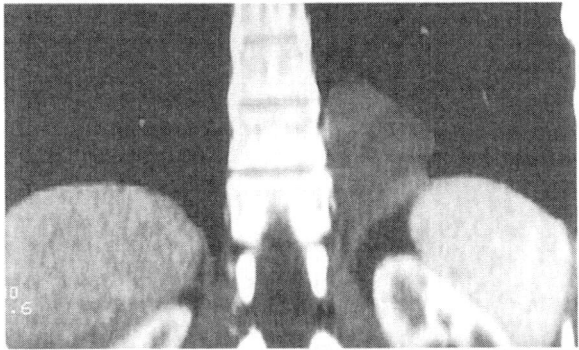

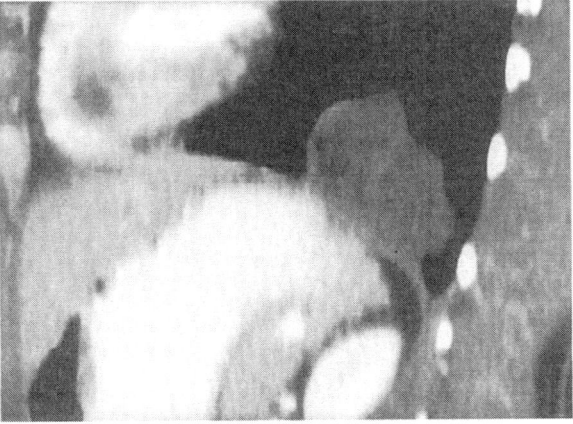

Fig. 14.4a–c. Loculated congenital cystic malformation (probably intradiaphragmatic sequestration) originating from the diaphragm. Axial scans (a) and especially the frontal (b) and sagittal reformations (c) very nicely show the close relationship between the mass and the diaphragm. Reformatted images show that the mass originates from the diaphragm. CT protocol: collimation 5 mm, table increment 5 mm, reconstruction interval for frontal and sagittal reformations 1 mm. Breath-hold at FRC. Intravenous contrast

as such is not visible (because of the absence of fat between the diaphragm and the subdiaphragmatic organ), contact between a mass and the diaphragm or diaphragmatic invasion by a tumor can often be diagnosed by looking at the expected contour of the diaphragm (Figs. 14.5–14.7).

14.1.4.4 Eventration

Eventration of the diaphragm is defined as an abnormally high or elevated position of one leaf or part of

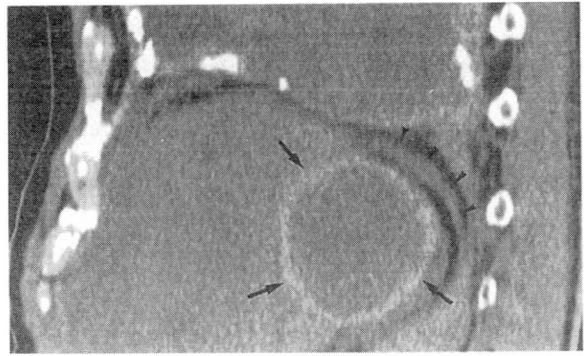

Fig. 14.5. Echinococcus cyst in the liver (*arrows*) of a patient who previously underwent pneumonectomy. Sagittal reconstruction shows that the cyst is located below the diaphragm. Note that the costal part of the diaphragm is visible because of the presence of fat immediately above and below (*arrowheads*). CT protocol: collimation 3 mm, table increment 3 mm, reconstruction interval for frontal and sagittal reformations 1 mm. Breath-hold at FRC. No contrast

one leaf of the intact diaphragm as a result of paralysis, aplasia, or atrophy (of varying degrees) of muscle fibers (BISGARD 1947). In the area of eventration the normal diaphragmatic muscle fibers are replaced by a thin layer of connective tissue and a few scattered muscle fibers. Eventration can be congenital, resulting from congenital failure of proper muscularization of a part or of the entire diaphragmatic leaf (TARVER et al. 1989; LINDSTROM and ALLEN 1966). Eventration can also be acquired and is then the result of long-lasting paralysis causing atrophy and scarring of the diaphragmatic muscle (McNAMARA et al. 1968; BOVORNKITTI et al. 1960; MICHELSON 1961). Total eventration of one hemidiaphragm is more often seen on the left side. Partial eventrations are usually right sided with a predilection for the anteromedian portion. However, diaphragmatic eventration may occur almost anywhere along the diaphragmatic surface and is commonly multifocal. Because, even in total eventration, there is usually some normal diaphragmatic muscle surrounding the layer of connective tissue, eventration is accentuated on CT scans performed at suspended deep inspiration when compared with CT scans performed at suspended deep expiration.

Since eventration is usually asymptomatic, the role of CT and spiral CT is usually limited to the differentiation of this entity from a tumoral mass in

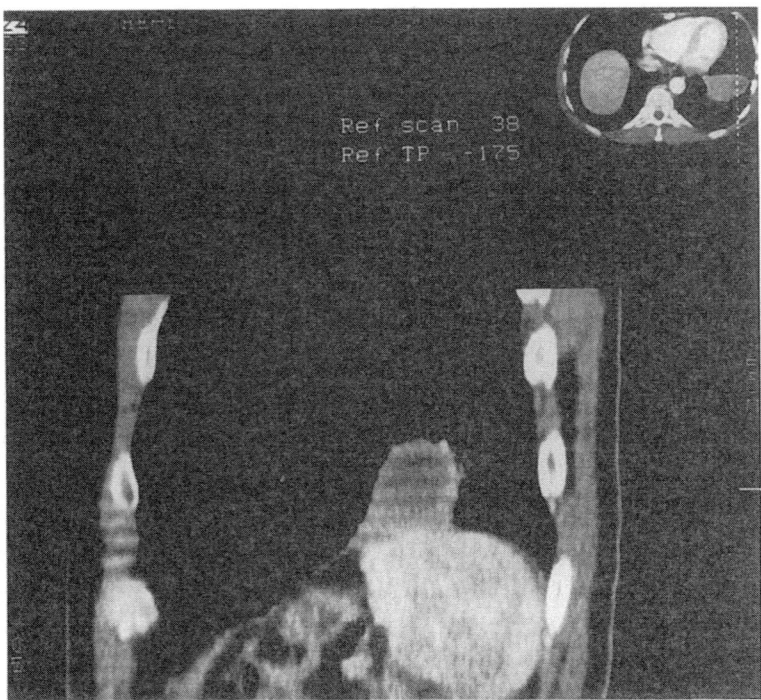

Fig. 14.6. Malignant lung tumor (squamous cell epithelioma) in contact with the diaphragm. In this case it is very difficult to decide whether the tumor is invading the diaphragmatic muscle or whether there is only contact between the mass and the diaphragm. CT protocol: collimation 5 mm, table increment 5 mm, reconstruction interval for sagittal reformations 1 mm. Breath-hold at FRC. Intravenous contrast

Fig. 14.7. Malignant lung tumor (squamous cell epithelioma) growing through the diaphragm and invading the liver. Although invasion was suggested on the axial scans, tumor extension was better appreciated on reformatted images. CT protocol: collimation 8 mm, table increment 8 mm, reconstruction interval for sagittal reformation 1 mm. Breath-hold at FRC. Intravenous contrast

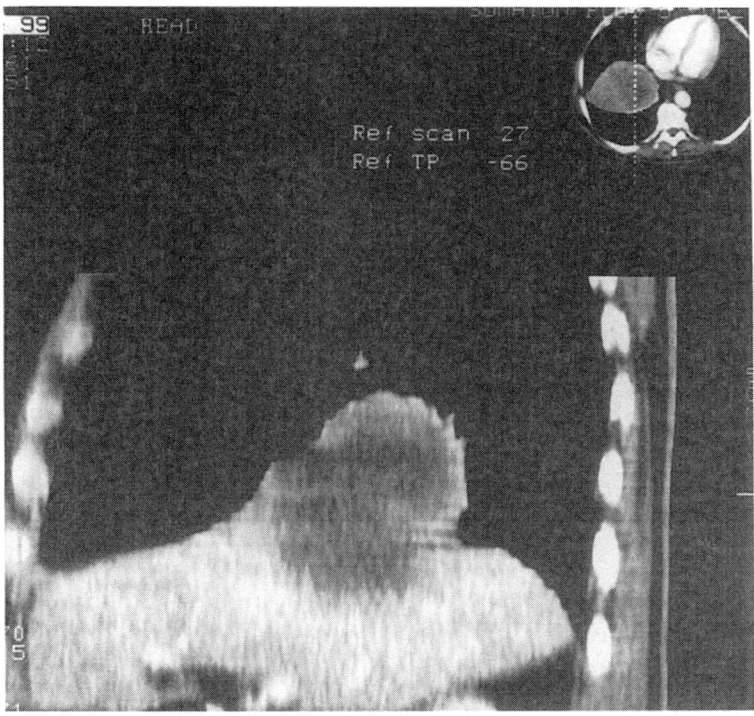

a patient presenting with a focal bulge on the diaphragmatic contour (Fig. 14.8). In contrast to a herniation, where there is a defect in the diaphragm and where abdominal fat or an abdominal organ protrudes into the chest, in eventration the diaphragm, although thin and only consisting of a thin layer of connective tissue, is not interrupted. Differential diagnosis is often possible because of typical localization of both congenital hernias and eventrations, but can be more difficult when herniation is the result of a postraumatic diaphragmatic tear. Differential diagnosis with focal, possibly reversible paralysis is, however, usually impossible.

14.1.4.5 Paralysis of the Diaphragm

The role of CT in the diagnosis of diaphragmatic paralysis is limited. The radiological evaluation of paralysis requires chest radiographs and adequate fluoroscopic tests or, when the latter are not possible, ultrasonography, together with a good knowledge of the clinical history of the patient. CT can be helpful in the diagnosis of intrathoracic causes of phrenic nerve injury (UJITA et al. 1993). CT and especially spiral CT can also be valuable in the differential diagnosis of a paralysed (hemi)diaphragm and

peridiaphragmatic pathology (subpulmonary pleural effusion, ascites, lung atelectasis, lung or liver mass adjacent to the diaphragm). As mentioned previously, the differential diagnosis with eventration can be difficult and is often impossible.

14.1.5 Conclusions

Because of its capability to scan the diaphragm and the peridiaphragmatic region during one breath-hold and especially because of the ability to perform high-detail multiplanar reformations, spiral CT has become very important in the study of the diaphragm and adjacent structures. Especially sagittal and coronal reformations are very important in localizing abnormalities to the diaphragm itself, the intra-abdominal viscera, the cardiophrenic space, the pleura, the lung, or the pericardium.

14.2 Chest Wall and Pleura

14.2.1 Introduction

The use of CT in the study of diseases of the chest wall is usually limited to the evaluation of tumor

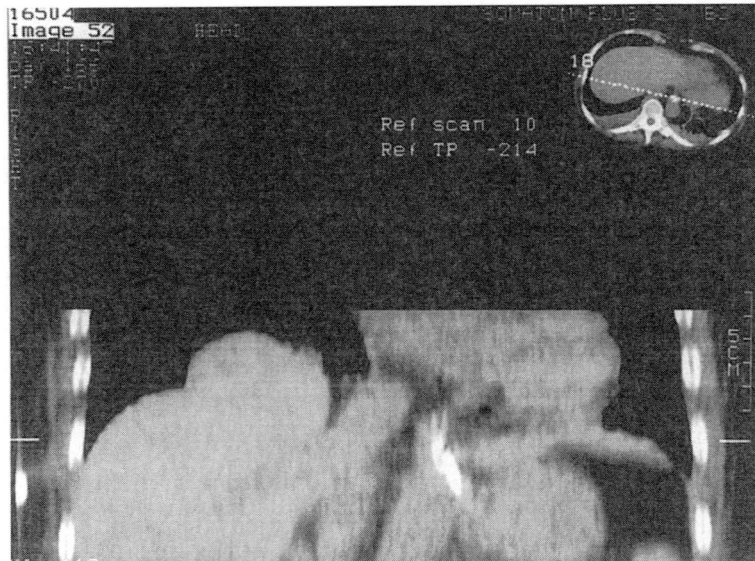

a

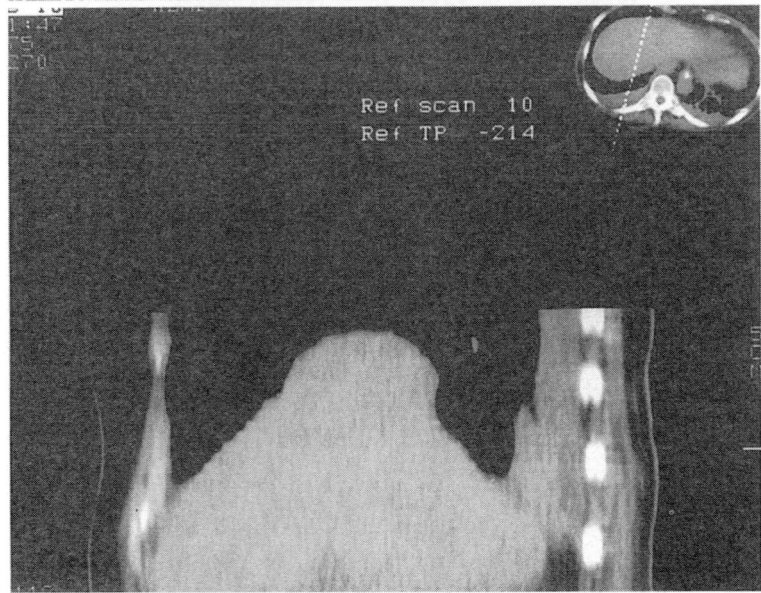

b

Fig. 14.8a,b. Focal eventration. Frontal (a) and sagittal (b) reformations. Focal bulge on the contour of the right hemidiaphragm. Because the diaphragm itself is not visible, differential diagnosis with focal diaphragmatic paralysis and herniation is difficult. However, diagnosis of eventration is based on the location, on the smooth contour, and on the fact that normal abdominal tissue (liver) is seen immediately below the elevated part of the diaphragm. CT protocol: collimation 5 mm, table increment 5 mm, reconstruction interval for frontal and sagittal reformations 1 mm. Suspended deep inspiration. No contrast

extension: detection of pleural and chest wall invasion by peripheral bronchogenic carcinoma or determination of tumor extension in patients with a tumor of the breast or with mesothelioma. However, it is well known that two-dimensional CT scans generally have a low sensitivity and specificity when invasion of the parietal pleura and chest wall by a lung tumor is examined (PEARLBERG et al. 1987; PENNES et al. 1985; WEBB et al. 1991; EPSTEIN et al. 1986; GRENIER et al. 1989). Although experience is limited, studies have shown that 2D or 3D reformations obtained with spiral CT can provide valuable additional information (KURIYAMA et al. 1994a). Moreover, the

ability of spiral CT to visualize a tumor during its phase of maximal contrast enhancement is presently used to study tumors of the breast (TEIFKE et al. 1994).

14.2.2 Acquisition and Injection Techniques

The value of spiral CT is related not only to the short examination time, which reduces motion artifacts, but also to the ability to perform reformations. For these reasons, but also because high detail is necessary, scans should be performed with a thin collimation (2–5 mm) and a pitch not exceeding 1 and be reconstructed with high overlap. Of course, these parameters have to be adapted to the scan volume and to the ability of the patient to stop breathing.

When intravenous contrast is given, an appropriate delay between the start of the injection and the scan should be chosen in order to allow enhancement of the tumor and also, when present, of the thickened pleura and atelectatic lung tissue.

14.2.3 Pathology of the Chest Wall and Pleura

14.2.3.1 Congenital and Acquired Deformations

In evaluating congenital disease of the chest wall, one needs to use CT only occasionally (TOOMBS et al. 1981; GOULIAMOS et al. 1980). However, conditions such as congenital absence of a pectoral muscle and deformities of the sternum, the ribs, and the vertebrae sometimes can be assessed to advantage on transaxial images. In addition, when surgical correction is considered, 3D reconstruction of the bony chest can in some cases help the surgeon to better understand the deformation of the chest and to choose the best surgical procedure to correct it (HALLER et al. 1989) (Fig. 14.9).

Computerized tomography can also be used to follow-up patients who have undergone therapeutic or reconstructive surgery of the chest wall. It has been shown that axial CT scans are accurate in depicting chest wall deformity after tissue expansion for breast reconstruction in women who have had mastectomy for breast cancer (SINOW et al. 1991). It can be expected that spiral CT-generated 3D surface images of these patients will yield additional information in some selected cases (HURWITZ et al. 1994).

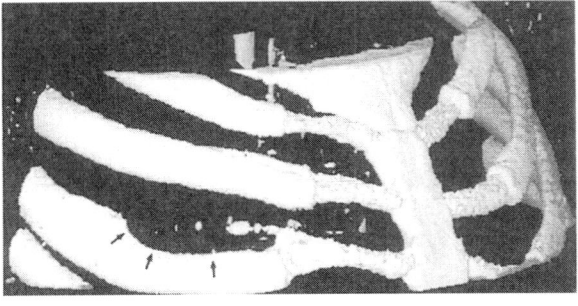

Fig. 14.9. Localized deformation of the rib cage. Three-dimensional reformatted image very nicely shows the localized deformation of the anterior part of the rib (*arrows*), which was not visible on transverse CT sections. (Courtesy of M. Rémy-Jardin, Lille, France)

CT also offers characteristic images in patients with pleural empyema treated with an Eloesser window thoracostomy (SHAPIRO et al. 1988).

14.2.3.2 Trauma

Most osseous injuries are easily evaluated on plain films but sometimes CT imaging adds significant information (MIRVIS and TEMPLETON 1992; STARK and JARAMILLO 1986; DEE 1992). Although the presence of life-support devices and orthopedic devices can make it difficult to position a traumatized patient and although cooperation of the patient is often limited, spiral CT has the advantage over conventional CT that scanning time can be reduced. In this way it can help to detect and locate multiple fragments of bones, hematomas in soft tissues, foreign bodies, subluxations, and damage to the spinal canal.

14.2.3.3 Invasion of the Chest Wall by Tumor

Assessment of pleural and chest wall invasion is an important component of lung cancer staging. However, the accuracy of axial CT in those cases where the tumor is adjacent to the chest wall without any bone destruction is low (PEARLBERG et al. 1987; PENNES et al. 1985; WEBB et al. 1991; EPSTEIN et al. 1986; GRENIER et al. 1989). A first reason for this is the axial format precluding evaluation of lesions in contact with the apex of the chest and with the diaphragm. A second reason is the fact that features such as a large contact (more than 3 cm) between the mass and the pleura, an obtuse angle between the tumor and the chest wall, an associated pleural thickening, and the presence of pleural tags, usually considered as signs of chest wall invasion, also occur with benign lesions. Three-dimensional techniques have been used successfully to study lung tumors, peripheral pulmonary vessels, and pleural surface (Fig. 14.10) (KURIYAMA et al. 1994a,b). In a study where they reviewed 2D and 3D images obtained with spiral CT in 42 patients with peripheral bronchogenic carcinoma, KURIYAMA and co-workers (1994b) found that 3D reconstruction imaging was superior to 2D CT in the assessment of pleural invasion. Three-dimensional reconstructions allowed them to correctly predict visceral pleural involvement in 92% of patients compared to only 17% of patients with the use of 2D CT imaging. According to their results it was possible in most but not in all patients to differentiate between simple pleural tags

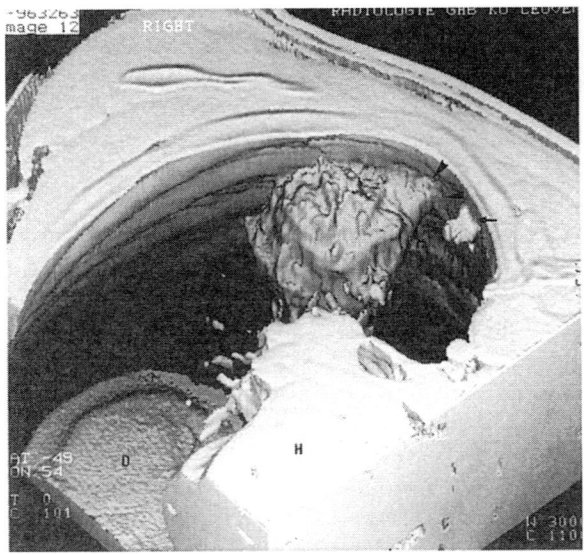

Fig. 14.10. Three-dimensional reconstruction of a malignant lung tumor in contact with the chest wall. Pleural puckering (*arrowheads*) suggested visceral pleural enhancement. This was confirmed at surgery. Note a second tumor localization immediately adjacent to the mass (*arrows*). *D*, diaphragm; *H*, heart. CT protocol: collimation 3 mm, table increment 3 mm, 3D reconstruction

(i.e., fibrotic bands extending from the lesion to the visceral pleura) and visceral pleural invasion presenting as pleural puckering associated with a locally thickened pleura. Another way of evaluating parietal pleural invasion of lung masses was proposed by SHIRAKAWA and co-workers (1994). These investigators performed spiral CT scans of the chest during deep inspiration and expiration in patients with peripheral lung tumors in contact with the chest wall. They found the presence of respiratory phase shift to be a reliable indicator of lack of parietal pleural invasion for tumors in middle and lower lung lobes.

In cases where tumor invasion in the chest wall or the diaphragm is obvious, 2D sagittal or frontal reformatted images can be helpful in ascertaining the extent of the mass (Fig. 14.11). It has not yet been determined whether these reformatted images provide more information than sagittal or frontal magnetic resonance images. MRI is at present considered the imaging modality of choice for studying superior sulcus tumors and their extension to the chest wall (TAKASUGI et al. 1989). In our experience, due to the lack of motion artifacts, spiral CT is a little more sensitive in showing invasion in the bony cortex of the ribs. In a study where tumor extension into the chest wall was examined with both spiral CT and

MIR, DESCHILDRE and co-workers (1994) found that the two techniques showed comparable sensitivity but that spiral CT had a higher specificity. Three-dimensional image reconstruction methods can also be used in selected cases to clarify a complex relationship between a tumor invading the chest wall and vascular structures of the thoracic inlet (MEIER et al. 1993; TELLO et al. 1993; RUBIN et al. 1995) (Fig. 14.11d).

Both conventional and spiral CT can also be helpful in the study of neoplasms of the bones and of the soft tissues of the chest wall. The most frequently occurring benign tumor-like condition of the bones of the chest wall is fibrous dysplasia. Giant cell tumor, hemangioma, enchondroma, osteochondroma, hemangioma, and aneurysmal cyst are less frequent (DE GAUTARD et al. 1981). Lipomas, together with hemangiomas, fibrous tumors, and neurogenic tumors, are the most frequently occurring benign soft tissue tumors. CT can yield additional important information to that provided by the conventional chest film; it is especially useful in showing the exact tumor extent but also, in some selected cases, in establishing the definitive diagnosis. In particular, CT can establish the diagnosis of lipomas by showing their low density (MENDEZ et al. 1979), and that of hemangiomas when contrast enhancement suggests a vascular tumor.

Metastases to bones or soft tissues are the most common malignant tumors involving the chest wall. Primary malignant chest wall tumors are: chondrosarcoma, multiple myeloma, fibrosarcoma, osteosarcoma, and Ewing's sarcoma. Conventional CT and spiral CT-generated reformations can help to show the bony destruction and the presence and amount of soft tissue infiltration and are indicated especially when percutaneous biopsy or surgery is considered (SCHAEFER and BURTON 1989).

14.2.3.4 Pleural Abnormalities

The combination of axial scans and 2D and 3D reformations can be helpful in some selected cases to establish the extent of pleural disease and to estimate the total surface that is involved (MEIER et al. 1993) (Fig. 14.12). Spiral CT can also be helpful in cases where it is difficult to differentiate pleural disease from lung or diaphragmatic abnormalities (Fig. 14.13). Sagittal reformations can better show the curvature of bronchovascular structures towards a pleural-based area of lung atelectasis (comet tail sign): an additional diagnostic feature of rounded

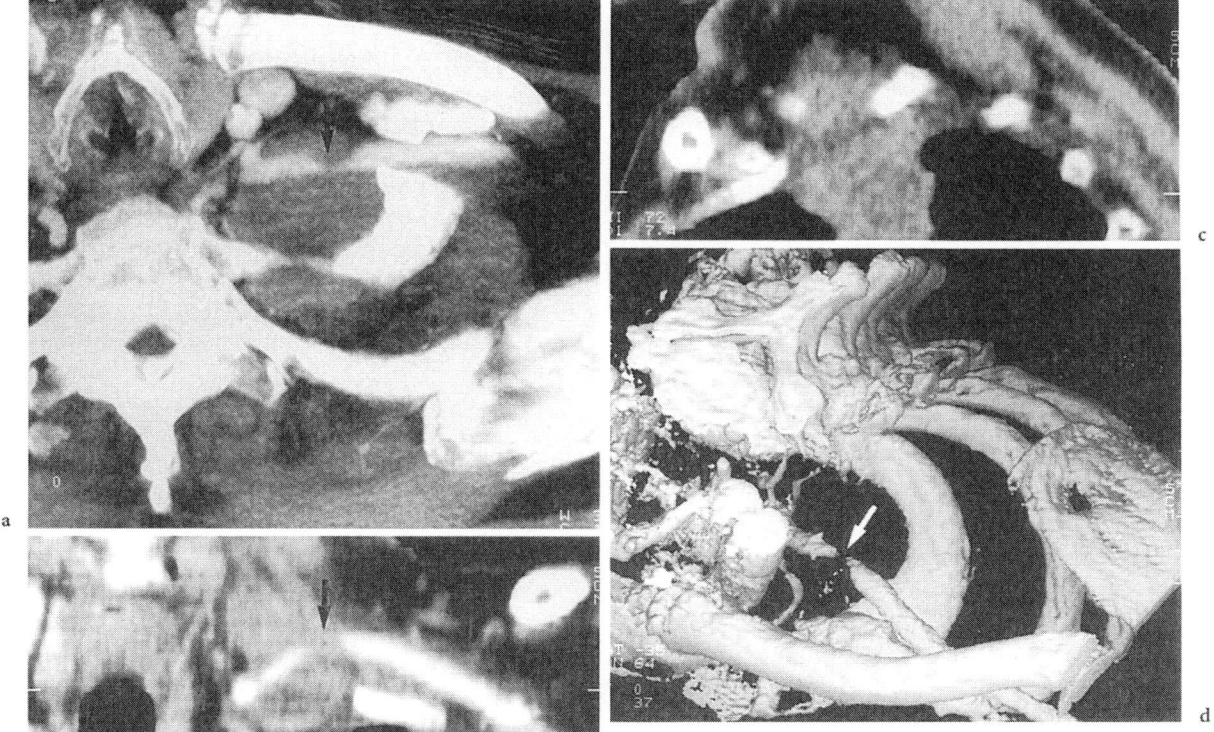

Fig. 14.11a–d. Superior sulcus tumor invading the chest wall. Maximal intensity projection (MIP) from transverse scans (a) and coronal oblique (b) and sagittal (c) reformations show the tumor extending into the apical soft tissues and surrounding the left subclavian artery, which is narrowed (*arrows*). This narrowing is also demonstrated on a 3D reformation of the left apex (d; *arrow*). CT protocol: collimation 3 mm, table increment 4 mm, reconstruction interval for frontal and sagittal reformations 1 mm. MIP and 3D reconstruction. Breath-hold at FRC. Intravenous contrast. (Courtesy of M. Rémy-Jardin, Lille, France)

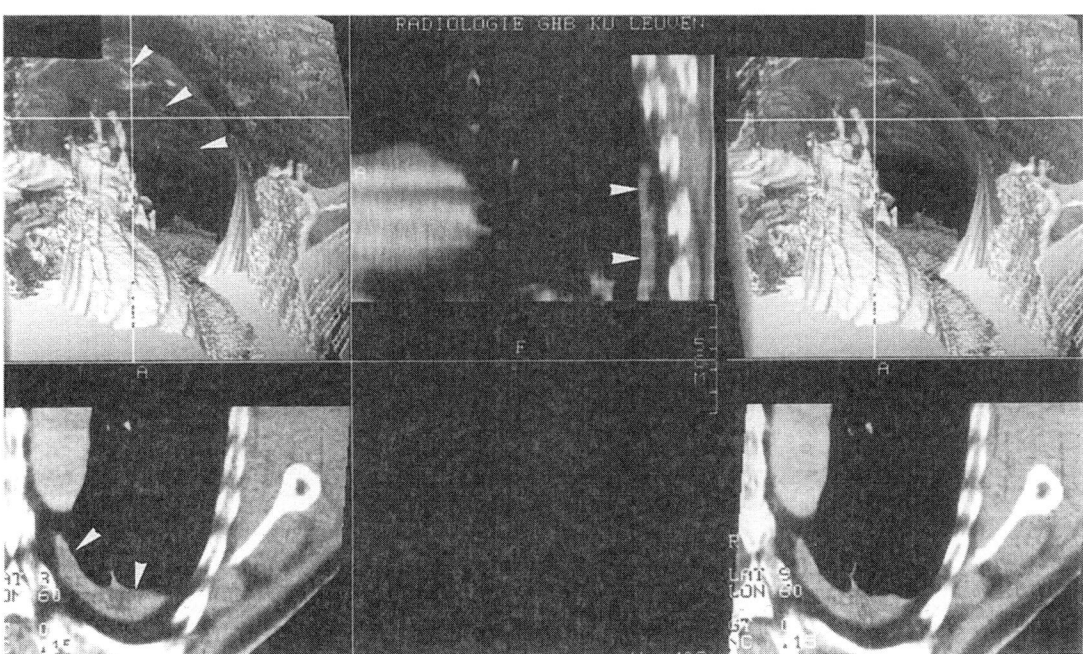

Fig. 14.12. Extensive pleural thickening related to asbestos exposure (*arrowheads*). Simultaneous evaluation of 2D and 3D reformations allows a better study of the extension of pleural disease. CT protocol (thoracic survey): collimation 8 mm, table increment 12 mm, reconstruction interval for reformations 1 mm. Breath-hold at FRC

atelectasis that previously could be shown only by sagittal conventional tomograms or MRI (VERSCHAKELEN et al. 1989a) (Fig. 14.14; see also Chap. 11).

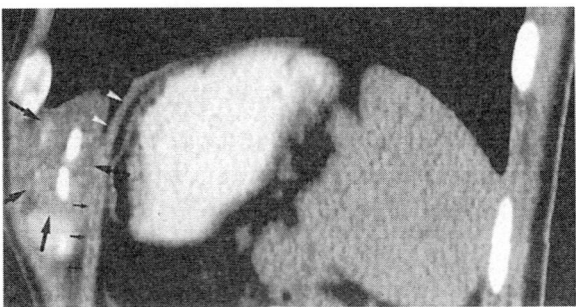

Fig. 14.13. Benign pleural mesothelioma (*large arrows*). Spiral CT allowed the diagnosis of a mass not originating from the diaphragm but located in the pleural space. Note the difference between the muscular part of the diaphragm, presenting as a double line (*small arrows*), and the central tendon presenting as a single line (*arrowheads*). CT protocol: collimation 3 mm, table increment 3 mm, reconstruction interval for sagittal reformation 1 mm. Breath-hold at FRC. Oral contrast

14.2.3.5 Tumors of the Breast

Despite a few reports in the late 1970s and early 1980s (CHANG et al. 1978, 1982; GISVOLD et al. 1979) of increased contrast concentration and demonstration of occult cancers by CT, this method has not replaced mammography, which has superior spatial resolution. Nevertheless, CT scan is often performed when tumor infiltration in the chest wall is suspected or to look for axillary, parasternal, and mediastinal adenopathy.

The development of spiral CT has renewed interest in use of this technique not only for staging but also for detection of breast carcinoma (TEIFKE et al. 1994; SARDANELLI et al. 1995). Spiral CT has the advantage that it can examine the breasts and axillary areas in a short time with high detail during optimal enhancement of the tumor. TEIFKE and co-workers (1994) found spiral CT very helpful for elucidating problems in the diagnosis of breast lesions. They appreciated especially the speed of the method, the comfort for the patient, the absence of movement artifacts, the easy standardization, and the wide applicability of the method, making it a good alterna-

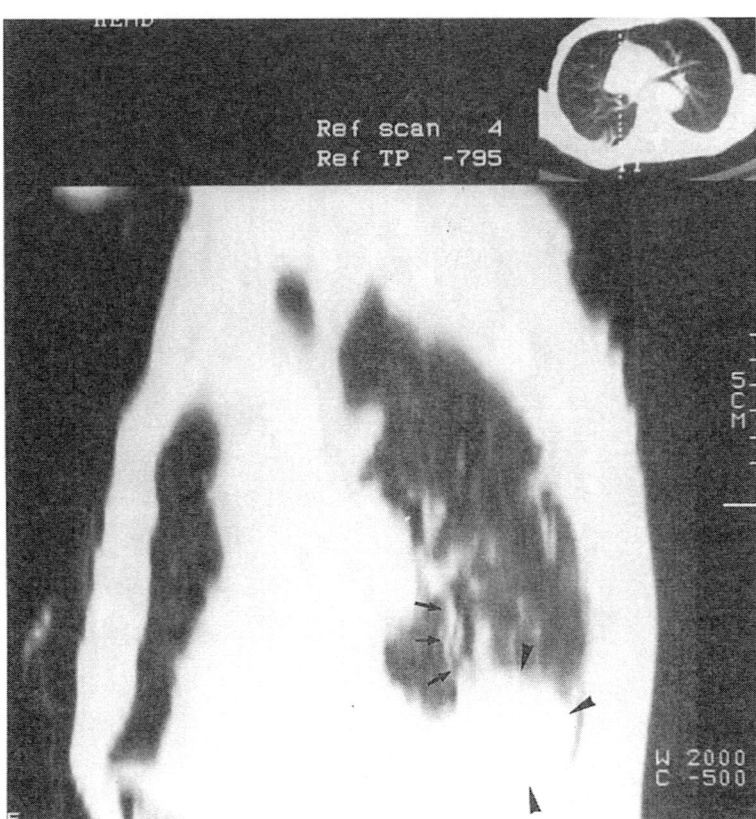

Fig. 14.14. Rounded atelectasis of the lung (*arrowheads*). Sagittal reformation showing curvation of bronchovascular bundles towards the mass (*arrows*). CT protocol (thoracic survey): collimation 8 mm, table increment 12 mm, reconstruction interval for sagittal reformation 1 mm. Breath-hold at FRC. Intravenous contrast

tive to MRI when the latter technique is not available. These authors compared spiral scans performed before and 50 s after injection of contrast. A mass showing an increase in density of less than 30 Hounsfield units (HU) proved very likely to be a benign lesion (fibroadenoma), while an increase in density of more than 60 HU was very suggestive of a malignant tumor. For lesions with an enhancement between 30 and 60 HU, the differential diagnosis between benign and malignant disease was difficult; in such cases the diagnosis should be based on other criteria such as delineation of the tumor. SARDANELLI and co-workers (1995) used a different technique based on protocols used in MRI of the breast. These authors studied the enhancement of the tumor after 1, 3, and 8 min with three consecutive spiral CT scans and cal-

culated the enhancement percentage. They found that the study of contrast uptake after 3 and 8 min yielded important additional information in the differential diagnosis between certain malignant tumors and breast dysplasia (Figs. 14.15, 14.16).

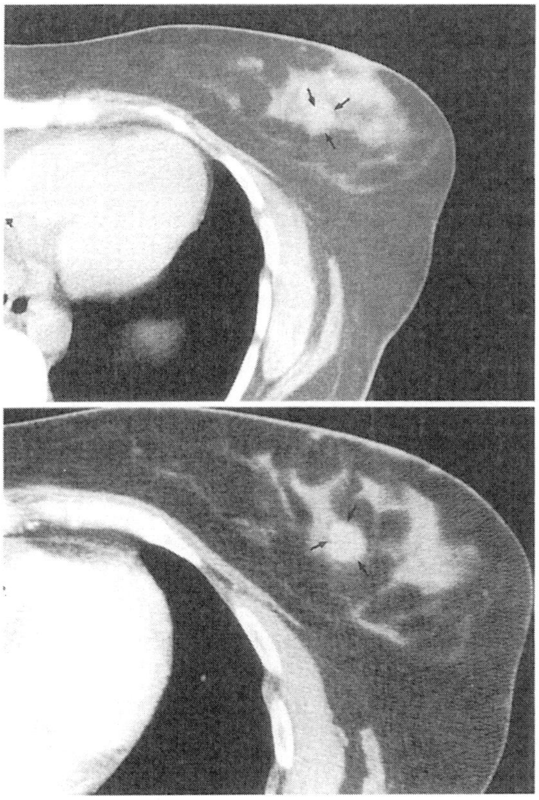

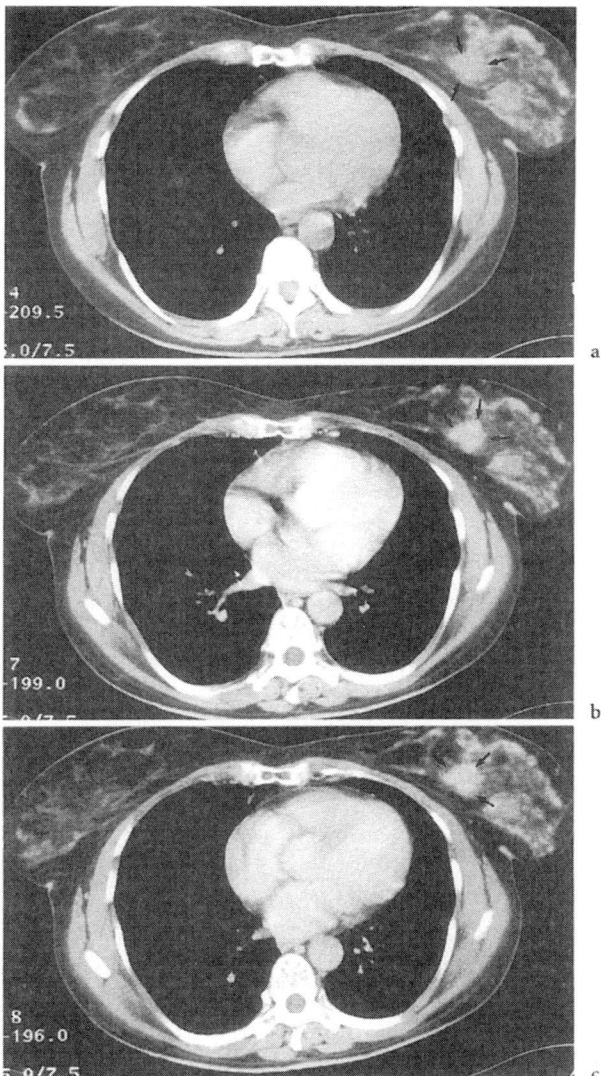

Fig. 14.15a,b. Benign fibroadenoma of the breast. Before administration of contrast (a) a retroareolar opacity with a density of 20 HU was seen (*arrows*). One minute after the start of injection of contrast (b) the lesion had reached a density of 73 HU (*arrows*). Density was 71 HU after 3 min (not shown) and showed slow enhancement thereafter, reaching a density of 102 HU after 8 min. CT protocol: collimation 5 mm, table increment 5 mm, reconstruction interval 3 mm. Breath-hold at FRC. Intravenous contrast. (Courtesy of C. Van Ongeval, Leuven, Belgium)

Fig. 14.16a–c. Poorly differentiated invasive adenocarcinoma of the breast. Because of dense breast tissue the mass was hardly visible on precontrast CT images (density = 27 HU) (a; *arrows*). After administration of intravenous contrast the mass showed rapid enhancement and density was 80 HU 1 min (b) after start of injection (*arrow*). Density then slowly decreased (*arrows*) and reached a value of 70 HU 3 min after start of injection (c). After 8 min density was still about 70 HU (not shown). CT protocol: collimation 5 mm, table increment 5 mm, reconstruction interval 3 mm. Breath-hold at FRC. Intravenous contrast. (Courtesy of C. Van Ongeval, Leuven, Belgium)

14.2.4 Conclusions

The advantage of spiral CT over conventional CT in the study of the chest wall and pleura is related to its ability to yield high-detail images in a very short time. In this way motion artifacts and respiratory misregistration, which often occur with conventional CT of these areas, can be avoided. The value of 2D and 3D reformations has not yet been fully determined.

References

Anderson LS, Forrest JV (1973) Tumors of the diaphragm. Am J Roentgenol 119:259–265

Bisgard JD (1947) Congenital eventration of the diaphragm. J Thorac Surg 16:484–488

Bogaert J, Weemaes K, Verschakelen JA et al. (1995) Spiral CT findings in a postoperative intrathoracic gastric herniation: a case report. Eur Radiol 5:192–195

Bovornkitti S, Kangsadal P, Sandvichien S, Chatikavanij K (1960) Neurogenic muscular aplasia (eventration) of the diaphragm. Am Rev Respir Dis 82:876–880

Brink JA, Heiken JP, Semenkovich J, Teefey SA, McClennan BL, Sagel SS (1994) Abnormalities of the diaphragm and adjacent structures: findings on multiplanar spiral CT scans. Am J Roentgenol 163:307–310

Carter B, Giuseffi J, Felson B (1951) Traumatic diaphragmatic hernia. Am J Roentgenol 65:56–71

Caskey CI, Zerhouni EA, Fishman EK, Rahmouni AD (1989) Aging of the diaphragm: a CT study. Radiology 171:385–389

Chang CHJ, Sibala JL, Fritz SL, Gallagher JH, Dwyer SJ III, Templeton AW (1978) Computed tomographic evaluation of the breast. Am J Roentgenol 131:459–464

Chang CHJ, Nesbit DE, Fisher DR et al. (1982) Computed tomographic mammography using a conventional body scanner. Am J Roentgenol 138:553–558

Cotter CP, Tyndal EC (1986) Traumatic diaphragmatic injuries. Arch Fr Pediatr 33:197–203

Dee PM (1992) The radiology of chest trauma. Radiol Clin North Am 30:291–306

de Gautard R, Dussault RG, Chahlaoui J, Duranceau A, Sylvestre J (1981) Contribution of CT in thoracic bony lesions. J Assoc Can Radiol 31:39–41

Demos TC, Solomon C, Posniak HV, Flisak MJ (1989) Computed tomography in traumatic defects of the diaphragm. Clin Imaging 13:62–67

Deschildre F, Petyt L, Rémy-Jardin M, Rémy J, Wannebroucq J (1994) Evaluation de la TDM par balayage spirale volumique (BSV) vs IRM dans le bilan d'extension pariétal des masses thoraciques. Rev Im Med 6(S):188

Epstein DM, Stephenson LW, Gefter WB, van der Voorde F, Aronchik JM, Miller WT (1986) Value of CT in the preoperative assessment of lung cancer: a survey of thoracic surgeons. Radiology 161:423–427

Fataar S, Rad FF, Schulman A (1979) Diagnosis of diaphragmatic tears. Br J Radiol 52:375–381

Gale ME (1985) Bochdalek hernia: prevalence and CT characteristics. Radiology 156:449–452

Gale ME (1986) Anterior diaphragm: variations in the CT appearance. Radiology 161:635–639

Gelman R, Mirvis SE, Gens D (1991) Diaphragmatic rupture due to blunt trauma: sensitivity of plain chest radiographs. Am J Roentgenol 156:51–57

Gisvold JJ, Reese DF, Karsell PR (1979) Computed tomographic mammography (CTM). Am J Roentgenol 133:1143–1149

Gouliamos AD, Carter BL, Enami B (1980) Computed tomography of the chest wall. Radiology 134:433–436

Grenier P, Dubray B, Carette MF, Frija G, Musset D, Chastang C (1989) Preoperative thoracic staging of lung cancer: CT and MR evaluation. Diagn Intervent Radiol 1:23–28

Gurney J, Harrison NL, Anderson JC (1985) Omental fat simulating pleural fluid in traumatic diaphragmatic hernia: CT characteristics. J Comput Assis Tomogr 9:1112–1114

Haller JA, Scherer LR, Turner CS, Colombani PM (1989) Evolving management of pectus excavatum based on a single institutional experience of 664 patients. Ann Surg 209:578–582

Heiberg E, Wolverson MK, Hurd RN, Jagannadharao B, Sundaram M (1980) CT recognition of traumatic rupture of the diaphragm. Am J Roentgenol 135:369–372

Holland DG, Quint LE (1991) Traumatic rupture of the diaphragm without visceral herniation: CT diagnosis. Am J Roentgenol 157:17–18

Hurwitz DJ, Stofman G, Curtin H (1994) Three-dimensional imaging of Poland's syndrome. Plast Reconstr Surg 94:719–723

Kleinman PK, Raptopoulos V (1985) The anterior diaphragmatic attachments: an anatomic and radiologic study with clinical correlates. Radiology 155:289–293

Kuriyama K, Hosomi N, Sawai Y et al. (1994a) Three-dimensional imaging of focal lung disease using spiral volumetric CT. Jpn J Clin Radiol 39:9–13

Kuriyama K, Tateishi R, Kumatani T et al. (1994b) Pleural invasion by peripheral bronchogenic carcinoma: assessment with three-dimensional helical CT. Radiology 191:365–369

Lewandowski B, Winsberg F (1983) Echographic appearance of the right hemidiaphragm. J Ultrasound Med 2:243–249

Lindstrom CH, Allen RP (1966) Bilateral congenital eventration of the diaphragm. Am J Roentgenol 97:216–218

McNamara JJ, Paulson DL, Urschel HC, Razzuk MA (1968) Eventration of the diaphragm. Surgery 64:1013–1021

Meier RA, Marianacci EB, Costello P, Fitzpatrick PJ, Hartnell GG (1993) 3D image reconstruction of right subclavian artery aneurysms. J Comput Asssis Tomogr 17:887–890

Mendez G Jr, Isikoff MB, Isikoff SK, Sinner WN (1979) Fatty tumors of the thorax demonstrated by computerized tomography. AJR 133:207–212

Michelson E (1961) Eventration of the diaphragm. Surgery 49:410–422

Mirvis SE, Templeton P (1992) Imaging in acute thoracic trauma. Semin Roentgenol 27:184–210

Naidich DP, Zerhouni EA, Siegelman SS (1991) Computed tomography and magnetic resonance of the thorax. Raven Press, New York

Oyen R, Marchal G, Verschakelen J et al. (1984) Sonographic aspect of hypertrophic diaphragmatic muscular bundles. J Clin Ultrasound 12:121–123

Panicek DM, Benson CB, Gottlieb RH, Heitzman ER (1988) The diaphragm: anatomic, pathologic and radiologic considerations. Radiographics 8:385–425

Paris F, Tarazona V, Casillas M, Blasco E, Canto A, Pastor J, Acosta A (1973) Hernia of Morgagni. Thorax 28:631

Pearlberg JL, Sandler MA, Beute GH et al. (1987) Limitations of CT in evaluation of neoplasms involving chest wall. J Comput Assis Tomogr 11:290–293

Pennes DR, Glazer GM, Wimbish KJ et al. (1985) Chest wall invasion by lung cancer: limitations of CT evaluation. Am J Roentgenol 144:507–511

Pery M, Kaftori J, Rosenberger A (1984) Causes of abnormal right diaphragmatic position diagnosed by ultrasound. J Clin Ultrasound 12:121–123

Rubin GD, Dake MD, Semba CP (1995) Current status of three-dimensional spiral CT scanning for imaging the vasculature. Radiol Clin North Am 33:51–70

Sardanelli F, Melani E, Calabrese M, Parodi RC, Giacchino M, Massa T, Vecchio C (1995) Dynamic spiral CT of suspected breast tumors. Eur Radiol 5(Suppl):280

Schaefer PS, Burton BS (1989) Radiographic evaluation of chest-wall lesions. Surg Clin North Am 69:911–945

Schwartz EE, Wechsler RJ (1989) Diaphragmatic and paradiaphragmatic tumors and pseudotumors. J Thorac Imaging 4:19–28

Shapiro MP, Gale ME, Daly BD (1988) Eloesser window thoracostomy for treatment of empyema: radiographic appearance. Am J Roentgenol 150:549–552

Shin MS, Berland LL (1985) Computed tomography of retrocrural spaces: normal, anatomic variants and pathologic conditions. Am J Roentgenol 145:81–86

Shirakawa T, Fukuda K, Miyamoto Y, Tanabe H, Tada S (1994) Parietal pleural invasion of lung masses: evaluation with CT performed during deep inspiration and expiration. Radiology 192:809–811

Sinow JD, Halvorsen RA, Matts JP, Schubert W, Letourneau JG, Cunningham BL (1991) Chest-wall deformity after tissue expansion for breast reconstruction. Plast Reconstr Surg 88:998–1004

Snyder WH, Greany EM (1965) Congenital diaphragmatic hernia; 77 consecutive cases. Surgery 57:576–588

Stark P, Jaramillo D (1986) CT of the sternum. Am J Roentgenol 147:72–77

Takasugi JE, Rapoport S, Shaw C (1989) Superior sulcus tumors: the role of imaging. J Thorac Imaging 4:41–48

Tarver RD, Cones DJ, Cory DA, Vix VA (1989) Imaging the diaphragm and its disorders. J Thorac Imaging 4:1–18

Teifke A, Schweden F, Cagil H, Kauczor HU, Mohr W, Thelen M (1994) Spiral-Computertomographie der Mamma. Fortschr Röntgenstr 161:495–500

Tello R, Scholz E, Finn JP, Costello P (1993) Subclavian vein thrombosis detected with spiral CT and three-dimensional reconstruction. Am J Roentgenol 160:33–34

Thomas GG, Clitherow NR (1977) Herniation through the foramen of Morgagni in children. Br J Surg 64:215–217

Toombs BD, Sandler CM, Lester RG (1981) Computed tomography of chest trauma. Radiology 140:733–738

Ujita M, Ojiri H, Ariizumi M, Tada S (1993) Appearance of the inferior phrenic artery and vein on CT scans of the chest: a CT and cadaveric study. Am J Roentgenol 160:745–747

Van Daele G, Joris L, Eyskens E (1987) Traumatische diafragmaruptuur. Tijdschr Geneesk 43:1649–1653

Verschakelen JA, Demaerel P, Coolen J, Demedts M, Marchal G, Baert AL (1989a) Rounded atelectasis of the lung: MR appearance. Am J Roentgenol 152:965–966

Verschakelen JA, Marchal G, Verbeken E, Baert AL, Lauweryns J (1989b) Sonographic appearance of the diaphragm in the presence of pleural disease: a cadaver study. J Clin Ultrasound 17:222–227

Webb WR, Gatsonis C, Zerhouni EA, Heelan RT, Glazer GM, Francis IR, McNeil BJ (1991) CT and MR imaging in staging non-small cell bronchogenic carcinoma: report of the radiologic diagnostic oncology group. Radiology 178:705–713

Wilbur AC, Gorodetsky A, Hibbeln JF (1994) Imaging findings of adult Bochdalek hernias. Clin Imaging 18:224–229

Worthy SA, Kang EY, Hartman TE, Kwong JS, Mayo JR, Müller NL (1995) Diaphragmatic rupture: CT findings in 11 patients. Radiology 194:885–888

Yamana D, Ohba S (1994) Three-dimensional image of Bochdalek diaphragmatic hernia; a case report. Radiat Med 12:39–41

Yamashita K, Minemori K, Matsuda H, Ohishi T, Matsunobe S (1993) MR imaging in the diagnosis of partial eventration of the diaphragm. Chest 104:328

15 Spiral CT in the Year 2000

W.A. KALENDER

CONTENTS

15.1 Introduction

X-ray computed tomography (CT) has played an important role in imaging the chest in the past due to the acceptably short scan times and the fact that the high-density differences in the lung provide high contrast on CT images. Other imaging modalities are available, and the potential for their use will certainly increase in the years to come. In particular, magnetic resonance imaging (MRI) may prove to be competitive or superior in a number of applications. Nevertheless, it can be safely assumed that CT will continue to play a dominant role in imaging of the chest. The advent of spiral CT in 1989 (KALENDER et al. 1989; VOCK et al. 1990) provided the basis for this expectation. The particular advantages of spiral CT and the advances in clinical examinations are presented in this textbook in great depth. But this positive development has by no means arrived at its endpoint. There are a number of potential improvements in technology, in data and image processing, and in special applications which will further enhance the role of spiral CT in chest imaging.

What can we expect from spiral CT in the coming decades? And what should be the aims of the various technical developments? Certainly, we wish for even faster scanning, we hope for improved and more isotropic spatial resolution, we expect that the operation of scanners and evaluation of data will become easier, and, last but not least, we would like patient dose to be reduced. In this chapter, we intend to discuss in detail the particular aims of further improvements in spiral CT, the state of the art, and the probable or necessary technical developments and new applications. The principles and performance characteristics of spiral CT have already been described in Chap. 1. As an additional review for the more technically oriented reader, a very recent textbook which resulted from the American Association of Physicists in Medicine (AAPM) 1995 Summer School can be recommended (GOLDMAN and FOWLKES 1995).

15.2 Scan Times: Very Fast Volume Scanning Is the Demand

There is no doubt: fast scanning is a clinical advantage or even a necessity. Physiologic motion is always present in the chest, and patient motion can never be reliably excluded. Subsecond scan times per 360° rotation are demanded in order to reliably exclude artifacts in the imaging of single slices. Even more important, gapless and artifact-free imaging of complete organs can only be achieved if very short volume scan times, i.e., scans within a single breathhold or within a few seconds, are possible. In addition, dynamic and functional examinations can only be performed in many cases if volume scans can be repeated in relatively short periods (see Sect. 15.6). Continued reductions in scan times and a definite reduction in volume scan times have to be a specific aim for spiral CT in the year 2000.

Today, subsecond scanning of single slices is already available; 0.75 s per full rotation is the best which conventional scanners can presently offer. Volumes are typically scanned in 20–60 s, but mostly with relatively thick slices. To scan a 35-cm thorax with thin slices is still not possible in a single spiral

W.A. KALENDER, PhD, Professor, Institut für Medizinische Physik, Universität Erlangen, Krankenhausstraße 12, 91054 Erlangen, Germany

scan. Electron beam scanning (BOYD and LIPTON 1983), a technical alternative which is not yet fully developed, offers very short scan times of typically 0.1 s per slice, but volume scan times are not reduced to the same degree. One reason for this, and the general problem in reducing scan times, is the fact that scan speed only is not enough for fast imaging. X-ray power has to be increased to the same degree that scan times are reduced in order to assure that the necessary dose or mAs values per 360° scan are maintained. Therefore solution of the mechanical problems which increase quadratically with scan speed is not the only task; rather, x-ray tube and generator technology equally presents challenges, and it appears mandatory in any case to make use of the available x-ray power in a more efficient way.

Increases in system efficiency will be limited since today's systems already operate close to the optimum. Therefore further increases in scanner rotation speed will demand adequate increases in peak x-ray power. The use of two-dimensional detectors in the form of multiple arrays or image plates may be a solution to the problem of achieving much faster volume scan times, however, since several slices are scanned per rotation. Resulting reductions in total scan time would imply that peak x-ray power has to be maintained only for this shorter time, with the total energy deposited in the x-ray tube reduced accordingly.

15.3 Spatial Resolution: Isotropic Imaging Is the Aim

High spatial resolution in the scan plane has been an established advantage of CT for quite some time and is documented by common terms like "high-resolution CT of the lung" (e.g., MAYO et al. 1987). Resolution of 0.5- to 1.0-mm structure elements is typically achieved. Perpendicular to the scan plane, i.e., along the body's longitudinal axis and the z-axis of the scanner, resolution is worse due to slice thicknesses of several millimeters and the fact that slices are taken adjacent or with gaps, but not overlapping. Therefore, in general, resolution is not isotropic in slice imaging modalities like CT.

Isotropic imaging, i.e., imaging with approximately the same spatial resolution in all directions, is the ideal we are striving for in 3D imaging – not only in cases where 3D displays are required, but in all cases where organs are assessed in total and not only by representative sections. Imaging modalities offering isotropic resolution would allow us to assess ana-

tomical structures in arbitrarily chosen planes with approximately the same image quality. What are the particular promises and practical implications of isotropic imaging? It would allow us to scan at an arbitrary gantry angle and to choose the optimal image plane retrospectively. And it would allow us to choose different planes or orientations from a single volume scan without a compromise in image quality and without renewed scanning and dose. Slice imaging modalities traditionally failed to provide isotropic resolution. CT started with an in-plane spatial resolution of 1–2 mm and section widths of 10 mm and more; volume elements represented by each pixel were closer to a rod than to a cube. Things have improved considerably over the years, but isotropic spatial resolution has never been claimed with conventional CT. When the principles and results of "spiral volumetric CT" were first presented they were introduced as a means of achieving rapid and continuous volume scanning, even accepting slight degradations in image quality due to the smoothing of section sensitivity profiles (SSPs) (KALENDER et al. 1990). Also the selection of scan parameters and the available x-ray power was very limited at that time.

This situation has changed dramatically since 1989. Spiral CT is now considered particularly suited for high-resolution 3D imaging, with respect to both the availability of scan parameters and the availability of advanced image reconstruction algorithms. Today's scanners allow longer scan times and thereby the use of thin slices; e.g., a scan of 80 revolutions with a 1-mm slice width and a feed of 1.5 mm per revolution, i.e., pitch = 1.5, will allow for a scan range of 120 mm in a single 60-s scan. The introduction of 180° algorithms (POLACIN et al. 1992) allowed the degradation of SSPs to be limited (see also Chap. 1). Nevertheless, the degradation of SSPs remains a disadvantage. However, spiral CT is based on continuous scanning along the z-axis, and it allows slices to be reconstructed at arbitrarily fine increments. This improved sampling along the z-axis is a clear advantage. How do these two effects balance out?

It has been shown in two independent studies that the positive effect of continuous sampling along the z-direction outweighs the disadvantage of SSP degradation with respect to z-resolution if many overlapping images are reconstructed (WANG and VANNIER 1994; KALENDER et al. 1994). While Wang and Vannier used an analytical model assumption for SSPs, Kalender et al. used the measured SSPs. Nevertheless, they both arrived at the same result, namely the finding of improved z-resolution in spiral CT. It has to be stressed, however, that this inherent sampling advantage of spiral CT can only be employed if a sufficient number of images has been reconstructed. In both studies the authors arrived at the optimum in resolution at a minimum of five images to be reconstructed per table feed d, the distance the table travels per 360° rotation. (It is equal to the section width for pitch = 1.) For most practical purposes, two to four images per distance d are recommended. The question of whether isotropic resolution is possible in CT was not addressed and not answered in the studies mentioned above; they only compared spiral CT and conventional CT at that time.

Closer evaluations of 3D spatial resolution using a perspex hole pattern are shown in Fig. 15.1 (KALENDER 1995a). Scans were taken with 1-mm

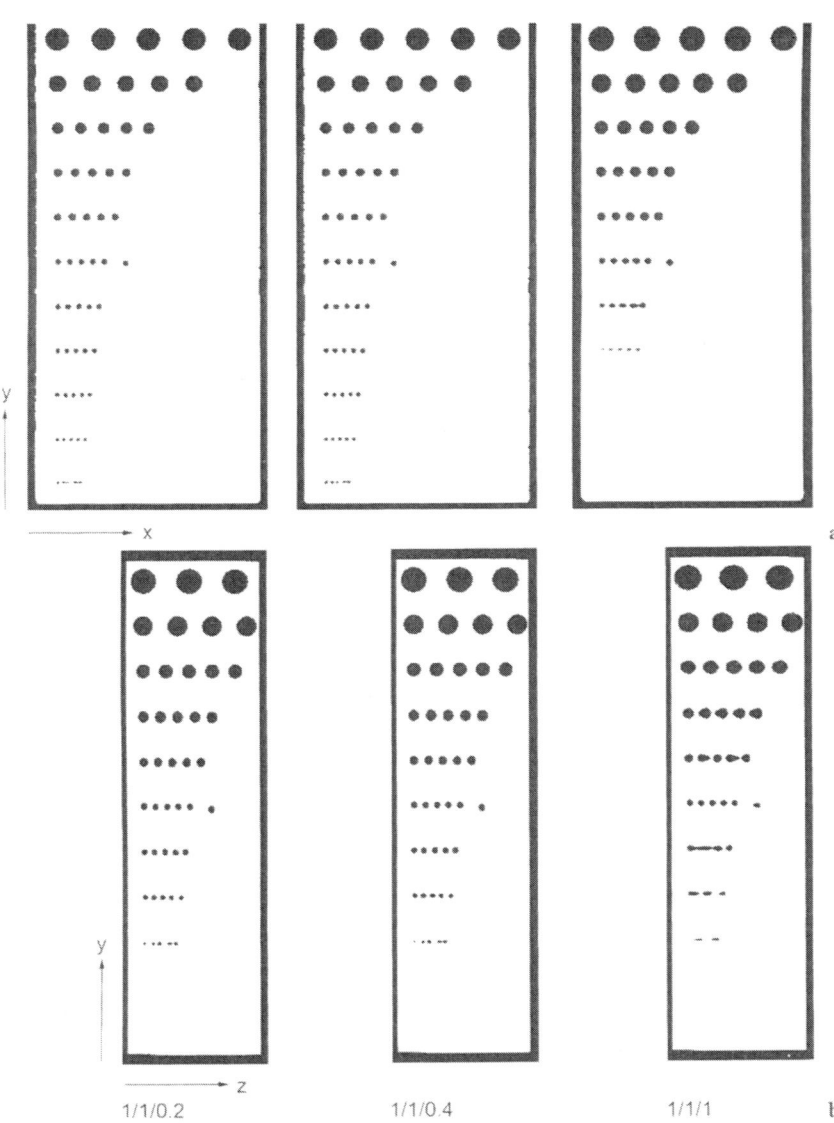

Fig. 15.1a,b. 3D spatial resolution: isotropic imaging appears possible. a Spatial resolution in the x/y scan plane is the same for conventional CT and for spiral CT if the same reconstruction parameters are chosen. 0.5-mm holes are resolved well with a "sharp" kernel (left and center). Reconstructions with a "standard" kernel, which are preferred for 3D SSD displays, do not provide the maximum of spatial resolution, here only 0.8 mm holes (right). b Spatial resolution in reformatted y/z plane images is lower than the maximum achievable in the directly scanned x/y plane. However, spiral CT scanning with adequate parameters (1-mm sections, 1-mm table feed per rotation) and images at fine reconstruction increments (RI) practically offers the same resolution in all principal planes for 3D displays (compare a, right, with b, left). (Number triples specify section width S / table feed d / reconstruction increment RI). (Reproduced with permission from (KALENDER 1995a)

section width and 1-mm table feed per rotation (Somatom Plus 4A, Siemens Medizinische Technik, Erlangen). In-plane measurements confirmed two well-known facts: (a) resolution is identical for conventional and for spiral CT (Fig. 15.1a, left and center); (b) spatial resolution in the image plane depends on the reconstruction algorithm (Fig. 15.1a, center and right). While "bone" or "high-resolution" algorithms are commonly used to assess bony and other high-contrast structures in CT images directly, it is common practice in preparing 3D SSD displays to use a "standard" or "body" algorithm which does not augment noise and thereby helps to avoid artifacts, e.g., "flying pixels." Thus, submaximal resolution of typically six to seven holepairs per cm is provided in-plane.

With the resolution test aligned perpendicular to the scan plane in the y/z plane, images are reconstructed at a given reconstruction increment (RI), and reformatted images are synthesized to display the y/z plane. The reconstruction increment has a strong influence on resolution, as has been pointed out previously (WANG and VANNIER 1994; KALENDER et al. 1994). The 0.8-mm holes are well resolved for image reconstruction at RI = 0.2 mm (Fig. 15.1b, left) and RI = 0.4 mm (Fig. 15.1b, center), but this is not the case when images are reconstructed at RI = 1.0 mm (Fig. 15.1b, right). RI = 0.2 mm offers only marginally higher resolution than RI = 0.4 mm. This confirms the earlier findings that the optimum is approximated well with five images reconstructed per nominal section width (RI = 0.2 mm) and that three images per nominal section width appear to be a good compromise for practical purposes. And, surprising to many, spatial resolution in the y/z plane is better or equal to that in the original x/y imaging plane (compare Fig. 15.1a, right, with Fig. 15.1b, left). Thus, although still limited to small volumes, physical measurements suggest that isotropic spatial resolution is available in 3D spiral CT imaging.

The situation looks different if thick slices of 3–5 mm are needed due to dose and noise considerations, as is typical in studies of the abdomen. Certainly, here we still do not achieve isotropic spatial resolution; rather, we actually intend to achieve good low-contrast resolution instead. Therefore standard or smooth reconstruction kernels are used to achieve favorable noise characteristics; low-contrast structures of a few millimeters can be resolved. And it does not appear impossible a priori to present small low-contrast lesions with the same clarity in direct scans and in multiplanar images. If this is achieved we can claim isotropic imaging, isotropic resolution independent of contrast.

Some improvement of spatial resolution in the scan plane is certainly possible and welcome, but the clear aim for spiral CT in the year 2000 has to be isotropic spatial and low-contrast resolution. Thin-slice volume scanning is the specific demand. To achieve this aim in spatial resolution, two-dimensional detectors may again be viewed as the technical basis for the necessary improvements. The arguments are very similar to those in the discussion of volume scan speed: obtaining several thin slices simultaneously reduces the total scan time and allows finer sampling and better use of the available x-ray power.

15.4 Necessary Technical Developments in Spiral CT Scanners

X-ray CT technology went through a phase of very rapid technical development in the 1970s, but went into a phase of saturation and relative rest in the 1980s. The introduction of slipring technology, which allowed for continuous data acquisition and for the reduction of scan times from typically between 2 and 10 s to 1 s, was one of the few major events in that decade. But it provided the necessary basis for spiral scanning. And the introduction of spiral scanning in 1989 triggered renewed interest in CT and efforts to achieve further developments in CT technology.

We have already monitored a number of amazing results in the first half of the 1990s which will be illustrated by two examples comparing scan parameter settings available in 1989 and in 1995.

1. The maximal spiral scan time was increased from 12 s to 60 s. Note that the scan time per 360° rotation only improved from 1.0 to 0.75 s during the same period.
2. The maximal x-ray power of 20 kW over 12 s was increased to 40 kW over 30 s or 25 kW maintained over 60 s. Note that the peak x-ray power per 1-s scan only improved from 40 kW to 60 kW during the same period.

Apparently, the most dramatic improvement was achieved in providing higher continuous x-ray power, the necessary prerequisite for spiral CT to become usable without any drawbacks as compared to conventional CT. This applies above all to neuroradiological applications, where high mA settings for low noise levels are required. Full equivalence of spiral CT and conventional CT for such applications is not yet established. In CT of the chest, which has lower power requirements, this is not a major problem for single scans or limited volumes. It will be a problem, however, for extended volumes scanned with thin slices and for repeated volume scans.

Further improvements in scan speed and x-ray power are necessary and to be expected, but they will mostly occur in the range of percentage points and not by factors of 2 and more. High voltage generators and x-ray tube technologies are already highly advanced and highly efficient, and breakthroughs are unlikely to occur. Yet, the demands for fast volume scanning and for isotropic spatial resolution require fast acquisition with thin slices translating into total mAs products which cannot be delivered in full by conventional scanners. However, there appears to be an intelligent alternative to the horsepower race of increasing scan speed and x-ray power, i.e., the more efficient use of available x-ray power by employing two-dimensional detectors. It is quite conceivable that the one-dimensional detector, a single array of detector elements, may be replaced by either several such arrays or by a plate detector similar in principle to those used in digital radiography. If we have an array of n detector lines, this would mean that we could reduce the volume scan time by roughly a factor of n. Above all, we would make much more efficient use of the x-ray tube's output. Incidentally, the same considerations caused the development of CT from first generation (single detector and pencil beam) to second generation (a few detectors with a small fan beam) to third and fourth generations (one complete detector array and a full fan beam). Also, in the early CT scanners, as for example the EMI Mark I and the Siemens Siretom 1000, dual detector arrays were already used. The first scanner with a two-dimensional array would deserve the claim to represent the fifth generation. Quite a number of technological problems have yet to be solved with respect to detector technology, however, and new approaches to image reconstruction from cone beam data will have to be investigated and developed. But we may consider these as challenges and not as insoluble problems.

Alternative approaches to CT scanning in the past involved electron beam tomography (EBT) and the use of plate detectors. The introduction of EBT (BOYD and LIPTON 1983) presented a breakthrough in cardiac imaging in the early 1980s, but that development was not continued to the degree that EBT became competitive with conventional CT. The use of image intensifier screens as an area detector was not successfully completed either, but some performance parameters were demonstrated by the "dynamic spatial reconstructor" (ROBB et al. 1983), which already set the aim for future developments as defined above: submillimeter slices with the complete volume scanned in a few seconds.

15.5 Improvements in Data and Image Processing

It is not surprising that one may predict further advances in computer technology and in image processing methods. The availability of higher computing power and of larger, directly accessible fast memory is certainly to be expected for the year 2000. Digital image processing is a specialty which is quickly progressing and which will profit further from improvements in technology. Where and how will these developments be set to use in spiral CT scanning and image evaluation?

In order to efficiently handle the data rates and the large data volumes which have to be expected from true volume scanning, advances in computer technology and storage devices will be necessary. It is easy to predict that the technologies will evolve. It will be harder, yet possible, to develop the necessary algorithms for data processing and image reconstruction. Reconstruction of cone beam data into images with few or no artifacts is one challenge; the development of new and improved z-interpolation algorithms for spiral CT is a further one. Active research is already being conducted. with respect to both topics. While cone beam reconstruction is still in a very early phase focusing on basic questions, efforts in spiral CT are directed at relatively subtle effects. One such effort which aims at reducing the artifacts still seen in 3D displays is shown in Fig. 15.2 (KALENDER 1995b). All these efforts at new or improved reconstruction schemes are still limited by long computing times and cannot yet be considered practical. But they will very likely be practical and routinely available in the year 2000.

Image segmentation has been successfully employed in a number of tasks involving relatively simple, but time-consuming and tedious work. Semiautomatic segmentation of the total lung, which exhibits high contrast to the surrounding soft tissues, and determination of density and histogram parameters is a common example. More complex tasks in image segmentation demand more sophisticated approaches and processing of 3D data volumes instead

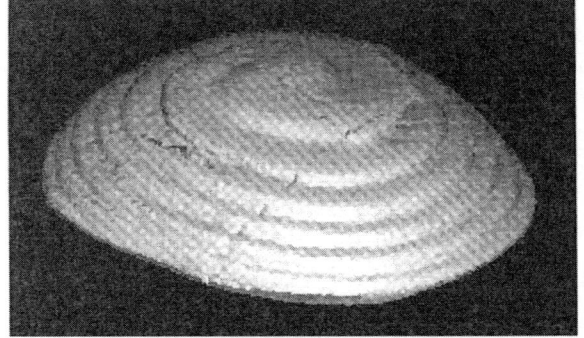

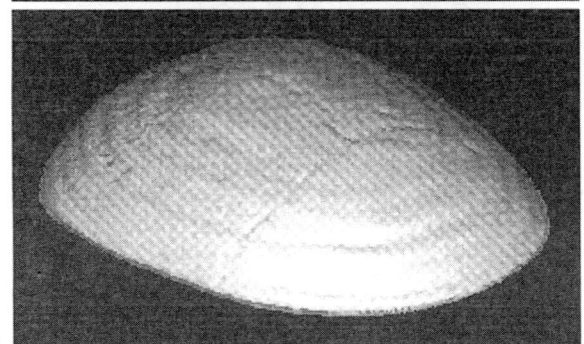

Fig. 15.2a,b. Advanced z-interpolation algorithms offer the potential to reduce artifacts and may allow scanning at higher pitch values. **a** In standard 180° linear interpolation, some inconsistencies may show up as artifacts in shaded-surface 3D displays. **b** Reconstruction of the same data with an experimental 180° object-adaptive 3D interpolator (KALENDER 1995b) reduces these effects without a loss in spatial resolution

lung during a single breathhold; the computer memory of today's typical workstations is too small to hold a complete data volume; computers are too slow to process the complete volume in acceptably short times; and computer scientists still have a lot to learn to provide automated segmentation of a quality comparable to that achieved by a trained human observer. It appears logical and reasonable to assume that the necessary developments will occur in parallel, with little doubt regarding the technical developments but with many open questions regarding the degree of success of image segmentation techniques and the development of expert systems to support diagnosis. Nevertheless, we may safely expect improvements which are relevant to the practice of radiology and new or advanced applications.

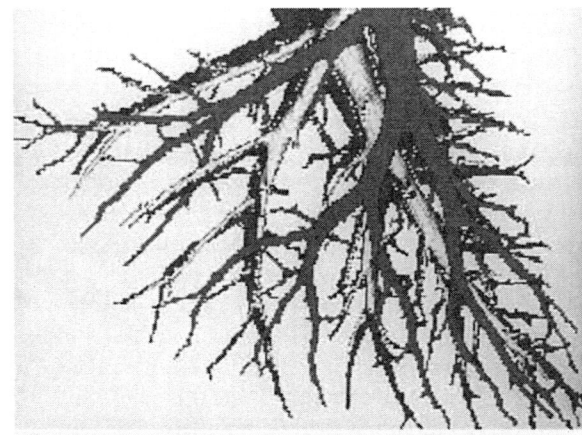

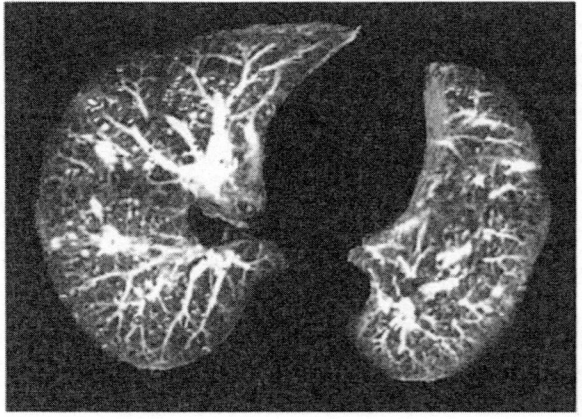

Fig. 15.3a,b. Advanced computer technology and image processing techniques will allow largely automatic segmentation of lung anatomy. While the examples shown here demanded excessive processing times, real-time 3D evaluations will become possible in the future. **a** Isolated displays of lung vessels and bronchi in an excised canine lung lobe (courtesy of S. Wood). **b** Automated finding of micronodules (depicted in *green*)

of successive processing of 2D images, however. Appropriate developments are already underway, but they are to some extent hampered by the limits of the available technology. A perfect example is automated segmentation of complete lung anatomy. It appears feasible to solve this task, and it certainly might help clinical diagnosis. The aim of segmentation would be to identify vasculature, i.e., arterial and venous structures separately, the bronchial tree, lung parenchyma and pathological structures, e.g., lesions. All this should preferably include assignment of structures to the respective lung lobes and segments and reference to normal anatomy offered in anatomical atlases. Efforts at segmenting lung vessels and bronchi in spiral CT data volumes have already been started (Fig. 15.3a) (WOOD et al. 1996); attempts at automated identification of micronodules were undertaken by our group in cooperation with the editors of this textbook (Fig. 15.3b). Both examples demonstrate the feasibility of such studies. But they also reveal the limitations and problems we are still facing: scanners are too slow to image the complete

15.6 Advanced Clinical Applications

CT angiography (CTA) of the chest and, inherently, the diagnosis of lung emboli is a primary example of a CT application which became available with the advent of spiral CT. As pointed out above, we expect that faster and repeated volume scans will become available with improved spatial resolution and that higher computing power and improved processing algorithms will be offered. This will make CTA an even more powerful application and probably the method of choice in the diagnosis of lung emboli. But further new and improved clinical applications of spiral CT in the chest will certainly arise. This will be illustrated by two examples of applications which appear very feasible under the assumed conditions.

The assessment of ventilation and perfusion of the lung is a very frequent task in diagnostic radiology. Today, it is approached routinely by nuclear medicine techniques. The possibility of repeated fast volume scans of the lung after intravenous administration of contrast medium or the inhalation of stable xenon gas mixtures may yield similar results to nuclear medicine with much improved anatomical and pathological detail. First efforts at ventilation imaging by dynamic CT with xenon inhalation have already been completed; these revealed the potential of such studies (Fig. 15.4a), but they were not successful routinely due to the limitation to a single slice and the disturbing effects of patient breathing motion. The extension to dynamic scanning of complete volumes will allow for corrections of the motion problem and, if scanning is sufficiently fast, reduce the further problem that xenon diffuses quickly into tissue and is transported away by blood circulation. The technique of dynamic volume scanning can similarly be applied after intravenous contrast medium injection to monitor bolus kinetics, which may be helpful in the diagnosis of perfusion defects and in the differential diagnosis of lesions. If successful, these applications would entail a large number of examinations.

Virtual bronchoscopy or, in more general terms, perspective volume rendering, is another advanced application which appears feasible with the predicted advances in technology. First demonstrations have already been given (Fig. 15.4b) (RUBIN et al. 1996), but we are still far from routine applications. The quality of the original image data, above all with respect to more isotropic 3D spatial resolution, and processing techniques still have to be improved. Most important, however, processing times are still prohibitive. We have to await the technical improve-

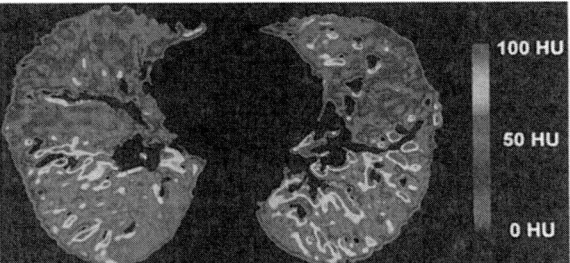
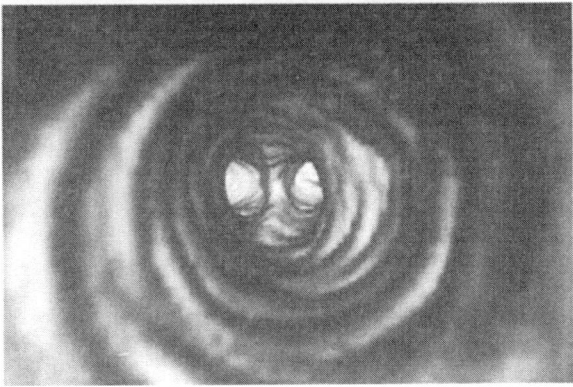

Fig 15.4a,b. New and improved spiral CT applications will become possible with faster scanning. a Dynamic functional studies of complete volumes will allow assessment of ventilation and perfusion of the lung. Inhalation of stable xenon provides displays and quantitative evaluation of regional ventilation patterns as shown here. b Virtual endoscopy of the chest will allow for new noninvasive approaches to bronchoscopy and angioscopy and "fly-through" views of all anatomical structures. A virtual bronchoscopy scene is shown here (courtesy of G. Rubin)

ments announced in earlier sections before routine applications will be feasible. Virtual bronchoscopy and angioscopy may become fascinating spiral CT applications, demonstrating the inherent quality of volume scanning in a very impressive way, yet very likely they will not have the same clinical impact as ventilation and perfusion measurements.

15.7 Patient Dose: What Are the Trends?

The benefits and the diagnostic power of CT have often been proved. The particular advantages of spiral CT in the chest have been presented in detail in this textbook. Yet, in all discussions of the advantages of CT in comparison to other competing modalities, there is always the important argument that ionizing radiation is used with an unknown risk to the patient. Public concern with respect to ionizing radiation has increased decisively in recent years. CT is at the center of this concern as it contributes about one-third of the total exposure of the population from medical applications in the western world. Furthermore, some sceptics claim that dose will increase further due to the advent of volume scanning. Is there hope that the dose levels in CT of the chest will be reduced?

In general, spiral CT has not increased dose in CT examinations. Rather, it offers the potential to reduce dose for several reasons:

1. mA settings in spiral CT are often necessarily reduced as the desired power levels are not available for extended scans. This may change in the future, but doses in spiral CT will not exceed those in conventional CT.
2. The need for overlapping scans, often taken for improved multiplanar or 3D displays, is rendered obsolete by spiral CT.
3. The possibility of using table feed values greater than the collimation width in spiral CT (pitch > 1) leads to an immediate reduction in dose by a factor equal to the pitch factor.

This potential for dose reduction is given under the assumption that the frequency of examinations is unchanged and that always the same volume is scanned. If the improved capabilities of spiral CT were to lead to an increase in CT scanning, the cumulative exposure would increase accordingly, but this would happen in the context of appropriate indications.

Also in general, it will not be easy to significantly reduce the dose per scan without a loss in image quality. The x-ray detectors used in CT are close to the optimum in detection efficiency, and this is also true of the whole system. There is only limited room for improvement. Intelligent measures such as automatic exposure control have not yet been introduced or established in CT. Together with patient-specific settings of parameters they may provide one key to dose reduction. Efforts to reduce dose will continue, but decisive breakthroughs will not be possible for reasons of physics. We will have to face continued discussions about dose. To give exact information about patient dose and to put these values into perspective by comparison with other exposure levels is one proposed strategy to reduce the "fear of the unknown." For example, a spiral CT scan of the complete chest (120 kV, 210 mA, 32-cm range) will cause an effective dose of about 7 mSv; this value may be put into perspective by comparison with the natural background radiation of 2.4 mSv per year (KALENDER 1995b).

15.8 Conclusions

"Predictions are particularly difficult when they are concerned with the future." This statement, phrased in various forms by many in the past – some intentional and some unintentional philosophers – has to be kept in mind. And, certainly, predictions with respect to technical and clinical developments in this chapter may prove to be wrong; some predicted developments might actually occur well before the year 2000. Wherever I failed I can only ask for the reader's understanding.

As a summary and conclusion to this chapter, having hinted at the uncertainties, I forecast the following performance for spiral CT of the chest in the year 2000:

1. Fast volume scans, with the complete thorax scanned in a single breathhold with thin slices
2. Only slightly increased in-plane resolution, but significant improvements towards isotropic resolution, i.e., above all improved spatial resolution in the z-direction
3. Improved image quality due to higher scan speed and improved volume reconstruction algorithms
4. New and advanced applications, primarily dynamic studies of ventilation and perfusion, automated search for and automated classification of lung nodules, and quantitative analysis of lung density and structure
5. Slight reduction in dose per single scan, but no significant reduction in effective dose as the complete lung will often be scanned with higher resolution, providing enhanced diagnostic information

References

Boyd D, Lipton MJ (1983) Cardiac computed tomography. Proc IEEE 71:298–308

Goldman LW, Fowlkes JB (1995) Medical CT and ultrasound: current technology and applications. Advanced Medical Publishing, Madison, Wisconsin

Kalender WA (1995a) Three-dimensional spiral CT: is isotropic imaging possible? Radiology 197:578–580

Kalender WA (1995b) Principles and performance of spiral CT. In: Goldman LW, Fowlkes JB (eds) Medical CT and ultrasound: current technology and applications. Advanced Medical Publishing, Madison, Wisconsin, pp 379–410

Kalender WA, Seissler W, Vock P (1989) Single-breath-hold spiral volumetric CT by continuous patient translation and scanner rotation. Radiology 173(P):414

Kalender WA, Seissler W, Klotz E, Vock P (1990) Spiral volumetric CT with single-breath-hold technique, continuous transport, and continuous scanner rotation. Radiology 176:181–183

Kalender WA, Polacin A, Suess C (1994) A comparison of conventional and spiral CT: an experimental study on the detection of spherical lesions. J Comput Assist Tomogr 18:167–176

Mayo JR, Webb WR, Gould R, Stein M, Bass I, Gamsu G, Goldberg HI (1987) High-resolution CT of the lungs: an optimal approach. Radiology 163:507–510

Polacin A, Kalender WA, Marchal G (1992) Evaluation of section sensitivity profiles and image noise in spiral CT. Radiology 185:29–35

Robb R, Hoffmann E, Sinak LJ, Harris LD, Ritman EL (1983) High-speed three-dimensional X-ray computed tomography: the dynamic spatial reconstructor. Proc IEEE 71:308–319

Rubin GD, Beaulieu CF, Argiro V et al. (1996) Perspective volume rendering of CT and MR images: application for endoscopic imaging. Radiology 199:321–330

Vock P, Soucek M, Daepp M, Kalender WA (1990) Lung: spiral volumetric CT with single-breath-hold technique. Radiology 176:864–867

Wang G, Vannier M (1994) Longitudinal resolution in volumetric X-ray computerized tomography. Analytical comparison between conventional and helical computerized tomography. Med Phys 21:429–433

Wood SA (1996) Analysis of three dimensional lung structure during inflation using computed tomography. J Appl Physiol (in print)

Subject Index

List of Contributors

JOHN E. ALDRICH, PhD
Department of Radiology
University of British Columbia and Vancouver
Hospital and Health Sciences Centre
855 West 12th Avenue
Vancouver, BC
Canada V5Z 1M9

ALEXANDER A. BANKIER, MD
Department of Radiology
University of Vienna
Währinger Gürtel 18-20
1090 Vienna
Austria

CATHERINE BEIGELMAN, MD
Department of Radiology
Hôpital de la Salpétrière
47, boulevard de l'Hôpital
75641 Paris Cédex 13
France

PHILIP COSTELLO, MD
Senior Director, Radiology
The Queen Elizabeth Hospital
28 Woodville Road
Woodville
5011 S. Australia

DOMINIK FLEISCHMANN, MD
Department of Radiology
University of Vienna
Währinger Gürtel 18-20
1090 Vienna
Austria

PHILIPPE GRENIER, MD
Department of Radiology
Hôpital de la Salpétrière
47, boulevard de l'Hôpital
75641 Paris Cédex 13
France

CHRISTIAN J. HEROLD, MD
Department of Radiology
University of Vienna
Währinger Gürtel 18-20
1090 Vienna
Austria

WILLI A. KALENDER, PhD, Professor
Institut für Medizinische Physik
Universität Erlangen
Krankenhausstr. 12
91054 Erlangen
Germany

JOHN R. MAYO, MD
Department of Radiology
University of British Columbia and Vancouver
Hospital and Health Sciences Centre
855 West 12th Avenue
Vancouver, BC
Canada V5Z 1M9

RETO MEULI, MD
Department of Radiology
University Hospital
CHUV Lausanne
1011 Lausanne
Switzerland

DAVID P. NAIDICH, MD
Department of Radiology
New York University Medical Center/
Bellevue Hospital
27th Street and 1st Avenue
New York, NY 10016
USA

MATHIAS PROKOP, MD
Department of Radiology I
Hannover Medical School
30623 Hannover
Germany

Jacques Rémy, MD
Department of Radiology
Hospital Calmette
Boulevard Jules Leclerc
59037 Lille Cédex
FRANCE

Martine Rémy-Jardin, MD, PhD
Department of Radiology
Hospital Calmette
Boulevard Jules Leclerc
59037 Lille Cédex
FRANCE

Geoffrey D. Rubin, MD, Assistant Professor
Department of Radiology, S 072B
Stanford University Hospital Medical Centre
300 Pasteur Drive
Stanford, CA 94305-5105
USA

Cornelia M. Schaefer-Prokop, MD
Department of Radiology I
Hannover Medical School
30623 Hannover
Germany

Pierre Schnyder, MD
Department of Radiology
University Hospital
CHUV Lausanne
1011 Lausanne
Switzerland

Michael W. Vannier, MD
Mallinckrodt Institute of Radiology
Washington University School of Medicine
510 South Kingshighway Blvd.
St. Louis, MO 63110
USA

Johny A. Verschakelen, MD
Department of Radiology
University Hospitals K.U. Leuven
Herestraat 49
3000 Leuven
Belgium

Peter Vock, MD
Department of Diagnostic Radiology
University Hospital
3010 Berne
Switzerland

Ge Wang, PhD
Mallinckrodt Institute of Radiology
Washington University School of Medicine
510 South Kingshighway Blvd.
St. Louis, MO 63110
USA

Stephan Wicky, MD
Department of Radiology
University Hospital
CHUV Lausanne
1011 Lausanne
Switzerland

MEDICAL RADIOLOGY – Diagnostic Imaging and Radiation Oncology

Titles in the series already published

Non-Disseminated Breast Cancer Controversial Issues in Management   Edited by G.H. Fletcher and S.H. Levitt

Current Topics in Clinical Radiobiology of Tumors   Edited by H.-P. Beck-Bornholdt

Practical Approaches to Cancer Invasion and Metastases
A Compendium of Radiation Oncologists Responses to 40 Histories   Edited by A.R. Kagan with the assistance of R.J. Steckel

Radiation Therapy in Pediatric Oncology   Edited by J.R. Cassady

Radiation Therapy Physics   Edited by A.R. Smith

Late Sequelae in Oncology   Edited by J. Dunst and R. Sauer

Mediastinal Tumors. Update 1995   Edited by D.E. Wood and C.R. Thomas, Jr.

Thermoradiotherapy and Thermochemotherapy
Volume 1: Biology, Physiology, and Physics
Volume 2: Clinical Applications
Edited by M.H. Seegenschmiedt, P. Fessenden and C.C. Vernon

Carcinoma of the Prostate. Innovations in Management   Edited by Z. Petrovich, L. Baert, and L.W. Brady

Springer
and the
environment

At Springer we firmly believe that an international science publisher has a special obligation to the environment, and our corporate policies consistently reflect this conviction.
We also expect our business partners – paper mills, printers, packaging manufacturers, etc. – to commit themselves to using materials and production processes that do not harm the environment. The paper in this book is made from low- or no-chlorine pulp and is acid free, in conformance with international standards for paper permanency.

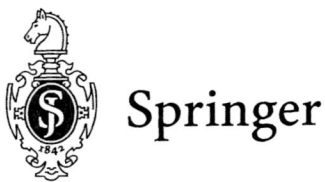